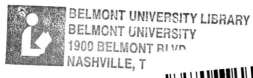

Practical
Electromyography
Third Edition

Practical Electromyography

Third Edition

Ernest W. Johnson, M.D.
*Professor, Department of Physical Medicine
and Rehabilitation
Associate Dean
College of Medicine and Public Health
The Ohio State University
Columbus, Ohio*

William S. Pease, M.D.
*Associate Professor and Chairperson
Department of Physical Medicine
and Rehabilitation
Medical Director
Dodd Hall Rehabilitation Program
The Ohio State University
Columbus, Ohio*

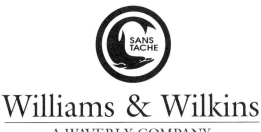

Williams & Wilkins
A WAVERLY COMPANY

BALTIMORE • PHILADELPHIA • LONDON • PARIS • BANGKOK
BUENOS AIRES • HONG KONG • MUNICH • SYDNEY • TOKYO • WROCLAW

Acquisition Editor: John P. Butler
Managing Editor: Linda S. Napora
Production Coordinator: Kimberly Nawrozki
Designer: Rita Baker-Schmidt
Illustration Planner: Ray Lowman
Typesetter: Bi-Comp
Manufacturer: Maple Press
Digitized Illustrations: Bi-Comp

Accurate indications, adverse reactions, and dosage schedules for drugs are provided in this book, but it is possible that they may change. The reader is urged to review the package information data of the manufacturers of the medications mentioned.

Printed in the United States of America

First Edition, 1980

Library of Congress Cataloging-in-Publication Data

Practical electromyography / [edited by] Ernest W. Johnson, William S. Pease. – 3rd ed.
    p.   cm.
    Includes bibliographical references and index.
    ISBN 0-683-04457-5
    1. Electromyography.   2. Neuromuscular diseases—Diagnosis.
I. Johnson, Ernest W., 1924-   . II. Pease, William S.
    [DNLM: 1. Electromyography.   2. Electrodiagnosis.   WE 500 P895 1997]
RC77.5.P7   1997
616.7'407547—dc20
DNLM/DLC
for Library of Congress   96-17610
                                                                                                          CIP

The publishers have made every effort to trace the copyright holders for borrowed material. If they have inadvertently overlooked any, they will be pleased to make the necessary arrangements at the first opportunity.

To purchase additional copies of this book, call our customer service department at **(800) 638-0672** or fax orders to **(800) 447- 8438**. For other book services, including chapter reprints and large quantity sales, ask for the Special Sales department.

Canadian customers should call **(800) 268-4178**, or fax **(905) 470-6780**. For all other calls originating outside of the United States, please call **(410) 528-4223** or fax us at **(410) 528-8550**.

Visit Williams & Wilkins on the Internet: **http://www.wwilkins.com** or contact our customer service department at **custserv@wwilkins.com**. Williams & Wilkins customer service representatives are available from 8:30 am to 6:00 pm, EST, Monday through Friday, for telephone access.

97 98 99 00 01
1 2 3 4 5 6 7 8 9 10

ISBN 0-683-04457-5

To our wives

Margaret E. Ginn-Pease and Joanne E. Johnson

Their love, encouragement, and zest for life make creative work possible.

Preface

Some would ask, "Why write a Third Edition?" Our considered reply is this: The practice of Medicine has changed markedly. Managed care is the magic phrase. Outpatient procedures are assuming primacy. The electrophysiologic extension of the neurologic examination is the efficient outpatient method to evaluate the nervous system.

Techniques to manage injuries and diseases more expeditiously are essential. Outcome measures are dictating management methods. Electrodiagnostic consultation is essential for evaluating neuromuscular diseases before, during, and after expensive treatment. More objective evaluation allows better measurement of severity and outcome.

Now it becomes even more important to individualize the electrodiagnostic studies and view the electrodiagnostic (EDX) medical consultation as a "Gestalt."

With the close association we've had with the American Association of Electrodiagnostic Medicine and the American Board of Electrodiagnostic Medicine, we decided to splice the text with contributions from some extraordinarily gifted colleagues.

The content has been expanded to include cutting-edge approaches to clinical electrodiagnosis. Older, well-established concepts have been updated and some eternal verities restated.

We emphasize the need to adjust the electrodiagnostic medicine consultation as the findings unfold—the entire procedure performed by a physician-specialist—who is performing a diagnostic evaluation and developing a management plan.

Our decision to drop the chapter on central evoked potentials was difficult, but we dropped it rather than duplicate well-known, easily available techniques in a shortened and, perhaps, superficial manner. We acknowledge the excellent monographs for these standard procedures of which most, if not all, are done by technicians with predetermined protocols much like the electroencephalogram (EEG). Somatosensory evoked potential (SSEP) techniques differ greatly from a physician-performed, dynamically varied electrodiagnostic consultation.

William S. Pease, M.D.
Ernest W. Johnson, M.D.

Contributors

JAMES W. ALBERS, M.D., Ph.D.
  Professor of Neurology and Director, Neuromuscular Program, Department of Neurology
  Professor, Department of Occupational Medicine and Environmental and Industrial Health,
    University of Michigan Medical Center, Ann Arbor, Michigan

ALBERT C. CLAIRMONT, M.D.
  Assistant Professor—Clinical, Department of Physical Medicine and Rehabilitation, The
    Ohio State University, Columbus, Ohio

DANIEL CLINCHOT, M.D.
  Assistant Professor, Department of Physical Medicine and Rehabilitation, The Ohio State
    University, Columbus, Ohio

DANIEL DUMITRU, M.D.
  Professor, Department of Rehabilitation Medicine, The University of Texas Health Science
    Center at San Antonio, San Antonio, Texas

WILLIAM J. HENNESSEY, M.D.
  Clinical Instructor, Department of Physical Medicine and Rehabilitation, The Ohio State
    University College of Medicine, Columbus, Ohio

ERNEST W. JOHNSON, M.D.
  Professor, Department of Physical Medicine and Rehabilitation, Associate Dean, College of
    Medicine and Public Health, The Ohio State University, Columbus, Ohio

CHARLES LEVY, M.D.
  Assistant Professor, Deparatment of Physical Medicine and Rehabilitation, The Ohio State
    University, Columbus, Ohio

SCOTT A. MURRAY, M.D.
  Clinical Instructor, Department of Physical Medicine and Rehabilitation, The Ohio State
    University, Columbus, Ohio

W. JERRY MYSIW, M.D.
  Associate Professor, Department of Physical Medicine and Rehabilitation, The Ohio State
    University, Columbus, Ohio

SANJEEV D. NANDEDKAR, PH.D.
  Clinical Application Manager, TECA Corporation, Pleasantville, New York

WILLIAM S. PEASE, M.D.
  Associate Professor and Chairperson, Department of Physical Medicine and Rehabilitation,
    Medical Director, Dodd Hall Rehabilitation Program, The Ohio State University,
    Columbus, Ohio

LAWRENCE R. ROBINSON, M.D.
  Associate Professor, Department of Rehabilitation Medicine, University of Washington,
    Physiatrist-in-Chief, Department of Rehabilitation Medicine, Harborview Medical Center,
    Seattle, Washington

PAULETTE A. SMART, M.D.
  Clinical Instructor, Department of Physical Medicine and Rehabilitation, The Ohio State
    University, Columbus, Ohio

ERIK STÅLBERG, M.D., PH.D.
  Professor, Department of Clinical Neurophysiology, University Hospital, Uppsala, Sweden

BORIS M. TEREBUH, M.D.
  Clinical Instructor, Department of Physical Medicine and Rehabilitation, The Ohio State
    University, Columbus, Ohio

ROBERT J. WEBER, M.D.
Professor and Chairman, Physical Medicine and Rehabilitation State University of New York Health Science Center, Syracuse, New York

ASA J. WILBOURN, M.D.
Director, EMG Laboratory, The Cleveland Clinic Foundation, Associate Clinical Professor, Case Western Reserve University, Cleveland, Ohio

Contents

Chapter 1

The Electrodiagnostic (EDX) Consultation Including EMG Examination

Boris M. Terebuh
Ernest W. Johnson

The electromyographic examination is a powerful diagnostic and prognostic tool; however, it is only part of the complete evaluation of a patient with weakness, pain, sensory disturbance, atrophy, fatigue, or a limp. This evaluation begins with a detailed history and neuromuscular examination to isolate those areas that should be investigated electrodiagnostically. A thorough functional screening examination helps to focus attention on muscle groups that warrant scrutiny. The lower limbs can be screened by asking the patient to assume and rise from a squatting position and then to walk on his or her heels and toes. Upper limb functional screening can be performed by placing the patient's arms in an adducted position with elbows flexed to 90° while the patient grasps two of the examiner's fingers in each hand. The patient is then asked to resist the examiner's attempt to abduct and adduct the arms and flex and extend the elbows. Sensory modalities and muscle stretch reflexes should also be evaluated.

After these preliminary activities have been completed, the electromyogram can be properly planned. This procedure should only be performed by a physician specifically trained in electrodiagnostic medicine. The process should be explained to the patient while avoiding technical and specific details. In most instances it is inadvisable to show the needle electrode to the patient because people often equate prospective pain with the length of the needle rather than its caliber. The discomfort associated with insertion of the needle elec-

trode can be minimized with a concomitant pinch of the skin. Often relaxation can be achieved by having the patient contract an antagonist muscle group slightly.

Most examinations, particularly those for the evaluation of radiculopathy, are facilitated by the patient being placed in the prone position. A pillow should be placed under the chest if the neck or upper limbs are being studied; it should be placed under the abdomen and pelvis if the lower limbs are the focus of attention. It is also helpful when a pillow is positioned under the ankles to keep the knees slightly flexed (Fig. 1–1).

Generally the weakest muscle is studied first to identify the specific problem. Because there are 434 skeletal muscles in the body, it is necessary to be intimately familiar with surface and functional anatomy to ensure that the appropriate muscle is being studied. A thorough understanding of neuromuscular anatomy will also promote a well-planned electromyographic examination with the fewest number of muscles studied. To confirm the proper needle electrode placement, the patient should be asked to move his or her limb so that the muscle is appropriately activated.

Each muscle under investigation should be explored proximally, centrally, and distally. Each penetration through the skin should include 10 to 20 needle insertions into the muscle tissue. Using the skin penetration site as the pivot point, the needle tip should be reoriented 15° to 30° with each insertion so that a circular area is sampled.

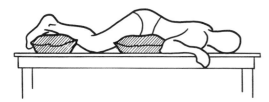

Figure 1-1. Place a pillow beneath the pelvis and lumbar spine to facilitate relaxation of the lumbar paraspinal musculature. Doing the same beneath the upper chest will promote relaxation of the cervical paraspinals. A pillow placed beneath the ankles provides comfort to the patient in a prone position.

FIVE STEPS TO THE EMG EXAMINATION

The five essential steps to the electromyographic examination are outlined below. These steps should be performed in sequence by the neophyte electromyographer (i.e., for the initial 2,000 to 3,000 studies performed). To use shortcuts prior to accumulating this level of experience can result in the overlooking of essential electrodiagnostic information.

Step 1: The Muscle at Rest

The first step in an electromyographic evaluation involves penetrating the tissue of the muscle being studied with the needle electrode and observing for spontaneous electrical activity on the electrodiagnostic instrument. This observation should be made after the penetrating needle has come to rest and there is no muscle movement. A normal muscle with intact neural innervation (with few exceptions) will be electrically silent at rest.

FIBRILLATION POTENTIALS AND POSITIVE SHARP WAVES

When an individual muscle fiber activates, its membrane depolarizes. This is electrodiagnostically characterized by a wave form with an amplitude of 50 μV to 400 μV, whereas the duration depends on the length of the muscle fiber. Muscle fiber membrane action potentials propagate at a rate of 4–5 m/s with a duration on 0.5–1.5 milliseconds. The origin of the discharge can be inferred from its amplitude and duration as well as its rate and rhythm. The indicator of a spontaneously dis-

charging single muscle fiber is a rate from 2 Hz to 20 Hz and generally a regular rhythm.

A fibrillation occurs from the spontaneous depolarization of a single muscle fiber (Fig. 1–2). Although it is usually characterized by a duration of 0.5–1.5 msec and an amplitude of 50 μV to 400 μV, the fibrillation potential is influenced by the distance from the recording electrode tip and the characteristics of the amplifier and the type of electrode. These potentials are usually di- or triphasic with the initial phase positive. The initial phase can be negative when the tip of the needle electrode is in contact with the site where the muscle cell membrane depolarization begins. The rate and rhythm of fibrillation potentials will identify the potentials as spontaneous. Discharges that occur at a slow rate (in the range of 2 Hz – 20 Hz) and regular rhythm should be considered spontaneous in origin.

The discharge of a single muscle fiber can be recorded in one of two locations: at the tip of the recording electrode outside the muscle fiber or in contact with the depolarized membrane. The former is referred to as fibrillation; the latter as a positive wave.

The discharge of a fibrillating single muscle fiber can be recorded as a positive "sharp" wave if the tip of the recording needle is in contact with the depolarized portion of the muscle fiber (Fig. 1–3B). The duration of a positive wave is longer than that of a fibrillation. Amplitudes are generally greater. A positive wave, as its name implies, has an initial positive spike that is followed by a slower neg-

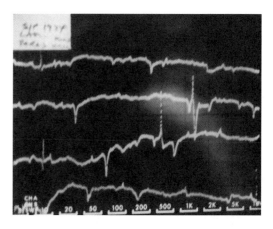

Figure 1-2. Fibrillation potentials and positive waves. (Caliber: 10 msec, 50 μV, Filter: 2Hz–10MHz)

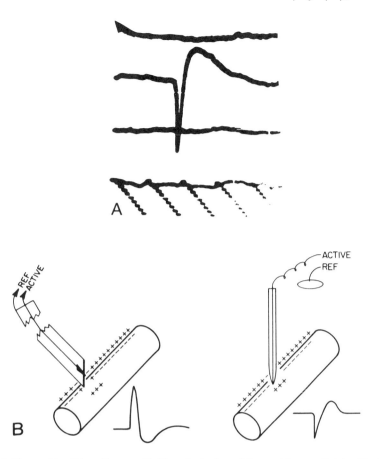

Figure 1–3. *A.* The positive "sharp" wave. (Caliber: Each slanted line = 10msec. Height: 50 μV, Filter: 2Hz–10KHz). *B.* Diagrammatic representation of hypothesis explaining recording differences between coaxial and monopolar needle electrodes (not drawn to scale). The barrel portion (reference) of the coaxial needle (left) is in contact with the depolarized zone, causing the positive wave to be negative. The hemispheric field also causes reduced numbers of potentials. The monopolar electrode (right) is in contact (180°) with the depolarized zone, causing more-frequently- and earlier-appearing positive waves.

ative phase and then a gradual return to the isoelectric baseline (Fig. 1–3A). Because the positive wave must be provoked by the needle electrode (i.e., it is really an artifactual potential), mild muscle cell membrane instability will be first manifested by positive waves. In addition, minimal membrane instability not yet unstable enough to result in fibrillations can manifest as positive waves (31). Fibrillations are presumably the result of altered excitability of the muscle cell membrane. This instability results in a spontaneous activation of the muscle fiber in a variety of ways, including denervation of the muscle fiber, loss of central nervous system (CNS) inhibition, and mechanical, chemical, and electrical stimulation. Fibrillation potentials are not an indica-

tor of any singular disease state and are seen in a variety of conditions in which the muscle cell membrane becomes hyperexcitable. One should view the muscle cell membrane as inherently prepared to depolarize but inhibited by the nerve twig and the neuromuscular junction. This control is lost through denervation of the muscle fiber (i.e., separation from its nerve supply), hypo- and hyperkalemia, local trauma, inflammatory states, certain stages of upper motor neuron diseases, and myopathies, among others. In some instances this intrinsic instability in the muscle cell membrane is present without any apparent disease. This may be a forme fruste of paramyotonia congenita (32) with increased insertional activity and positive waves seen often in a family constellation-presumably autosomal dominant.

FASCICULATION POTENTIALS

A fasciculation potential is the electromyographic manifestation of the spontaneous and involuntary discharge of a motor unit or a portion thereof. Characteristically, these potentials occur at a slow (less than 5 Hz) and irregular rate (Fig. 1–4). 5 Hz is the lowest frequency at which a low-threshold volitional motor unit is recruited.

Fasciculation potentials also appear in a variety of sizes and configurations. Fasciculation potential configurations may be classified as simple or complex. Simple fasciculations are described as bi- or triphasic. All complex fasciculations, however, are polyphasic and are classified as either typical polyphasic potentials or iterative or repetitive discharge polyphasic potentials. A typical or usual polyphasic fasciculation potential crosses the isoelectric line more than four times. An iterative

or repetitive polyphasic potential represents a motor unit that discharges two or three times. These are seen in alkalotic states, e.g., in a hyperventilating patient or with incipient tetany. Early in the alkalosis the volitional potentials are iterative; as the process progresses these volitional iterative discharges become spontaneous and appear as fasciculation potentials. The first sign of an alkalotic state or incipient tetany, however, is a repetitive discharge motor unit potential under volitional control.

Studies have attempted to distinguish those fasciculation potentials that can be seen in motor neuron disease from those fasciculations found in normal individuals (29). The rate of firing is not necessarily a characteristic of the type of fasciculation seen in motor neuron disease. Frequently, fasciculation potentials seen in neuron disease are of very short duration and low amplitude, indicating that the discharge originates in the most peripheral portion of the motor unit. Other fasciculations seen in motor neuron disease can be of large amplitude and polyphasic.

It is conventional wisdom that fasciculation potentials seen by themselves are not necessarily pathologically significant. Exceptions occur: for example, myokymic discharges.

MYOKYMIC DISCHARGES

The myokymic discharge is a special type of fasciculation potential (Fig. 1–5). This dis-

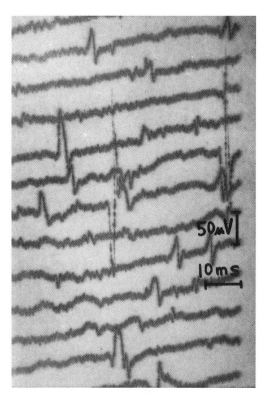

Figure 1–4. Fasciculations recorded from the anterior tibial muscle of an ALS patient. (Caliber: 50 μV, 10 msec. Filter: 2Hz–10KHz)

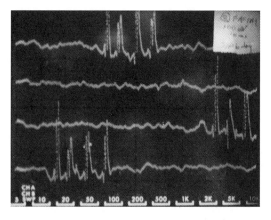

Figure 1–5. Myokymic discharge recorded from the frontalis muscle with a monopolar needle six days after onset of Bell's Palsy. (Caliber: 50 μV, 10 msec. Filter: 2Hz–10KHz)

charge most likely is the result of spontaneous activation and transmission across segments of injured or diseased nerves. This process results in synchronous or grouped discharges of motor unit potentials on the electromyogram. Myokymia is clinically recognizable as continuous "wormy" quivering of the muscles. Facial myokymia is seen in brainstem tumors and multiple sclerosis. Neuromyotonia is similar clinically but is distinguished on electromyogram by a higher frequency and an almost-musical tone.

For the first step of the electromyogram, the gain setting should be 50 μV/cm and the sweep speed 5 msec/cm to 10 msec/cm. Although recommendations of other gain settings have been made, it is necessary in this step to use sufficient gain to ensure the visualization of fibrillation potentials that may be remote or old and therefore as small as 20 μV. A filter setting in the range of 20 Hz to 10 KHz is necessary. The use of 100 μV/cm is a carry-over from the use of instruments that were supplied with a 5-inch oscilloscope with a gain setting of 100 μV/inch (which equals 40 microvolts/cm). All of the electromyograms today employ metric measurements. One can measure the rate of tremor in Step One by reducing the sweep speed to 100 msec/cm (one second/10cm trace) and the gain to 500 μV/cm. Grouped discharges (e.g., with myokymia) are also best recognized at slow sweep speeds of 20–50 msec/cm.

STEP TWO: INSERTIONAL ACTIVITY

To evaluate insertional activity, the electromyographer moves the needle electrode briskly through the muscle tissue, causing bursts of electrical activity. These bursts are referred to as "injury potentials" because they result from mechanical disruption of a group of muscle cell membranes. If there is no muscle tissue present in the region that the needle electrode is exploring, there will be no electrical activity. The evaluation of insertional activity is the most misinterpreted portion of the electromyogram. Insertional activity is best characterized as normal, reduced, or increased.

With normal insertional activity, the duration of the insertional activity results from the movement of the electromyographer's hand. Some electromyographers, whose hands move quickly, may produce a burst of injury potentials having a duration of 75 msec to 100 msec of insertional activity. Other electromyographers, who move the needle slowly and for a somewhat longer period of time, may produce a burst of 300 msec or 400 msec of insertional activity. Thus, the characterization of insertional activity by duration is entirely inappropriate and relates only to the specific technique of moving the needle through the muscle.

If much of the muscle has been replaced with fibrous tissue or edema, the insertional activity will be reduced.

An increase in insertional activity occurs when muscle cell membranes are extraordinarily hyperirritable. This condition exists in such disease states and disorders as acute polymyositis, muscular dystrophy, denervated muscle, myotonic disorders, and in neuropathic and myopathic processes. In these instances the electrical activity will persist long after needle movement has ceased.

END-PLATE NOISE AND END-PLATE SPIKES

When the tip of the needle is in the end-plate zone, some rather characteristic discharges occur (Fig. 1–6). Initially, the tip of the needle provokes the release of acetylcholine quanta that migrate across the synaptic cleft and depolarize the postsynaptic membrane, resulting in an increase of miniature end-plate poten-

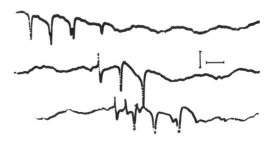

Figure 1–6. Endplate spikes being recorded as positive waves as needle electrode is advanced through endplate zone. (Caliber: 100 μV, 10 msec. Filter: 2Hz–10KHz)

tials. They are nonpropagated and thus monophasic; negative in polarity; and fire at high frequencies (up to 1,000 Hz). Formerly this sound was described as a "seashell murmur". A more meaningful description, however, is an increase in the noise level of the oscilloscope trace, perhaps doubling or tripling it from 5 μV at a gain setting of 50 MV/cm to 15–20 μV. As these miniature end-plate potentials reach the threshold of activation of the cell membrane, the muscle fiber discharges, resulting in a biphasic spike with an initial negative phase. This has the same characteristics as a fibrillation potential except that, because it originates at the end-plate, the initial de-flection is negative instead of positive. If the needle electrode is advanced slightly and its tip samples from the depolarized zone, the end-plate spikes will be recorded as positive waves (Fig. 1–7). Caution should be exercised when considering the following distinction: positive waves recorded from fibrillating muscle fibers are pathologic, and those recorded from the end plate zone are not (Fig. 1–8). The distinguishing characteristics are their rhythm and rate of firing. The endplate spike discharges irregularly at 20 Hz to 150 Hz. Additionally, the presence of the needle in the end-plate zone usually provokes the patient to complain of a characteristic dull ache.

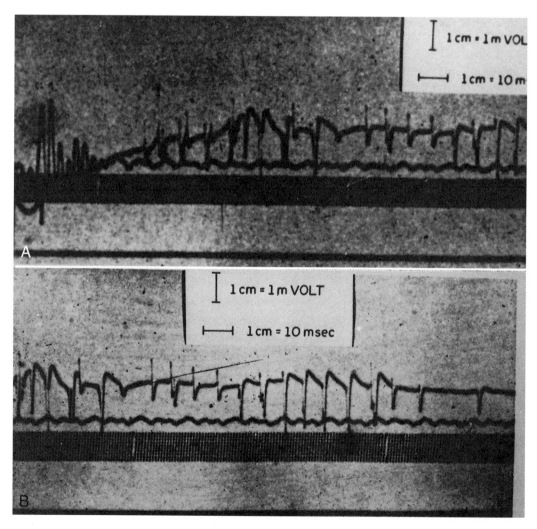

Figure 1–7. A continuous tracing in two parts. Endplate spikes evolving into positive waves as the needle electrode is advanced through the endplate zone and into the depolarized zone. (Caliber: on photo. Filter: 2Hz–10KHz)

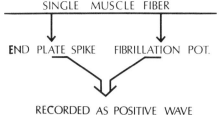

Figure 1–8. Origin of the positive "sharp" wave.

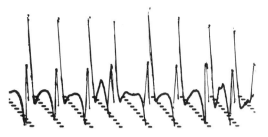

Figure 1–9. Cramp. Monopolar needle electrode in soleus. (Caliber: Each slanted line = 10 msec. Height = 500 μV, Filter: 2Hz–10KHz)

CRAMP

Should the needle be in the presence of a cramp, high-frequency (up to 150 Hz) synchronous motor unit discharges would be seen (Fig. 1–9).

COMPLEX REPETITIVE DISCHARGES

In areas affected by motor unit diseases of various types including muscular dystrophy, amyotrophic lateral sclerosis, and chronic radiculopathy, the needle electrode occasionally records a discharge that has been termed a complex repetitive discharge (Fig. 1–10). Other names used in the past to describe these potentials include bizzare high-frequency discharges and pseudomyotonic discharges; the latter term is inappropriate because these potentials lack the waxing and waning qualities of myotonic discharges.

A complex repetitive discharge is spontaneous muscle fiber activity that appears as a continuous train of spikes at a regular frequency of 5 Hz to 150 Hz. The waveform is complex and is relatively uniform from one discharge to another. The discharge begins and ends abruptly, sounding like a motor boat.

The potentials seem spontaneous; they appear to be provoked readily by movements of the needle electrode or percussion of the muscle. They are a nonspecific finding seen in conditions of chronic denervation (e.g., with motor neuron disease, long-standing radiculopathy, chronic polyneuropathy) and in myopathies (e.g., muscular dystrophy, polymyositis). Complex repetitive discharge potentials result from ephaptic activation of hyperexcitable muscle fibers, which usually have lost their innervation (30). When studied with single fiber electromyography, the discharges are seen as complex potentials containing up to ten or more distinct single fiber action potentials. Complex repetitive discharges with low repetition rates (less than 45 Hz) occasionally had highly irregular interdischarge intervals but showed no other differences from higher frequency discharges.

Jitter between individual spikes is less than 5 msec and is never seen when impulse transmission occurs across a motor end-plate. Therefore, the low jitter between individual spike components and consecutive discharges

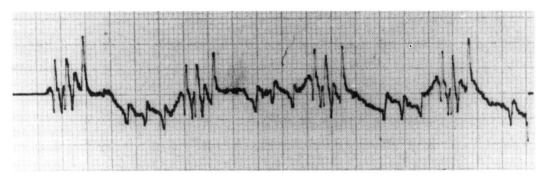

Figure 1–10. Complex repetitive discharge in Duchenne dystrophy. Monopolar needle electrode in extensor digitorum longus. (Caliber: Each square = 5 msec, 50 μV. Filter: 2Hz–10KHz)

is considered evidence of ephaptic or direct electrical activation of muscle fiber to muscle fiber. The discharge is initiated by a fibrillating pacemaker muscle fiber, which activates one or several adjacent fibers. One of these fibers then reactivates the principal pacemaker, creating a closed loop. This cycle continues until the pacemaker fibers become subnormally excitable and block the propagation. The electromyographer must be careful to distinguish these discharges from similar findings of myotonia, neuromyotonia, and cramp syndrome.

By using single fiber EMG studies, Stålberg showed this to be the activation of a denervated pacemaker or a very hyperirritable single muscle fiber that acts by ephaptic transmission to discharge neighboring hyperirritable fibers (30). This discharge begins abruptly and discontinues abruptly. When the complex repetitive discharges occur at rates that exceed the highest frequency of normally recruited motor units (45 Hz), they are referred to as high-frequency complex repetitive discharges.

For Step 2, the gain setting should be 50–100 μV/cm with a sweep speed of 5–10 msec/cm. Note that the gain setting should always be adjusted so that the entire potential is seen. The low filter frequency setting can be moved up to 20 Hz so that needle electrode movement will not cause the trace to move excessively.

Step 3: Minimal Contraction of a Muscle

When the recording needle is in the desired muscle, the patient is asked to begin contracting that muscle. In so doing, the lowest threshold motor units will be activated at approximately 5 Hz. These motor units are generally smaller and arise from Type I muscle fibers. Although it is traditional to refer to motor unit potentials, actually only a small portion of the entire motor unit is recorded with the tip of the needle electrode. The spike of the motor unit potential may represent as few as one or two muscle fiber action potentials. In normal muscle, the first recruited motor unit begins to fire more rapidly as the strength of contraction increases. As contraction strength continues to increase, additional

motor units are recruited. These motor units have a different morphology than the original motor unit. The moment at which the second motor unit appears is designated the recruitment interval (Fig. 1–11). Specifically, the recruitment interval is the time interval between successive discharges of the initial motor unit immediately preceding the appearance of the second recruited motor unit. The reciprocal of the recruitment interval is the recruitment frequency. Most of the commercially available electromyograms have digital memory with the capability of storing 500 msec or more of discharges so that the recruitment frequency and interval can be easily determined.

The recruitment interval is actually a sensitive diagnostic index of weakness. In neuropathic disease, the recruitment interval would be shortened; that is, because there are fewer motor units available when the strength of contraction increases, the first unit will be firing more rapidly at the moment that the second unit is recruited. Shortening the recruitment interval increases the recruitment frequency. Conversely, in early myopathic disease, the recruitment interval would be lengthened (Fig. 1–12); that is, the first motor unit would be firing more slowly at the moment that the second unit is recruited because each motor unit has fewer muscle fibers functioning and therefore is weaker.

In reinnervation, the motor unit potential (MUP) may be prolonged in duration, have low amplitude, and be highly polyphasic. As the new axon sprouts mature, the muscle fibers discharge more synchronously, thus making the MUP larger and less polyphasic. Ulti-

RECRUITMENT INTERVAL (RI)

Time between succeeding contractions of 1st MU at moment of 2nd MU recruited

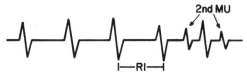

= Reciprocal of firing rate of 1st MU at moment of 2nd MU recruitment /

Figure 1–11. Recruitment interval (reciprocal of recruitment frequency).

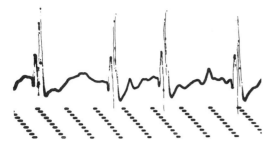

Figure 1–12. Reduced recruitment in severe axonal neuropathy. (Monopolar needle in extensor digitorum longus.) Note firing rate is 36 Hz. (Caliber: Each slanted line = 10 msec. Height = 200 μV. Filter: 2Hz–10KHz)

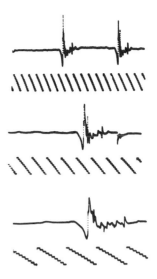

Figure 1–13. Complex motor unit potential recorded in reinnervating peripheral nerve injury (s/p 5 months). Monopolar needle electrode in deltoid. The satellite potential is evident in the bottom tracing 10 msec after the main complex. (Caliber: Each slanted line = 10 msec. Height = 200 μV. Filter: 2Hz–10KHz)

mately, a reinnervated motor unit will be only larger than normal, particularly if it adopted more muscle fibers than in the original motor unit.

Type II motor units are generally recruited later and are larger in amplitude and of longer duration. The Type II motor units are activated in a vigorous contraction (see Step 4) that is referred to as ballistic recruitment. Note that the amplitude of the recorded motor unit potential is measured peak to peak. A trigger-and-signal delay line can help make accurate measurements of the motor unit potentials.

In some chronic reinnervation states, a satellite potential will occur 10–15 msec later than the major potential but is time-locked. This presumably is due to incomplete myelination of an immature twig (Fig. 1–13).

The gain setting for Step 3 should be 50–100 μV/cm and a faster sweep at 2 to 5 msec/cm. These changes provide an opportunity to examine in detail the amplitude, duration, number of phases, and stability of the motor unit potential. The polyphasic motor unit potential has more than five phases because it crosses the isoelectric line more than four times (Fig. 1–14).

Step 4: Maximal Effort

In order that maximal effort be exerted by the patient, the electrode should be placed superficially in the muscle so that making a maximal contraction will not be painful. The muscle should be a single joint muscle because it is extraordinarily difficult to generate maximal effort with a two-joint muscle when the

patient is in a recumbent position. For example, the vastus medialis (a single-joint muscle) should be used instead of the rectus femoris, which crosses both hip and knee.

With neuropathic conditions, during the maximal contraction, there is a reduced number of motor units in relation to strength of contraction (Fig. 1–12). The effort of the patient can be gauged by the rate of firing. One should not indicate that there is a reduced number of motor units or a reduced recruit-

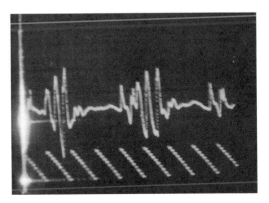

Figure 1–14. Polyphasic motor unit potential. The center waveform represents the sum of the first and third potentials. (Caliber: Each slanted line = 10 msec. Height = 200 μV. Filter: 2Hz–10KHz)

ment pattern unless there is a maximal rate of firing. It has been estimated that the tip of the electrode can record, at a maximum, portions of eight or ten motor units; therefore, if only two motor units are present on the screen, one could assume that there is a substantial degree of weakness present. Because a grade of 4 out of 5 or greater on manual muscle tests has been shown when only 40% to 50% of the motor units remain, it will be difficult for the manual muscle test to detect degrees of weakness representing a loss of 30% or fewer motor units during Step 4 of the electromyographic examination.

This difficulty in detecting weakness suggests that the recruitment interval or frequency is a more sensitive electromyographic technique than Step 4 by itself. When one sees considerable notching at the peaks of the motor unit during maximal contraction, one should return to Step 3 for further estimation of the proportion of polyphasic potentials (Fig. 1–13). If the polyphasic potentials have increased more than 10%, they should be reported as "an increased proportion of polyphasic potentials." The audio signal can suggest a reduction of the motor unit potentials in Step 4.

With so-called "hysterical weakness," Step 4 reveals the electrical correlate of the ratchety response that is characteristic; that is, groups of motor unit potentials discharge separated by a space, similar to a tremor.

Step 4 gain settings should be set at 200–1,000 μV/cm. Sweep speed should be 10 msec/cm. It is essential that all of the potentials be visualized on the screen; thus, the gain setting should be adjusted to see the entire motor unit potential.

Step 5: Diagnostic Electromyography

When an abnormality has been detected, one must then explore other muscles to determine if the disease or injury is limited to a branch of a peripheral nerve or an entire root level, or if the abnormality is more generalized. This must be accomplished by a systematic needle exploration of the limb and paraspinal muscles. A detailed knowledge of surface, functional, and neuromuscular anatomy is necessary for appropriate completion of this step. Usually, if a generalized disease process is suspected, at least three of five limbs should be explored. For purposes of electrodiagnosis, the head is considered a limb. In a motor unit disease, such as ALS, the tongue and soft palate should be explored.

Knowledge of the clinical patterns of disease is also essential in order to explore those regions of muscle that are most likely to be involved early in the disease process. An example is the upper trapezius in facioscapulohumeral muscular dystrophy.

An important consideration is the fact that muscles located in various parts of the body have substantially different electrodiagnostic characteristics. Motor unit action potentials differ in duration, amplitude, and firing rates depending on the anatomic function and physiology of a given muscle (Table 1–1). The extrinsic eye muscles, for example, have very tiny, short-duration potentials (perhaps 100–200 μV in amplitude, one msec in duration) and firing rates of up to 100 Hz. The vastus medialis represents the other extreme. Its motor unit potentials may be 1,500–2,000 μV and 12 msec in duration. As a rule, the more-centrally located muscles have smaller amplitudes and shorter duration potentials.

SPECIAL CONSIDERATIONS OF ANATOMY

Accessible muscles for needle exploration include most of the 434 skeletal muscles in the body. The trapezius and the facial muscles are extraordinarily thin, so that an exploring electrode may penetrate through these muscles unless meticulous care is taken. This is

Table 1–1
Normal Amplitudes of MUP 1st Recruited/ Monopolar Electrode

Muscle	Microvolts (μV)
Pectoralis major	429 ± 12
Biceps brachii	490 ± 11
Gluteus maximus	533 ± 17
Abductor digiti	926 ± 63
Gastrocnemius	1133 ± 34
Triceps brachii	1157 ± 45
Quadriceps femoris	1217 ± 43

particularly true with certain diseases, for example, facioscapulohumeral muscular dystrophy in the trapezius, or trauma to the 11th cranial nerve with subsequent atrophy of this muscle.

There have been reports of penetration of the pleural space by careless electromyographers who are unfamiliar with surface anatomy. This has occurred when exploring the proximal portion of the supraspinatus muscle or the lateral extent of the paraspinal muscles in the cervical region of thin individuals. The abdominal muscles should also be explored extremely carefully so that the peritoneal cavity is not compromised. When evaluating the intercostal and abdominal muscles, it is wise to insert the needle at a sharply acute angle to the skin rather than at a right angle.

The serratus anterior is easily explored in the midaxillary line. Because its attachments are on the rib, the examiner's fingers can be placed in the intercostal space above and below a rib, inserting the needle in between. This is also the proper site to place a surface electrode when recording the compound muscle action potential of the serratus anterior muscle.

Electromyographic evaluation of the diaphragm elicits anxiety in many examiners. By applying the Koepke technique (2, 12, 13) carefully, the adverse sequela of pneumothorax and hepatic, splenic, or colonic penetration can be minimized. The diaphragm can be accessed between the tenth and eleventh ribs in the left midaxillary line or in the anterior axillary or medial clavicular lines by inserting the needle electrode over the lower costal margin. The diaphragm attaches on the cartilage of the lower costal margin. With this technique, the needle electrode is introduced sufficiently caudal to the lung parenchyma. Care must be taken not to penetrate the peritoneum, which is located just deep to this position. Gentle respirations by the patient will confirm placement of the needle in the diaphragm by ensuring that accessory respiratory muscles are not activated. Motor unit potentials of the diaphragm characteristically are more numerous and have smaller amplitudes and shorter durations than those of other chest wall muscles (2, 13).

The external anal sphincter is skeletal muscle and can be explored easily with a needle. It is difficult to get it to relax, however. In it there is usually activity present; so more important diagnostically is the presence of a full recruitment pattern or whether fibrillation potentials and positive waves are easily seen (1). These are the findings if there is substantial compromise of the pudendal nerve or the roots (S3 and S4) that innervate that muscle.

The inferior oblique muscle of the eye is explored without penetrating the conjunctiva because it is accessible through the skin in the inferior medial aspect of the orbit. This would be a useful muscle to explore with ocular paresis of various types.

The tongue is best evaluated by penetrating inferior and posterior to the base of the mandible, through the mylohyoid, and into the base of the genioglossus (Fig. 1–15). To evaluate Steps 1 and 2, the tongue should be relaxed within the mouth (Fig. 1–16). To evaluate Steps 3 and 4 on one side, the tongue should be protruded in the opposite direction.

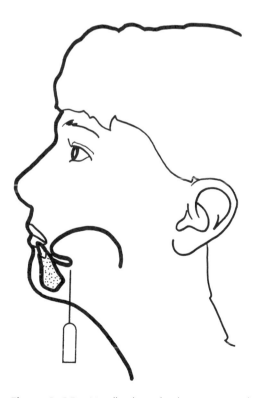

Figure 1–15. Needle electrode placement to evaluate the tongue.

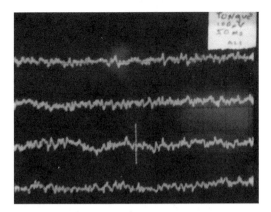

Figure 1–16. Tongue recording in ALS patient. Note the small fasciculation. (Caliber: 100 μV, 50 msec. Filter: 2Hz–10KHz)

GENERAL COMMENTS

The needle examination can be better accomplished with a monopolar electrode because it has been shown that the area of recording of a monopolar needle is about twice that of the coaxial needle. Furthermore, because of its dimensions and configuration, the monopolar needle electrode has been experimentally and clinically shown to record more profuse positive waves and at an earlier time than the coaxial needle (if disease or injury is present)(6). Theoretically, this difference could be explained by the beveled tip of a coaxial needle that records only a hemispheric field. Furthermore, the advancing tip of the coaxial needle is the barrel (i.e., reference) (Fig. 1–3) rather than the recording electrode. As a result, the positive wave should be recorded as an initial negative deflection with a subsequent low-amplitude, long-duration positive deflection and may not be recognized as a positive wave. It is generally believed that the monopolar needle is less painful; however, it does have the disadvantage of insulation retraction at the tip with a reduction in the amplitude of the motor unit potential. This requires frequent needle inspection, but this problem is nearly eliminated with the use of disposable needle electrodes.

Electromyography should only be performed by a physician specifically trained in this science. A well-planned electromyogram is essential for several reasons. First, a well-planned study implies consideration of information gathered from a detailed neuromuscular history and physical examination. Second, it implies a thorough knowledge of neuromuscular anatomy, which is essential and fundamental to the appropriate application of electromyographic technology. Third, it implies a thorough understanding of the pathophysiology of neuromuscular diseases. The necessary condition of a well-planned EMG study is the flexibility to make alterations should unexpected findings arise. Fourth, and most pragmatically, a well-planned examination minimizes the discomfort experienced by apprehensive patients, especially children, by shortening the length of the examination and minimizing the number of needle penetrations. This is the most efficient time utilization of electromyographer and patient alike. If the electromyogram is regarded as anything but an extension of a detailed history and neuromuscular physical examination, it will at best provide extensive data that has marginal clinical significance, but at worst can become misleading to diagnostic and prognostic pursuits.

References

1. Bailey J, et al.: A clinical evaluation of electromyography of the anal sphincter. Arch Phys Med Rehabil 1970;51:403.
2. Bolton C: AAEM Minimonograph #40: Clinical neurophysiology of the respiratory system. Muscle Nerve 1993;16:809–818.
3. Buchtal F, et al.: Motor unit territory in different human muscles. Acta Physiol Scand 1959;45:72.
4. Buchtal F, Pinelli P: Action potentials in muscular atrophy of nuerogenic origin. Neurology 1953;3:591–603.
5. Denny-Brown D: Interpretation of the electromyogram. Arch Neurol Phychiatry 1949;61:99.
6. Jasper H, Ballem G: Unipolar electromyograms of normal and denervated human muscle. J Neurophysiol 1949;12:231–244.
7. Jensan SF: Spontaneous electrical activity in denervated extraoccular muscles. Acta Ophthalmol 1972;50:827.
8. Johnson E, et al.: EMG abnormalities after intramuscular injections. Arch Phys Med Rehabil 1971;52:250.
9. Johnson E, et al.: Sequence of electromyographic abnormalities in stroke syndrome. Arch Phys Med Rehabil 1975;56:468.
10. Johnson E, et al.: Use of electrodiagnostic examination in a university hospital. Arch Phys Med Rehabil 1965;46:<pp?>.

11. Kimura J, et al.: Reflex response of orbicularis oculi muscle to supraorbital nerve stimulation. Arch Neurol 1969;21:193.

12. Koepke GH: The electromyographic examination of the diaphragm. Bullitin Am Assoc EMG EDX 1960;7:8.

13. Koepke GH, et al.: Sequence of action of the diaphragm and intercostal muscles during respiration: I. Inspiration. Arch Phys Med Rehabil 1958;39:426–430.

14. Kugelberg E: Electromyograms in muscular disorders. J Neurol Neurosurg Psychiatry 1947;10:122.

15. Kugelberg E, Cobb W: Repetitive discharges in human motor fibers during post-schaemic state. J Neurol Neurosurg Psychiatry 1954;14:88.

16. Kugelberg E, Petersen I: "Insertional Activity" in electromyography. J Neurol Neurosurg Psychiatry 1949;12:268–273.

17. Lambert E, McMorris R: Size of motor unit potentials in neuromuscular disorders. Fed Proc 1953;13:263.

18. Lambert E, et al.: Studies on the origin of the positive wave in electromyography. Newsletter Am Assoc EMG EDX 1957;3:3.

19. Landau W: The essential mechanisms in myotonia: An electromyographic study. Neurology 1952;2:369–388.

20. Lederman RJ, Wilbourn AJ: Brachial plexopathy: Recurrent cancer or radiation? Neurology 1984;24:1331–1335.

21. Mechler F: Changing electromyographic findings during the chronic course of polymyositis. J Neurol Sci 1974;23:237–242.

22. McMorris R: Amplitudes and durations of first recruited motor unit potentials. Thesis, Mayo Foundation, Graduate Education, University of Minnesota, 1952.

23. Petajan J: Clinical electromyographic studies of diseases of the motor unit. Electroencephalogr Clin Neurophysiol 1974;36:395.

24. Petajan J, Philip B: Frequency control of motor unit action potentials. Electroencephalogr Clin Neurophysiol 1969;27:66.

25. Rosen J, et al.: Electromyography in spinal cord injury. Arch Phys Med Rehabil 1969;50:271.

26. Schwartz M, et al.: The reinnervated motor unit in man. J Neurol Sci 1976;27:303.

27. Stohr M: Benign fibrillation potenials in normal muscle and their correlation with endplate and denervation potentials. J Neurol Neurosurg 1977;40:765.

28. Taylor RG, Kewalramani LS, Fowler WM: Electromyographic findings in lower extremities of patients with high spinal cord injury. Arch Phys Med Rehabil 1974;55:16–23.

29. Trojabrg W, Buchthal F: Malignant and benign fasciculations. Acta Neurol Scand 1965;41(suppl 13):251.

30. Trontelj J, Stålberg E: Bizare repetitive discharges recorded with single fiber EMG. J Neurol Neurosurg Psychiatry 1983;46:310–316.

31. Weichers D: Mechanically provoked insertional activity before and after nerve section in rats. Arch Phys Med Rehabil 1977;58:402.

32. Weichers D, Johnson E: Diffuse abnormal electromyographic insertional activity: A preliminary report. Arch Phys Med Rehabil 1979;60:419–422.

33. Wiederholt W: "End-plate noise" in electromyography 1970;20:214.

Chapter 2

Quality Improvement for the Electrodiagnostic Consultation

Scott A. Murray
Ernest W. Johnson
William S. Pease

In the current healthcare environment, delivering high-quality and high value patient care is paramount. Hospital systems, third party organizations, and healthcare providers are scrutinizing the delivery of services more than ever. In evaluating quality of care, stronger emphasis has been placed on cost effectiveness, patient perceptions, appropriateness, and efficacy of care. The care administered by an electrodiagnostician is no exception to this emphasis.

The premise of this chapter is that there is always room for improving the quality and performance in an electrodiagnostic medicine clinic. The authors' goal is to help the electrodiagnostician to develop an appreciation of ways to improve aspects of clinical practice.

The chapter is divided into three main sections, including the following: 1) introducing quality improvement concepts; 2) improving electrodiagnostic medicine consultations, including ways to improve delivery of care unrelated to the actual electrodiagnostic examination; and 3) ways to specifically improve electrodiagnostic medicine reports. Critiques of sample reports and a summary conclude the chapter.

GENERAL CONCEPTS OF QUALITY IMPROVEMENT

What is High Quality Health Care and Why is it Important?

The Joint Commission on Accreditation of Healthcare Organizations (JCAHO) is a government-funded unit whose mission is to improve the quality of health care provided to the public (25). Many hospitals and other healthcare organizations have adopted their policies, and some have made them requirements. Philosophies embraced by this organization have evolved with catch phrases including medical audits, quality assurance, quality improvement, continuing quality improvement, total quality improvement, and recently, performance improvement (24).

JCAHO defines performance as what is done and how well it is done to provide health care (i.e., doing the right thing and doing it well). The level of performance is the degree to which what is done is effective and appropriate for the individual patient. Other dimensions of performance include the degree to which health care is safe, efficient, caring, and respectful of the patient, available in a timely manner to patients who need it, and continuous with other care providers. The effect of an organization's performance of these functions is reflected in patient outcomes, cost of its services and, sometimes, on patients' perceptions of what was done and how it was done (24).

Performance improvement is a philosophy of organizational management whose goal is to design a mechanism for ongoing, comprehensive, performance-based self-assessment and improvement. It is based on the premise that healthcare organizations exist to maximize the health of the people they serve while using resources efficiently, involving users in decision making, and making decisions based on data. This approach shifts the primary focus from the performance of individuals to the performance of the organization's systems and processes, while continuing to recognize the importance of the individual competence of medical staff members and other employees (24).

Three issues must be considered by any organization dedicated to excellence. The first issue is the organization's relationship with its external environment. Today, successful healthcare organizations must be able to anticipate, understand, and flexibly respond to changes in the dynamic healthcare environment. The second issue is the organization's internal characteristics and functions. Excellence in patient care requires state-of-the-art professional knowledge; clinical, management, governance, and support expertise; and competent technical skills integrated and coordinated organizationwide to respond effectively and efficiently to patient and family needs. The third issue is a methodology for systematically assessing and improving important functions and work processes and their outcomes (24).

An example of a systematic approach for implementing this strategy is JCAHO's Ten-Step Model (25). The model can be used when designing a new process, redesigning an existing process, or acting on an opportunity for incremental improvement in an existing process.

Step 1: Assign responsibility for overseeing the performance improvement plan.
Step 2: Delineate the scope of care (i.e., all services provided by the organization).
Step 3: Identify important aspects of care.
Step 4: Identify objective indicators.
Step 5: Establish thresholds.
Step 6: Collect and organize data.
Step 7: Initiate evaluation.
Step 8: Take actions to improve care.
Step 9: Assess the effectiveness of actions.
Step 10: Communicate results to relevant individuals and groups.

Burwick said that "fully implementing quality improvement is an extended process.

It requires leadership, commitment, and resources such as time and expertise. The experience of organizations who have begun the implementation suggests that these efforts also have accompanying satisfactions: the pleasure of taking constructive action, improvement in performance, and savings of time and money" (12).

Implementing Performance Improvement in an Electrodiagnostic Medicine Clinic: Examples

Many processes must be done correctly to reach a satisfactory outcome in an electrodiagnostic medicine clinic. Something could go wrong in any of the steps, resulting in an unsatisfactory outcome. Determinants of how the clinic is managed vary according to the setting in which the laboratory functions. For example, a clinic in an academic setting has different goals because of the presence of residents and medical students. In this situation, key functions include resident supervision and education (33).

Aspects of the JCAHO's Ten-Step Model (25) can be used in a clinic to design, measure, assess, and improve work processes. Several specific examples are given below.

EXAMPLE 1. ELECTRODIAGNOSTIC EVALUATION OF PERIPHERAL NEUROPATHY: IMPROVING PERFORMANCE

Potential Aspects of Care to Monitor
1) The presence of a provisional diagnosis, based on adequate history and physical examination; 2) Testing of appropriate* nerves and muscles for a given diagnosis; 3) Interpretation of the findings of nerve conduction and needle electromyography; 4) Education of the patient and the family regarding diagnosis, possible treatment options, and prognosis; and 5) Timely reporting of the results to the referring physician.

---

*These terms need to be defined before monitoring has started and should be consistent with the AAEM Guidelines in Electrodiagnostic Medicine (2).

Possible Indicators

1) Is there evidence that an adequate* history was taken?; 2) Are relevant* physical examination findings documented?; 3) Are appropriate* and adequate* number of nerves examined by nerve stimulation studies?; 4) Were appropriate* muscles examined with a needle electrode?; 5) Are interpretations consistent with the electrodiagnostic data?; 6) Is there documentation of patient and family education?; 7) Was timely* reporting of the results to the referring physician carried out?

Acceptable Thresholds

All the above indicators have a 90% threshold.

Data Collection

Data collection is ongoing.

Data Analysis

Data analysis is carried out quarterly or monthly.

Actions Taken

Opportunities to improve care are identified. Actions are recommended and the effect of actions taken is examined.

Communication

Results and conclusions are reported at appropriate medical staff meetings and to the leaders of the organization. (33)

EXAMPLE 2. IMPROVING PATIENT SATISFACTION

Potential Aspects of Care to Monitor

Patients should be satisfied with the timeliness of the service provided, the courtesy with which the services were provided, the environment, and the physician's attitude.

Possible Indicators

1) Are the services provided in a timely* manner?; 2) Is the staff courteous?; 3) Is the environment safe and accessible?; 4) Does the patient see the physician without undue wait* in the reception area?; 5) Is the procedure explained to the patient before starting?; and 6) Does the physician explain the results at the end of the procedure?

Acceptable Thresholds

1) Ninety percent of services are provided in a timely manner; 2) The staff is reported as courteous by 75% of the patients; 3) The environment is reported to be accessible by 80% of the patients; 4) Seventy-five percent of the patients are seen within 30 minutes of their scheduled time; 5) The procedure is explained to 100% of the patients; and 6) The results of the testing are explained in 100% of the cases.

Data Collection

Data is collected using a questionnaire. The questionnaire (with a stamped addressed return envelope) is mailed to 20% of the patients (a minimum of ten) seen during the past month. Data collection is carried out quarterly.

Data Analysis

Data analysis is carried out quarterly.

Actions Taken

Opportunities to improve care are identified and actions recommended. The effects of actions on patients are evaluated.

Communications

Findings are communicated to the referring physicians, other healthcare providers, and the leaders of the organization (33).

EXAMPLE 3. PROCESS EVALUATION: SCHEDULING OF PATIENTS

Possible Indicators

1) Is there adequate staff to answer all the incoming requests for scheduling?; 2) Is there a need to have a 24-hour answering system?; and 3) Are the patients seen in a timely manner after they request an appointment, and is there a provision to respond to an emergency request? (33)

EXAMPLE 4. UTILIZATION MONITORING AND EVALUATION

Possible Indicators

1) Are the patients being referred appropriately?; 2) How many patients have failed to keep their appointments?; 3) What actions are taken if patients do not show up for their scheduled appointments?; and 4) What percentage of the patients referred to the clinic have positive findings? (33)

IMPROVING ELECTRODIAGNOSTIC MEDICAL CONSULTATIONS

In this section, we describe many areas involved with the completion of high-quality electrodiagnostic medicine consultations.

What is an Electrodiagnostic Medical Consultation?

An electrodiagnostic medicine consultation is a medical consultation in which neurophysiologic techniques are applied to diagnose, evaluate, and treat patients with impairments or disabilities of the neurologic or muscular systems (6). As with any other specialty, this medical consultation should include a directed history and physical examination, electrodiagnostic examination (as an extension of the physical exam), clear and concise summary, diagnostic impressions, recommendations to the referring physician, and appropriate interventions. When completed correctly, the electrodiagnostic medicine consultation is an invaluable resource for the referring physician that will assist with the care of the patient, ideally toward an accurate diagnosis and successful outcome. As an expert in the neuromuscular system, the electrodiagnostician is well trained to provide this service.

Qualifications of the Electrodiagnostic Medicine Consultant

It is the position of the American Association of Electrodiagnostic Medicine (AAEM) [+] that "the electrodiagnostic medicine consultant must be a physician who has special training in the diagnosis and treatment of neuromuscular diseases and is also an expert in the application of particular neurophysiologic techniques to

study these disorders" (2). Recommended minimal educational requirements are 1) the completion of an accredited postgraduate medical specialty training program in neurology, physical medicine and rehabilitation, or their equivalent and 2) completion of a period of preceptorship in electrodiagnostic medicine during or after residency training (2). To assess mastery in electrodiagnosis, the American Board of Electrodiagnostic Medicine offers a voluntary certification process requiring that the clinician meet the above educational requirements, obtain at least one year of experience following residency, undergo training, performing, and interpreting electrodiagnostic examinations on an additional 200 or more patients, and pass an examination consisting of waveform recognition, videotape anatomy, and written and oral sections (6).

The knowledge and expertise gained from such specialized medical training maximizes the ability of the consultant to consider appropriate differential medical diagnoses from the patient's preliminary history and physical examination. The course of the electrodiagnostic examination can then be appropriately planned and modified as the findings unfold. Improper performance or interpretation of the electrodiagnostic examination may be dangerous to the patient and misleading to the referring physician (2). For these reasons, electrodiagnostic examinations should be done only by physicians fully trained in electrodiagnostic medicine. This AAEM position is endorsed by the American Medical Association (10), American Academy of Neurology (8), American Academy of Physical Medicine and Rehabilitation (9), American Neurological Association, Department of Veterans Affairs (43), and many state medical examination boards (40).

Equipment

Electrodiagnostic instrumentation is an important factor in performing high-quality electrodiagnostic medicine consultations. Not only must consultants have the appropriate equipment, but they must know how to use it and ensure that the test is safe and the results obtained are accurate and reliable. General points of how instrumentation contributes to

---

[+]The American Association of Electrodiagnostic Medicine (AAEM, formerly the American Association of Electromyography and Electrodiagnosis) was founded in 1953 and incorporated as a nonprofit organization in 1959 to increase and extend the knowledge of electromyography and electrodiagnostic medicine, improve the quality of patient care, and promote the professional association of physicians interested in electromyography and electrodiagnostic medicine. The American Board of Electrodiagnostic Medicine (ABEM) is an organization whose goal is to enhance the quality of patient care through a voluntary certification process.

the performance of a high-quality consultation will be discussed in this section. More detailed technical aspects of equipment, its usage, and errors can be found in Chapter 4 of this text and in the AAEM Minimonograph 16 (20).

1. INSTRUMENTS

Almost all modern electrodiagnostic instruments meet the specifications recommended by the American Association of Electrodiagnostic Medicine (2), including both analog and digital models (16). Newer digital instruments allow the use of trigger delay lines, automatic cursor placement, averaging, amplitude and area measurements, frequency analysis, interference pattern analysis, and the ability to change the sweep and display sensitivity after waveform capture (20). "Embedded" computers are also used for more sophisticated functions such as identifying individual motor units, counting turns, and report generation; computer-based "expert system" programs give guidance in test planning and data interpretation (23, 38, 44).

Many other equipment variables contribute to the performance of high-quality electrodiagnostic studies, but these have not been objectively tested. Factors that should influence the type of instrument employed or purchased include user-friendliness of the system; ease of appropriate report generation; efficiency of testing allowed; and the availability of technical support. It is especially important for the instrument to be flexible and for its specialized features not to impair a skilled examiner's ability to produce a high-quality electrodiagnostic medicine consultation. Although there is not a study or report that objectively compares features of different instruments, clinicians from several prominent electrodiagnostic medicine clinics have described their likes and dislikes of instruments used in their specific clinical situations (41).

Another equipment variable is whether monopolar or concentric needle electrodes should be used. Because of their different electrical responses, the electrodiagnostic medicine consultant must appreciate that separate reference databases are established and should be used for the two types of electrodes (19). In general, monopolar needle electrodes produce larger amplitudes, greater phasicity, similar durations, and less pain, and are less expensive when compared to concentric electrodes (19, 37).

Disposable needle electrodes have become much more popular than reusable electrodes mainly because of lower maintenance, patients' concerns of infection, and reasonable costs for disposable electrodes. Also, the quality of modern manufactured disposable needles is comparable to reusable ones (15). Several studies have shown minor, if any, electrical response differences between disposable and reusable electrodes (7, 28, 34). More consistent differences were seen in the properties of needle electrodes from different manufacturers, reflecting differences in materials, design, and construction (7, 14).

There are several concerns with reusable needle electrodes. When needles are bent, dirty, corroded, or barbed, or if the Teflon coating is frayed or excessively thinned, polarization potentials are unstable. Unstable polarization potentials can sometimes cause artifacts that resemble abnormal membrane potentials (19). With repeated sterilization, the exposed area can increase up to 20% even without obvious Teflon fraying. Because a monopolar needle records the average potential over its exposed tip, cracked, chipped, or frayed Teflon coating will cause a reduction in the amplitude of motor unit potentials. If breaks or cracks in the Teflon coating exist along the shaft of the electrode, the signal received at the tip will be "short-circuited" back into the tissue, further reducing the amplitude. Because the Teflon does not extend fully to the hub in many monopolar needles, the needle should not be inserted its entire length (19).

2. KNOWLEDGE OF EQUIPMENT

Data acquisition systems can be very complex. To obtain accurate data, the electrodiagnostic medicine consultant must be familiar with the sources and magnitudes of the various equipment errors and the techniques that can be used to reduce their effects (see Chapter 4). Knowledge of these technical limitations can prevent overinterpretation of subtle and borderline abnormalities that could merely represent artifacts or "experimental" errors (20).

With the integration of computer analysis, the electrodiagnostic medicine consultant must know how and when to override the computer. The computer can fail or make errors (e.g., inappropriately placed takeoff or peak amplitude markers). The electrodiagnostician must be an expert in the principles of analysis and, therefore, be in control of the latest technology rather than being controlled by it (38).

3. EQUIPMENT SAFETY

The electrodiagnostic medicine consultant should be aware of the few health risks to patient and self when exposed to electrodiagnostic equipment (2). Besides transmission of infectious diseases and bleeding complications from needle electrodes, there are three rare instances when electrical injury may occur: in patients with cardiac pacemakers, with leakage current or direct stimulation in "electrosensitive" patients, and with needle stimulation hydrolysis.

Electrodiagnostic studies can be performed on patients with implanted cardiac pacemakers with little risk (31). In general, the closer the stimulation site is to the pacemaker and pacing leads, the greater the chance that voltage of sufficient amplitude will inhibit the pacemaker.. It is especially important that patients with cardiac pacemakers be properly grounded. Nerve conduction studies are not recommended for any patient with an external conductive lead terminating in or near the heart (2).

Certain individuals are more susceptible to electrical injury. These are mostly frail individuals and those in which the bodies' natural barriers have been compromised. An example is the use of central venous or arterial catheters. Electricity directly conducted by the catheter may reach the heart, leading to arrhythmias. Leakage of fluid or moisture can further decrease the skin's electrical resistance. Several safeguards to prevent this from happening include avoiding stimulation next to areas with percutaneous catheters and excess moisture; performing routine electrical checks for leakage current; and using proper grounding and "isolated" patient leads (2).

Leakage current is current that leaks to the instrument chassis or recording electrodes that can be released as an electrical shock when contacted by the patient or the electrodiagnostic medicine consultant. The three-prong power cord "ground" basically solves the problem of leakage current if no components of the system fail. "Isolated" leads and amplifiers, which use nonconductive coupling methods or current-limiting devices, are standard features in contemporary instruments and make it extremely unlikely that a dangerous level of leakage current can "shock" the patient (20). Common faults that could result in loss of ground or in excessive leakage current include faulty wires, the use of two-pin extension cords, and fluid spills (See Ref. (29), pp. 610–615).

To promote patient safety, standards have been established for the maximum allowable leakage currents (5, 35, 39, 42). The JCAHO Accreditation Manual for Hospitals requires that protocols and procedures be established for routine equipment inspections to ensure compliance with the standards, and that records of the periodic tests be kept (24). In our institution, the frequency of safety checks of all hospital-based electrical equipment is determined by its rank on a scale that weighs how the instrument is used, how frequent maintenance is expected, and the risk if the instrument should fail. Following these criteria, our electrodiagnosis instruments receive safety inspection annually by a qualified biomedical equipment technician. It is the responsibility of the electrodiagnostic medicine consultant to ensure that the particular instrument in use meets the minimum safety specifications. Currently, the AAEM does not have a stated position regarding the frequency or types of safety and accuracy checks (21).

Hydrolysis or ionization may occur at the tip of a needle electrode used for nerve stimulation. The greater the needle tip surface area, the greater the voltage and pulse duration required for damage. While it is not known what tissue damage may result from hydrolysis or ionization, monopolar electromyograpy (EMG) needles can be used with a greater margin of safety if the Teflon insulation is stripped back 3 mm to 4 mm to distribute the current over a larger area. Concentric EMG electrodes should not be used because the small area of the central electrode core leads to much higher current densities (20).

4. EQUIPMENT ACCURACY/RELIABILITY

Unlike safety standards, no established guidelines specify the frequency with which the electrodiagnostic instruments should be checked for precision or calibration (21). All common contemporary amplifiers and electrodiagnosis instruments are manufactured with the ability to measure accurately and precisely the signals required for an appropriate electrodiagnostic examination (16). However, assessment of performance after the equipment arrives in the clinic is left to the electrodiagnostic medicine consultant or equipment technician. Loss of calibration is more easily recognized on digital instruments because large errors usually occur as compared to small gradual changes possible with analog-type instruments. Still, the most significant variable regarding the accuracy of electrophysiologic testing is the skill with which the examination is performed (11).

Appropriate Management of Referrals

Many physicians are familiar with the clinical value of electrodiagnosis; however, the electrodiagnostician can further educate the physicians on how to improve the appropriateness of referrals and prepare the patient for the examination. This can maximize the electrodiagnostic consultation's contribution to the administration of high-quality care. Ways to accomplish this include arranging a meeting or lecture with potential or current referral sources and distributing an information brochure, e.g., the AAEM Resource Guide for Referring Physicians (3).

This interaction can help clarify which services and assistance the electrodiagnostic medicine consultant can provide. It should be emphasized that electrodiagnosis is extremely valuable in the contemporary practice of medicine and involves objective assessment

reflecting, but not directly measuring, biochemical and morphologic aspects of central and peripheral motor and sensory functions. The electrodiagnostic medicine consultation is most helpful to patients with problems of weakness, paresthesia, pain, or fatigue. These can usually be diagnosed with respect to anatomic localization, severity, and nature of the dysfunction (3). Not only can electrodiagnostic studies support or confirm clinical diagnoses, but they have an important role in prognosis and guiding management of a variety of neuromuscular conditions (30).

Electrodiagnosis is especially helpful with carpal tunnel syndrome, ulnar nerve entrapment, peroneal nerve compression at the fibular neck, polyneuropathy, and cervical and lumbosacral radiculopathies. It is also useful in evaluating weakness caused by myasthenia gravis, Lambert-Eaton myasthenic syndrome, botulism, polymyositis, myopathy, motor neuron disease, and polyradiculoneuropathy (3).

If surgical correction of nerve or root compromise is being considered, the referring physician should realize that the benefits of surgery parallel the degree of physiologic compromise shown by electrodiagnosis, not the anatomic defect revealed by imaging (30).

The referring physician must understand when a patient should be referred to get the most benefit from the study. Some information can be obtained any time during the course of a disease or injury to a motor unit. For example, after four to five days, a neuron that is dying from an acute peripheral nerve injury will lose excitability because of wallerian degeneration. Thus, at one week after injury or onset of the disease, prognostic information can be obtained. The referring physician should approach the electromyographer with any questions about the timing of the referral or a follow-up examination (30).

Because the patient's anxiety about the test is often worse than the test itself, the referring physician can have a significant influence on their emotional well-being when they arrive for the examination. It can be helpful if the patients know beforehand that electrodiagnosis is a diagnostic test—not a treatment—that can detect whether there are problems involving nerves or muscle and that does not require any preparation by the patient. Routine activities such as eating, exercise, and going back to work will not affect the test and can be resumed immediately following the procedure. The patients should know that the procedure has no side effects except, occasionally, some mild discomfort or a small amount of ecchymosis or bleeding at the needle electrode insertion site. It is also useful to provide the patient with a pamphlet, such as "What is Electrodiagnosis?" by the AAEM (4).

Timely processing of referrals, testing, reporting of the test results, and dealing with emergency cases can significantly influence patient care. For example, the timeliness with which the consultation is completed can positively influence patient care outcomes as it provides information needed to develop an effective treatment plan (33). There are few emergency indications for an electrodiagnostic consultation. An exception to this is differentiating between tetanus, botulism, inflammatory neuropathy, or other acute process versus hysterical paralysis in the emergency department. Otherwise, nearly all procedures can be scheduled in advance for the mutual convenience of the patient and examiner so that an adequate amount of time is allowed for unhurried, appropriate consideration of the clinical problem.

Patient Satisfaction

Patients and others judge the quality of health care based on patient health outcomes, the cost of healthcare services, and sometimes their perceptions of what was done and how it was done (33). Several factors can significantly affect patient satisfaction, including whether the services provided are timely, the staff is courteous, the environment is comfortable and meets their needs, and the physician is perceived as caring. Patients appreciate being scheduled for the examination shortly after the referral is made and then being seen at their scheduled appointment time. Ideally, the clinic environment is safe, easy to locate and access, with ample parking facilities. A comfortable reception area is preferable with easily located beverage and bathroom facilities and easily accessible magazines and health information leaflets. Most patients also prefer an

explanation of the test from the referring physician or a brochure sent before the test, and they appreciate further explanation of the test by the electrodiagnostic medicine consultant at the time of the examination (13, 33).

Staff awareness and education have also been shown to improve patient satisfaction. A questionnaire administered to the patient after the test can be helpful in assessing whether patient needs are being met (22).

Aspects of Patient Comfort

The requirements of the room selected for the consultation should be carefully considered. If possible, the room should be shielded from electrical sources that may interfere with the procedure and be comfortably warm so that the patient may be undressed without shivering (a source of artifacts). The room should contain an examination table for the patient to lie on in a relaxed position with adequate cushioning available (32). If the table is powered by electricity, it may need to be unplugged to avoid 60-cycle interference.

As mentioned previously, patients appreciate being educated about the electrodiagnostic examination by the referring physician, through information leaflets, and by the electrodiagnostic medicine consultant at the time of the examination (36). This information should be delivered in simple language, avoiding technical jargon. It should include a breakdown of the basics of the electrodiagnostic examination, a warning about physical discomfort that may be experienced, and an explanation of why the test is being conducted and how it will contribute to their medical treatment. A completely informed, and thus more relaxed, patient can cooperate more with the examination and help the practitioner collect the data required to formulate an appropriate diagnosis and prognosis (15).

Anxiety can be further relieved if the electrodiagnostic medicine consultant gains the patient's confidence during the taking of the history and the physical examination that addresses the patient's main complaints. It can also be helpful to allow the patient to view the electrodiagnostic instrument's screen and be given a simple explanation of the waveforms that appear. Friendly conversation during the procedure can distract the patient from the test's discomfort.

Although it is very difficult to predict which patients will tolerate the electrodiagnostic examination poorly, electrodiagnostic physicians tend to be good judges of the degree of pain that patients are experiencing (18). If a patient becomes anxious and requests that the examination be stopped, this wish should be honored. The practitioner may decide to stop the portion of the test causing patient discomfort and offer to proceed with another part of the investigation (15). Sometimes it is better to stop the examination altogether and resume it on another day than to continue in the face of diminishing cooperation. If further EMG study is necessary, the patient can return and might be even more cooperative than on the first visit. Analgesic or sedating medication can also be considered.

History and Physical Examination

By themselves, electrodiagnostic procedures usually are not diagnostic. Unless combined with a focused patient history and physical examination done by the electrodiagnostic medicine consultant, the electrodiagnostic examination may at best be unrewarding and at worst misleading (17). Based upon the history and the physical examination, which focuses on the neuromusculoskeletal system as it relates to the patient's history and chief complaint, the physician can formulate preliminary clinical diagnoses and determine the appropriate electrodiagnostic procedures.

Electrodiagnostic Examination Approach/Techniques[++]

The guiding principle to high-quality electrodiagnostic examinations is that there are no set protocols for evaluating patients' signs and symptoms. The first steps in the electrodiagnostic examination are determined by the directed history and physical examination. Example guidelines have been presented elsewhere for these initial steps (2, 15). The exam-

ination proceeds in a direction dictated by the initial electrodiagnostic findings and the examiner's medical knowledge and experience. In this manner, appropriate data are collected and the proper conclusions drawn. Techniques used should be consistent with those of standard textbooks, cited journal articles, or publications of generally recognized organizations. An adequate number of techniques should be used for each specific question investigated. The number of studies should be limited to those that allow a reasonable differential diagnosis and are pertinent and thorough but neither excessive nor superficial (2).

Consultation Report

The next section presents an in-depth view of the aspects of high-quality electrodiagnostic medicine reports.

Determining What to Charge

Fees should be reasonable, commensurate with the difficulty of the study, time involved, and number of procedures performed. It is our belief that a single global fee, perhaps at two levels stratified by case type, could minimize the seductive opportunity for increasing the number of procedures to increase the charges. Whatever the schedule, the fees should be disclosed upon the request of a patient or referring physician.

ELECTRODIAGNOSTIC MEDICINE CONSULTATION REPORT

The written report/summary of the electrodiagnostic medicine consultation serves an obviously important purpose. As mentioned previously, completing an appropriate electrodiagnostic study is only part of the physician's responsibility to the patient. Without clearly communicating the procedure results to the patient and treating physician, the study is useless. The electrodiagnostic medicine report serves as the communication between the electrodiagnostician and referring physician and is a permanent record of the complex diagnostic procedure to allow comparison with future tests. It not only has obvious medicolegal implications, but most important, it

---

[++]Details of specific electrodiagnostic techniques are presented in their respective chapters earlier in this book.

fills a vital role in the management of the patient.

Although it may take many acceptable forms, the electrodiagnostic medicine report should be complete and precise with logical and reasonable diagnostic inferences. Therefore, the report is a summary of the anatomic and neurophysiologic data translated into probable clinical diagnoses. All reports should include the following components:

- Demographic data;
- Pertinent history and physical examination;
- Tabulation of data including nerve stimulation studies and needle electromyographic investigation;
- Summary of the neurophysiologic findings;
- Translation of that summary into a probable clinical diagnosis (or list of differential diagnostic probabilities); and
- If appropriate, a plan, recommendations, and follow-up.

Demographic Data

This section should include the date the electrodiagnostic medicine consultation was completed, the name, address, age, and sex of the patient, and the source of referral (the name of the referring physician). It should also include whether the test was done on an inpatient or outpatient basis and whether previous electrodiagnostic studies have been done.

History and Physical Examination

Completing a focused history and physical examination is essential, but the number of findings that need to be recorded remains personal preference. The referring physician knows the patient but usually does not have the neuromusculoskeletal expertise of the electrodiagnostic medicine consultant. Therefore, recording detailed information may benefit the referring physician, but it is intended primarily as a permanent record in the medical file. The pertinent positive aspects of the examination should be documented, just as they would

be on any other medicine consultation. If dictated, it takes little time to record the patient's history and physical examination; however, hand writing the report can be time consuming. At the least, the temporal and topographic summary of the complaint or reason for the referral should be included (e.g., foot drop for one month). Again, whether recorded in detail or not, a pertinent history and physical are essential to planning and executing an appropriate electrodiagnostic examination.

Tabulation of Data

1. NEEDLE ELECTROMYOGRAPHY

List all of the muscles examined without listing any additional muscles. Avoid using a preprinted list of muscles; this promotes the habit of studying a "routine" set of muscles without considering the most time-efficient or appropriate muscles for the individual patient. Appropriate root levels and peripheral nerve innervation should also be recorded. This provides an excellent educational exercise for both the electrodiagnostician and the referring physician and helps the referring physician to follow the process of anatomic localization.

Several columns designating the activity investigated should be included next to the muscles examined: insertional activity, spontaneous (rest) activity (positive sharp waves, fibrillation potentials, fasciculations, etc.), motor unit recruitment, and motor unit action potential (MUAP) morphology (phases, amplitude, duration, rise time, etc.).

In normal muscle, "injury potentials" are noted during the needle insertion, but in various disease states, positive waves persist after needle electrode movement stops (e.g., with denervation, active myopathies, etc.). This finding is properly listed under "insertional activity." If needle insertion fails to evoke many injury potentials (e.g., in fibrotic muscle), it is proper to describe the activity as "reduced." However, if a few positive waves are produced, it is neither proper nor useful to describe insertional activity as "increased" when the more appropriate description is "a few positive waves" or "unsustained trains of positive sharp waves." Positive waves should, therefore, be reported as being occasional, few, many, or trains. (See also Chapter 1.)

Spontaneous activity can include fasciculations, positive sharp waves, and fibrillation potentials. Description of fibrillation potentials should include numbers, e.g., grades 1+ to 4+. Atypical potentials such as complex repetitive discharges and myokymic potentials can be noted in an accompanying paragraph describing the abnormality at the bottom of the columnar data (15).

Many reports include the percentage of polyphasic motor units (a potential crossing the isoelectric line more than four times). However, it is best to simply report an "increased proportion of polyphasics." Generally, 15% of MUAPs in normal muscle are polyphasic. One should indicate the type of needle electrode that was used to examine the patient. This has obvious implications when one is considering MUAP parameters, particularly amplitude and number of phases (15).

Reliable quantitative motor unit assessment requires a trigger and delay line associated with proper filter settings. Motor unit parameters should be determined after the recording electrode is placed so as to minimize the rise time, which by convention should be less than 0.5 msec. These parameters include motor unit configuration [peak-to-peak amplitude (μV or mV); total duration (msec); number of phases; number of turns; variation of shape, if any, with consecutive discharges; presence of satellite (linked) potentials, if any]; and recruitment characteristics [threshold of activation (first recruited, low threshold, high threshold); onset frequency (Hz); recruitment frequency (Hz), and interval (msec) or ratio of individual potentials]. (See Chapter 1.)

If evaluated qualitatively, the recruitment pattern should be reported as normal (full), reduced, or increased. Normal or full recruitment implies that for a given level of patient effort, there is an appropriate number of motor units firing at appropriate rates. Reduced or decreased recruitment is used when there are fewer than anticipated motor units firing at rapid rates with minimal to moderate force of contraction. "Single unit pattern" is used to describe a single MUAP firing at a rapid rate (usually at greater than 30 Hz; it should be specified) during maximal voluntary effort

in the absence of additional motor unit recruitment. At the other extreme, increased or early recruitment means that multiple motor units are firing at rapid rates at relatively low levels of force.

Descriptive terms implying diagnostic significance (e.g., myopathic, neuropathic, regeneration, nascent, giant, BSAP, and BSAPP) should be avoided in the tabulation of data, as these implications could be incorrect and offer no objective information for comparison studies.

2. NERVE STIMULATION STUDIES

Tabular data should include the nerve being examined and the stimulation site and recording electrode locations (including distances). The action potential latency, peak amplitude, duration of negative spike, conduction velocity, and any change in shape or size from proximal to distal stimulation should be determined and recorded. The direction of the conducted impulses (antidromic or orthodromic) and whether the latency measure is to the takeoff or the peak should also be indicated. Any occasions in which needle stimulation or recording is used or unusual stimulus intensity is required (e.g., a duration of 0.5 msec) should be noted. Limb temperature should be recorded if outside the normal range. Amplitude and duration measurements are essential in assessing conduction block; unfortunately, these parameters are frequently absent from reports (27). With late responses, limb length should be measured. Technical or physical problems, such as local swelling or deformity, should be documented in the summary of findings or comments section.

All repetitive stimulation results should be included in this section of the report. Specifically, a convenient table should document both pre- and post-exercise increment and decrement data. The percentage of amplitude decrement between the first and fourth response is typically described for postsynaptic neuromuscular junction defects. For presynaptic neuromuscular junction abnormalities, the difference between the first and ninth response should be recorded. Single fiber jitter and fiber density data can also be included in this section of the report (15).

Report Format

A tabular format of collected data with space provided for the summary and interpretation is usually the best way to document information, convey it to the referring physician, and use it for comparison with later electrodiagnostic medicine reports. Some electrodiagnosticians use a narrative form without tabular presentation of the data, presumably with a work sheet kept in a file with the patient's record. Both report types are satisfactory, but many electrodiagnosticians find the former presentation most useful.

In our opinion, reference values can be misleading to referring physicians and invite unproductive discussion about what is "normal" for individual nerves. Only a qualified electrodiagnostician can determine whether nerve conduction parameters are normal. On many EMG reports, inappropriate space is occupied by listing "normal values" and implies that other values are abnormal and diagnostically significant. For example, to suggest that the normal distal latency of the median nerve is less than a specific value is not only incorrect, but is conceptually misleading. Latencies and conduction velocities are generally meaningless without amplitudes and durations of evoked potentials and precise surface measurements. Values outside a reference range should serve as "red flags" to alert the electrodiagnostician to consider them in relation to other data collected. The significance of these values should then be addressed in the comments that follow the tabulation of data.

Preprinted lists of muscles or nerves and word processing packages with preprogrammed report comments should be used with caution. Although preprinted forms and reports can save time, they may be unnecessarily restrictive, stereotypic, and misleading to both the referring physician and the electrodiagnostician. Conducting an electrodiagnostic examination is a dynamic process and should not be performed stereotypically. Blank areas of the preprinted report, indicating muscles or nerves not examined, may confuse the referring physician and unnecessarily distract one from the important data obtained. A legend for abbreviations and grading scales should be included in the final report for the benefit of physicians who are not familiar with the terminology.

Summary of Electrodiagnostic Data/Comments

After listing data in the report, it is good practice to summarize pertinent aspects of the information. This short paragraph should include precise anatomic and neurophysiologic descriptions. Portions of the examination that directly relate to the patient's symptoms and any findings that suggest additional disease entities should be noted. This is an important aspect of the consultation, as it substantiates investigating muscles or nerves that may not directly correspond to the original reason a consultation was requested. Summarizing the data obtained also allows one the opportunity to consider all of the information as a whole and how it is interrelated to the patient's presentation. At times, the practitioner may consider additional investigations inspired by the summarized results. Once the electrical studies have been structured in an organized way, the process of formulating an impression is made considerably easier (15).

Impressions/Diagnoses

The correct interpretation of results depends largely on the experience and knowledge of the electrodiagnostician. The interpretation must be made in conjunction with the history and physical examination because electrodiagnostic findings are usually not specific and few, if any, are pathognomonic.

The impression should be clearly and concisely worded to disclose as much information as possible and avoid confusion. It should be written with terms understandable to both the referring physician and, ideally, the patient. It should attempt to explain how the electrodiagnostic findings fit or do not fit the clinical picture. Often, electrodiagnosis can be diagnostic of a definite anatomic or physiologic abnormality but not of a definite clinical disease. In such cases, a brief explanatory paragraph listing of the differential diagnoses and suspected etiologies is appropriate. If the examination findings allow, prognosis and severity of the pathology affecting the patient's neuromuscular system should be estimated. If a musculoskeletal etiology is suspected, this information should be documented as a clinical diagnosis. Noting that, given the electrodiagnostic findings, the specific referring diagnosis is either excluded or unlikely is helpful to the referring physician.

When the electrodiagnostic study is negative there are several alternatives for reporting (27). "No electrodiagnostic abnormalities in the muscles and nerves sampled" is satisfactory. Avoid generalizations such as "no motor unit disease present" or "no evidence of muscle or lower motor neuron disease." It is useless and inappropriate to include "clinical correlation is suggested" on the report. For a consultation report to be complete, a clinical diagnosis or list of differential diagnoses is required. Simply stating "no lower motor neuron disease" as the only conclusion is incomplete and does not provide the referring physician with all that the electrodiagnostic medicine consultation has to offer.

Recommendations, Treatment, and Follow-up

The content of this section depends on the specialization of the referring physician. Because the electrodiagnostician is an expert in the neuromuscular and skeletal systems, the referring physician likely will welcome recommendations for treatment options, tests, or additional consultation to narrow the differential diagnoses. If additional electrodiagnostic studies are needed, a proposed time frame should be stated at this point.

In nearly all cases, the electrodiagnostician should inform the patient of the examination findings. Suggestions for changes in clinical management should be made to the referring physician and should not be discussed with the patient unless the referring physician has requested that the electrodiagnostic medicine consultant participate in clinical management.

Timely Communication with the Referring Physician

Timely communication of the consultation results to the referring physician can positively affect the quality of patient care. If the elec-trodiagnostic medicine consultant disagrees with the referring physician's preliminary diagnosis, the results imply a serious illness, the results suggest that a surgical treatment is indicated, or the surgery already planned is not indicated, then the referring physician should be directly contacted by phone. Confirmation of the diagnosis and discussion of the next steps in management can then be accomplished in a shorter period of time. Most facilities have capabilities to electronically communicate the report to the referring physician, avoiding the unfortunate circumstance in which the written report arrives after the patient returns to the referring physician.

Report-Writing Errors and Suggestions for Higher Quality Reports

The most important function of the electrodiagnostic medicine report is to clearly convey the results of the consultation to the referring physician and to serve as documentation for future comparison or review. Because an incomplete or erroneous report can negatively affect patient care, it is important that the report be clear, complete, precise, accurate, and logical to serve the intended functions (27).

Johnson et al. reviewed 112 EMG reports submitted for a continuing education course and found that the majority were incomplete or erroneous in some way. The main categories of errors were anatomic, terminologic, technical, and interpretive (27).

Anatomic errors include noting imprecise locations of the electrodes and listing incorrect root levels and inaccessible muscles. Knowing functional anatomy is required to precisely locate a muscle. For example, the opponens pollicis is frequently recorded as the only explored muscle in the thenar group when the needle electrode was most probably in the abductor pollicis brevis (APB), because the opponens pollicis lies underneath the APB. The electrodiagnostic medicine consultant's knowledge of anatomy should ensure that precise needle electrode locations are listed on the electromyographic report; e.g., extensor carpi ulnaris, semimembranosis, vastus medialis, and medial gastrocnemius should be used instead of the imprecise and unacceptable terms "forearm muscle," "wrist extensor," "hamstrings," "quadriceps," and "calf muscles." The posterior tibialis and rhomboids are examples of muscles that are not accurately accessible. There also is frequent confusion concerning upper limb digits, i.e., five digits: four fingers and a thumb. Descriptions such as thumb, index, long, ring, and little finger leave little room for misunderstanding. Also, "upper limb" indicates the arm, forearm, and hand; "lower limb" indicates the thigh, leg, and foot; and, "extremity" should be used only to indicate the hand or foot.

HELPFUL NERVE ROOT AND MUSCLE GENERALIZATIONS:

- The only C_6 root distribution on the volar surface of the forearm is the brachioradialis ($C_{5,6}$) and the pronator teres ($C_{6,7}$).
- The only C_6 root distribution on the extensor surface below the elbow is in the supinator ($C_{6,7}$) and the extensor carpi radialis longus and brevis ($C_{6,7}$).
- The only muscle below the knee supplied by L_4 is the anterior tibialis.
- It is extremely difficult to identify the location of the posterior tibialis muscle; instead, the usual needle location is in the flexor digitorum longus or the flexor hallucis longus.
- In the hand, the opponens pollicis lies deep to the abductor pollicis brevis; therefore, an examiner who lists the opponens pollicis as having been explored without listing the abductor pollicis brevis is probably in error.
- There is no S_2 contribution in paraspinal muscles or in the anal sphincter ($S_{3,4}$).

Terminology used in electrodiagnostic medicine reports should be consistent with the AAEM Glossary of Terms in Clinical Electromyography (1). This publication makes a strong plea for discarding diagnostic terms (e.g., denervation, nascent, myotonic, giant, myopathic potentials) to describe biologic electrical activity. Therefore, it is improper to use "denervation potential" when clearly these potentials are nonspecific and appear in a variety of motor unit diseases and in upper motor neuron conditions. The electrical activity observed should be described in terms of amplitude, duration, shape, and rate of firing instead of with diagnostic labels (27). Proper terminology needs to be reinforced.

Aspects of the report that imply technique or procedural errors include conduction velocities miscalculated from the data presented, unrecorded duration and amplitude of evoked potentials, unperformed conduction studies although the diagnosis requires it, distal motor latencies too short (less than 2 msec), incompatible motor and sensory latencies, omissions in noting distances on distal latencies, and erroneous conclusions when copies of actual recordings of evoked potentials and stimulating artifacts are included with the report.

Using preprinted lists of nerves and muscles or using standard phrases is also considered a technical (or technique) error. The printed lists tend to limit and thus stereotype the electrodiagnostic examination. Incorrect interpretation can be a problem for "cookbook-style" electrodiagnosticians. When a clinical situation falls outside the usual and expected, an analytic approach to the full range of possibilities is beyond the scope of the individual who does everything in routine fashion. This person is best recognized by stereotypic reports that include the same list of muscles and nerves, the same jargon, and the same phrases, none of which is individualized to a particular patient (26).

Interpretation errors are suggested when conclusions are not supported by the included electrodiagnostic data or the examination is incomplete. Overinterpretation can occur if electrodiagnosticians adhere to a rigid set of reference values, as there is a wide range of normal electrophysiology that varies according to patient age, the temperature of the tissues, the anatomic location, the type of electrode, and many other factors. Underinterpretation occurs if subtle abnormalities are overlooked or if too few or the wrong muscles are examined.

Perhaps the greatest electrodiagnostic medicine pitfall occurs when the examination is performed by persons not expertly trained in the diagnosis of neuromuscular diseases or in the diseases' electrophysiologic appearance (15). Only a practicing physician with both theoretic and clinical knowledge of neuromuscular diseases, including their differential diagnoses, is an appropriate electromyographer.

Preparation of written reports in the previously described manner will allow accurate data presentation and maximize the benefit to patient care. To monitor the quality of the electrodiagnostic medicine report, it is encouraged that reports are reviewed by peers at regular intervals (e.g., ten reports each month). In a training program, it is suggested that resident reports should be regularly reviewed anonymously with a group of the residents (15). Questions to ask when reviewing reports include 1) Is the report legible?; 2) Is the report written in language that the referring physician should understand?; 3) Is the final diagnosis supported by the electrodiagnostic findings?; and 4) If the final diagnosis is ambiguous, are there additional diagnostic procedures suggested to help the referring physician?

REPORT EXAMPLES

The following actual electrodiagnostic medicine cases help demonstrate both desirable and undesirable report features. The first example was presented as part of a clinical conference case presentation; the remainders were submitted by attendees of electrodiagnosis continuing education courses as samples of their work. Several areas for improvement will be mentioned in each critique.

There are many acceptable forms that the report can take; however, all should include the basic elements that comprise a medical consultation report: demographic data, history and physical examination, tabulation of data (needle electromyography and nerve stimulation studies), summary of data, impression/diagnoses, and recommendations, treatment, and follow-up if indicated.

Example 1

Report for EMG Examination

(Fig. 2–1) Critique

- This report demonstrates appropriate content of the electrodiagnostic medicine consultation. It includes all the de-

mographic data (erased for purposes of confidentiality), including patient identification, referring physician, and date of the study. The described history and physical examination are focused, yet encompassing enough to provide pertinent positive and negative aspects. This allows a clinical diagnosis before the testing begins and serves as a record for comparison at future appointments. The clinical diagnosis is then used to formulate an appropriate strategy for collecting electrodiagnostic data. Data are clearly presented in table form. A data summary, comments, impressions, and recommendations are included. By including all these aspects, this report typifies a medical specialist's consultation and can optimize the contribution to patient care.

- All examined muscles are listed with specific and correct anatomic names, complete with peripheral nerve and appropriate nerve roots. (However, "Quadriceps" should be more precisely listed as "vastus medialis" if this was the muscle examined.)

- Nerve stimulation sites, muscles used for pickup, and length of measured segments are clearly reported. F-wave parameters are also appropriately provided.

- Conclusions are stated in terms easily understood by the referring physician.

- Data tables should be organized with adequate space allocated for appropriate description of data (which is not the case with the example here). Motor units and recruitment should be described with objective terms if possible. If units are abnormal and a trigger and delay line is used, parameters of motor unit amplitude, duration, and shape can be quantified (i.e., quantitative electromyography). The amplitude and frequency of the first recruited motor unit, the number of units recruited as compared to the strength of contraction, the amplitude during maximal contraction, and the recruitment frequency or interval are also appropriate measures to report.

EMG Examination

Patient Name:	**Address:**
Social Security:	**Phone:**
Date Of Birth:	**Status**
Referring MD:	**Date of Exam:**
Street Address:	
City State Zip:	

Dear Dr. _____ ,

_____ was seen today on _____ . As you know, he is a 59 year old who presents with complaints of lower limb weakness and leg cramps for the past couple of months. He relates the onset to "around Labor Day." He states the cramps have occurred primarily at night and feels the weakness has been slowly progressive since onset. He has had increasing difficulty climbing stairs and problems walking on carpeted surfaces. He feels these symptoms have involved both lower limbs but seems to be affecting the left more severely. He denies back or neck pain. He has had cramping sensations in his hands more recently. He denies any recent trauma. He states he was formerly very healthy and active. He had been doing aerobics and walking on a treadmill. He has discontinued his normal exercise due to the severe leg cramps. He is unaware of any swallowing or visual difficulties or bowel or bladder disturbances.

PMH: Significant for hypertension. Has been treated with Calan for several years. He has recently been switched to a new medication for the last 2-3 weeks. He has had surgical removal of polyps from the area of his rectum. His medical history has otherwise been essentially unremarkable.

Social History: His job entails primarily computer work. He denies the use of tobacco or EtOH.

Physical Examination: In general he is a very pleasant elderly white male in NAD. He is able to ambulate independently without difficulty but somewhat slowly. He is unable to heel or toe walk successfully. He is able to perform multiple full squats without difficulty. There are periodic observable fasciculations seen in all four limbs but not overly prominent. There are more significant fasciculations seen in his tongue. His cranial nerve examination is normal. ? mild dysarthria. He has essentially full ROM of all 4 limbs and neck and trunk without discomfort. He has a negative Spurlings and SLR bilaterally. He has mild palpable tenderness over his lumbar paraspinal muscles but none elsewhere. There is mild weakness bilaterally with ankle dorsiflexion, plantar flexion, eversion as well as EHL extension. Knee flexion and extension is -5/5. He has 4+/5 strength in his hand intrinsics bilaterally. Wrist extension and flexion is also 4+/5. The remainder of his upper limb MMT is -5/5 to normal. MSR's are 3+/4 and symmetrical throughout all 4 limbs. He has a positive Hoffman's on the left. His toes are downgoing.

Laboratory: EMG/NCV study

Muscles Studied		Root	Nerve	Insertional	Fibs	Fasc	Motor Unit
	Tongue	CNXII	Hypoglossal	1+ pos	1+	few	Mod neuropathic
Right	Deltoid	C56	Axillary	0	0	0	Mild neuropathic
"	Biceps	C56	Musculocutaneous	0	0	0	"
"	Brachiorad	C56	Radial	occ pos	0	0	"
"	Triceps	C567	Radial	0	0	0	moderate neuropathic
"	Ex Dig Comm	C78	Radial	occ pos	0	0	"
"	1st Dorsal	C8-T1	Ulnar	2+ pos	1+	few	"
R&L	Paracervical	C3-T1		0	0	0	
"	Quadriceps	L234	Femoral	2+ pos bilat	0	many	"
"	Ant Tibialis	L45	Peroneal	2-3+ pos	0	few	"
"	Peron Long	L5-S1	Peroneal	"	0	"	"
"	Ex Hal Long	L5-S1	Peroneal	"	0	"	"
"	Flx Dig Long	L5-S1	Tibial	"	0	"	"
"	Gastroc	L5-S12	Tibial	"	0	many	"
Right	1st Dorsal	S12	Tibial	"	0	0	"
R&L	Paraspinal	T8-S1		2+pos multiple levels	0	0	

Figure 2–1. Report for EMG examination (Example 1).

Peroneal Study	**Motor Latency**	**Amplitude**	**Motor NCV**
Normal	<6.0ms	2-8K	42-60m/s
Right (8 cm to EDB)	5.4ms	1.2K	
Right (Fibula to Ankle)		1.1K	48m/s
Left (8 cm to EDB)	6.8ms*	360μV*	
Left (Fibula to Ankle)		350μV	48m/s
Left (Across Knee)		350μV	56m/s
Peroneal F-Wave	Fastest: 51.6ms	Avg: 55.4ms*	Response: 6/10*
Right (at ankle)			

Tibial Study	**Motor Latency**	**Amplitude**	**Motor NCV**
Normal	<6.0ms	3-9K	42-60m/s
Left (med mall to Abd Hall)	6.6ms*	2.3K	
Left (pop fossa)		2.3K	45m/s
Tibial F-Wave	Fastest 44.4ms	Avg: 47.8ms	Response: 10/10
Left (at ankle)			

Sural Study	**Sensory Latency**	**Sensory Amplitude**
Normal	<4.2ms	10-30μV
Right (14cm)	3.8ms	12μV
Left (14 cm)	3.7ms	16μV

Ulnar Study	**Motor Latency**	**Amplitude**	**Sensory Latency**	**Amplitude**	**Motor NCV**
Normal	<3.8ms	4-12K	<3.8ms	20-50μV	45-70m/s
Right (8cm to ADM)	3.2ms	7K			
Right (below elbow)		7K			56m/s
Ulnar F-Wave	Fastest: 28.6ms	Avg: 29.9ms	Response: 7/10		
Right (at wrist)					

10-18-95 CPK: 416 u/L   (>50% incr)

EMG Summary/Comments: There is significant membrane irritability seen in multiple muscle groups in both lower limbs with somewhat of a distal gradient as well as the hand intrinsics in the right upper limb. Additionally, there is membrane irritability seen in multiple areas tested in the more caudal paraspinal muscles diffusely in somewhat of a non-localizing fashion as well as the tongue. The motor unit recruitment is mild to moderately neuropathic in many of the areas tested as above. There are some mild chronic motor unit changes of increased duration and mildly increased polyphasicity. There are mild to more steady fasciculations seen in multiple muscle groups as above including the tongue. Some of the distal motor latencies are mildly prolonged as above with increased motor late response blocking. Some of the CMAP amplitudes are mildly diminished, compatible, to some extent, with the degree of muscle atrophy seen clinically. The sural sensory responses are normal.

Impression: Evidence of motor neuron disease (e.g., ALS)

Comments: At this point I would recommend evaluation by one of the neurologists for what I suspect is a progressive motor neuron disease. I will call you to discuss these findings. We will be happy to see him for any rehabilitation needs following this if you so desire.

Thank you for this referral.

Figure 2-1. (continued)

- Terms that imply diagnostic significance (e.g., myopathic, neuropathic, regeneration, nascent, giant, etc.) should be avoided as their implications could be incorrect and they offer no information for comparison studies. These interpretations are more appropriately stated in the comments or impressions sections.
- Fasciculation potentials should be reported as rare, occasional, few, or many, and include descriptions of shape, rate, and rhythm.
- Normal values in the report are probably not helpful as they could be misleading to readers who are unfamiliar with the technical variations that can affect electrodiagnostic data. Values outside the "normal" values could therefore be misinterpreted as indicating pathology. "Reference values" is the preferred term; these values should be used only if the amplifier, instrument, and settings in the current study are similar to those used to obtain the reference values. If reference values are used to draw attention to specific patient data, the values should be placed off to the side to be less obtrusive.
- Injury potentials are normal insertion findings with each advance of the needle electrode; therefore, it is proper to use "normal" to describe an absence of abnormal discharges. Labeling insertional activity as "zero" suggests absence of activity as is seen when the muscle is fibrotic and electrically silent.

Example 2

Report for EMG Examination

(Fig. 2–2) Critique

- Pertinent positive and negative history and physical examination findings should be reported. In this example, "weakness of right dorsiflexion" is the only clinical information provided and it is not clear whether this was determined by history or physical examination. Documenting normal or weak foot inversion would help in differentiating between the two entities highest on the differential diagnosis list. It is not essential that a complete history and physical examination be recorded. However, it is recommended that findings be reported that support the clinical diagnoses and conclusions and that can be used for comparison with future studies.
- The types of potentials listed under the Insertional Activity heading should be clear. If positive waves are noted, they should be listed as occasional, few, many, or trains of positive waves. This allows distinction from the nonspecific label, "increased insertional activity," which is frequently meant to imply longer than normal bursts of injury potentials with needle electrode movement. Because positive waves are produced by mechanical irritation from the needle, they vary by how the examiner moves the needle electrode. Therefore, quantitative grading of insertional positive waves or of injury potentials is not useful. If needle insertion fails to evoke many injury potentials in fibrotic muscle, it is proper to describe the activity as "reduced." If a few positive waves are produced, it is neither proper nor useful to describe insertional activity as "increased" when the more appropriate description is "a few positive waves" or "unsustained trains of positive sharp waves."
- For each muscle examined by EMG, the appropriate peripheral nerve and commonly contributing nerve roots should be listed. The nerve roots are provided to help the reader and electromyographer decide which branches or roots are involved in a lesion. Muscles should be listed by their specific anatomic names: e.g., specify either the gastrocnemius or soleus muscle (not gastrocsoleus); specify which quadriceps muscle or medial hamstring muscle was examined. Only the most common, major nerve root in-

ELECTROMYOGRAPHIC EXAMINATION

PATIENT_____   AGE_____ DATE_____

PROBLEM_____ weakness of (R) dorsi flexion _____   REFERRING PHYSICIAN_____

_____   HOSPITAL_____

MUSCLE	INNERVATION	INSERTIONAL ACTIVITY	FIBRILLA-TION	FASCICULA-TION	MOTOR UNIT ACTION POTENTIALS
QUADRICEPS	L2-4, femoral	Normal	0	0	Normal number, amplitude, and duration
TIBIALIS ANTERIOR	L4-SI, peroneal	++	++		↓ recruitment, ↓ #, ↑ rate
PERONEUS LONGUS	L4-SI, peroneal	+	+		↓ recruitment, ↓ #, ↑ rate
EXT. HALLUCIS LONGUS	L4-SI, peroneal	+	+		I-2 rapidly firing motor units
EXT. DIG. LONGUS	L4-SI, peroneal	+	+		↓ recruitment, ↓ #, ↑ rate
GASTROCSOLEUS	L5-S2, tibial	Normal	0		Normal number, amplitude, and duration
GLUTEUS MAXIMUS	L5-S2, inf. gluteal				
GLUTEUS MEDIUS	L4-SI, sup. gluteal				
BICEPS FEMORIS long & short head	L5-SI, tibial				
ADDUCTOR LONGUS	L2-4, obturator				
PARAVERTEBRAL	LI-L4, SI				
	L5	+			
TENSOR FASCIAE LATAE	L4-SI, s.g.	Normal			
MEDIAL HAMSTRINGS	L5-SI, tibial				
(R) ABD. HALLUCIS	L5-SI, tibial (medial plantar)				
EXT. HALLUCIS LONGUS					
PERONEUS LONGUS					
TIBIALIS ANTERIOR					
(L) PARAVERTEBRALS	L5 & SI				

(R) Sural distal sensory latency antidromically over I4cm -- 3.5 ms (6 mcV amp)
over I7cm -- 4.2 ms (5 mcV amp)

NCV of the left peroneal nerve is 43 M/sec below fibular head to ankle with a distal motor latency of 4.0 ms. The amplitudes are 6.2 mv at the fibular head and 6.5 mv at the ankle.

F-wave utilizing the left tibial nerve with stimulation at the ankle and pick up over the abductor hallucis with I0 responses obtained:
FASTEST RESPONSE -- 57.2 ms (NL is 58.0 ms or less)
SLOWEST RESPONSE -- 58.8 ms

	RIGHT	LEFT
Peroneal distal motor latency to the extensor digitorum brevis muscle	4.8 ms (6.7 amp)	4.0 ms (6.5 mv amp)
Peroneal distal motor latency to the tibialis anterior from above fibular head	6.6 ms (0.7 mv amp)	4.8 ms (3.I mv amp)
below fibular head	3.0 ms (2.8 mv amp)	2.8 ms (3.3 mv amp)
Superficial peroneal distal sensory latency antidromically over I4 cm	5.2 ms (7 mcV amp)	4.5 ms (7 mcV amp)

IMPRESSIONS: 1) Statistically these findings would still be most consistent for a right L5 radiculopathy but nevertheless there is very strong evidence, and in my opinion he most likely has a common peroneal mononeuropathy consisting primarily of a partial conduction block pattern at the right fibular head. As mentioned above, this latter type of lesion does generally have an excellent prognosis.
2) Based on the electrodiagnostic studies today, there is no evidence for a generalized axonal or demyelinating neuropathy.

Figure 2–2. Electromyographic examination report (Example 2).

nervations should be listed, because the inclusion of minor and variant innervations will lead to confusion. It is not helpful to include all roots. For example, the anterior tibialis muscle could receive a minor contribution from S_1; however, the major contributions are from L_4 and L_5. Variations

and minor innervations should be discussed in the comments section to avoid this difficulty.
• Impressions should be clearly stated. In this example, common peroneal nerve palsy at the fibular neck appears to be a correct diagnosis. Comparing right to left side distal peroneal nerve motor

unit action potential (MUAP) amplitudes, there is an approximately 15% loss of fibers secondary to axonal loss. MUAPs proximal and distal to the right fibular neck suggest that approximately 75% of the remaining fibers have experienced conduction block. If the cause of the neurapraxic lesion is removed, the fibers experiencing conduction block should recover with small residual deficits. Therefore, there is a good prognosis for patient recovery. Radiculopathy of the L_5 nerve root is not well supported as membrane irritability is seen only in the right lower limb in the peroneal nerve distribution. Stimulation of the peroneal nerve proximal to the right fibular head with pickup over the extensor digitorum brevis muscle would have helped clarify the diagnosis. F waves are not needed in this study. Documenting a more-thorough history and physical examination would have allowed formulation of a clinical impression to more accurately clarify this patient's problem.

- In this report, ample space was allocated for each column in the data table. This allowed for suitable qualitative descriptions of MUAPs and recruitment.
- Note that the inclusion of prognostic information is appropriate in the impressions section and helpful for improving the quality of patient care by the referring physician.

Example 3

Computer-Generated Report

(Fig. 2–3) Critique

- This example was produced with a report-generating computer program. At first glance, this type of report can appear very orderly and easy to read. However, the program may need to be fine-tuned before it will produce acceptable reports. This specific example is very sloppy in regard to completeness, data presentation, support of the

conclusions, and the provision of useful information to the referring physician.
- The report format should include space for all the components necessary for a complete electrodiagnostic medicine consultation, i.e., pertinent history and physical examination, data tables, data summary, comments, impressions, and recommendations. Many of these aspects are missing from the current report, including the history, physical examination, and reason for the consultation. Any technical difficulties should be mentioned in a comments section.
- Muscle names should be specific, e.g., semimembranosis instead of medial hamstrings. Space should be allocated for a list of innervating peripheral nerves and nerve roots to allow better understanding of the anatomic localization by the referring physician.
- Data tables should be arranged with adequate room for complete description of responses, e.g., motor unit and recruitment parameters. Unnecessary data should be omitted from the tables to avoid distraction from meaningful data; e.g., P-P amplitude and sensory onset latency values should be omitted from this report. Also, the number of reported digits to the right of a decimal point should be limited to that allowed by the precision of the measurements made — e.g., it is usually appropriate to describe distal latencies only to the tenth of a millisecond.
- Many report-generating programs allow for the insertion of generic comments or results. This could save time at the expense of more accurate individualized reports. In this example, it is doubtful that MUAP amplitude, duration, and phases were assessed for all twenty-four muscles reported.
- Uncommon abbreviations should be defined in a key or legend.
- The electrodiagnostic medicine consultant must have an appreciation of common nerve anomalies. In this report, the possibility of an accessory peroneal

nerve should have been considered and tested for when responses were absent with stimulation of the anterior ankle.

- Proper technique and experience are necessary when trying to minimize voluntary muscle contraction during needle electromyography. In this study, many of the muscles important for making appropriate diagnoses were described as "unable to relax." Maneuvers should have been attempted that would cause contraction of antagonist muscles, thereby allowing the investigated muscle to relax, e.g., applying pressure to the abdominal muscles to affect paraspinal muscle relaxation. If the study cannot be completed because of a lack of muscle relaxation, a second visit to evaluate paraspinal muscles, for example, might be needed and recommended in the report text.

- Avoid testing muscles that are difficult to accurately localize. For example, the tibialis posterior muscle is the deepest-lying muscle in the leg and needle examination should be avoided unless necessary (e.g., if the posterior tibialis is being considered for tendon transfer). Also, localization is not very reliable because the needle could instead easily be in the flexor digitorum longus (FDL) or flexor hallucis longus (FHL) muscles, which are also activated by plantar flexion (FDL, FHL) and inversion of the foot (FDL).

- Report conclusions should be supported by the patient history, physical examination, and electrodiagnostic data (as an extension of the physical ex-

Name (L,F)			
ID #		DOB	/ /
Referring Physician		Date of Test	/ /

Motor Nerve Conduction					
Nerve	Amplitude	Velocity	Latency	Distance	Comment
	mv	m/s	ms	cm	
L.Peroneal Ankle-EDB	NR	–	–	–	
L.Tibial Ankle-AHB	0.9		5.85		
L.Tibial Knee-AHB	0.8	34.0	17.6	40.0	
R.Peroneal Ankle-EDB	NR				

Sensory Nerve Conduction					
Nerve	Amplitude (uV)		Velocity m/s	Latency (ms)		Comment
	peak	P-P		onset	peak	
L.Sural	NR	–	–	–	–	
R.Sural	NR	–	–	–	–	

NR= No Response Recorded

Conclusion:
1. The nerve conduction studies are compatible with a sensorimotor peripheral neuropathy.

2. The denervation pattern is compatible with a left L5 <u>ventral</u> radiculopathy.

Figure 2–3. Computer-generated EMG report (Example 3).

Muscle	Root	PSW	Fib	Fasc	MUAP			Rec	Dis
					Amp	Dur	Phases	Pat	Charge
R.Iliopsoas		0	0	0	Nl	Nl	Nl	Full	
R.Gluteus medius		0	0	0	Nl	Nl	Nl	Full	
R.Quadriceps		0	0	0	Nl	Nl	Nl	Nl/eff	
R.Tibialis Ant.		0	0	0	Nl	Nl	Nl	Nl/eff	
R.Lat Hamstring		0	0	0	Nl	Nl	Nl	Nl/eff	
R.Adductors		0	0	0	Nl	Nl	Nl	P.Act	
R.Med Gastroc		0	0	0	Nl	Nl	Nl	P.Act	
R.Int Hamstrings		0	0	0	Nl	Nl	Nl	P.Act	
R.Tibialis Post.		↑Irr	0	0	Nl	Nl	Nl	Nl/eff	
R.Lat Gastroc		Un able	to	re lax	Nl	Nl	Nl	Full	
R.Lumbosacral Paras		Un	abl e	to	re	lax	to	test	
R.Peronei		Un able	to	re lax	Nl	Nl	Nl	Full	
L.Quadriceps		0	0	0	Nl	Nl	Nl	Nl/eff	
L.Lat Hamstring		0	0	0	Nl	Nl	Nl	Nl/eff	
L.Iliopsoas		0	0	0	Nl	Nl	Nl	P.Act	
L.Adductors		0	0	0	Nl	Nl	Nl	P.Act	
L.Lat Gastroc		Un Able	to	re lax	Nl	Nl	Nl	Full	
L.Tibialis Ant.		Sev	0	0	Nl	Nl	Nl	Nl/eff	
L. Tibialis Post.		1+	Sev	0	Nl	Nl	Nl	Nl/eff	
L.Peronei		Sev -1+	Sev	0	Nl	Nl	Nl	Nl/eff	
L.Med Gastroc		↑Irr	0	0	Nl	Nl	Nl	Nl/eff	
L.Int Hamstrings		Sev	0	0	Nl	Nl	Nl	Nl/eff	
L.Lumbosacral Paras		Un	abl e	to	re	lax	to	test	
L.Gluteus medius		Un able	to	re lax	Nl	Nl	Nl	Full	

Key:
NT *Not*
Tolerated   P.Act *Poor Activation*   NAS   *No Abnormality Seen*

Figure 2–3. (continued)

amination). This example is a case of overinterpretation. Insufficient data were reported to answer any question potentially posed by the referring physician. The diagnoses of sensorimotor peripheral neuropathy and L$_5$ ventral radiculopathy are not objectively supported. EMG abnormalities are few and do not allow distinction between L$_5$ and S$_1$ root compromise. Because no paraspinal muscles were reliably tested, it is not possible to localize the lesion to the root level if it is not known. Also, tibial nerve MUAP durations could have helped support the conclusion of a neuropathy. This paucity of collected data could be the result of poor technique, lack of knowledge, lack of practical experience, or all of the above.

Example 4

REPORT FOR NERVE CONDUCTION STUDY

A nerve conduction study was requested to rule out bilateral carpal tunnel syndrome for S.H., a 43 year old gentleman who complains of numbness and pain in his palms and thumb, index and ring fingers. Onset was approximately one year ago with symptoms worsening mid-summer, this year. His work requires repetitive hand/wrist motion.

A nerve conduction study was performed on the above date on the upper extremity, bilaterally. The left median motor distal latency was quite prolonged at 7.00, with very low amplitudes and abnormal conduction velocities. The left median F waves were quite prolonged. The left ulnar nerve showed normal values. The left median sensory was quite prolonged at 6.16, mid-palm conduction velocity across the wrist was quite prolonged at 16.50, and median/radian sensory delta was extremely prolonged at 3.08. The right median motor distal latency was prolonged at 4.50, with better amplitudes and normal conduction velocities. The right median F-waves were mildly prolonged. The right ulnar motor distal latency was mildly prolonged at 3.40, with normal amplitudes and conduction velocities. Right ulnar F-waves were mildly prolonged. Right ulnar sensory was normal at 2.77, median sensory was prolonged at 4.41, mid-palm conduction velocity across the wrist was prolonged at 22.20, and median/radian sensory delta was prolonged at 1.25.

Impression: Findings of the nerve conduction study are compatible with severe left median nerve compromise at the wrist level with axonal loss; less severe right median nerve compromise at the wrist level without axonal loss and moderate right ulnar nerve compromise at the wrist level.

Report for EMG examination (Example 4)

CRITIQUE

- This example uses the paragraph or dictated form of reporting. It was assumed that the electrodiagnostic medicine consultant kept a worksheet in the office files to use for future reference; however, these three paragraphs are all that were communicated to the referring physician.

- There are many forms of reporting, but all require the basic components of the electrodiagnostic medicine consultation. In this report, a brief history and reason for the study are mentioned, but pertinent physical examination findings are absent. Electrodiagnostic data are presented in paragraph form. Impressions are stated; however, comments and recommendations are not included.

- Clearly, it is much easier to locate data and compare specific measurements when all of the collected data are presented in tables than when in paragraph form. In this report, it appears that only abnormal values were reported. Some recordings were specific, but others were listed only as abnormal. No distances or locations of stimulation or recording were stated. This makes it impossible to know which studies were actually done and not practical to use for comparison with a future consultation completed by another electrodiagnostic medicine consultant.

- All impressions and diagnoses should be supported by the reported data. Again, this report is an example of overinterpretation. MUAP amplitudes distal to the site of the suspected lesions were not recorded; therefore, axonal loss and neurapraxia could not be assessed. The F waves reported did not contribute to the stated diagnosis, but may have been suggestive of a more proximal or general neuropathic process. Prolonged distal latency recordings proximal to the wrist are not diagnostic for compromise at the wrist because all F waves were reported as being abnormal. Therefore, presented data do not objectively support ulnar nerve compromise at the wrist.

- Reported values should be only as precise as those surface measurements actually made. When calculating numbers (e.g., conduction velocities), the reported values should have been rounded to the same number of significant digits as the operand with the fewest significant digits. For example, segment distances measured over skin are, at most, precise to the tenth of a centimeter. Therefore, if reporting a conduction velocity using a distance of 22.5 cm and a latency difference of 4.4 msec, the velocity should be reported with two significant digits, which would be 51 m/sec. Digital instruments can precisely measure latencies to the hundredth of a millisecond; however, because the latencies are based on surface distance measurements that are significant only to the tenth of a centimeter, we recommend that distal latencies be reported only to the tenth of a millisecond.

SUMMARY

- Many hospitals, insurance companies, and other healthcare organizations have adopted policies that require continuous monitoring and improvement in all aspects of healthcare delivery. All members of the electrodiagnostic medicine team must understand and be prepared to practice these principles to continuously improve the quality of patient care.
- **Performance Improvement** principles involve doing the right things and doing them well. Appropriate care must be timely, effective, safe, efficient, and coordinated with other medical professionals. Caregivers must be caring and respectful of the patients. The effects of performance are reflected by patient outcomes, costs of services, and patients' perceptions of what was done.
- An **electrodiagnostic medicine con-**

sultation is a medical consultation in which neurophysiologic techniques are applied to diagnose, evaluate, and treat patients with impairments or disabilities of the neurologic or muscular systems. Because it is a medical consultation, it should include a focused patient history and physical examination, an electrodiagnostic examination (as an extension of the physical examination), a clear and concise summary, diagnostic impressions, recommendations to the referring physician, and appropriate interventions. All of these elements should be present for the consultation to maximally contribute to patient care.

- The **electrodiagnostic medicine consultant** must be a physician who has special training in the diagnosis and treatment of neuromuscular diseases and is an expert in the application of neurophysiologic techniques to study these disorders.
- Components of a **high-quality electrodiagnostic medicine consultation** include: an appropriately referred and informed patient; a timely appointment; a focused history and physical examination; the collection of appropriate electrodiagnostic data; the formulation of appropriate medical impressions, recommendations, and treatment if indicated; and the timely communication of the diagnostic impressions and recommended plan to the patient and referring physician.
- Many other factors contribute to the completion of a high-quality electrodiagnostic medicine consultation including knowledgeable and courteous clinic staff; comfortable reception and examination areas; a knowledgeable and technically skilled electrodiagnostic medicine consultant; safe and accurate equipment; and a high-quality electrodiagnostic medicine consultation report that the referring physician can understand.
- A **high-quality electrodiagnostic medicine consultation report** should include demographic data, pertinent pa-

tient history and physical examination, tabulation of data with appropriate objective descriptions, summary of neurophysiologic findings, translation into probable clinical diagnoses, and, if appropriate, a plan, recommendations, and follow-up.

- Needle electromyography data tables should include a list of all muscles examined with appropriate root levels and peripheral nerve innervation and columns to describe insertional and spontaneous activity, motor unit recruitment, and morphology.

- Nerve stimulation study data tables should include the nerve being examined, the stimulation site, and the recording electrode locations, including distances. The action potential latency, peak amplitude, duration of negative spike, conduction velocity, and any change in shape or size from proximal to distal stimulation should also be determined and recorded.

- Timely communication of a clear, complete, precise, and logical consultation report can positively influence the quality of patient care. Conversely, an incomplete or erroneous report can negatively affect patient care. The most common report errors relate to anatomy, terminology, technique, and interpretation.

- Consultation reports should be reviewed by peers regularly. Questions to ask when reviewing reports, include: 1) Is the report complete, legible, and written in language that the referring physician should understand?; 2) Were appropriate tests and number of tests done?; 3) Is the final diagnosis supported by the electrodiagnostic findings?; and 4) If the final diagnosis is ambiguous, are there additional diagnostic procedures suggested to help the referring physician?

References

1. AAEM: Glossary of terms in clinical electromyography. Muscle Nerve 1987;10(8 Suppl):G1–60.
2. AAEM: Guidelines in electrodiagnostic medicine. Muscle Nerve 1992;15:229–253.
3. AAEM: Resource guide for referring physicians: Electrodiagnostic medical consultation. Rochester, Minnesota: Am Assoc Electrodiagnostic Med, June 1991.
4. AAEM: What is electrodiagnosis? Rochester, Minnesota: Am Assoc Electrodiagnostic Med, May 1993.
5. AAMI: Safe current limits for electromedical apparatus. Arlington, Virginia: Assoc for Advancement of Medical Instrumentation, 1993.
6. ABEM: 1995 Information for candidates. Rochester, Minnesota: Am Board Electrodiagnostic Med, 1994.
7. Ackmann JJ, Lomas JN, Hoffmann RG, et al.: Multifrequency characteristics of disposable and nondisposable EMG needle electrodes. Muscle Nerve 1993;16(6):616–623.
8. American Academy of Neurology: Minutes of executive board meeting 11.9(1). December 2, 1981.
9. American Academy of Physical Medicine and Rehabilitation: Statement: Clinical diagnostic electromyography. November 1983.
10. American Medical Association: House of Delegates, Resolution: G2, I-83. 1983.
11. Bigos SJ, Bowyer OR, Braen GR, et al.: Acute low back problems in adults. Clinical Practice Guideline No. 14. AHCPR Publication No. 95–0642. Rockville, Maryland: Agency for Health Care Policy and Research, Public Health Service, U.S. Department of Health and Human Services, 1994.
12. Burwick DM: Curing health care: New strategies for quality improvement. San Francisco: Jossey-Bass Publishers, 1990.
13. Clarke T: An audit of patient perceptions. J Electrophysiol Technol 1992;18:207–213.
14. Dorfman LJ, McGill KC, Cummins KL: Electrical properties of commercial concentric EMG electrodes. Muscle Nerve 1985;8(1):1–8.
15. Dumitru D: Electrodiagnostic medicine. Philadelphia: Hanley & Belfus, 1995.
16. ECRI: Evoked potential units; Electromyographs. Healthcare product comparison system. Plymouth Meeting, Pennsylvania: ECRI, 1995.
17. Felsenthal G: Electrodiagnosis: Clinical examination or laboratory test? Maryland State Med J 1975;24(1):66–67.
18. Gans BM, Kraft GH: Pain perception in clinical electromyography. Arch Phys Med Rehabil 1977;58:13–16.
19. Gitter AJ, Stolov WC: AAEM Minimonograph #16: Instrumentation and measurement in electrodiagnostic medicine-Part I. Muscle Nerve 1995;18:799–811.
20. Gitter AJ, Stolov WC: AAEM Minimonograph 16: Instrumentation and measurement in electrodiagnostic medicine-Part II. Muscle Nerve 1995;18:812–824.
21. Haig AJ: AAEM Chairperson: Equipment and computer committee. Personal communication. December 1995.
22. Hamilton-Bruce MA, Black AB, Stratos K: Quality assurance in a neurophysiology laboratory. Aust Phys Eng Sci Med 1994;17(2):94–95.
23. Jamieson PW: Computerized interpretation of electromyographic data. Electroencephalography Clin Neurophysiol 1990;75(5):392–400.

24. JCAHO: Management of the environment of care. In: 1995 Accreditation manual for hospitals. Oakbrook Terrace, Illinois: Joint Commission on Accreditation of Healthcare Organizations, 1994;(1:Standards):45–48.

25. JCAHO: The Transition from QA to CQI: An introduction to quality improvement in health care. Oakbrook Terrace, Illinois: Joint Commission, 1991.

26. Johnson EW: Why and how to request an electrodiagnostic examination and what to expect in return. In: MacLean IC, ed. Electromyography: A guide for the referring physician. Philadelphia: WB Saunders, 1990:149–158. (Kraft GH, ed. Physical medicine and rehabilitation clinics of North America; 1:1).

27. Johnson EW, Fallon TJ, Wolfe CV: Errors in EMG reporting. Arch Phys Med Rehabil 1976;57(1):30–32.

28. Joynt RL: The selection of electroyographic needle electrodes. Arch Phys Med Rehabil 1994; 75(3):251–258.

29. Kimura J: Electrodiagnosis in diseases of nerve and muscle: Principles and practice. 2nd ed. Philadelphia: FA Davis, 1989.

30. Kraft GH: Electromyography: Doctors' questions answered. In: MacLean IC, ed. Electromyography: A guide for the referring physician. Philadelphia: WB Saunders, 1990. (Kraft GH, ed. Physical medicine and rehabilitation clinics of North America; 1:1).

31. LaBan MM, Petty D, Hauser AM, et al.: Peripheral nerve conduction stimulation: Its effect on cardiac pacemakers. Arch Phys Med and Rehabil 1988;69:358–362.

32. Láhoda F, Ross A, Issel W: EMG primer: A guide to practical electromyography and electroneurography. Heidelberg: Springer-Verlag, 1974.

33. Monga T: AAEM: Guidelines for establishing a quality assurance program in an electrodiagnostic laboratory. Rochester, Minnesota: Am Assoc Electrodiagnostic Med, (in press) 1995.

34. Nandedkar SD, Tedman B, Sanders DB: Recording and physical characteristics of disposable concentric needle EMG electrodes. Muscle Nerve 1990;13(10):909–914.

35. NFPA: Standard for health care facilities, Chap. 7: Electrical equipment (99:7); and Chap. 12: Hospital requirements (99:12). In: National Fire Codes, vol. 5. Quincy, Massachusetts: National Fire Protection Association, 1993.

36. O'Neill L, Timson L: A simple and effective way of monitoring quality assurance in a neurophysiology department. J Electrophysiol Technol 1991;17:81–93.

37. Sherman HB, Walker FO, Donofrio PD: Sensitivity for detecting fibrillation potentials: A comparison between concentric and monopolar needle electrodes. Muscle Nerve 1990;13(11): 1023–1026.

38. Stålberg E: The value to the clinical neurologist of electromyography in the 1990s. Clin Experimental Neurol 1990;27:1–28.

39. Standards: What's new in NFPA 99–1993? Health Devices 1993;22(8–9):413–415.

40. State Medical Board of Ohio. Ohio Revised Code, Section 4731.34.

41. Technology and equipment review: Electromyographs. J Clin Neurophysiol 1994;11(2):264–273.

42. Underwriters Laboratories Inc: Standard for medical and dental equipment, UL 544. 3rd ed. Northbrook, Illinois: Underwriters Laboratories Inc, 1993.

43. Veterans Administration: Professional services letter: Professional qualifications for performing electromyographic examinations. January 4, 1980.

44. Vingtoft S, Fuglsang-Frederiksen A, R<as>onager J, et al.: KANDID—an EMG decision support system—evaluated in a European multicenter trial. Muscle Nerve 1993;16(5):520–529.

Chapter 3

"Objective EMG": Quantitation and Documentation In The Routine Needle Electromyographic Examination

Sanjeev D. Nandedkar

The routine electrodiagnostic (EDX) examination consists of two parts: nerve conduction study (NCS) and needle electromyographic (EMG) examination. The NCS is performed very objectively. The responses are recorded under standardized conditions of electrode placement, temperature, distance, etc. The measurements of the response are compared against a well-defined set of reference values. As a result, the NCS provides quantitative data that can be used for electrodiagnosis and assessment of disease severity. Measurements from serial studies can be compared to assess disease progression and the underlying pathophysiology (1, 13).

In contrast, the needle EMG examination remains very subjective. The EMG abnormalities are recognized by observing signal waveforms on the display screen and by listening to their sound on an audio monitor. Although a variety of quantitative techniques are commercially available, they are seldom used as a part of the routine needle EMG examination. Quantitative analysis (QA) is almost synonymous with a specialized procedure that is rarely performed. The lack of quantification in EMG results from a variety of reasons, as follows:

1. QA is very time-consuming. For analysis of motor unit action potentials (MUAPs), it is recommended that 20 or more MUAPs be recorded from the tested muscle. This can require 20 to 30 minutes for a single muscle.

2. Patient cooperation is essential for good-quality recordings of MUAPs.

3. The reference values depend on the muscle, patient's age and gender, type of recording electrode (concentric versus monopolar), recording technique (use of trigger delay line, manual analysis, etc.), and other factors (3,12,15,17). As a result, it is not possible for every laboratory to develop reference values even for the most commonly tested muscles. Lack of reference values will make it difficult to justify QA.

4. When the EMG abnormalities are obvious on the subjective assessment, the time-consuming QA will not add to electrodiagnosis.

In light of these practical problems, one asks what the usefulness of QA is in the routine EMG. QA has been most useful in demonstrating the sensitivity and specificity of various EMG features in electrodiagnosis. Muscle biopsy studies, computer simulations, and QA have allowed us to establish the relationship between the EMG signals and their generators, i.e., motor units (4, 10, 17). This permits us to make better assessments and interpretations of the EMG signals. Finally, QA has provided impetus to develop better, faster, and more robust techniques. With access to faster computers, QA will become less demanding as a technique (6, 9, 12). **Thus, the knowledge and techniques of QA can easily be** incorporated within the routine EMG examination to recognize and document EMG abnormalities. Documenting abnormalities will make routine needle EMG an objective test procedure.

QA is unfortunately associated with computer-aided EMG. Although computers make it easier to manipulate, calculate, and store quantitative data, they are not necessary for quantifying EMG signals. Furthermore, QA is time-consuming only when the EMG signals are normal. When abnormalities are obvious, one need not spend time in acquiring 20 different MUAPs. Quantifying a few abnormal MUAPs is quite adequate to objectively demonstrate the EMG abnormalities and thus assist electrodiagnosis. This is called the "outlier" principle and mimics the subjective assessment of EMG abnormalities (2, 14). (For objective comparisons in serial studies, one must record a large number of MUAPs in each study.)

This chapter describes simple protocols for acquiring and displaying EMG signals on most commercially available electromyographs. The emphasis will be on "reading" the display. By reading the display in an objective fashion, one can recognize EMG abnormalities easily. A hardcopy of the display will document the abnormalities and thus add objectivity to EMG.

HOW TO READ THE EMG DISPLAY

An EMG instrument makes a plot of voltage values (Y axis) versus time (X axis). On the display, each axis is divided into 10 (or more) bins, called divisions (Fig. 3–1). The "sensitivity" or "display gain" on the instrument defines the voltage change corresponding to one division along the Y axis. Similarly, the "time base" or "sweep speed" defines the time corresponding to one division along the X axis. The EMG signal measurement is a two-step process. To measure signal amplitude, one measures the vertical deflection (i.e., along the Y axis) as a number of divisions. Multiplying the number of divisions by the display gain gives the signal amplitude. As an example, the potential in Figure 3–1A has a peak-to-peak deflection of about three divisions. With the sensitivity setting of 100 μV, the signal amplitude is equal to 300 μV. The measurements of time are done in a similar way.

The display of the EMG signal begins at the left edge of the screen. When it reaches the right edge, the instrument has acquired and displayed one sweep. The next sweep is again initiated at the screen's left edge. This is called a "free running" sweep (Fig. 3–1A). Most of the EMG examination is performed in this mode of EMG acquisition and display.

Modern instruments can acquire and display several consecutive sweeps on the screen. This is called the "cascaded sweep" mode. In Figure 3–1B, the top sweep is the earliest acquired sweep. The second sweep is initiated at the end of first sweep, and so on. Thus, time interval can be measured between events on different sweeps. For example, in Figure 3–1B, there are six divisions after the potential on the top trace and three divisions before the potential on the second trace. With the time base set to 10 msec/division, the nine divisions correspond to a time interval of 90 msec.

In the **amplitude triggered** mode, the operator defines an amplitude level. When the EMG signals are less than this level, they are not displayed. When the signal amplitude exceeds the set level, the signal display is initiated and one sweep is shown on the screen. To view signals before the trigger levels, the instrument can show delayed EMG signals (Fig. 3–1C). This mode of display is used in most techniques of QA.

With access to digital technology, it is now possible to acquire and display signals at multiple time bases. A combination of fast (e.g., 10 msec/div) and slow sweep (e.g., 100 msec/div) will show the details of the signal and also the repetitive patterns (Fig. 3–1D). A portion of the long sweep can also be reviewed to study waveforms' details after signal acquisition. This is called a dual or long sweep display.

QA PROTOCOLS

The routine needle EMG examination (5) can be divided into four different assessments: insertional activity (IA), spontaneous activity (SA), EMG at minimal force of contraction, and analysis of the interference pattern (IP). The typical settings for the filters are 3 Hz to 20 Hz for low frequency and 5 kHz to 10 kHz

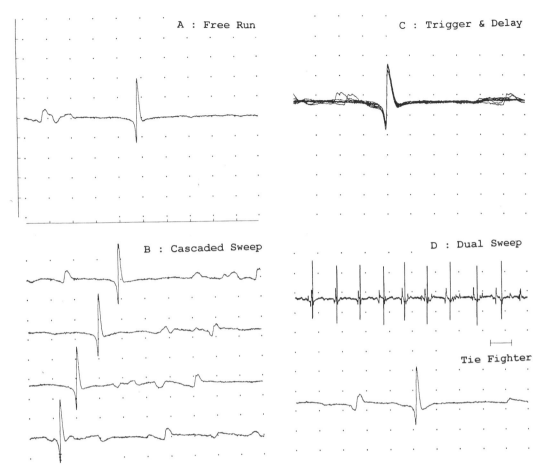

Figure 3–1. EMG signals recorded from the biceps brachii muscle of a normal subject are shown using different types of displays: *A*, Free running, *B*, Cascaded sweep, *C*, Trigger and delay, and *D*, Dual sweep (short and long sweep). The sensitivity is 100 μV/division and the sweep duration is 100 msec. In *C*, four consecutive triggered sweeps are superimposed. In *D*, the duration of upper sweep is 1 second, i.e., long sweep. The bottom trace is the live EMG signal, i.e., short sweep. The bottom trace can also be used to review a portion of the long sweep. The portion of the long sweep selected for review is defined by the "H" symbol (called the "Tie Fighter" from the motion picture "Star Wars") under it.

for high frequency. The sensitivity is adjusted as necessary. The sweep duration is usually 100 msec (i.e., 10 msec/div). The IA and SA are graded on a subjective scale such as 0–4+, or increased/decreased. The details of this assessment are discussed elsewhere. Abnormal activity can be documented by making a hardcopy of the EMG display screen (Fig. 3–2).

EMG AT MINIMAL FORCE OF CONTRACTION

A **motor unit** (MU) consists of all muscle fibers innervated by a single motor neuron. When the motor neuron discharges, all fibers in the MU respond by producing an action potential. This electrical event is registered as a motor unit action potential (MUAP) in the EMG recordings. The shape of the MUAP waveform depends upon the MU architecture, i.e., the number, size, and distribution of muscle fibers in the MU, the geometry of the end- plate zone, etc. (10, 15). When the MU architecture changes because of disease processes such as loss of fibers and reinnervation, the MUAP waveform also changes. This forms the basis for analyzing the MUAPs.

At minimal force of contraction, only a few MUs are activated. Hence, the EMG signal contains discharges of only a few MUAPs. This allows recognition of individual MUAPs and their abnormalities. The MUAP is usually

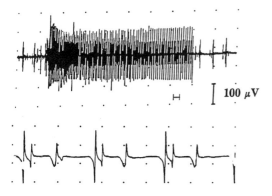

100 μV

Figure 3–2. A dual sweep display documents a spontaneous high frequency discharge. The long sweep (top trace) has a duration of 3 seconds. The discharge starts and stops suddenly and is made of three action potentials (bottom trace, sweep duration = 100 msec), repeating at roughly 30 msec intervals. The firing rate of these three potentials is slightly higher just at the beginning of the discharge.

assessed with the time base set to 10 msec/div. The sensitivity is usually 100–500 μV/div, but can be changed as necessary in order to view the MUAPs well. The MUAP abnormalities are assessed from their peak-to-peak

amplitude, the duration and phases of the waveform, and the firing rate of the MU.

QA (1,4,6,17) demonstrates that the MUAP duration is increased in neurogenic diseases and reduced in myopathy (Fig. 3–3). The duration measurements are relatively constant with slight movement of the recording electrode (7). This constancy makes duration a robust measurement that is suitable for differentiating between myopathy and neuropathy. Absence of short duration MUAPs will rule out myopathic disease processes, whereas short duration MUAPs will be consistent with myopathy.

The MUAP amplitude is increased in neurogenic conditions. Although the MUAP amplitude is usually normal or reduced in myopathy, it can be mildly increased in some patients with myopathy (Fig. 3–3). Therefore, a slight increase in MUAP amplitude is a nonspecific abnormality. A significant increase in amplitude (more than twice the mean value) is rarely seen in myopathy. Such measurements can be considered as specific of neurogenic diseases.

The incidence of **polyphasic** MUAPs is increased with neurogenic and myopathic dis-

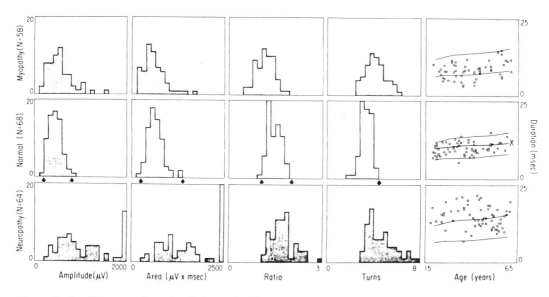

Figure 3–3. QA was performed in the biceps brachii muscle of 68 control subjects, 64 patients with neuropathy, and 58 patients with myopathy. The histograms of mean values of amplitude, area, area/amplitude ratio, and turns are shown. The arrows under the histogram for normal subjects define the normal limits. The duration values are plotted against the patient's age and the horizontal lines define the upper and lower limits of mean MUAP duration. (Reprinted with permission from Stewart C, Nandekar S, Massey J, et al.: Evaluation of an automatic method of measuring features of motor unit action potentials. Muscle Nerve 1989;12:141–148.)

eases. Therefore, increased polyphasia is also a nonspecific abnormality (Fig. 3–3). Polyphasic MUAPs in myopathy frequently have long duration. This results from an increase in the variability of fiber diameter rather than an increase in the number of muscle fibers. Therefore, polyphasic MUAPs should be excluded from documenting abnormalities of duration. It should be emphasized that normal muscles also have a few polyphasic MUAPs. Hence, occasional polyphasic MUAPs should not be considered as abnormal.

The MUAP area:amplitude ratio (7) is reduced in patients with myopathy (Fig. 3–3). This corresponds to a "thin" and spiky appearance of MUAPs. This ratio is normal or increased in neurogenic conditions.

Abnormalities of any MUAP feature can be documented to demonstrate EMG abnormalities. The normal values of MUAP amplitude and duration described in literature have been defined for their mean values obtained from 20 or more MUAPs. These limits should not be used to identify individual abnormal MUAPs. Although the mean MUAP durations for the large muscles of the upper and lower extremities (e.g., biceps brachii, triceps, quadriceps, tibialis anterior, etc.) are in the range of 7 msec to 14 msec, individual MUAPs can have durations from 5 msec to 20 msec (2, 14). It is the latter range that should be used to document abnormal individual MUAPs. These limits correspond to one-half and two divisions on the display with the typical time base setting of 10 msec/div. Small muscles of the hand and facial muscles have smaller MUs. Hence, their MUAPs have shorter durations. The aforementioned limits should not be used to assess duration abnormalities in these muscles.

The MUAP amplitude changes significantly with slight changes in the electrode position. Therefore, the range of normal MUAP amplitude is large. Manipulation of needle position to minimize MUAP rise time will result in large MUAP amplitudes. Nevertheless, at minimal force of contraction, MUAPs with amplitudes greater than 2 mV can be considered abnormal (14). Waveforms of such MUAPs will often be clipped on the display when the sensitivity is set at 200 μV/div. MUAPs with amplitudes greater than 4 mV or

5 mV are specific of neurogenic abnormality. Unlike the MUAP duration, the MUAP amplitude in small normal muscles can be similar to the amplitude in large muscles. Hence, MUAPs with a 1-mV to 2-mV amplitude in small muscles should not be interpreted as evidence of neurogenic abnormality.

The above patterns of abnormalities derived from QA (1,4,6,7,14,17) can be used in the routine needle examination to recognize and document MUAP abnormalities. However, one might ask, how can we identify and extract individual MUAPs without adding significantly to the time of the EMG examination?

When the position of the recording electrode is maintained, each active MU has a unique MUAP waveform in the EMG signals (Fig. 3–4A). Every time the MU discharges, its MUAP will be seen on the display. Sometimes two MUAP waveforms will superimpose on each other. The resulting waveform may not resemble the component MUAPs. Unlike individual MUAPs, the waveforms from MUAP superimpositions do not repeat at a regular rate in the EMG signal (Fig. 3–4B). As a rule of thumb, if a waveform can be seen three or more times, it is a MUAP.

At minimal force of contraction, a MU discharges roughly 10 times each second. This should give one MUAP waveform during each 100 msec sweep interval (i.e., 10 msec/division), as in the routine EMG examination (Fig. 3–1A). This can make the recognition of MUAPs rather tedious, especially when there are three or four active MUs. A cascade display of three to four sweeps on the screen should contain three or four MUAP discharges of each MU. This will make it very easy to recognize MUAPs and their abnormalities (Fig. 3–1B). By measuring the time interval between successive discharges of the identified MUAP, its firing rate can be calculated. When the aforementioned abnormalities are recognized, a printout of the signal will document them.

The EMG signals in Figure 3–5A were recorded from the biceps brachii muscle at a sensitivity of 200 μV/division and a sweep duration of 100 msec. We can recognize two waveforms that occur four times. Hence, they are considered to be MUAPs. Their peak-to-

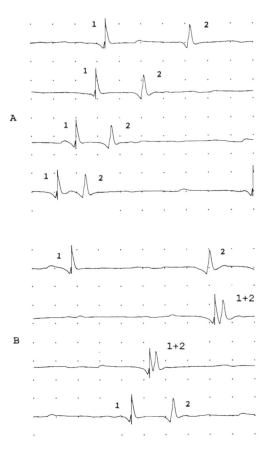

Figure 3-4. EMG signals recorded in the biceps brachii muscle of a normal subject are shown using a cascaded sweep display. Four consecutive sweeps are shown. The sweep duration is 100 msec and the sensitivity is 200 μV/division. *A.* Two distinct waveforms (labeled as *1* and *2*) can be seen four times, once on each trace. Hence, each waveform is an MUAP discharge. *B.* Another portion of the same recording is shown. The waveforms on the second and third trace look similar. However, they occurred only twice. These represent superimposition of the two MUAPs and not a different MUAP.

peak deflection is roughly two divisions, i.e., roughly 400 μV. Their duration is roughly 1 division, i.e., about 10 msec. Finally, they have two to three phases, i.e., the MUAPs are simple. These are normal MUAPs (from a healthy subject).

When viewing the EMG signals in Figure 3–5B, we can recognize a complex MUAP from its three occurrences, one on each sweep. Polyphasicity is a nonspecific abnormality. We can also recognize four discharges of a very "thin" MUAP. Its duration is less than half a division (less than 5.0 msec). These ob-

servations are consistent with a myopathic abnormality in this muscle. (This patient had polymyositis).

Another recording from the biceps brachii muscle at a sensitivity of 1 mV/div and a sweep duration of 100 msec is shown in Figure 3–5C. Visual inspection reveals three different MUAPs. The peak-to-peak deflection of one and three are close to two divisions, i.e., the MUAP amplitude is roughly 2 mV. The MUAPs are triphasic; i.e., the MUAPs are simple. It is difficult to assess their duration owing to a shifting baseline and waveform superimpositions. At this sensitivity setting, it appears to be about 1.5 divisions (i.e., 15 msec). At a setting of 200 μV/div, these MUAPs would appear to have much longer durations. These observations are consistent with a chronic neurogenic abnormality. (This patient had old polio).

The technique of cascaded sweeps (previously called raster) is very easy to use in the routine EMG examination. The only drawback of this method is that the user must stop acquisition and review the traces. When the baseline is not stable or when there is a partial overlap of MUAPs, measurement of duration can be difficult (Fig. 3–5C). Use of the amplitude triggered delay line allows us to timelock discharges of a single MU on the display screen (Fig. 3–6). When three triggered sweeps are superimposed, we have a valid MUAP. This mode of EMG display is used to assess waveforms of one MUAP at a time. Reducing the sweep duration permits observation of the details of the waveforms, such as turns and serrations. One can then average such time-locked discharges to obtain MUAPs with a clean baseline. However, in routine studies, this is not usually necessary. It is easy to visually discriminate between the MUAP of interest and other background signals.

Triggered discharges in Figure 3.6A show good superimposition. The sensitivity is 200 μV/division and the sweep duration is 5 msec/division. The faster sweep speed allows more details of the MUAP to be observed. By subjective assessment, the MUAP is triphasic with an amplitude of 900 μV and a duration of 10 msec. This represents a normal MUAP.

Recordings from the biceps brachii muscle of a patient with myopathy are shown in Fig-

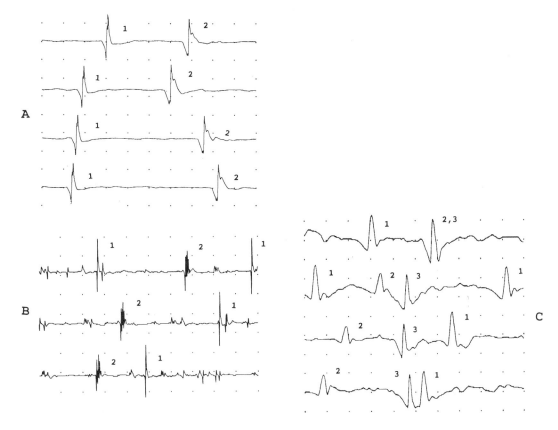

Figure 3–5. Concentric needle EMG recordings from the biceps brachii muscle of a normal subject, *A*, a patient with myopathy, *B*, and a patient with neuropathy, *C*, are shown using a cascaded sweep display. Discharges of individual MUAPs recognized by subjective assessment are labeled. Note the higher sensitivity setting for the patient with neuropathy.

ure 3–6B. Note that the sweep duration is 2 msec/division. At this setting, the MUAP duration is about 1 division (i.e., 2 msec). The MUAP amplitude is normal and the waveform is biphasic. This represents a simple, short-duration MUAP, which is consistent with myopathic abnormality. Note that a very fast sweep speed was required in order to view this short-duration potential.

Triggered discharges of a MUAP in the biceps brachii muscle of a patient with polio are shown in Figure 3–6C. We quantify these waveforms as a triphasic MUAP with a 3-mV amplitude and at least a 20-msec duration. This is consistent with a neurogenic abnormality.

This technique requires the operator to manipulate the needle position to record sharp MUAPs and to adjust the trigger level on the instrument. Ideally, the signal should contain discharges of only one or two MUAPs. This technique can be tedious and difficult. However, once a good trigger has been obtained, the MUAP can be recognized very easily. The late-appearing satellite potentials, which are difficult to recognize during a free-running sweep, can also be detected.

When MUAPs are viewed using an amplitude triggered delay line, one can easily perform a little bit of single fiber EMG (16) during the routine EMG. Action potentials (APs) of muscle fibers of the MU that are away from the recording electrode contribute to the low-frequency components of the MUAP. By increasing the low filter frequency from 10 Hz to 500 Hz (Fig. 3–7A&B), the activity from distant fibers is significantly attenuated. As a result, the MUAP represents mainly the action potentials of the closest few muscle fibers; individual single muscle fiber APs can be rec-

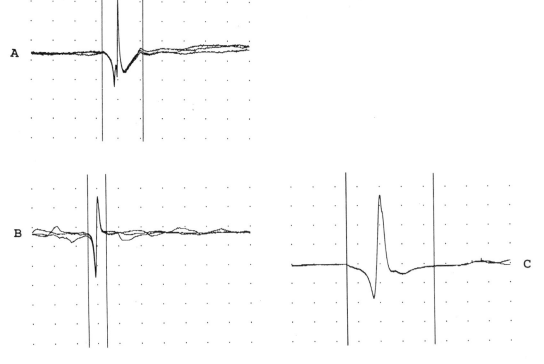

Figure 3–6. An amplitude-triggered delay line and a superimposed cascaded sweep display are used to assess single MUAP waveforms in the biceps brachii muscles of a normal subject, *A*, a patient with myopathy, *B*, and a patient with neuropathy, *C*. Three consecutive sweeps are superimposed. Note the faster sweep in *B* and lower amplifier sensitivity in *C*. The MUAP duration is reduced in myopathy and increased in neuropathy. All MUAPs have a simple waveform. The MUAP amplitude is increased in neuropathy.

ognized. At faster sweep speeds (Fig. 3–7B), one can recognize that successive discharges of the MUAP do not superimpose. Normal MUAPs show only a slight variability (Fig. 3–7B). When the MUAP variability is increased significantly (Fig. 3–8), the MUAP is called "unstable." This corresponds to increased jitter on the single fiber electromyography (SFEMG).

Unstable MUAPs indicate abnormalities of neuromuscular transmission. Abnormal neuromuscular transmission is not diagnostic of myasthenia gravis or myasthenic syndrome. During reinnervation, the newly formed end-plates are immature and produce unstable MUAPs. When the reinnervation is complete and the end-plates mature, the MUAPs become stable. Thus, assessment of stability can be extremely useful in any condition in which reinnervation occurs, i.e., all kinds of neuropathies.

The firing rate of the MU is a clinically valuable feature (11) that is often underutilized in electrodiagnosis. It can quickly be assessed by observing the position of MUAP waveforms in a cascaded display. When the MU discharges at less than 10 Hertz (Hz), the interdischarge interval will be more than 100 msec, i.e., one sweep length. Hence, the MUAP discharges will appear to shift right (Fig. 3–9A). Conversely, when the MU discharges at more than 10 Hz, the MUAP discharges will appear to shift left on the display (Fig. 3–9B). When the MUAP appears twice on **each** sweep, the firing rate is 20 Hz or more. Note that a MUAP discharge will occasionally appear twice on a single sweep when the firing rate is greater than 10 Hz (Fig. 3–9B).

Using these rules, the MUAPs in Figure 3–5A have a firing rate of about 10 Hz or less. The complex MUAP and the thin spiky of the second MU is called the "recruitment frequency" (RF). The clinical usefulness of the RF is discussed elsewhere in this book.

Displays of long sweeps are useful to assess firing rates as well as firing pattern. A recording from the diaphragm of a patient with neuropathy is shown in Figure 3–10. The ten-second long sweep (top trace) shows three bursts of EMG activity corresponding to respiration (middle trace). Review of a small section of the long sweep (bottom trace) shows MUs firing at roughly 10 Hz.

ANALYSIS OF RECRUITMENT PATTERN

At minimal force of contraction, the EMG signal contains discharges of only a few MUs (Fig. 3–11B and C). As described earlier, individual MUs and their firing rates can be assessed by visual inspection of cascaded or triggered sweeps. When the force of contraction is increased, the firing rate of the MUs increases and new MUs are recruited (Fig. 3–11D). The EMG waveforms now contain

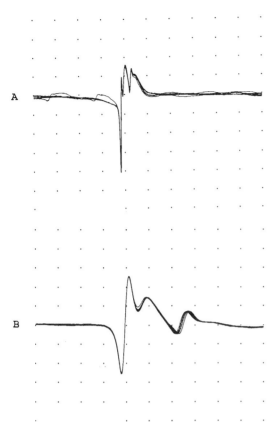

Figure 3–7. An amplitude-triggered delay line and a cascaded sweep display are used to assess discharges of a single MUAP recorded from the biceps brachii muscle of a normal subject. Five consecutive discharges are superimposed. The sensitivity is 100 μV/division. *A.* Sweep: 30 msec. Low filter: 10 Hz (normal setting). *B.* Low filter frequency increased to 500 Hz. Sweep: Reduced to 5 msec (SFEMG setting). Note the reduced amplitude and duration owing to change in filter setting and the variability of the MUAP waveform.

MUAP in Figure 3–5B are firing at more than 10 Hz. The MUAPs in Figure 3–5C are also firing at 10 Hz or more.

At minimal force of contraction of a normal muscle (Fig. 3–9A), the EMG signal contains repeated discharges of a single MU. When the force of contraction is increased, the firing rate of the MU increases (Fig. 3–9B). When the active MU cannot generate the desired force of contraction, a new MU is recruited. The recruitment can be recognized by a sudden change in the sound of the EMG signal and the appearance of a new MUAP waveform in the EMG signal (Fig. 3–9C). The firing rate of the first MU just before the recruitment

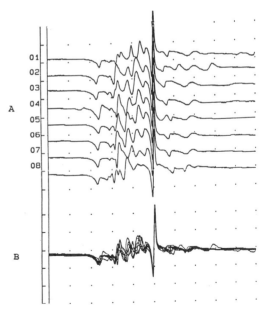

Figure 3–8. Successive discharges of an MUAP were recorded using an amplitude-triggered delay line and a cascaded sweep display. A concentric needle was used for recording. Sweep: 20 msec. Low filter: 500 Hz. The instability of the MUAP in this patient with polio can be seen in both cascaded and superimposed displays of sweeps.

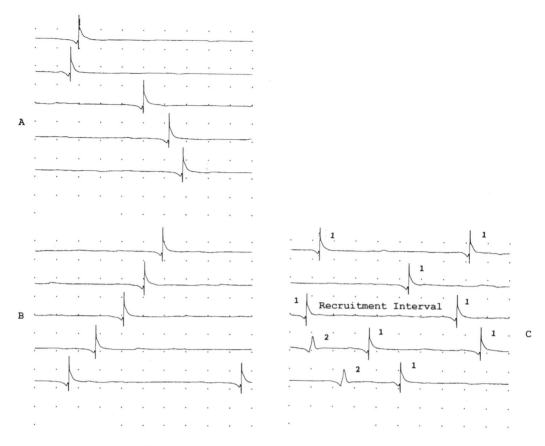

Figure 3–9. Firing rate and recruitment frequency measurement from a cascaded sweep display. Concentric needle EMG signals were recorded from the biceps brachii muscle of a normal subject at minimal force of contraction. Sweep: 100 msec. Sensitivity: 200 μV/division. *A.* Initially, the signal contained discharge of a single MU firing at less than 9 Hz. *B.* With a slight increase in the force of contraction, the firing rate of the MU increased to 11 Hz. With further increase in force, the MU firing rate increased and a new MU was recruited (labeled as *2*) in *C*). The recruitment interval is 70 msec, giving a recruitment frequency of 14 Hz.

discharges of several MUAPs that superimpose on one another repeatedly. The EMG signal, called **interference pattern** (IP), appears complex, and individual MUAPs can no longer be recognized (Fig. 3–11E).

In general, when several MUs are recruited, the baseline cannot be recognized and the IP is said to be "full" (Fig. 3–11F). At maximum force in a normal muscle, a full IP is usually recorded (Fig. 3–11F). If the IP contains discharges of only a few MUs, it is described as "reduced," "incomplete," or "discrete." At maximum force, such a pattern reflects lack of MU recruitment owing to loss of MUs or lack of maximum effort, perhaps owing to pain or central nervous system dysfunction.

The MU recruitment can be recognized from changes in the signal amplitude (Fig. 3–11A). Recognizing the MU recruitment is easy when the newly recruited MUAP has the largest amplitude in the signal (Fig. 3–12A). It must be emphasized that the MUAP amplitude is significantly affected by the distance between the recording electrode and the muscle fibers of the MU (10). Hence, many recruited MUs will have smaller amplitude MUAPs; these will not be recognized easily from signal amplitude changes (Fig. 3–13). However, the MUAPs will alter the signal baseline and thus contribute to the fullness of the IP signal. What one recognizes upon subjective assessment of the signal is the change in the amplitude of the largest spikes

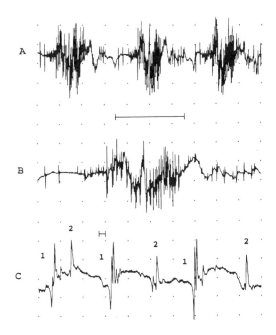

Figure 3-10. EMG signals were recorded from the diaphragm of a neuropathic muscle. The EMG activity occurs in bursts, corresponding to respiration (top and middle traces). This is recognizable on the long sweep of 10 seconds (top trace). A small portion of this recording is reviewed in the lower trace. Discharges of individual MUAPs recognized by subjective assessment are labeled *1* and *2* and show a firing rate of 10 Hz.

in the IP signal, i.e., the EMG envelope amplitude (Fig.3–11A). The envelope is defined by connecting together the positive peaks and the negative peaks (Fig. 3–11F) (4, 8). Solitary large-amplitude peaks should be excluded from this measurement.

The definition of "solitary" is subjective. Excluding one most-positive and one most-negative peak per 100 msec epoch (8) gives fairly good estimations for the envelope measurements (Fig. 3–11F; see Figs. 3–15B, 3–16B, 3–17B later in the chapter). In some cases, a single large-amplitude MUAP will discharge at high rates, which requires excluding more peaks than suggested above (see Fig. 3–16C).

The **sound** of the IP signal on an audio monitor is also helpful for "listening" for the abnormalities. The sound reflects the frequency spectrum of the IP. In patients with myopathy, the IP sound has a higher pitch, i.e., the spectrum shifts to higher frequencies. With neurogenic diseases, the IP has a dull

sound, indicating a shift to lower frequencies. The higher the signal frequency, the greater the number of peaks in the signal. This relationship led to the concept of measuring "turns" of the IP signal (18). With myopathy, the number of turns (or signal reversals) is increased. Most techniques of quantitative IP analysis are based on measuring turns and some form of amplitude measurement. These details are beyond the scope of this chapter. The IP measurements are much more tedious than the MUAP measurements. As a result, IP quantification is best performed using an automated technique.

So, how can one add objectivity to IP analysis in routine EMG? Surprisingly, the documentation of IP abnormalities is much simpler than that of MUAPs. There is no need to assess individual waveforms and their multiple occurrences. From a simple printout of the IP epoch (or sweep) recorded at maximum force, it is easy to recognize the amplitude of the envelope and fullness of the signal. It is characteristic of myopathy if, in a weak or wasted muscle, the IP is full with its envelope amplitude reduced. Conversely, a reduced or discrete IP with increased envelope amplitude reflects a neurogenic disease process.

On instruments that can display long-duration epochs of EMG, it is easy to see these abnormalities (Fig. 3–14). In normal muscles, the IP becomes full and the envelope amplitude increases when the force of contraction is increased. In patients with myopathy, the IP becomes full at moderate effort and the envelope amplitude fails to reach high values even at maximum force. In patients with neuropathy, the IP contains discharges of large-amplitude MUAPs even at minimal force of contraction. With increasing force, the number of spikes in the IP does not increase significantly.

The IP abnormalities can also be documented by viewing cascaded sweeps. At a 100-msec sweep duration, the fullness of the IP can be assessed (Figs. 3–15A, 3–16A, 3–17A). Superimposing these sweeps allows one to assess the envelope amplitude (Fig. 3–15B, 3–16B, 3–17B). In patients with myopathy, one can occasionally record large-amplitude thin MUAPs. These contribute to the so-called "solitary" or "occasional" large

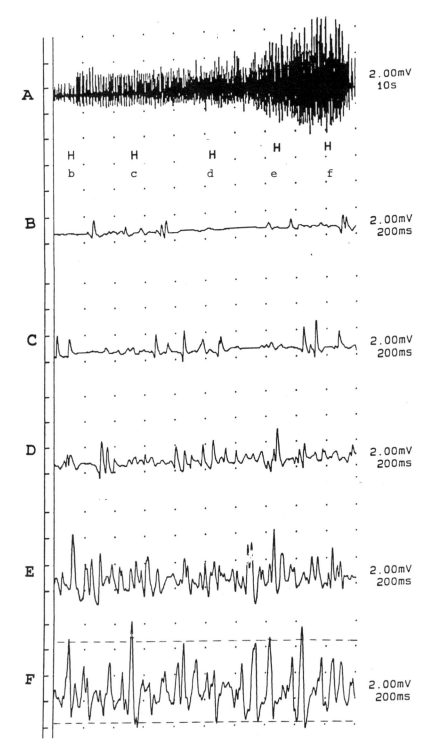

Figure 3-11. EMG signals recorded from the biceps brachii muscle of a normal subject when the force of contraction was increased from minimum to maximum. The sensitivity was 2 mV/division. A long sweep recording of 10 seconds is shown in A. Two-hundred-msec sections of this signal, defined by the position of the "H" symbol underneath, are shown in B through F. Note the increase in envelope amplitude and disappearance of signal baseline with increased force of contraction. At maximum effort (F), the IP is full. The horizontal dashed lines on the signal exclude the two most positive and two most negative peaks (i.e., one peak per 100 msec). The amplitude difference between them is the EMG envelope amplitude (6 mV).

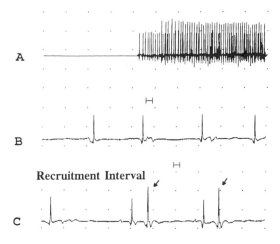

Figure 3–12. EMG signals recorded from the biceps brachii muscle of a normal subject using a dual sweep display. The long sweep in *A* has a duration of 10 seconds. Two portions of this recording, corresponding to the duration of the "H" symbol, are reviewed in *B* and *C*. Initially, the signal contained discharges of a single MUAP (*B*). When the force of contraction was increased, a new MUAP with larger amplitude is recruited (*C*). The recruitment can easily be recognized by a sudden change in the signal amplitude in the long sweep (*A*). The recruitment frequency (equal to 1000/recruitment interval (ms)) in this recording is about 9 Hz.

amplitude spikes, which may correspond to hypertrophic fibers. Including them in envelope measurements would falsely give normal IP envelope amplitude. For the recording in Figure 3–16C, the envelope amplitude reduced from 2.5 mV (normal) to 1 mV (reduced) by excluding discharges of a single MUAP. This recording also shows that large-amplitude MUAPs can sometimes be recorded in patients with myopathy.

When the IP signals are recorded at 0.5 mV/div or higher sensitivity and 10 msec/div sweep speed, the high frequency nature of the signal can be documented. At this setting, voltage changes smaller than 100 μV cannot be recognized by visual inspection, and all measured peaks are also the "turns" of the IP. One can count the number of upward-turned peaks in two divisions of signal (i.e., 20 msec). Multiplying this measurement by 100 gives an estimate of the number of turns/second (Fig. 3–16A). In the large muscles of the upper and lower extremities (i.e., biceps brachii, extensor digitorum communis, quadriceps, tibialis anterior, etc.), the number of turns/sec is

rarely greater than 1000. In other words, if the IP contains more than 10 upward-going peaks within 2 divisions of signal (at the aforementioned settings), it is indicative of myopathy.

An IP can be incomplete or discrete owing to the loss of MUs or lack of maximum effort. In these situations, MUAP firing rates are useful to document neurogenic abnormalities. Although it is easy to control the force of contraction, it is almost impossible to increase the firing rate of an MU without recruiting other MUs. A discrete IP in patients with neuropathy will usually have fast-firing MUs (Fig. 3–17C).

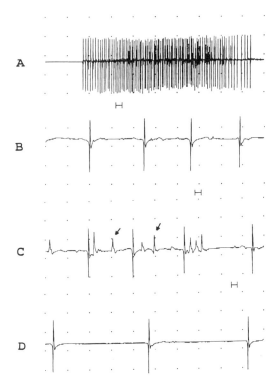

Figure 3–13. A long duration sweep display was used to record EMG signals from the biceps brachii muscle of a normal subject (*A*). Three sections of this recording, marked by the "H" symbol are shown in *B* through *D*. Initially, the signal contained discharges of a single MU (*B*). With increased force of contraction, additional MUs are recruited (indicated by arrows). However, their MUAP amplitudes are smaller than the first recruited MU (*C*). When the force was reduced, the last recruited MUs were first to be released (i.e., stopped discharging). As a result, the signal contained discharges of only the first recruited MU (*D*).

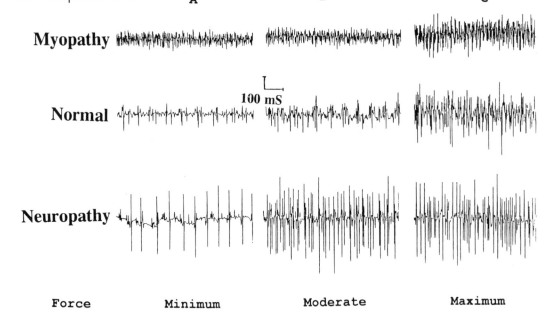

A **B** **C**

Myopathy

Normal

100 mS

Neuropathy

Force   Minimum   Moderate   Maximum

Figure 3–14. A long duration sweep (1 second) display was used to record IP signals from the biceps brachii muscles of a normal subject, a patient with myopathy, and a patient with neuropathy. Signals were recorded when the force of contraction was minimal, moderate, and maximum. The amplitude calibration is 500 μV for the patient with myopathy and the normal subject and 1 mV for the patient with neuropathy. At maximum force in myopathy, the IP is full with envelope amplitude of 1 mV to 1.5 mV. At the same force level, the patient with neuropathy has a reduced IP with envelope amplitude of about 6 mV.

Figure 3–15. IP assessment using cascaded sweep display. The sensitivity is 500 μV/div and the sweep duration is 100 msec. At maximum force, this normal subject shows a signal with no baseline (A), indicating a full pattern. Excluding the four most positive and four most negative peaks (1 peak per 100 msec) from the superimposed sweeps (B), the envelope (defined by dashed lines) amplitude is estimated to be 2.5 mV.

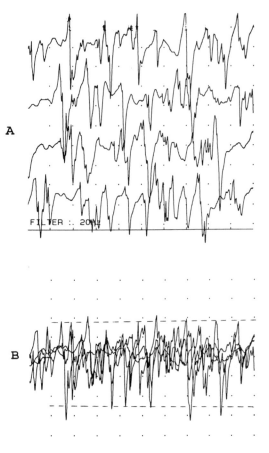

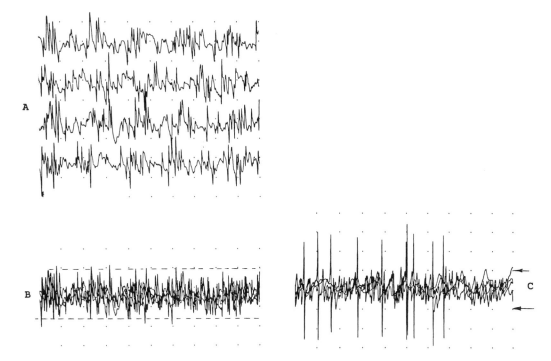

Figure 3-16. Cascaded sweep display is used to document IP at maximum force in a patient with myopathy. The sensitivity is 500 μV/division and sweep duration is 100 msec. The absence of horizontal baseline (*A*) indicates a full pattern. Most sections of 20 msec (two divisions), have more than 10 upward-turned peaks. This corresponds to more than 1000 turns/sec on QA. Upon superimposing the sweeps (*B*), the envelope (defined by dashed lines) amplitude is less than 1.5 mV (reduced). At another site, the IP contained discharges of a single MUAP with large thin amplitude spike (*C*). This results in solitary spikes in the IP. By excluding these spikes, the envelope amplitude reduced from roughly 2.5 mV (normal) to approximately 1 mV (reduced).

WHAT CAN GO WRONG IN DOCUMENTING ABNORMALITIES?

What we observe and document are EMG signals and their measurements. Based on the findings in other muscles and other tests, the underlying pathophysiology should be assessed. As much as possible, the terms "myopathic" and "neurogenic" should not be used to describe the EMG signals. For example, in severely weak muscles of patients with neuropathy, one can record abnormalities similar to those in myopathy. The best diagnostic information can usually be found in moderately weak muscles (strength grades 3 and 4).

Polyphasicity of MUAPs can be one of the earliest abnormalities in neuromuscular diseases. However, because normal muscles can have up to 20% polyphasic MUAPs (17), assessment of polyphasic MUAPs should be

done with caution. When two or more simple MUAPs superimpose by chance, the resulting waveform can be polyphasic. Recordings in Figure 3–18A show 12 sweeps recorded at a 100-msec sweep duration. Two simple MUAPs firing at 11 Hz to 12 Hz can be recognized. In another portion of the same recording (Fig. 3–18B), we can see 10 consecutive sweeps, i.e., duration of one second, when the MUAP waveforms superimpose giving complex waveforms. However, none of the waveforms occur three times. Therefore, there are no polyphasic MUAPs in this recording. We want to emphasize that polyphasic MUAPs must be validated by observing at least three discharges.

Using a triggered delay line can also assist in identifying and documenting polyphasic MUAPs. When MUAPs have satellite potentials, they can appear before or after the main MUAP spike. If the sweep duration is too

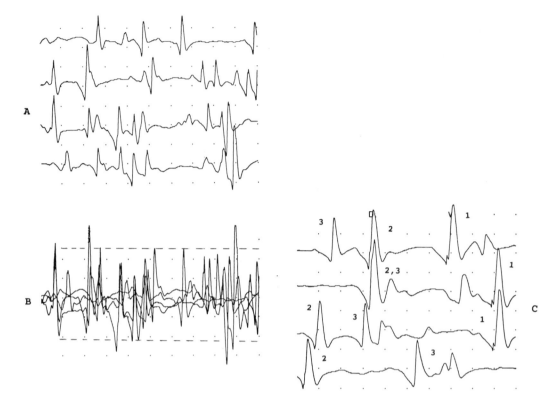

Figure 3–17. EMG IP abnormalities in the biceps brachii muscle of a patient with neuropathy are documented using cascaded sweep display. The sensitivity is 1 mV/division in *B* and 2 mV/division in *A*, and the sweep duration is 100 msec. Even at maximum effort, the signal baseline can be seen clearly, i.e., the IP is reduced in *A*. When the sweeps are superimposed, the envelope (defined by dashed lines) amplitude is more than 4 mV. In *C*, the sweep duration is 50 msec and the sensitivity is 2 mV/division. At maximum effort, discharges of individual MUAPs can be recognized. The MUs are firing at approximately 20 Hz. The MUAP amplitude is more than 5 mV. All of these features are characteristic of neurogenic abnormalities.

short, these potentials may be missed. This is likely to occur in patients with dystrophy where the MUAPs can be short as well as very long with complex waveforms. Therefore, polyphasic MUAPs should be excluded from documenting abnormalities of MUAP duration.

When MUAP stability is assessed from triggered discharges recorded at a 500-Hz low filter setting, the MUAP amplitude and duration are reduced. If the filter setting is not changed back to the default value of 3–20 Hz, the remaining study will appear myopathic. Although "unstable" waveforms are found with diseases of the neuromuscular junction, other abnormalities can also make MUAP appear unstable. The MUAP in Figure 3–19 appears to be blocking. However, there appears to be little jitter in the blocking poten-

tial. This contradiction (normal jitter with blocking) indicates that the MUAP "instability" is not from neuromuscular transmission. In this recording, sometimes the MU discharges twice within a short period of time. When the extra discharge does not occur, the MUAP appears to block.

By viewing the EMG signals in different ways, one can observe many of the MUAP features that are considered quantitative. Although one should use these tricks and develop new protocols to assess features that are not discussed in this chapter, it is important to know the limitations of the instruments. Digital instruments offer the facility of acquiring, storing, and reviewing long epochs of EMG. However, when digital instruments are not properly configured, they can distort waveforms. This distortion

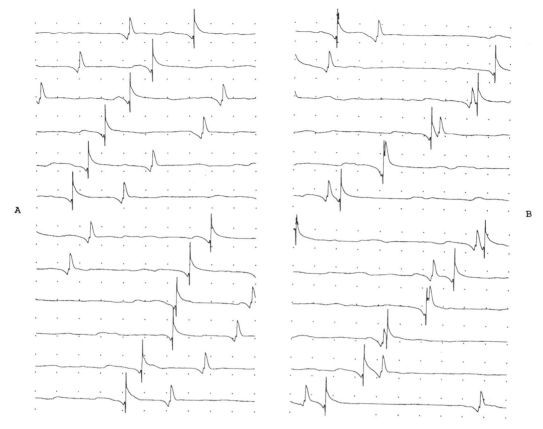

Figure 3-18. Polyphasic waveforms can result from superimpositions of simple MUAPs. EMG signals were recorded from the biceps brachii muscle of a normal subject. The sweep duration was 100 msec and the display gain is 400 μV/division. In one section of the recording (A), individual MUAP discharges can be recognized easily. The MUAPs have a biphasic waveform. In another portion of the recording (B), superimposition of MUAPs result in complex waveforms. However, each waveform is seen only once. Therefore, these should not be considered as polyphasic MUAPs.

is called aliasing, and the user may not realize it is occuring.

As described earlier, a cascaded display of 300 or 400 msec epoch of EMG signals can be quite useful in identifying individual MUAPs. **If the instrument does not permit cascaded sweeps, do not change the sweep duration to a higher value, e.g., 200 to 500 msec.** At this slow sweep setting, the main spike of the MUAP will not be well recognized, thus defeating the goal of waveform comparisons. On digital instruments, longer sweeps are likely to distort the EMG signals by changing the effective digital display resolution without the operator realizing it. All digital instruments sample the EMG signals at regular intervals and then plot the "sampled" amplitude values on the screen. Many digital instruments plot one sweep of the EMG by acquiring and plotting a fixed number of samples, e.g., 1000. If the sweep duration is 100 msec, the machine displays the signal every 100 μS (100 msec divided by 1000). This interval is short enough that important waveform details are not missed. If the sweep duration is now changed to 200 msec, the EMG will be displayed at a 200-μS interval. At this setting, it is possible that sharp peaks in the MUAP will be missed in some discharges.

The recording in Figure 3–20A was made from the biceps brachii muscle of a healthy subject. It shows discharges of a single MUAP. The MUAP amplitude in successive discharges is relatively constant. The same signal recorded at 500 msec (Fig. 3–20B) shows a few discharges with a smaller amplitude. The

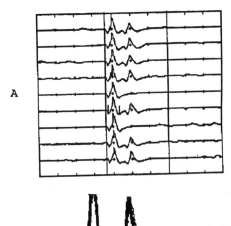

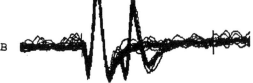

Figure 3-19. In a patient with neuropathy, amplitude-triggered delay line and cascaded sweep was used to record discharges of a single MU. In *A*, the sweep duration is 50 msec. The MUAP showed blocking in cascaded mode. However, on changing the sweep duration to 30 msec and superimposing sweeps (*B*), the jittering potential appeared identical to the main MUAP and showed no jitter. This represents an extra discharge generated in the nerve fiber and not abnormal neuromuscular transmission.

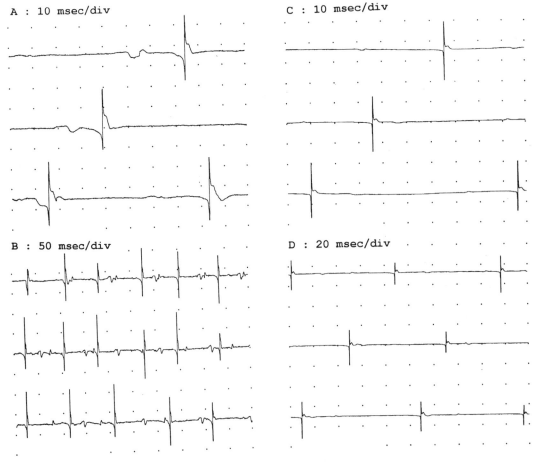

Figure 3-20. On digital instruments, long sweep durations can result in signal distortion by aliasing. All sweeps in this figure are obtained by plotting 1000 samples. Sweeps in *A* and *C* were recorded with a sweep duration of 100 msec. This gives a display resolution of 100 μsec. Note the loss of waveform details (e.g., duration assessment) and the variability of MUAP amplitude at longer sweep durations; 500 msec in *B* (500 μsec display resolution) and 200 msec in *D* (200 μsec display resolution).

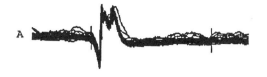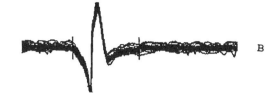

MUAP	Amplitude (μV)	Duration (mS)	Phases	Firing Rate (Hz)
A	451	16.3	3	15.4
B	841	9.2	3	13.1

Figure 3–21. A multi-motor MUAP analysis algorithm was used to document abnormalities in a patient with early radiculopathy. Two MUAPs from two different sites are shown. The MUAP amplitude, duration, and phases are normal. They have a high firing rate and there is no other active MU. This documents increased recruitment frequency without increased number of MUAPs.

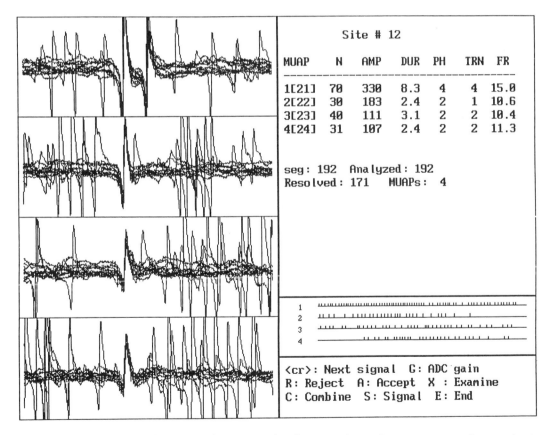

Figure 3–22. A multi-muscle MUAP analysis was used to document abnormalities in a patient with myopathy. A six-second epoch of EMG recorded at one side was analyzed. On the left side, discharges of four different MUAPs are shown in a triggered mode. The simple MUAPs show normal amplitude and reduced duration. The MUAP with two spikes (top left) has normal duration. The firing pattern of the MUs is shown below the MUAP measurements on the right. The horizontal line represents 10 seconds. Each vertical tick represents one firing of the MU. The firing rates are normal.

same amplitude variability is seen in Figures 3–20C and 3–20D when the sweep duration was changed from 100 msec to 200 msec. This may be misinterpreted as an unstable MUAP or irregularly firing MUs. Hence, the amplitude variability seen on digital instruments should be assessed with caution and, if possible, should be validated at faster sweep speeds using a triggered delay line. To further emphasize the point, consider a sweep made of 500 samples and a sweep duration of 200 msec. The instrument will display signals every 400 μS. At this setting, one could miss fibrillations or considerably underestimate their frequency of occurrence or their amplitudes. All of the long EMG epochs shown in this chapter were acquired at a 100-μS sampling interval. The display was then adjusted by a computer algorithm to reveal sections of the long epoch.

SUMMARY

The EMG signals are observed at a 100-msec sweep duration so that one can recognize the waveform details. However, the events within the EMG recordings require analysis of much longer epochs. For example, the spontaneous discharges frequently last for several seconds. To assess recruitment, firing rates and recruitment frequencies, firing patterns, etc., long epochs of EMG can be convenient. A display of EMG at a slow sweep can add significantly to the EMG assessment. Many modern instruments are capable of generating such a display without compromising the signal resolution (i.e., without long intervals between successive samples). A combination of a slow and fast sweep will make it much easier to recognize and document EMG abnormalities as shown.

In the age of powerful and cheap computers, "smart" EMG analysis algorithms can be "built in" to the clinical instrument. In the so called multi-MUAP analysis technique (2, 9), the computer can break down EMG recordings at minimal force into discharges of component MUAPs. The entire process can be performed in only a few seconds and can occur simultaneously with and without interrupting the routine EMG examination. Such techniques will permit a quick documentation of EMG abnormalities in several muscles

without adding significantly to the time of examination (Figs. 3–21, 3–22).

There is a lot of useful information in EMG that does not get analyzed because of a variety of factors. Insufficient understanding of the instrument is probably the most significant problem in quantification. By using simple maneuvers to acquire signals and common sense to "view" the signal, one can recognize and document quantitative EMG abnormalities in day-to-day clinical EMG practice; i.e., one can make the routine needle EMG examination "objective."

ACKNOWLEDGMENTS

I would like to thank TECA Corporation (Pleasantville, NY) for providing support for this project. The EMG recordings for the illustrations were provided by Dr. Paul Barkhaus, Dr. Donald Sanders, and Dr. Salil Tiwari. Their help is greatly appreciated.

References

1. Barkhaus P, Nandedkar S, Sanders D: Quantitative EMG in inflammatory myopathy. Muscle Nerve 1990;13:909–914.
2. Bischoff C, Stålberg E, Falck B: Reference values of motor unit action potentials obtained with multi-MUAP analysis. Muscle Nerve, 1994;17:842–851.
3. Buchthal F, Pinelli P, Rosenfalck P: Action potential parameters in normal human muscles and their physiological determinants. Acta Physiol Scand 1954;22:219–229.
4. Buchthal F, Kamieniecka Z: The diagnostic yield of quantified electromyography and quantified muscle biopsy in neuromuscular disorders. Muscle Nerve 1982;5:265–290.
5. Daube J: Needle examination in electromyography. AAEM Minimonograph #11. Rochester, Minnesota: American Association of Electrodiagnostic Medicine, 1979.
6. Dorfman L, McGill K: Automatic quantitative electromyography. Muscle Nerve 1988;11:804–818.
7. Nandedkar S, Barkhaus P, Sanders D, et al.: Analysis of amplitude and area of the concentric needle EMG motor unit action potentials. Electroencephalogr Clin Neurophysiol 1988;69:561–567.
8. Nandedkar S, Sanders D: Measurement of the amplitude of the EMG envelope. Muscle Nerve 1990;13:933–938.
9. Nandedkar S, Barkhaus P, Charles A: Multimotor unit action potential analysis (MMA). Muscle Nerve 1995;18:1155–1166.
10. Nandedkar S, Sanders D, Stålberg E, et al.: Simulation of concentric needle EMG motor unit action potentials. Muscle Nerve 1988;11:151–159.

11. Petajan J: Motor unit recruitment. AAEM Mini-monograph #3, Muscle Nerve 1991;14:489–502.

12. Stålberg E, Chu J, Bril V, et al.: Automatic analysis of the EMG interference pattern. Electroencephalogr Clin Neurophysiol 1983;56:672–681.

13. Stålberg E: Electrodiagnostic assessment and monitoring of motor unit changes in disease. Muscle Nerve 1991;14:293–303.

14. Stålberg E, Bischoff C, Falck B: Outliers: A way to detect abnormality in quantitative EMG. Muscle Nerve 1994;17:392–399.

15. Stålberg E, Andreassen S, Falck B, et al.: Quantitative analysis of individual motor unit action potentials. A proposal for standardized terminology and criterion for measurement. J Clin Neurophysiol 1986;3:313–348.

16. Stålberg E, Trontelj J: Single fibre EMG: Studies in healthy and diseased muscles. New York:Raven Press, 1994.

17. Stewart C, Nandedkar S, Massey J, et al.: Evaluation of an automatic method of measuring features of motor unit action potentials. Muscle Nerve 1989;12:141–148.

18. Willison R: Analysis of electrical activity in healthy and dystrophic muscle in man. J Neurol Neurosurg Psychiatry 1964;27:386–394.

Chapter 4
Practical Aspects of Instrumentation
Daniel Dumitru

The electrophysiologic instrument's components and the manner in which those components process biologic signals are important to understand so as to avoid artifactual data collection leading to erroneous diagnostic conclusions. This chapter presents a practical approach to the electrophysiologic instrument. The instrument is considered from the perspective of its various constituent subcomponents and the way a biologic signal is processed on its way to being displayed both visually and acoustically (Fig. 4–1). Recording electrodes are located on or in the body to detect the nerve or muscle signal of interest. An amplifier then magnifies the signal because biologic potentials are measurable in microvolts or millivolts. Low and high frequency filters then extract extraneous artifacts. The resultant signal is both fed into a loudspeaker and additionally processed by an analog-to-digital converter. A cathode ray tube (CRT) then displays the processed signal for visual analysis. A stimulator delivers a neural depolarizing current to induce action potential propagation for motor and sensory nerve evaluation. Inadequate knowledge of any of the above processing steps can lead to faulty signal interpretation, resulting in an erroneous diagnosis.

RECORDING ELECTRODES

Recording electrodes can be subdivided into two basic types: 1) surface electrodes, and 2) needle electrodes. Each of these electrodes can be further subdivided into several different types of electrodes for specific recording situations. The practitioner should be familiar with the type of electrode discussed in order

to apply the best electrode for individual recording needs.

Three electrodes are used to record a biologic waveform: 1) active; 2) reference; and 3) ground electrodes. The active electrode, also referred to as E-1 or G-1, is positioned in the vicinity of the electrical generator of interest. A reference electrode (E-2 or G-2) is typically positioned in a location of relative electrical silence, except for sensory nerve recordings, with respect to the signal recorded by the active electrode. In the body, there is no place of true electrical silence but only regions of relatively more or less electrical potential. Finally, a ground electrode is placed in proximity to the active electrode to essentially serve as a reference "zero" or ground potential.

Surface Electrodes

As the name implies, surface electrodes are located on the skin's surface and can record either nerve or muscle action potentials. The general advantage of all surface electrodes is that they can be secured simply to the patient's skin with tape or in a self-retaining manner with little or no discomfort. A major disadvantage of surface electrodes is that the skin offers a considerable resistant barrier, lessening the biologic signal's ability to reach the recording electrode. Also, an electrode located on the skin is frequently at some distance from the biologic generator of interest. This is important because the amplitude of a biologic signal diminishes rapidly over short distances.

The resistance offered by biologic tissues to potentials traveling within the body is referred to as impedance. Skin impedance can be reduced by gently abrading the stratum

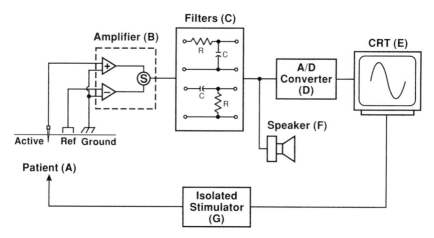

Figure 4–1. Schematic representation of the electrophysiologic instrument's component parts. Electrodes in or on the patient (A) detect action potentials and transmit them to a differential amplifier (B). The differential signal is filtered (C) and then fed to the loudspeaker (F) for aural analysis and the analog-to-digital converter (D) for a digital representation of the analog signal. The signal is then ready for visual display on the cathode ray tube (E). Excitation of the peripheral nervous system is possible with the stimulator (G). (Reprinted with permission from Dumitru D, Walsh NE: Electrophysiologic instrumentation. In: Dumitru D, ed. Clinical electrophysiology: Physical medicine and rehabilitation state of the art reviews. Philadelphia: Hanley & Belfus, 1989.)

corneum with commercially available pumice solutions or fine sandpaper. If sandpaper is used, it should be discarded after each patient to avoid cross contamination of body fluids. Abrasion of the skin is usually only necessary when sensory nerve action potentials (SNAPs) or somatosensory evoked potentials (SEPs) are elicited because of their relatively small size (tens of microvolts to several tenths of a microvolt). Compound muscle action potentials (CMAPs) are typically several millivolts and easily recorded with surface electrodes, provided an electrolyte paste is located between the electrodes and the skin's surface.

When using surface electrodes, a small amount of electrolyte cream or paste must always be placed between the electrode and the skin (39). The practitioner should use only enough electrolyte to just cover the recording electrode's surface because excess cream can form a conducting pathway between recording electrodes or between recording and stimulating electrodes, forming a short circuit. The electrolyte serves to decrease the impedance and mediate the biologic signals' transmission from the subcutaneous tissues across the skin, so as to be detected by the electrodes' metal surface. Electrodes can be made of any metal, provided they are good conductors

such as stainless steel, tin, gold, platinum, lead, silver, etc. A number of different types of surface electrodes are commercially available (Fig. 4–2).

DISC ELECTRODES

Disc electrodes are routinely used in electrodiagnostic medicine and consist of several types. A few disc electrodes are essentially flat and round; however, most electrodes have a central depression and give the appearance of a cup, thus defining the term "cup electrode." The cup or small central depression is specifically designed to reduce artifactually induced electrode bias potentials from interfering with the signal of interest (13).

Some manufacturers offer two disc electrodes imbedded in a plastic bar. Note that each manufacturer varies the interelectrode separation between 2.5 cm and 3 cm. This interelectrode separation can have profound consequences on the morphology of biologic waveforms (see below).

RING ELECTRODES

Ring or self-retaining clip electrodes are commonly used during the recording of antidromically elicited digital SNAPs, but they also can

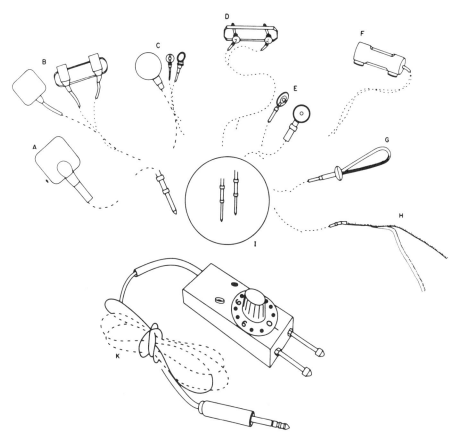

Figure 4–2. Various types of surface electrodes available. *A.* Square ground electrode. *B.* Lead strips mounted in a plastic bar. *C.* Circular ground electrode. *D.* Nonlead plastic bar electrode. *E.* Flat 1-centimeter disc electrodes. *F.* Flat disc electrodes mounted in a plastic bar. *G.* Wire ring electrodes. *H.* "Pipe cleaner" electrodes. *I.* 1-millimeter tip plug (2- millimeter tip plug: left of *I*). *K.* bipolar surface stimulator. (Reprinted with permission from Braddom RL, Schuchmann J: Motor conduction. In: Johnson EW, ed. Practical electromyography. Baltimore: Williams & Wilkins, 1980.)

be used as stimulating electrodes. There is usually a region where a portion of the electrode does not contact the skin. This region should be positioned so as not to affect the desired signal. For example, if a median nerve SNAP from one of the first four digits is required, that region of no-skin-contact should be positioned posteriorly where the radial nerve innervates the digit's dorsum. Also, the bare metal of the ring can contact adjacent digits, leading to noise when the hand moves following median or ulnar nerve stimulation. A dry tissue or gauze placed around the ring electrodes provides a convenient insulation that precludes this movement artifact from interfering with the intended signal. It is also

a good practice to rotate the ring partially around the digit several times in order to spread the paste and reduce the skin's impedance thus improving signal detection.

Electrode Separation

Surface electrodes are positioned at specific locations to record biologic signals unique to the activated nerve or muscle. This implies that the active electrode is located as close as possible to the biologic signal's source, whereas the reference electrode is at a relatively quiet area. Implicit in the electrode location is the concept of distance and what is considered an optimal interelectrode separation. The separation between active and reference electrodes is best considered separately for SNAP and CMAP recordings.

SNAP RECORDINGS

The location of active and reference electrodes is important for both antidromic and orthodromic SNAP studies with the same principles applicable to both techniques. A SNAP's amplitude is one of the important parameters used for diagnostic purposes. It is directly dependent on the distance separating the active and reference electrodes. The "optimal" interelectrode separation for recording SNAPs can be addressed from a theoretical and practical standpoint (20).

The approximate rise time (the time from SNAP's onset to the negative spike's maximum amplitude) for a normal SNAP is 0.8 msec or less. If we assume a conduction velocity of 50 meters/second (m/s), the rise time portion of the SNAP will have a physical expanse along the nerve of 4 cm (nerve conduction velocity {NCV} = distance {D} · time; 50 m/s = D · 0.8 ms; D = 4 cm). This means that the leading edge of the SNAP extends 4 cm along the nerve before its maximal amplitude is reached at any one point on the nerve. As a result, if the active and reference electrodes are located within this zone of electrical activity (4 cm of interelectrode separation or less) they will record similar information, which is cancelled by the instrument (Fig. 4–3). Cancellation of similar data leads to a reduction in the waveform's amplitude because it is not permitted to fully resolve. This "early" potential truncation leads to a shortening of the potential's peak latency. The onset latency remains unaffected as the active electrode detects the SNAP's onset prior to any information reaching the reference electrode. Placing the active and reference electrodes too close can result in SNAPs with reduced amplitudes, negative spike duration, and shortened peak latencies, giving the false impression of a possible axonal loss lesion.

CMAP RECORDINGS

When recording CMAPs, the above-noted distance of 4 cm is no longer relevant. The most important aspect of CMAP interelectrode separation is to locate the active elec-

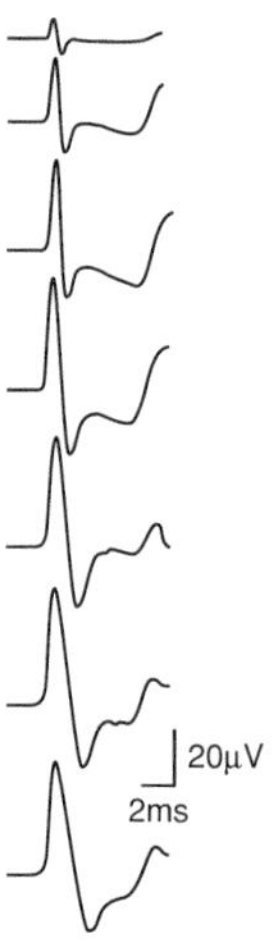

		Electrode Separation (cm)	Onset Latency (ms)	Peak Latency (ms)	Amplitude (μV)	Negative Spike Duration (ms)	Rise Time (ms)
A		0.5	2.8	3.2	8	0.7	0.4
B		1.0	2.8	3.4	23	1.0	0.6
C		2.0	2.8	3.5	34	1.2	0.7
D		3.0	2.8	3.6	39	1.4	0.8
E		4.0	2.8	3.7	41	1.8	1.0
F		5.0	2.8	3.7	41	2.0	1.0
G		6.0	2.8	3.7	41	2.2	1.0

Figure 4–3. An antidromic median SNAP is recorded with a separation of 14 cm between the cathode and active recording electrode. A series of seven recording montages is used with increasing interelectrode separations between the active and reference electrodes (A through G). As the interelectrode separation increases, so do the peak latency, negative spike duration, rise time, and amplitude while the onset latency remains unchanged. The onset latency defines a maximal conduction velocity of 50 m/s. An optimal interelectrode separation of 4 cm should maximize the SNAP parameters of interest, as with maximum peak latency and amplitude. (Reprinted with permission from Dumitru D: Electrodiagnostic medicine. Philadelphia: Hanley & Belfus, 1995.)

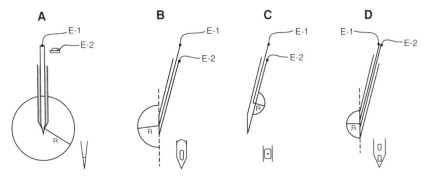

Figure 4–4. Pictorial depiction of the different needle recording electrodes available and their uptake areas. *A.* Monopolar needle electrodes require a separate reference and ground electrode. *B.* A standard concentric needle electrode, which uses the cannula as a reference but needs a separate surface ground. *C.* Single fiber electrode with E-1 as a side port pickup. The cannula serves as the reference. Again, a separate ground electrode is required. *D.* Bipolar concentric needle electrode with two recording ports close to each other. The cannula is the ground and the two central wires are the active and reference electrodes. (Reprinted with permission from Dumitru D: Electrodiagnostic medicine. Philadelphia: Hanley & Belfus, 1995.)

trode on the muscle's motor point and position the reference electrode off the muscle activated. A good location for the reference electrode is over the muscle's distal tendon near the tendon's insertion, which should be a relatively silent electric area. If the reference electrode is positioned 4 cm from the active electrode, it could still be on muscle tissue, particularly with large muscles. The net effect of situating the reference electrode on active muscle tissue is to reduce the CMAP's amplitude, possibly yielding a false positive result that suggests axonal loss.

Needle Electrodes

Four types of needle electrodes are commonly used in electrodiagnostic medicine: 1) monopolar; 2) standard concentric; 3) single fiber; and 4) subcutaneous electroencephalographic needles (Fig. 4–4). The main purpose of using any form of needle as opposed to surface recording electrodes is to position the electrode as close as possible to the biologic generator, particularly if the generator is located at some distance beneath the skin surface. The first three needle types are used to record the electrical activity arising from muscle tissue, whereas the fourth needle-electrode type is used to record cortical somatosensory evoked potentials. Of note, the monopolar needle can also be used to stimulate peripheral nerves (see stimulators), whereas the electroencepha-

lographic needle may also be used to perform subcutaneous SNAP and CMAP recordings. CMAPs are best recorded with surface electrodes to ensure detecting as much electrical activity from the muscle as possible. Needle-recorded CMAPs have a very restricted recording territory and the ensuing amplitude does not accurately reflect the entire muscle's activity. When recording CMAP's, therefore, surface electrodes should be used (Fig. 4–5).

When explaining the above needle electrodes to patients prior to their use, it may be a good idea to refer to the electrodes as pins and not needles to allay any anxiety associated with "needles." Stating that a small pin electrode is placed under the skin can be of benefit in gaining patient cooperation and enhancing the efficient collection of data.

MONOPOLAR NEEDLE

The monopolar needle is a solid stainless steel shaft 12–75 mm in length and 0.3–0.5 mm in diameter. It is coated in Teflon except for the distal 0.5 mm to 0.75 mm (10, 11, 24). Its recording surface is a cone shape with an exposed metal surface, approximating 0.17 mm^2 (15, 49). The electrical recording territory approaches that of a sphere surrounding the exposed needle tip (41, 42). Patients tolerate needle insertion relatively well because the Teflon permits easy tissue passage. Separate reference and ground electrodes are required

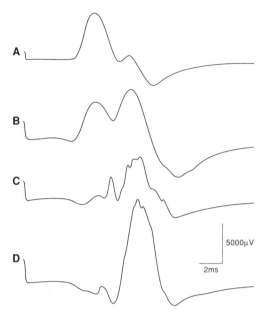

A

B

C

5000μV

D

2ms

Figure 4–5. The type of electrode used (surface vs. needle) to record a waveform can have significant effects on the CMAP. *A.* A surface electrode is used to record a CMAP from the abductor pollicis brevis following median nerve stimulation at the wrist. *B.* Placing a bare one-half inch needle electrode subcutaneously over the surface electrode location used in *A* results in a waveform with a different onset latency and waveform morphology. *C.* Locating a monopolar needle within the muscle at the same location as that used for the surface electrode in *A* results in a unique waveform different from either the surface or subcutaneous electrode recordings. *D)* Positioning the monopolar needle deeper into the tissue results in a larger amplitude potential than that recorded in *C.*

on the skin surface with the reference electrode placed in proximity of the needle insertion site (25). One could also use a second monopolar needle as a reference, especially with infants.

Prior to the use of disposable monopolar electrodes, there was considerable concern regarding the durability of the Teflon (10). Repeated usage eventually leads to the Teflon cracking and peeling back from the recording surface, increasing its surface area. The increased area of exposed metal adversely affected motor unit action potential (MUAP) parameters. Specifically, the MUAP amplitude and duration decreases with increasing loss of Teflon. With the advent of high-quality disposable monopolar needle electrodes,

concern regarding Teflon damage has been minimized. Disposable electrodes should be used when there is concern regarding transmissible diseases (26). It is imperative to not attempt to resterilize disposable needle electrodes, but to dispose of them immediately upon completion of the examination.

The monopolar needle has rather characteristic MUAP parameters compared to the concentric needle electrode (5, 6, 9, 11, 22, 46). The spherical recording territory of the monopolar needle, and its relatively large exposed area, permits recording from a comparatively large number of single muscle fibers belonging to a single motor unit. Also, the geometric configuration of the conical shape permits the needle tip to detect electrical activity close to the biologic generator; hence, it is located in a region of high voltage. The combination of relatively large numbers of muscle fibers and regions of high voltage result in MUAPs with larger amplitudes and more phases than comparable MUAPs recorded with a concentric needle. Interestingly, MUAP duration is the same whether recorded with monopolar or concentric needle electrodes (23, 27, 28, 34).

STANDARD CONCENTRIC NEEDLE

The term "standard" is used to distinguish the type of concentric needle routinely used from a concentric bipolar needle. The standard concentric (coaxial) needle consists of a stainless steel metal cannula with a centrally located platinum or nichrome wire (1). The bipolar concentric needle has two centrally located wires that serve as the active and reference electrodes. For this discussion, we do not discuss the bipolar electrode as it is rarely used for clinical purposes; hence, the term concentric needle is understood to refer to the standard type of concentric needle.

The metal cannula is 0.3–1.0 mm in diameter with a length similar to the monopolar needle (9, 33, 37). A concentric needle electrode's tip is beveled to 15°–20° with a central recording wire 150 μm in diameter insulated from the cannula. The recording surface is oval shaped, 150 μm by 580 μm, with an area of 0.08 mm^2. This internal wire is the active electrode, whereas the cannula serves as the reference electrode. A separate ground electrode is required. The lack of Teflon plus the beveled cutting edge can result in the concentric needle's insertion being slightly more painful for patients.

The concentric needle's recording territory is believed to approximate a hemisphere with the cannula acting to shield the electrical activity adjacent to it from the active recording surface (5, 7, 15, 30). The fact that the active (centrally located wire) and reference (cannula) electrodes are close to each other increases the instrument's common mode rejection. This means that the similar activity recorded by both the active and reference electrodes is eliminated to a certain degree, resulting in less noise detection. Some signal continues to be recorded because the electrical activity detected by the cannula is "averaged out" over its larger recording surface, tending to decrease its amplitude considerably. As a result, compared to a monopolar needle, the same MUAP has a smaller amplitude and fewer phases. As noted above, the duration of MUAPs is the same for both monopolar and concentric needle electrodes. Because the active recording surface and cannula are different, it may be possible for this difference to be sufficient to adversely affect differential amplification, as both recording electrodes do not record the same signal from a near or distant source. Also, that portion of the cannula protruding from the skin can act as an antenna and record more of an external signal than the active recording surface buried in the muscle. This finding is not usually a problem but can occasionally occur.

MONOPOLAR COMPARED TO CONCENTRIC NEEDLES

There continues to be discussion about the advantages and disadvantages of monopolar compared to concentric needle recordings. It must be understood that one needle is not "better" than the other but simply different. The practitioner should become familiar with both types of needle recordings and the way MUAPs as well as spontaneous activity appears. In the final analysis, both needles are comparable and usage depends upon personal preference.

SINGLE FIBER ELECTRODE

The single fiber electrode can be considered a modified concentric needle electrode (43, 48). A metal cannula is still used but the central wire is 25 μm in diameter and it exits the cannula about 0.5 cm proximal and opposite to the beveled tip. The small recording surface permits a very selective recording from one or two single muscle fibers with a hemispherical recording territory having a radius approximating 300–500 μm (40). A separate ground electrode is required (see Chapter 2).

SUBDERMAL ELECTROENCEPHALOGRAPHIC ELECTRODE

The subdermal electroencephalographic needle is 10–20 mm long with a diameter of 0.8 mm; it is made of stainless steel or a platinum/iridium alloy (39). These needles are primarily used to record evoked potentials but can also be employed to record near-nerve sensory or mixed nerve action potentials. There is no difference in the surface compared to needle-recorded cortical somatosensory evoked potentials (18, 51).

AMPLIFIERS

As previously noted, the small size of biologic signals requires a device to increase their magnitude for visual analysis (27). An amplifier is a device with the ability to significantly increase the size of recorded signals. Those aspects of amplifiers relevant to electrodiagnostic medicine examinations requiring explanation include 1) amplification with respect to sensitivity and gain; 2) input impedance; and 3) differential amplification.

Amplification

The amplification of biologic signals can be expressed in two different but related ways known as gain or sensitivity. Gain is defined as the ratio of the amplifier's output signal to its input signal. For example, if a 1-μV signal input emerges from an amplifier as 1 mV, the gain is 1,000 (Gain = Output ÷ Input = 1.0 mV ÷ 0.001 mV = 1,000). Because gain is a ratio of output to input voltage, no units are expressed. Sensitivity, unlike gain, is a ratio of the input voltage to the size of a CRT deflection. The CRT's vertical deflection is measured in centimeters (cm), and 1 cm is typically referred to as 1 CRT division. As a result, an amplifier with a setting of 1 μV/cm (1 μV/division) implies that every 1 μV of a signal generates a CRT deflection of 1 cm. A signal of 5 μV will produce a waveform on the CRT with an amplitude of 5 cm or 5 divisions.

It is important to understand that the gain or sensitivity has important consequences with respect to measuring sensory, and in particular, motor action potential parameters. As the gain or sensitivity is increased, initial waveform deflections from the CRT's baseline are visually detected earlier in time. This is because smaller aspects of the waveform's initiation are magnified, and hence more readily seen. The net result is to shorten the poten-

tial's onset latency. For example, an amplifier with a sensitivity of 500 μV/cm compared to 10,000 μV/cm records the same waveforms with onset latencies of 3.4 msec and 3.8 msec, respectively (Fig. 4–6). Both latencies are equally valid. The normal reference values, however, are quite different for the same population when the two sensitivities are used. This implies that the practitioner must reproduce the parameters under which the reference values were developed if those reference values are to be used. It is equally valid to develop one's own reference values with a different amplifier sensitivity, provided that the sensitivity is used for all patients.

Input Impedance

Amplifiers and electrodes have an inherent impedance to current flow. The biologic signal can be considered the current source of interest, whereas the electrode and amplifier in combination form a simple series circuit that obeys Ohm's law. Ohm's law states that the detected voltage (V) of a source generating a current flow (I) is equal to the current times the resistance (R) or, in biologic systems, the impedance (Z): $E = IR$ or $E = IZ$ (14, 38, 44). The biologic signal must first be recorded by the electrode, which means a certain amount of the voltage is lost or dropped across the electrode because of its intrinsic impedance. In other words, the current flowing from the patient into the electrode has to lose a portion of its associated voltage prior to reaching the amplifier.

The electrode and amplifier constitute a voltage divider as they form a series circuit. This means that the voltage not lost at the electrode remains to be amplified and hence displayed to the practitioner. Obviously, we would prefer to have as little signal voltage lost at the electrode as possible so that most, if not all, of the voltage reaches the amplifier and then is accurately presented to the practitioner. The amplifier and electrode are the only two components sharing the biologic signal's voltage; therefore, as long as the amplifier's impedance is significantly larger than the electrode's, only a small portion is divided or lost at the electrode. This important concept can be expressed through simple mathematical

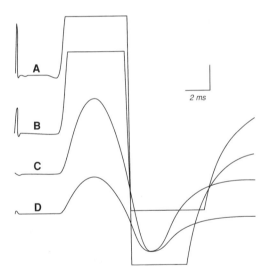

Trace	Sensitivity (mV/div)	Latency Onset (ms)	Amplitude (mV)
A	500	3.4	
B	1,000	3.5	
C	5,000	3.7	23
D	10,000	3.8	23

Figure 4–6. Effect of amplification on compound motor action potential onset latency. A sequential reduction in amplifier amplification results in a prolongation of the potential's onset latency. (Reprinted with permission from Dumitru D, Walsh NE: Practical instrumentation and common sources of error. Am J Phys Med Rehabil 1988;67:55–65.)

terms by arranging and applying Ohm's law several times.

As noted above, the biologic signal's voltage (E_{total}) loses a portion of its voltage across the electrode (E_{elec}), with the remaining voltage left to be amplified (E_{amp}) and subsequently observed. This means that the biologic signal can be represented as the sum of that voltage lost at each of the instrument's components:

$$E_{total} = E_{elec} + E_{amp}$$

Because the current is the same across each component in a series circuit, we can express each of the above component voltage drops according to Ohm's law:

$$E_{elec} = IZ_{elec}$$

$$E_{amp} = IZ_{amp}$$

These equivalent component terms can be substituted into the above voltage equation:

$$E_{total} = IZ_{elec} + IZ_{amp}, \text{ or}$$

$$E_{total} = I(Z_{elec} + Z_{amp})$$

Because we are interested in knowing what amount of voltage remains at the amplifier, we can substitute the rearranged Ohm's law equation for the amplifier subcomponent into the above equation ($I = E_{amp}/Z_{amp}$):

$$E_{total} = \frac{E_{amp} \cdot (Z_{elec} + Z_{amp})}{Z_{amp}}$$

The above equation can now be solved for that portion of the biologic signal's total voltage detected and hence amplified by the amplifier:

$$E_{amp} = \frac{E_{total} \cdot Z_{amp}}{Z_{elec} + Z_{amp}}$$

This final equation is merely a mathematical expression of the concept that the voltage presented to the amplifier depends upon the impedance of the amplifier and electrode. According to the above equation, if the amplifier's impedance is considerably greater than that of the electrode's, most of the biologic signal's voltage will remain for the amplifier. In other words, if the impedance of the electrode (Z_{elec}) is comparatively insignificant, it can be ignored and the equation simplifies to:

$$E_{amp} = \frac{E_{total} \cdot Z_{amp}}{Z_{amp}} \text{ or}$$

$$E_{amp} = E_{total}$$

It can now be appreciated that the amplifier's impedance, also known as input impedance, must be greater than the electrode's impedance. When this is the case, the voltage associated with the biologic signal of interest loses an insignificant portion to the electrode, permitting the amplifier to magnify most or all of the signal for its clinical analysis. If the electrode's impedance increases, less of the signal remains for the amplifier, and waveform distortion occurs. If an electrode's impedance is relatively high, it is possible for a small-amplitude potential to result, giving the false impression of axonal loss. Dirty electrodes can, therefore, result in false positive studies.

DIFFERENTIAL AMPLIFICATION

All commercially available electrophysiologic instruments use two amplifiers: one amplifier for the signal detected by the active electrode and the other for the reference electrode's signal (19, 32). These amplifiers are manufactured with the same specifications, however, it is impossible for them to be identical. The amplifier connected to the active electrode is also known as the "positive" amplifier; it simply magnifies the signal by the desired amount. The amplifier connected to the reference electrode ("negative" or inverting amplifier) not only magnifies the detected signal by the same amount as the positive amplifier, but also inverts the signal. These two signals are then electronically summated with the net result being displayed on the CRT.

If similar signals are detected by each electrode and the inverting amplifier reverses this signal's polarity, then like signals are elimi-

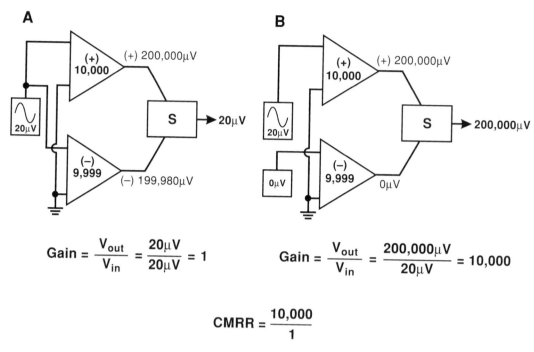

$$\text{Gain} = \frac{V_{out}}{V_{in}} = \frac{20\mu V}{20\mu V} = 1 \qquad\qquad \text{Gain} = \frac{V_{out}}{V_{in}} = \frac{200,000\mu V}{20\mu V} = 10,000$$

$$\text{CMRR} = \frac{10,000}{1}$$

Figure 4–7. The results of differential amplification are depicted. A. A signal is connected to both amplifiers in a common mode (same signal to each amplifier) manner. The gain is one. B. In the difference mode montage, the gain is 10,000. The common mode rejection ratio (CMRR) is 10,000 to 1. (Reprinted with permission from Dumitru D, Walsh NE: Electrophysiologic instrumentation. In: Dumitru D, ed. Clinical electrophysiology: Physical medicine and rehabilitation state of the art reviews. Philadelphia: Hanley & Belfus, 1989.)

nated (Fig. 4–7). The combination of similar amplifiers in which both amplify, but one inverts the signal, is known as differential amplification. It is named thus because it is really the difference between the signal recorded by each electrode that is amplified. The difference-mode signal (the signal present at one but not both electrodes) is what in actuality is amplified, whereas the common-mode signal (similar signals recorded at both electrodes) is cancelled.

As noted above, it is impossible to build identical amplifiers. In addition, no two electrodes are identical. These small amplifier and electrode impedance differences result in a good but less than perfect handling of similar signals. The ability of an instrument to amplify a signal present at one electrode (difference-mode signal), compared to its ability to eliminate the same signal when present at both electrodes (common-mode signal), is known as its common mode rejection ratio (Fig. 4–7). This value should be greater than 10,000:1 and is a rough guide to the amplifier's quality.

FILTERS

Filters can be thought of as devices that have the ability to extract portions of any signal detected by the two recording electrodes. These recording electrodes are nonselective; they present to the amplifier not only the desired biologic signal, but any environmental and undesired biologic signals as well. The signal of interest, therefore, is contaminated with undesirable signals. For the purpose of this discussion, noise is defined as unwanted signals arising within the instrument, whereas interference is considered to consist of unwanted signals arising outside the instrument. The main purpose of filters is to reduce the noise or interference contained in the signal and to distort the desired signal minimally. All signals can be thought of as consisting of relative amounts of arbitrarily defined high and low frequencies. As a result, filters can be divided into high and low frequency filters. The manner in which filters function may be understood by first considering the concept of subcomponent frequencies.

Subcomponent Frequencies

All signals, including biologic waveforms, can be thought of as composed of multiple time-varying sinusoidal waveforms with different amplitudes, phases, and frequencies summated together. The observed waveform, therefore, is really a net result of the summations and cancellations of multiple waveforms producing a composite or summated potential. This concept can be demonstrated by considering a series of five waveforms with different frequencies and amplitudes (Fig. 4–8). Summating all five waveforms produces a composite waveform that resembles a square wave. This net square wave potential bears absolutely no resemblance to any of the five subcomponent waveforms, yet is the result of all of them added together. Similarly, altering each subcomponent waveform slightly can re-

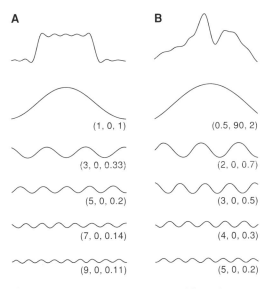

Figure 4–8. *A.* A square wave and five subcomponent sine waves, which when added together result in the square wave. *B.* A more "biologic"-appearing potential and its subcomponent sine waves. The frequency, phase shift, and relative amplitude are described below each subcomponent waveform. (Reprinted with permission from Dumitru D: Electrodiagnostic medicine. Philadelphia: Hanley & Belfus, 1995.)

sult in a potential that begins to resemble a biologically recorded potential.

A filter has the ability to extract these individual subcomponent waveforms from the signal detected at the two recording electrodes. Filters are powerful and important devices because they can profoundly affect a waveform's appearance by altering the subcomponent frequency content of the detected signal. Understanding the effects that filters can have on biologic waveforms is important to avoid false positive or negative results and hence erroneous diagnoses.

Low Frequency Filters

All commercially available instruments have adjustable low frequency filters. An equivalent term for a low frequency filter is a high pass filter, as the filter restricts low frequencies but permits high frequencies to pass through unaltered. For the purposes of this discussion, low frequencies are arbitrarily defined as those frequencies between 0 Hz and 500 Hz.

The best manner to appreciate the effects a low frequency filter can have on biologic signals is to evoke a SNAP or CMAP waveform multiple times and alter the low frequency filter while keeping the high frequency filter constant. As the low frequency filter is elevated from 1 Hz to 300 Hz for both the SNAP and CMAP, the following changes occur: 1) a shortening of the peak latency; 2) a reduction in the negative spike duration; 3) a decrease in amplitude; 4) the creation of an additional phase; and 5) no alteration in onset latency (Figs. 4–9 and 4–10) (8, 20, 36). Elevating the low frequency filter can also alter MUAP parameters. Specifically, increasing the low frequency filter from 2 Hz to 500 Hz results in a shortening of the MUAP's duration and a decrease in its amplitude (Fig. 4–11).

The above-described waveform changes can be understood by again considering the concept of subcomponent frequencies. When the low frequency filter is sequentially elevated, an increasing amount of low frequencies are extracted from the signal. It stands to reason that if data is removed from the waveform, the amplitude should decrease.

	High Frequency Filter (Hz)	Low Frequency Filter (Hz)	Onset Latency (ms)	Peak Latency (ms)	Amplitude (µV)	Negative Spike Duration (ms)
A	10,000	1	2.9	3.4	28.0	1.3
B	10,000	10	2.9	3.4	28.5	1.2
C	10,000	100	2.9	3.3	21.5	1.0
D	10,000	300	2.9	3.3	11.5	0.8

20µV
2ms

Figure 4–9. Recording an antidromic median nerve SNAP with different low frequency filters reveals a number of interesting waveform alterations (*A* through *D*). As the low frequency filter is elevated from 1 Hz to 300 Hz, the SNAP's onset latency is unaffected; however, the amplitude, peak latency, and negative spike duration decrease. The potential recorded at a low frequency filter of 300 Hz appears triphasic. (Reprinted with permission from Dumitru D: Electrodiagnostic medicine. Philadelphia: Hanley & Belfus, 1995.)

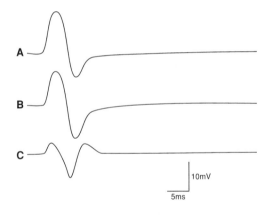

10mV
5ms

Trace	Low Frequency Filter (Hz)	Latency		Amplitude (mV)
		Onset (ms)	Peak (ms)	
A	1	3.5	6.7	1
B	10	3.5	6.3	10
C	100	3.5	5.0	100

Figure 4–10. A CMAP recorded with different low frequency filter settings results in waveform distortion similar to that documented for a SNAP. (Reprinted with permission from Dumitru D: Electrodiagnostic medicine. Philadelphia: Hanley & Belfus, 1995.)

Also, the waveform has a comparatively increased content of high frequencies because the low frequencies have been removed. Higher frequencies occur more rapidly in time than lower frequencies, thereby shifting the entire potential to occur sooner in time, i.e. to have a shorter latency. The comparatively higher frequency content similarly shortens the negative spike duration. A reduction in the waveform's low frequency content implies that the remaining higher frequencies become more manifest, demonstrating more phases per unit time than a signal dominated by low frequencies; hence, the addition of a third phase to the SNAP and CMAP. Finally, the onset latency is not affected because it rapidly rises from the baseline and is dominated by high as opposed to low frequencies.

High Frequency Filters

A high frequency or low pass filter is defined to affect frequencies between 500 Hz and 20,000 Hz. As for low-frequency filter waveform alterations, high frequency filters can also distort the potential of interest. Removing high frequency subcomponents from a waveform with a significant high frequency content tends to 1) delay the onset latency; 2) prolong the peak latency; 3) decrease the amplitude; and 4) increase the negative spike duration (Fig. 4–12). Similarly, lowering the high frequency filter can also affect MUAP parameters (Fig. 4–13).

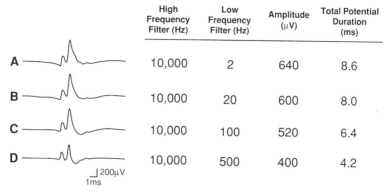

	High Frequency Filter (Hz)	Low Frequency Filter (Hz)	Amplitude (μV)	Total Potential Duration (ms)
A	10,000	2	640	8.6
B	10,000	20	600	8.0
C	10,000	100	520	6.4
D	10,000	500	400	4.2

Figure 4–11. Elevating the low frequency filter from 2 Hz to 500 Hz can have profound effects on a MUAP's duration and amplitude. Reprinted with permission from Dumitru D: Electrodiagnostic medicine. Philadelphia: Hanley & Belfus, 1995.)

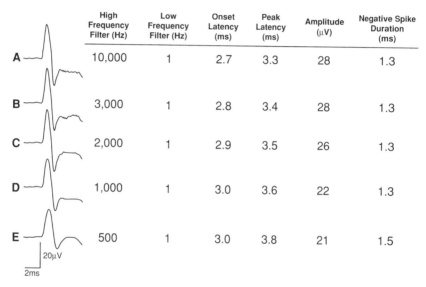

	High Frequency Filter (Hz)	Low Frequency Filter (Hz)	Onset Latency (ms)	Peak Latency (ms)	Amplitude (μV)	Negative Spike Duration (ms)
A	10,000	1	2.7	3.3	28	1.3
B	3,000	1	2.8	3.4	28	1.3
C	2,000	1	2.9	3.5	26	1.3
D	1,000	1	3.0	3.6	22	1.3
E	500	1	3.0	3.8	21	1.5

Figure 4–12. A median nerve antidromic SNAP can be recorded with a constant low frequency filter of 1 Hz and a variable high frequency filter from 10,000 Hz to 500 Hz (A through E). As the high frequency filter is serially reduced, the SNAP's amplitude declines and the onset and peak latencies increase. The negative spike duration increases only slightly. (Reprinted with permission from Dumitru D: Electrodiagnostic medicine. Philadelphia: Hanley & Belfus, 1995.)

Extracting an increasing amount of subcomponent high frequencies from a potential results in less data contained in the waveform, tending to reduce its amplitude. This ensuing waveform is predominated by low frequencies that take longer to occur in time than high frequencies, thereby prolonging the entire potential, including the onset and peak latencies. These same factors result in a comparatively longer negative spike duration.

Suggested Filter Parameters

A universal consensus on optimal filter settings for any type of electrodiagnostic medicine study does not exist. The main goal for high and low filter cut-offs is to include all of the desired signals' subcomponent frequencies and eliminate all of the undesired signals. Of course, it is impossible to reach this goal and all investigators compromise to different degrees (Table 4–1). Prior to using any reference

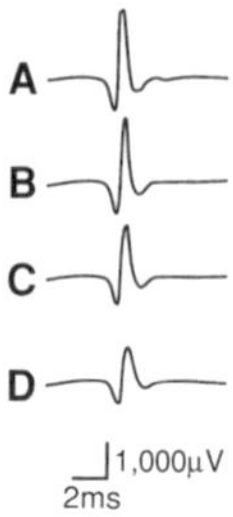

	High Frequency Filter (Hz)	Low Frequency Filter (Hz)	Amplitude (μV)	Total Potential Duration (ms)
A	10,000	20	2,900	3.2
B	2,000	20	2,600	3.2
C	1,000	20	2,100	3.6
D	500	20	1,500	3.8

1,000μV
2ms

Figure 4-13. A reduction in the high frequency filter from 10,000 Hz to 500 Hz reduced a MUAP's amplitude and increased its duration. (Reprinted with permission from Dumitru D: Electrodiagnostic medicine. Philadelphia: Hanley & Belfus, 1995.)

Table 4-1
Suggested Filter Parameters

Examination	Low Frequency (Hz)	High Frequency (Hz)
NCV (motor)	2–10	10,000
NCV (sensory)	2–10	200–10,000
EMG (qualitative)	20–30	10,000
EMG (quantitative)	2–5	10,000
SFEMG	500–1,000	10,000–20,000
SEP	1–10	500–3,000

NCV: nerve conduction velocity; EMG: needle electromyography; SFEMG: single fiber electromyography; SEP: somatosensory evoked potential. Note: Use as little filtering as possible so as not to distort the desired potentials recorded.

data, all of the parameters under which the reference data was collected (amplifier sensitivity, high/low frequency filter settings, etc.) must be exactly reproduced. If at all possible, a wide-open bandpass should be used.

SOUND

The energy contained within a biologic signal can be appreciated aurally as well as visually. The acoustic interpretation of normal and abnormal biologic signals is an intricate part of the needle electromyographic examination. Frequently, normal and abnormal needle electromyographic potentials can be appreciated aurally before they are observed. Because of the importance for this aspect of the electrodiagnostic medicine examination, the instrument must have the ability to reproduce and present acoustically the complete frequency content of the investigated waveform.

ANALOG-TO-DIGITAL CONVERSION

The amplified real time or analog signal is converted into a digital signal by a process known as analog-to-digital (A/D) conversion. This process can be conceptualized by considering the CRT to be divided into multiple vertical and horizontal points of resolution, forming a fine grid similar to a sheet of graph paper. Each aspect of the amplified waveform is assigned a digital or binary code for amplitude and time latency with respect to the grid and essentially "graphed" onto the CRT for visual analysis. In effect, the analog signal is sampled both vertically and horizontally. The less time between the horizontal points, the finer the resolution of the horizontal grid. Similarly, the less amplitude between each of the vertical points, the finer the vertical resolution. The vertical and horizontal resolution is important because a portion of the waveform can occur between resolution points and never be displayed. This means that a portion of the desired potential is lost, which can affect the waveform's amplitude and morphology. The above qualitative description of A/D conversion is frequently defined by a number of technical terms. An epoch or sweep is the total analysis time of the CRT; it is assigned by the practitioner. One sweep of the CRT extends from the left to the right margins of the screen and is divided into equal time increments known as bins or sample points. The amount of time required by the instrument's computer to sample the waveform and assign each sample point is called the dwell time, and its reciprocal is the sampling frequency. Sampling the amplified waveform and assigning both a horizontal and a vertical digital resolution point eventually produces a digital representation of the analog waveform. Inappropriately assigned horizontal (sweep speeds) or vertical (amplifier sensitivities) can result in a digital distortion of the analog waveform because it was poorly sampled. This can be illustrated by considering some simple examples of poor amplitude and time assignments.

Vertical Resolution

The height of the CRT screen can be thought of as consisting of a finite number of vertical resolution points. There are at least 256 points of vertical resolution for commercially available electrophysiologic instruments (12). The practitioner assigns these fixed points to represent millivolts or microvolts by adjusting the amplifier's sensitivity. Therefore, the instrument's ability to resolve a potential's amplitude is directly dependent upon the practitioner's knowledge of what to anticipate for waveform size (i.e., how large or small the waveform is). Assigning all of the vertical resolution points to represent 10 μV, for example, (the total vertical screen equals 10 μV) when evaluating a signal with a total amplitude of 15 μV, results in the potential's peaks occuring off the CRT. In this case, the instrument's sensitivity is too high for the given potential. Similarly, not assigning enough vertical resolution points can distort the wave-

form. If a potential has a maximal peak-to-peak amplitude of 20 μV but the amplifier's sensitivity is set to represent a total vertical resolution of 400 μV, the waveform will represent only a small portion of the CRT, resulting in a poorly resolved potential. The relationship of the desired waveform to the vertical resolution and hence the amplifier's sensitivity should approximate the situation where the signal fills about one-third to two-thirds of the CRT's vertical capacity (Fig. 4–14).

Horizontal Resolution

When considering the instrument's optimal horizontal or time analysis of a waveform, two requirements must be considered: 1) sufficient time must be assigned to the CRT to encompass the entire waveform; and 2) the most rapidly changing portion of the waveform must be provided sufficient dwell time (amount of time the instrument devotes to that aspect of the waveform) to resolve these high-frequency subcomponent waveforms. A CRT screen's horizontal portion can be considered a time scale measuring milliseconds and divided into 10 equal divisions. The total number of horizontal resolution points is set into the instrument by the manufacturer and is either 512 or 1024 data points, with more expensive instruments having the higher number of points. It is the practitioner, however, who decides how much of a time interval each of these points represents by adjusting the sweep speed. In general, the more time assigned to the total screen with slower sweep speeds, the less ability there is to resolve rapidly changing aspects of the waveform (Fig. 4–15). This occurs because each individual resolution point must be expected to represent a greater portion of the waveform. A reduction in the total amount of time represented by the entire CRT with faster sweep speeds means there is more time allotted by the instrument to examine each portion of the waveform, permitting many points to be assigned and increasing the capability of tracking rapid changes. In short, briefer time intervals can be more accurately analyzed because there are more points per millisecond capable of repro-

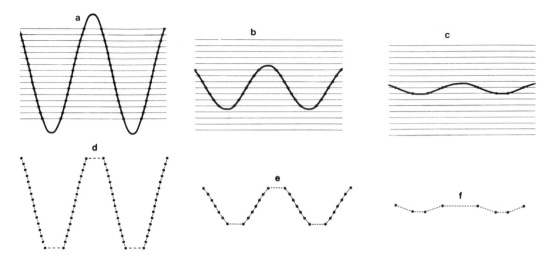

Figure 4–14. The effect of analog-to-digital conversion on signals of different amplitude. Sine waves of three amplitudes (*a,b,c*) are digitized using vertical intervals of equal size. At each step, the amplitude, marked by a dot, is measured. These measures are shown at the bottom (*d,e,f*) where the dots are connected by straight dashed lines. The signal in trace *a* exceeds the vertical range of the digitizer and is distorted in the digital representation in trace *d*. The signal in trace *b* fills about one-half of the digitizer range and is fairly well resolved in trace *e*. The signal in trace *c* fills only a small portion of the total vertical range and is poorly resolved in trace *f*. (Reprinted with permission from Spehlmann R: Evoked potential primer. Stoneham, MA: Butterworth, 1985.)

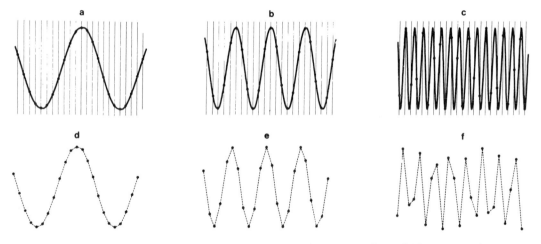

Figure 4–15. The relationship between sampling rate and signal frequency; effects of different signal frequencies at the same sampling rate. Sine waves at three different frequencies (traces *a,b,c*) are sampled at the same rate. At each sampling interval, their amplitude is marked by a dot. These dots, connected by straight dashed lines are shown as a digital display at the bottom (traces *d,e,f*). The sine wave in trace *a* is sampled about 14 times per cycle and is well depicted in the digital representation in trace *d*. The sine wave in trace *b*, being sampled at a rate only 6 times higher than its own frequency, is depicted with less but still fair detail after digitization as shown in trace *e*. In contrast, the sine wave in trace *c*, being slightly above the critical value of one-half the sampling rate, is not resolved adequately in the digital representation in trace *f*. It shows fewer peaks than the analog waveform and is an example of aliasing. (Reprinted with permission from Spehlmann R: Evoked potential primer. Stoneham, MA: Butterworth, 1985.)

ducing those quickly changing aspects of the waveform.

The sweep speed, like sensitivity, should be set with the goal of placing the waveform near the middle of the screen with maximum detail necessary. If a portion of the waveform changes rapidly, it is necessary for the instrument to accurately reproduce this portion of the waveform. Rapidly changing aspects of the waveform can only be reproduced if there are sufficient points of resolution to register every change in the signal. The waveform must be sampled very rapidly to accomplish an accurate reproduction. The rate at which a signal is sampled is referred to as the sampling frequency. A minimum sampling frequency of twice that of the signal's fastest changing components must be provided to characterize the signal accurately. In other words, it takes at the very least two resolution points to determine a change in the waveform. As noted above, each instrument is manufactured with a set number of horizontal resolution points. The time over which these resolution points are spread out over the CRT, however, is determined by the practitioner. As a result, the instrument's ability to track rapidly changing portions of a waveform is directly dependent upon the sweep speed.

Sampling frequency can best be understood with an example. Suppose a motor unit action potential has a rise time of 1 msec. This portion of the waveform occurs once in 1 msec and has an occurrence frequency of 1000 Hz (1/1 msec $\times$ 1000 msec/1 second = 1000 times/1 second, i.e., 1000 Hz). The instrument must sample this portion of the waveform with a sampling frequency of at least 2000 Hz. At least four to five times this sampling frequency is commonly used to ensure waveform reproduction. If the instrument has 1000 points of resolution, a sweep speed must be assigned that generates a minimum sampling frequency of 2000 Hz. In this example, a sweep speed of 50 msec/cm suffices to barely resolve the rise time (1 msec/2 points $\times$ 1,000 points/10 cm = 50 msec/cm). Clinically, a sweep speed of 10 msec/cm is typically used, which is five times the necessary sampling frequency (1000 points/100 msec $\times$ 1000 msec/ 1 second = 10,000 Hz).

Averaging

Some biologic signals such as somatosensory, brainstem auditory, and visual evoked potentials, as well as pathologic SNAPs, may be rather small and lost in the environmental and instrument baseline noise (3). In order to properly evaluate these potentials, the signal's amplitude compared to the enveloping noise's amplitude must be improved. This can be accomplished by using an averager.

Most, if not all, commercially available instruments use essentially the same principles with respect to averaging. The desired signal is surrounded by a time window specified by the practitioner. For example, responses occurring at the same time following a stimulus can be extracted from the surrounding noise by taking advantage of the fact that the desired waveform occurs at essentially the same time after each stimulation, whereas the noise impeding signal detection occurs randomly. The instrument places the signal and whatever time surrounding it into digital memory storage. The second response with an identical time frame is gathered and added point-for-point with the first response. Because the noise occurs randomly, peaks and troughs of noise cancel somewhat while the desired response summates to a small degree. The summated result is divided by two because two traces were added, and the final waveform is displayed (Fig. 4–16). If three traces or more were evoked, then the number of collected traces are all summated and divided by the number of gathered responses to generate an averaged response. The number of averages required to optimize a waveform is variable and dependent upon the size of the noise compared to the signal of interest.

The process of increasing the desired waveform's amplitude compared to the surrounding noise is referred to as improving the signal-to-noise ratio (S/N ratio). Improving the S/N ratio occurs through a square root of the number of averages performed. The S/N ratio can be expressed mathematically as the signal of interest (S) multiplied by the square root of the number of averages (n), with this quantity divided by the amplitude of the surrounding noise (A):

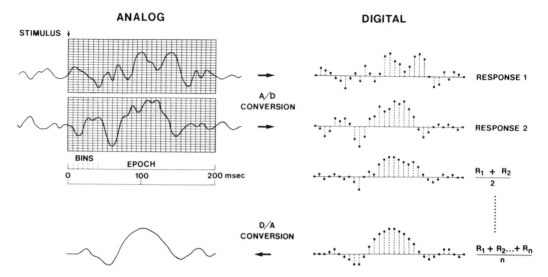

Figure 4-16. Two "noisy" analog signals are digitized through analog-to-digital conversion. The two digital responses are then summated. Random signals phase cancel while similar signals summate. The summated response is then divided by 2 and the process is repeated. For each average calculated, the composite signal is divided by the total number of waveforms so that each waveform has equal weight in the final averaged waveform. The final digital waveform is then converted back into an analog signal. This sequence of events depicts the manner in which potentials are averaged to improve the signal-to-noise ratio. (Reprinted with permission from Spehlmann R: Evoked potential primer. Stoneham, MA: Butterworth, 1985.)

$$S/N = \frac{S \times \sqrt{n}}{A}$$

This equation can be related to clinical practice by assuming that a desired signal has an amplitude of 2 μV and the noise amplitude is 4 μV. If a single stimulus is delivered, the S/N ratio is 0.5 (S/N = $\{2 \times \sqrt{1}\} \div 4 = 0.5$). Performing four averages generates an S/N of 1.0. If 16 averages are obtained, an S/N of 2 results. In each case, the S/N improved by a factor of the square root of the number of averages compared to the previous result. Specifically, four averages generated an S/N ratio of 1, which is twice the S/N ratio (0.5) of a single average, whereas 16 averages increased the S/N to 4, which is four times the S/N ratio of four averages. This process can be generalized by stating that regardless of the number of averages used to generate a particular S/N ratio, that ratio will be increased by the desired factor (Y) when the previous number of averages are multiplied by this factor squared (Y^2). [$\{X^2\}\{n\}$ = number of averages to increase S/N by a factor of X.] For example, if 10 averages generated a waveform with an S/N ratio of Z, then 40 total averages, (4 times

as many), are required to generate a waveform with an S/N ratio of 2Z. This is formulated by S/N = Z = $\{S\sqrt{10}\} \div A$, or Z = 3.16S/A; Then, to double the S/N, we would take $2^2 \times 10$, which equals 40 averages. Verification is provided by S/N = $\{S\sqrt{40}\} \div A$ = 6.32S/A or 2Z. Similarly, 90 total averages or 80 more than the original 10 are necessary to triple the original S/N ratio.

CATHODE RAY TUBE (CRT) DISPLAY

The CRT is an electronic device that generates electrons and directs them to a phosphorescent screen. This screen glows momentarily when the electrons contained in the phosphor material are excited by the electron beam. Magnetic deflection plates permit the electron beam to be directed at any portion of the screen. The electrophysiologic instrument directs the electron beam to begin at the top of the CRT and sweep across along a straight line until one edge of the CRT is reached. The electron beam then quickly returns to the original portion of the CRT but displaced slightly inferiorly. This process repeats until the entire screen has been covered. In effect, the process repeats so rapidly that by the time the phosphorescence begins to decline, the trace has reached each spot again, replenishing the screen. Combining the instrument to place a waveform in its digital memory and continually reproducing the waveform on the screen results in the waveform being "frozen" on the CRT screen. This occurs when a single stimulus is delivered but the ensuing SNAP or CMAP remains on the CRT until the next stimulus is delivered.

Trigger and Delay Line

An interesting device known as a trigger and delay is now incorporated into most instruments. This feature is primarily used during the needle electromyographic examination. The CRT sweep is triggered by some portion of a waveform reaching an amplitude level defined by the practitioner. Once this level has been achieved, there is a predetermined, finite amount of time before and after the triggering potential is displayed from the instrument's digital memory, such that the waveform is relatively delayed or appears in the same place on the CRT every time it is displayed. A trigger and delay line permits a "leisurely" evaluation of potentials that may be firing too rapidly to appreciate on a freely running CRT trace. Some instruments permit the practitioner to engage the averager so that motor unit action potentials can be averaged to better define baseline departure and return as well as other diagnostic parameters like amplitude, phases/turns, and duration.

STIMULATORS

A stimulator is composed of a cathode and an anode, which produces neural depolarization. The cathode is the stimulator's negative pole and attracts positive ions (cations), whereas the anode is the positive pole and attracts negative ions (anions). Current flow is defined to originate at the anode and terminate at the cathode equating to the direction of positive ion flow. Neural stimulation occurs when the cathode is located over the nerve of interest and enough current is generated to reach the nerve's threshold value. Once an action potential is induced, it travels both proximal and distal to the site of excitation. In electrodiagnostic evaluations, supramaximal currents are employed and defined as a current or voltage intensity 10% to 20% above an intensity that is sufficient to generate a maximal motor or sensory response.

Anodal Block

The anode is also of interest. Previous clinical neurophysiologic teaching assumed that the nerve is hyperpolarized beneath the anode, thereby precluding either action potential generation at this site or neural propagation past the anode, creating anodal block. The concept of anodal block appears to be valid with animal preparations using special current generators; however, anodal block has not been demonstrated to occur during the routine electrodiagnostic medicine evaluation within tolerable current limits (16). In fact, given sufficient current, the anode can actually cause the nerve to depolarize and generate a propagating action potential. The potential delay that occurs when the cathode and anode stimulation sites are reversed is entirely accounted for by the increased distance between the active electrode and cathode; it is not a result of anodal block.

Stimulator Types

Two basic types of stimulators can be used for neural conduction assessment: 1) constant current; and 2) constant voltage. A constant current stimulator delivers the desired amount of current with each stimulation even though the skin resistance may change (21). The same amount of current is delivered each time because the voltage with each stimulation changes in exactly the amount necessary to deliver the same current with a given alteration in resistance. This concept can be understood by considering Ohm's law: $E = IZ$. If the impedance (Z) of the skin changes, for example, then the driving voltage (E) must change accordingly to keep the current (I) constant. Suppose the skin impedance doubled. In order for the stimulator to deliver the same amount of current as it did prior to the impedance change, the voltage emanating from the stimulator must also double. Conversely, a constant voltage stimulator delivers the same amount of voltage with each stimulation even if the impedance changes. In this case, the current must vary inversely with the impedance. If the impedance increases, then the current must decrease to maintain the same voltage.

Stimulator type also varies by surface versus needle. Although the most commonly used stimulator in clinical practice is a surface cathode and anode, it is also valid to use a needle cathode and anode (4, 35, 47, 50). The best type of needle cathode to use is a monopolar needle with a pulse duration of 0.05 msec unless H-reflex studies are performed, in which case a duration of 1000 msec should be used. No neural injury should occur with a near-nerve cathode location, as the current density is insufficient to create temperatures detrimental to neural tissues (Fig. 4–17) (35). A needle cathode can be used with either a needle or a surface anode. The main purpose of using a needle cathode is to position the cathode beneath the skin's high impedance and in close proximity to the nerve, thereby requiring less current to depolarize the nerve. This results in less voltage used, reduced discomfort resulting from neural activation, and less stimulus artifact. Also, a more exact location of neural depolarization can be assured by reducing the amount of current spread across

the top of the skin (which might activate the nerve at a location other than intended, as can occur with surface stimulators). The disadvantages of using a needle cathode include needle phobia and neural insult.

Stimulus Artifact

One of the more annoying technical problems during the electrodiagnostic medicine examination is the generation of stimulus artifacts that interfere with the desired response. In some cases, the stimulus artifact can be of sufficient magnitude to obliterate the waveform under investigation, precluding analysis. In order to minimize stimulus artifact, the following should be performed: 1) Remove any perspiration between the cathode and active electrode; 2) Use only a small amount of electrolyte paste; 3) Position the ground electrode next to the active (E-1 or G-1) electrode; 4) Deliver enough stimulus to just achieve a supramaximal response; 5) Reduce skin impedance at all recording and stimulating sites (31, 45); and 6) Rotate the anode around the cathode in small increments until the stimulus artifact no longer interferes with the waveform (29).

Some investigators recommend elevating the low frequency filter as the stimulus artifact

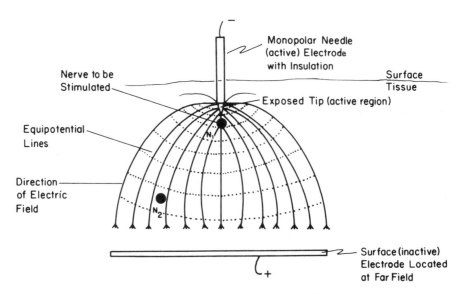

Figure 4–17. Electric field (–) and equipotential surfaces (...) generated during electric stimulation when using a needle electrode. N_1 and N_2 are nerves located within the field. (Reprinted with permission from Pease WS, Fatehi MT, Johnson EW: Monopolar needle stimulation: Safety considerations. Arch Phys Med Rehabil 1989;70:412–414.)

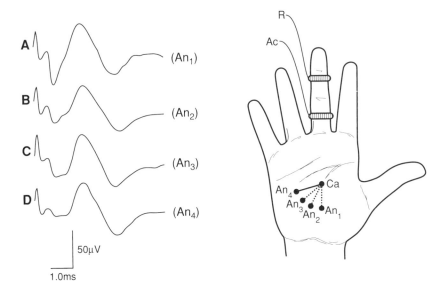

Figure 4–18. An antidromic median SNAP is recorded with the cathode (Ca) located 7 cm from the active recording electrode (Ac) and with the reference electrode (R) located 4 cm distal to the active electrode. The anode (An₁) is 2.5 cm proximal to the cathode. Trace A reveals the SNAP with an ill-defined onset latency as it is clearly affected by the stimulus artifact. Rotating the anode around the cathode in 0.5-cm increments (An₂ through An₄) eventually results in suppression of that portion of the stimulus artifact interfering with the SNAP's onset, permitting measurement of this parameter (Traces B through D). (Reprinted with permission from Dumitru D: Electrodiagnostic medicine. Philadelphia: Hanley & Belfus, 1995.)

contains a significant amount of low frequencies. Although this approach may diminish the artifact, it concomitantly affects the waveform. Rotating the anode around the cathode is a good way to reduce stimulus artifact after all of the above recommendations have been implemented (Fig. 4–18). Finally, to avoid the above complications, the use of a needle cathode can be successful in minimizing stimulus artifact when a large surface anode is positioned opposite the needle cathode.

SAFETY CONSIDERATIONS

It is the practitioner's responsibility to ensure the electrophysiologic instrument is properly maintained to manufacturer standards (32). This requires periodic electrical safety checks in which leakage current is evaluated. All electrodes and power cords must also be scrupulously maintained. One if the major concerns regarding electrical safety is the prevention of dangerous leakage current flows from the instrument into the patient. It is a good idea to prevent the patient from coming into contact with metal objects or other electrical devices during the examination. A functioning ground plug must be used to assist in preventing stray current flows from reaching the patient. The maximal amount of leakage current acceptable is 100 μA or less from the instrument's chassis to ground and 50 μA or less from the input leads to ground. Current frequencies of concern range from 0 to 1000 Hz because the heart is susceptible to depolarization at these frequencies. Less than 10 μA of leakage is tolerable when examining electrically sensitive patients: those persons with arterial lines or intravenous catheters. Patients with pacemakers can tolerate peripheral nerve stimulation but all stimulation should be performed away from the thorax. The skin must be thoroughly dried in all possible electrically sensitive patients and must not contact other metal objects such as side rails.

Whenever operating the instrument, it is good practice to periodically have the electrical outlet checked. An isolated earth spike and dedicated circuit help to diminish electrical noise. The instrument should be turned on prior to attaching any electrode to the patient and turned off only after the patient has been disconnected from the electrode leads to avoid power surges into the patients. Extension cords should not be used as they encourage leakage currents. An electrical device attached to the patient (e.g., a ventilator) should share the same ground circuit as the electrophysiologic instrument. Only one ground electrode should be attached to the patient. Following the above simple suggestions and ensuring routine electrical maintenance will result in the delivery of electrically safe electrodiagnostic medicine evaluations.

Additional safety considerations relate to the situation in which the patient's skin integrity must be breached either with a needle electrode or during the application of surface electrodes following aggressive skin abrasion. As previously noted, a needle electrode can be used to record voluntary MUAPs or apply an electrical stimulus. It is this author's recommendation that disposable needle electrodes should be used whenever possible. Universal precautions regarding infectious disease transmission should be followed. Disposable gloves should be worn at all times whenever there is a possibility of being exposed to the patient's blood or serum constituents. It is inappropriate to reuse gloves under any circumstances. Hands should be washed prior to starting and after completing the electrodiagnostic medicine evaluation. Any electrodes to be reused after exposure to the patient's body fluids (needle or surface: EMG or somatosensory evoked potential electrodes) should be soaked in a solution of sodium hypochlorite (household bleach) in dilutions of 1:100 to 1:10 for 15–20 minutes, thoroughly rinsed in tap water, and then either gas-sterilized or autoclaved for 1.0 to 1.5 hours at 120°C at 20 pounds per square inch.

Persons who have a medically (heparin or sodium warfarin) induced or pathologic coagulopathy should be examined only with needle electrodes or have aggressive skin abrasion if there is an absolute necessity for electrophysiologic data. A propensity for significant bleeding following needle induction occurs when a patient's platelet count falls below approximately 50,000/mm^3 or has a prothrombin time 1.5 to 2 times control values. Once the decision to explore muscle tissue has been made, a minimal number of muscles should

be examined and needle insertions per muscle employed to arrive at the diagnosis. Persons with clinically significant lymphedema should be examined with caution because of the potential for infection. In these patients, the skin should be thoroughly cleaned with an antimicrobial agent capable of killing surface bacteria prior to needle insertion.

Whenever a needle electrode is used around the supraclavicular region, thorax, or abdominal area, care must be exercised with respect to underlying structures. A detailed knowledge of anatomy is required to insert a needle electrode into any body region, particularly those overlying hollow viscera. Examining patients with a needle electrode in the thorax can result in a pneumothorax if the needle electrode is inserted too deeply without concern for lung tissue. Also, examining the abdominal muscles can result in puncture of the peritoneal cavity.

INTERFERENCE

A common form of interference arises from the poorly relaxed muscles in the form of surface-recorded MUAPs. Turning up the volume control on the speaker during a nerve conduction study can confirm inadequate patient relaxation, and appropriate measures can be taken to relax the patient. Also, a loose surface electrode can shift during the examination and generate an electrical potential capable of interfering with the waveform of interest. Performing a needle electromyographic examination around the chest region can result in a relatively large, regularly recurring potential. This is the electrocardiogram (EKG) and should be ignored. If a patient has a pacemaker a second type of regularly recurring potential in the form of a sharply delineated spike potential can be observed.

Perhaps the most commonly observed types of electrical interference arise from environmental sources in the form of 60 Hz interference. A 60-Hz signal can be recognized by noting that the time of recurrence is regular at intervals of 16.7 msec (60 cycles/1000 ms = 1 cycle/16.7 ms). If a regularly occurring (every 16.7 msec) potential abruptly occurs during the course of the examination, a dislodged electrode or broken electrode lead

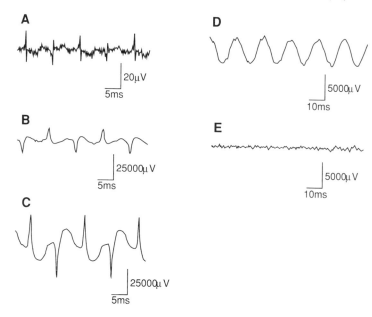

Figure 4–19. Examples of common forms of interference observed on a CRT screen. A. Fluorescent light during an electromyographic examination. B. Pure fluorescent light interference revealing details of its usual alternating spike appearance. C. Combination of fluorescent light and 60-Hz interference. D. Almost pure 60-cycle interference. E. Same trace as that in D except a 60- Hz notch filter has been introduced into the recording system. (Reprinted with permission from Dumitru D: Electrodiagnostic medicine. Philadelphia: Hanley & Belfus, 1995.)

should be suspected. If this type of interference is noted at the beginning of the examination, similar problems should be suspected. Also, if two different types of recording electrodes are used if or one of the electrodes is covered with foreign material, common mode rejection is compromised resulting in the appearance of 60-Hz interference. The electrodes should be of the same material and meticulously cleaned after each use to avoid interference. Fluorescent lighting can also be a strong source of a characteristic type of 60-Hz interference (Fig. 4–19). This type of interference can usually be eliminated by turning off the fluorescent lights and using daylight from windows if available or a small incandescent light bulb in a table lamp. It is possible to purchase fluorescent lights with low noise condensers, which may eliminate some of the noise problem.

Interference can be suppressed by using a dedicated circuit and earth spike for the ground. A dedicated circuit is a wall plug originating from the powerlines with no other associated wall plugs. In this way, the instrument does not share the power line with any other instruments or electrical appliances. This same wall plug uses a wire that connects to a metal spike driven into the ground, creating an isolated or dedicated ground. The combination of these two electrical factors can help reduce most environmental interference. Some investigators recommend the use of a Faraday box, in which the room is encased in a copper wire mesh. This type of arrangement can be expensive and defeated if a dedicated circuit is not used. It is possible to use a 60-Hz notch filter to suppress 60-Hz interference. This practice can result in waveform distortion secondary to filter effects and should not be routinely employed.

References

1. Adrian ED, Bronk DV: Discharge of impulses in motor nerve fibers. J Physiol 1929;67:119–151.
2. Braddom RL, Schuchmann J: Motor conduction. In: Johnson EW, ed. Practical electromyography. Baltimore: Williams & Wilkins, 1980.
3. Braddom RL: Somatosensory, brainstem, and visual evoked potentials. In: Johnson EW, ed. Practical electromyography. Baltimore: Williams & Wilkins, 1988.
4. Brown WF: The physiological and technical basis of electromyography. Boston: Butterworth, 1984.
5. Buchthal F, Guld C, Rosenfalck P: Action potential parameters in normal human muscle and their de-

pendence on physical variables. Acta Physiol Scand 1954;32:200–218.

6. Buchthal F, Rosenfalck P: Action potential parameters in different human muscles. Acta Psychiatr Neurol Scand 1955,30:125–131.

7. Butler BP, Ball RD, Albers JW: Effect of electrode type and position on motor unit action potential configuration. Muscle Nerve 1982;5:S95-S97.

8. Chu J, Chan RC: Changes in motor unit potential parameters in monopolar recordings related to filter settings of the EMG amplifier. Arch Phys Med Rehabil 1985;66:601–604.

9. Chu J, Chan RC, Bruyninckx F: Effects of the EMG amplifier filter settings on the motor unit action potential parameters recorded with concentric and monopolar needles. Electromyogr Clin Neurophysiol 1986;26:627–639.

10. Chu J, Chan RC, Bruyninckx F: Progressive Teflon denudation of the monopolar needle: Effects on motor unit potential parameters. Arch Phys Med Rehabil 1987:68:36–40.

11. Chu J, Johnson RJ: Electrodiagnosis: An anatomical and clinical approach. Philadelphia: JB Lippincott, 1986.

12. Cole JL: Equipment parameter determinants in evoked potential studies. Bull Am Soc Clin Evoked Potentials 1984;3:3–11.

13. Cooper R: Electrodes. Am J EEG Tech 1963;3:91–101.

14. Diamond SR: Fundamental concepts of modern physics. New York: AMSCO School Publications, 1970.

15. Dorfman LJ, McGill KC, Cummins KL: Electrical properties of commercial concentric EMG electrodes. Muscle Nerve 1985;8:1–8.

16. Dreyer SJ, Dumitru DD, King JC: Anodal block versus anodal stimulation: Fact or fiction. Am J Phys Med Rehabil 1993;72:10–18.

17. Dumitru D: Electrodiagnostic medicine. Philadelphia: Hanley & Belfus, 1995.

18. Dumitru D, Lester J: Comparison of SEP surface and needle electrodes. Arch Phys Med Rehabil 1991;72:989–992.

19. Dumitru D, Walsh NE: Electrophysiologic instrumentation. In: Dumitru D: ed. Clinical electrophysiology: Physical medicine and rehabilitation state-of-the-art reviews. Philadelphia: Hanley and Belfus, 1989.

20. Dumitru D, Walsh NE: Practical instrumentation and common sources of error. Am J Phys Med Rehabil 1988;67:55–65.

21. Dumitru D, Walsh NE, Porter LD: Electrophysiologic evaluation of the facial nerve in Bell's palsy. Am J Phys Med Rehabil 1988;67:137–144.

22. Guld C: On the influence of the measuring electrodes on duration and amplitude of muscle action potentials. Acta Physiol Scand 1951;25(Suppl 89):30:30–32.

23. Howard JE, McGill KC, Dorfman LJ: Properties of motor unit action potentials recorded with concentric and monopolar needle electrodes. Muscle Nerve 1988;11:1051–1055.

24. Jasper H, Ballem G: Unipolar electromyogram of normal and denervated human muscle. J Neurophysiol 1949;12:231–244.

25. Johnson EW: The EMG examination. In: Johnson EW, ed. Practical electromyography. 2nd ed. Baltimore: Williams & Wilkins, 1988.

26. Karam DB: AIDS and the electromyographer. Arch Phys Med Rehabil 1986;67:491.

27. Kimura J: Electrodiagnosis in diseases of nerve and muscle: Principles and practice. Philadelphia: FA Davis, 1983.

28. Kohara N, Kaji R, Kimura J: Comparison of recording characteristics of monopolar and concentric needle electrodes. Electroencephalogr Clin Neurophysiol 1993;89:242–246.

29. Kornfield MJ, Cerra J, Simons DG: Stimulus artifact reduction in nerve conduction. Arch Phys Med Rehabil 1985;66:232–235.

30. Kosarov D, Gydikov A: The influence of the volume conduction on the shape of the action potentials recorded by various types of needle electrodes in normal human muscle. Electromyogr Clin Neurophysiol 1975;15:319–335.

31. Lawler JC, Davis MJ, Everton CG: Electrical characteristics of the skin. J Invest Derm 1960;34:301–308.

32. Misulis KE: Basic electronics for clinical neurophysiology. J Clin Neurophysiol 1989;6:41–74.

33. Nandedkar SD, Sanders DB, Stålberg EV, et al.: Stimulation of concentric needle EMG motor unit action potentials. Muscle Nerve 1988;11:151–159.

34. Pease WS, Bowyer BL: Motor unit analysis: Comparison between concentric and monopolar electrodes. Am J Phys Med Rehabil 1988;67:2–6.

35. Pease WS, Fatehi MT, Johnson EW: Monopolar needle stimulation: Safety considerations. Arch Phys Med Rehabil 1989;70:412–414.

36. Pease WS, Pitzer NL: Electronic filter effects on normal motor and sensory nerve conduction tests. Am J Phys Med Rehabil 1990;69:28–31.

37. Pollack V: The waveshape of action potentials recorded with different types of electromyographic needles. Med Biol Eng 1971;9:657–664.

38. Reiner S, Rogoff JB: Instrumentation. In: Johnson EW, ed. Practical electromyography. Baltimore: Williams & Wilkins, 1980.

39. Spehlmann R: Evoked potential primer. Stoneham, MA: Butterworth, 1985.

40. Stålberg EV: Macro EMG, a new recording technique. J Neurol Neurosurg Psychiatry 1980;43:475–482.

41. Stålberg EV: Personal communication.

42. Stålberg EV, Chu J, Bril V, et al.: Automatic analysis of the EMG interference pattern. Electroencephalogr Clin Neurophysiol 1983;56:672–681.

43. Stålberg EV, Trontelj J: Single fiber electromyography. Woking, U.K.: Mirvalle Press, 1979.

44. Stolov W: Instrumentation and measurement in electrodiagnosis. AAEM Minimonograph #16. Rochester, Minnesota: American Association of Electromyography and Electrodiagnosis, 1981.

45. Swain ID, Wilson GR, Crook SC: A simple method of measuring the electrical resistance of the skin. J Hand Surg 1985;10-B:319–323.

46. Thage O, Trojaborg W, Buchthal F: Electromyographic findings in polyneuropathy. Neurology 1963;13:273–278.

47. Weber RJ, Piero D: Entrapment syndromes. In: Johnson EW, ed. Practical electromyography. Baltimore: Williams & Wilkins, 1980.

48. Wiechers DO: Single fiber electromyography. In: Johnson EW, ed. Practical electromyography, 2nd ed. Baltimore: Williams & Wilkins, 1988.

49. Wiechers DO, Blood JR, Stow RW: EMG needle electrodes: electrical impedance. Arch Phys Med Rehabil 1979;60:364–369.

50. Wongsam PE, Johnson EW, Weinerman JD: Carpal tunnel syndrome: Use of palmar stimulation of sensory fibers. Arch Phys Med Rehabil 1983;64:16–19.

51. Zablow L, Goldenshohn ES: A comparison between scalp and needle electrodes for the EEG. Electroencephalogr Clin Neurophysiol 1969;26:530–533.

Chapter 5

Needle Electromyography
Erik Stålberg

The organization of muscle fibers within the motor unit (MU) changes in typical ways in different nerve and muscle disorders. Many forms of neurogenic conditions are characterized by collateral sprouting from intramuscular nerve branches of surviving MUs. This increases the number of muscle fibers in individual motor units (8, 10). In the reinnervated MU, the muscle fibers are typically clustered instead of being randomly distributed as in the healthy patient. In muscle biopsy, this is seen as "fiber type" grouping, (17, 19).

In primary myopathies, on the other hand, degeneration of individual fibers causes a reduced number of muscle fibers within an MU. Muscle fiber regeneration and splitting will tend to increase the number of muscle fibers, now occurring in small clusters (30, 46). Fibrosis will further change the local topography of muscle fibers within a motor unit.

These types of MU changes can be studied not only with morphologic techniques, as referred to here, but also by electrophysiologic methods. The electromyographic signals are dependent upon the number of muscles fibers and their local concentration and sizes and upon neuromuscular and neuronal transmission. The electromyographic signal is also affected by the type of electrode used for recording (Fig. 5–1).

CONVENTIONAL EMG RECORDINGS

In conventional electromyography (EMG), concentric or monopolar electrodes are used. With some differences in the shape and size of the active recording zone, they record electrical signals from active muscle fibers within a radius of 2 mm to 3 mm (24). This recording zone is small compared to the size of the entire motor unit, because its territory is typically 3 mm to 10 mm in diameter. On the other hand, it is too large a recording volume to allow the selective recording from just one or a few muscle fibers for detailed analysis. The amplitude of the normal motor unit potential (MUP) is determined by only one to four fibers closest to the tip, and the duration of the MUP is determined by 30 to 60 fibers. Still, this technique is of great value in the study of motor unit characteristics, which differentiate normal from myogenic and neurogenic disorders. The MUP analysis is becoming quantitative and automatic. We have developed a technique by which up to six different MUPs are recorded from each recording site. The method is therefore called Multi-MUP recording (36) (Fig. 5–2). The method is based on decomposition algorithms. This algorithm extracts the individual elements (MUPs) that occur repeatedly, each time with the same shape. In this way a given MUP can be identified even when superimposed with activity from other motor units. The decomposition can be more or less complete, depending upon clinical or experimental application. If an exact firing (recruitment) pattern should be studied, a complete decomposition is necessary. If the aim is to quantitate MUP parameters, it is not necessary that each discharge be identified. Our Multi-MUP method is optimized in speed and accuracy for daily routine use. Similar methods have been developed by others (22). New parameters have been added to improve the detection of pathology (28, 43); reference values have been collected for a number of muscles (2); and a new way to express

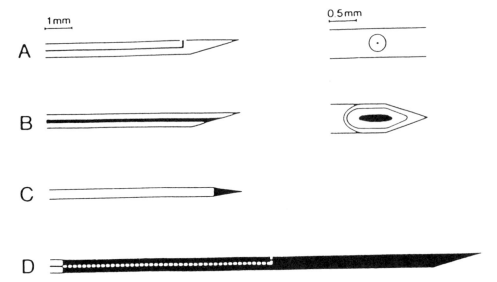

Figure 5-1. Different types of EMG electrodes. A. Single fiber EMG electrode with one recording surface. B. Concentric needle electrode. C. Monopolar electrode. D. Macro electrode.

abnormality has been defined (33). In neurogenic conditions, the MUPs are typically of increased duration and amplitude because of the grouping of muscle fibers within the motor unit, and they often change in shape at consecutive discharges (jiggle) (43). In myopathies, there is a reduction of duration owing to loss of muscle fibers and fibrosis (4). Furthermore, in both neurogenic and myopathic conditions, there is often an increased number of complex or polyphasic MUPs. These complex MUPs are due to an increased variation among pathologic muscle fiber diameters, causing a wider range of conduction velocities (along muscle membranes) and, to some degree, are due to the scattered positions of end-plates after reinnervation. These two phenomena produce increased temporal dispersion among individual single fiber action potentials, causing the typical changes in MUP shape. Recordings with conventional needle electrodes do not provide information about the size of the motor unit in terms of number of fibers or territory.

Other EMG methods, both more and less selective, have been developed to complement the conventional recordings. This chapter describes three of these special techniques. The classical EMG method is presented in other chapters of this book.

SINGLE FIBER ELECTROMYOGRAPHY (SFEMG)

In certain cases, essential information may be obtained by the detailed study of just one or a few muscle fibers from one motor unit. Examples of this include the study of neuromuscular transmission in individual end-plates and investigations of the distribution of muscle fibers in the motor unit. For this purpose, single fiber electromyography (SFEMG) was developed. After being proven valuable in these situations, SFEMG has taken a place in clinical routine work and will be described briefly here. The interested reader is referred to additional literature on the topic (47).

SFEMG is based on extracellular recordings of single muscle fiber action potentials with a small electrode, 25 μm in diameter, exposed in a side port of a steel canula 0.5 mm in diameter. Because of the small area of the recording surface and to the amplifier filter bandwidth, set to 500 Hz to 10 KHz, the average uptake area is limited to a hemisphere with a radius of about 300 μm, resulting in a high spatial resolution. On consecutive discharges, a given single fiber action potential has a well-defined and reproducible shape that

normal

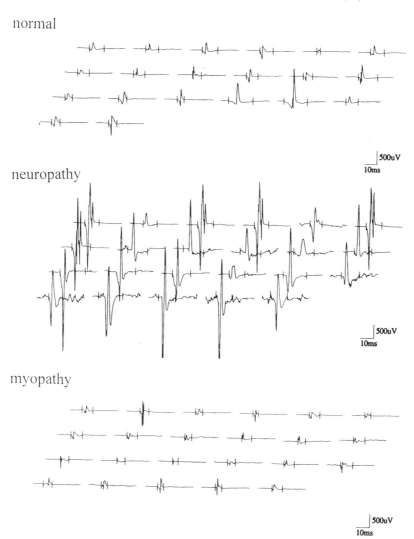

Figure 5–2.   MUP recordings from normal, neuropathic, and myopathic muscles using multiMUP analysis technique.

justifies time measurements with an accuracy as high as 0.1 μsec.

These recording advantages have been used over the years to study a number of morphologic and functional details in the motor unit. These studies range from studies of propagation along single muscle fibers, membrane characteristics, neuromuscular transmission of individual motor end-plates, local organization of muscle fibers in a motor unit, discharge characteristics of ventral horn cells, and conduction in cortico-spinal tract axons. This chapter describes studies of the neuromuscular transmission and of local muscle fiber distribution.

Neuromuscular Transmission

METHODS

Voluntary Activation

Most commonly the neuromuscular transmission is studied during slight voluntary contraction. The electrode is inserted into the muscle and a position is sought where two muscle fibers from the same motor unit (i.e., discharging synchronously) are recorded. When triggering the oscilloscope sweep on one of the spikes in the potential pair, the latency to the other varies during consecutive discharges. This phenomenon is called jitter. This is due to the summated variability of neuromuscular junction transmission time in the two motor end-plates involved in the recordings (Fig. 5–3).

Intramuscular Stimulation

Also used for these studies is microstimulation of individual muscle fibers and motor axons, either inside the muscle or in the nerve trunk. By means of a small monopolar electrode used as cathode and a surface electrode used as an anode, intramuscular stimulation is obtained. Stimulation strength is usually kept below 10 mA and stimulus pulse duration is typically 0.05 msec. Recording is through a SFEMG electrode about 20 mm away from the stimulation point. If a muscle fiber is directly stimulated, the jitter is less than 4 μsec; but if an intramuscular axon is stimulated, the jitter is more than 4 μs because of the involvement of the synapse at the motor end-plate (Fig. 5–4). Using this method, the neuromuscular junction can be studied under well-standardized conditions and over long periods of time. The method can also be used with uncooperative patients; comatose patients; patients with

movement disorders; infants; or in other situations in which voluntary patient activation is difficult. The technique can also be used in animal experiments.

Calculation of the Jitter

Jitter is expressed as the mean value of the difference between consecutive interpotential intervals (in absolute values). In stimulation studies, the interval between stimulus artifact and the resulting single fiber action potential is used for calculations. The jitter may be obtained from superimposed filmed recordings, but modern EMG instruments have the capability of automatic calculation of the jitter.

NORMAL FINDINGS

The Jitter During Voluntary Activity

The jitter during voluntary activation is approximately 5–60 μsec, depending on the muscle and the patient's age (Table 5–1). Motor end-plates within the same motor unit have different jitter values. The jitter does not show any appreciable change for up to 10 minutes of continuous activity with a mean

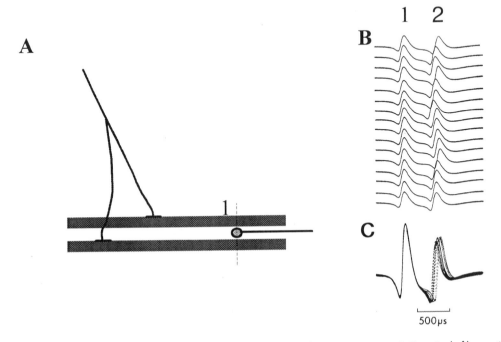

Figure 5–3. *A.* Schematic presentation of jitter recording during voluntary contraction. *B.* Two single fiber action potentials from fibers of the same motor unit recorded at high speed. The sweep is triggered by the first action potential. Several discharges superimposed demonstrating the variability of the interpotential interval, the neuromuscular jitter.

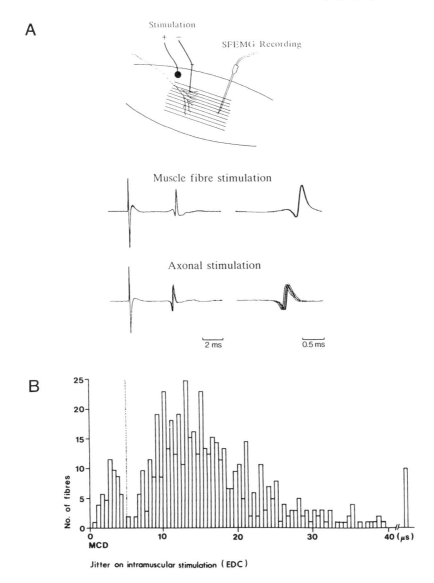

Figure 5-4. Intramuscular stimulation. A. Stimulating and recording electrodes (*upper*). Examples of typical responses with direct muscle fiber stimulation (low jitter) and with axonal stimulation (jitter greater than 4 μsec) [*middle*]. B. Dual distribution of jitter values in the EDC muscle corresponding to direct and axonal stimulation. Dividing line is at 5 μsec. (Reprinted with permission from Stålberg E, Trontelj JV: Single fiber electromyography in healthy and diseased muscle. New York: Raven Press, 1994.)

rate of about 10 Hz. In a study of the safety factor (27) of individual end-plates using regional curare, it was found that those with higher jitter were more sensitive to curare than those with initially low jitter. Thus, it seems justified to say that the jitter reflects the safety factor of transmission in individual motor end-plates.

It has been discussed whether neuromuscular blockade owing to local ischemia might be one of the reasons for muscular fatigue in normal muscle, developing during prolonged activity. In a study with ischemia after the inflation of a sphygmomanometer cuff around the upper arm, the jitter was measured in the extensor digitorum communis muscle activated voluntarily (6) (Dahlbäck et al. 1970). Following a few minutes of continuous activity during ischemia, the jitter started to increase fairly rapidly and one or the other of

Table 5–1
Fiber Density Results for the Extensor
Digitorum Communis Muscle, per Laboratory*

Lab.	Age < 60	60 < Age < 70	Age > 70
A	1.46 ± .15 (N = 119)	1.54 ± .17 (N = 21)	2.00 ± .41 (N = 31)
B	1.45 ± .14 (N = 20)	—	—
C	1.38 ± .08 (N = 69)	1.55 ± .18 (N = 18)	1.69 ± .18 (N = 7)
D	1.41 ± .16 (N = 3)	—	—
E	1.46 ± .10 (N = 17)	1.53 ± .11 (N = 2)	1.70 (N = 1)
H	—	1.58 ± .15 (N = 22)	1.74 ± .28 (N = 7)
All	1.43 ± .16 (N = 228)	1.56 ± .16 (N = 63)	1.91 ± .38 (N = 46)

*Mean ± SD; N = Number of subjects studied.
Upper reference limits (95% confidence) of jitter and fiber density for different muscles and ages as suggested by a collaborative study (13). The jitter limits are given both for individual muscle fiber pairs (i.e., the value above which no more than two of 20 muscle fiber pairs are accepted as normal) and for the mean value in a muscle.
Comment: Most of the above values agree very well with our own material and the previously suggested upper normal limits. The exceptions are the limits for individual MCD values in frontalis, biceps, and tibialis anterior, which appear to us slightly too high. The limits we use for these muscles are 45, 35, and 60's, respectively, for ages 10 to 70 years. Moreover, we accept only a single rather than two outliers as normal. The difference between our own and the multicenter value may reflect the minor differences in performance of different investigators. Therefore, we suggest the multicenter limits for those who do not have their own reference material. (Reprinted with permission from Stålberg E, Trontelj JV: Single fiber electromyography in healthy and diseased muscle. New York: Raven Press, 1994.)

the action potentials showed intermittent blocking, at first rarely and then more frequently until total block occurred. The time to blocking was shorter with higher innervation rates. Approximately 2000 to 4000 discharges were required before the onset of blocking. After release of the cuff, the transmission recovered quickly and the jitter became close to normal within a few minutes (6).

Jitter During Electrical Stimulation

The method is described in detail elsewhere (47). Because only one motor end-plate is involved, normal jitter during electrical stimula-

tion is lower than that with voluntary activation (Table 5–2). Theoretically, the values are reduced on average by a factor of $\sqrt{2}$ lower. This is in accordance with experimental results. In muscles in which separate reference values at electrical stimulation are missing, those from voluntary activation can be used after dividing by $\sqrt{2}$ (see Table 5–2).

Most normal end-plates display a rather constant jitter at different stimulation rates within the range of physiologic firing frequencies, reflecting a high safety factor. This has been studied in some detail (47). At a 50-Hz stimulation rate, a substantial increase in jitter occurred in comparison to the jitter values at 10 Hz in over two-thirds of the studied motor end-plates of healthy subjects. However, it still did not exceed the upper normal limit for 10 Hz (40 μs) in any of the tested end-plates. This suggests a remarkable ability of the presynaptic terminals to cope with the increased demand for acetylcholine (ACh) synthesis and mobilization even at these high rates. Similar to the results obtained with curare during voluntary activation (27), these results indicate

Table 5–2
Mean MCD Results For The Extensor
Digitorum Communis Muscle, per Laboratory*

Lab.	All ages	Age < 60	Age > 60
A	28.3 ± 5.5 (N = 160)	27.9 ± 5.5 (N = 141)	31.0 ± 4.4 (N = 19)
B	27.6 ± 3.2 (N = 26)	27.6 ± 3.2 (N = 26)	—
C	27.3 ± 4.5 (N = 55)	26.4 ± 3.8 (N = 45)	31.3 ± 5.7 (N = 10)
D	27.3 ± 5.6 (N = 4)	27.3 ± 5.6 (N = 4)	—
E	26.5 ± 4.3 (N = 26)	26.4 ± 4.5 (N = 22)	26.9 ± 3.7 (N = 4)
H	26.5 ± 3.8 (N = 25)	—	26.5 ± 3.8 (N = 25)
All	27.7 ± 4.9 (N = 296)	27.5 ± 4.9 (N = 238)	28.9 ± 4.9 (N = 58)

*Mean ± SD; N = Number of subjects studied.
Jitter values on axonal stimulation (means and upper limits for individual end-plates and a complete study) in EDC and orbicularis oculi. The values are derived from 90 (EDC) and 120 (orbicularis oculi) subjects. (Reprinted with permission from Stålberg E, Trontelj JV: Single fiber electromyography in healthy and diseased muscle. New York: Raven Press, 1994.)

that the jitter value can be used as an index of the safety factor of neuromuscular transmission.

NEUROMUSCULAR TRANSMISSION IN DISEASE

Myasthenia Gravis (MG)

The neurophysiologic mechanisms underlying the transmission defect in MG are well known (9). The end-plate potential (EPP) amplitude is reduced because of blocked or destroyed postsynaptic ACh receptors, whereas the number of ACh quanta released from the presynaptic terminal per nerve impulse is normal. The resulting reduction of safety factor for neuromuscular transmission with slowly rising EEPs causes increase in jitter values (Fig. 5–5B). When the EPPs are insufficient to reach the firing threshold, impulse blockings occur, thus giving rise to clinical weakness (Fig. 5–5C).

SFEMG findings in a patient with myasthenia include recordings with normal jitter values; jitter values above the normal range but without impulse blocking; and, depending on the severity of the disease, recordings with increased jitter and intermittent impulse blocking, the latter usually first appearing in association with a jitter of about 100 μs (Fig. 5–6).

In a large group of patients with MG investigated with SFEMG during voluntary activation (40), the extensor digitorum communis muscle was abnormal in 99% of those with moderate or severe generalized disease and in 75% of the patients in clinical remission.

The stimulation method can be used to study in detail rate-dependent changes of the efficiency of neuromuscular transmission at the individual end-plates. Indeed, myasthenia may be regarded as a natural model to study the normal function of the motor nerve terminal. In a recent study (48), 58 end-plates of 10 myasthenic patients were observed at different stimulation rates. A majority of the end-plates showed lower jitter and reduced incidence of blocking at the lowest stimulation rates followed by an increase in both measures at 2 Hz, 5 Hz, or 10 Hz. The normal presynaptic depression in the early phase of activity combined with a low safety factor is the basis of the decrement during repetitive stimulation and increased jitter. Stimulation rates of 20 Hz resulted in a return to lower jitter values, associated with a decreased incidence of blocking. This improvement is considered to be due to an increase in acetylcholine (ACh) released per stimulus, i.e., intratetanic potentiation (Fig. 5–6). The size of the response in the repetitive nerve stimulation test represents the net result of these two opposing processes.

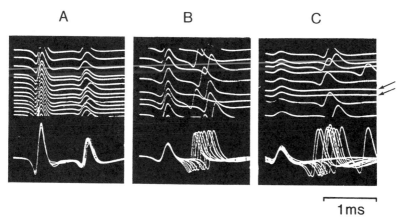

A   B   C

1ms

Figure 5–5. SFEMG jitter recordings from extensor digitorum communis muscle of a patient with myasthenia gravis. The oscilloscope sweep is triggered by the first action potential and the interval variability between the single fiber action potentials (the neuromuscular jitter) is shown as a variable position of the second potential. In the upper part the sweeps are moving downward, and below the recordings are superimposed. A. Normal jitter. B. Increased jitter without impulse blocking. C. Increased jitter and occasional blocking. (Reprinted with permission from Stålberg E, Trontelj JV: Single fiber electromyography in healthy and diseased muscle. New York: Raven Press, 1994.)

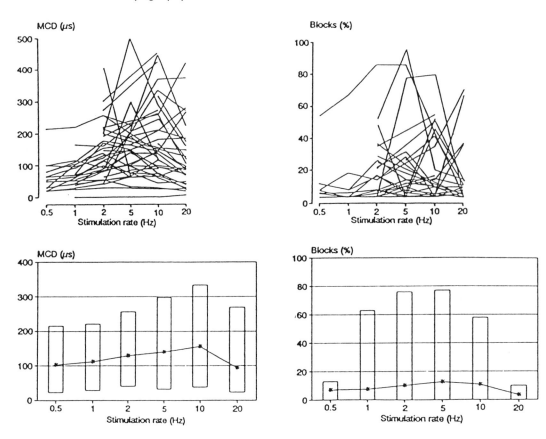

Figure 5-6. *Top*: Jitter and frequency of blocking in a sample of 40 myasthenic end-plates at different stimulation rates. The values belonging to individual motor end-plates are connected with lines. Twelve end-plates did not show any blocking. *Bottom*: Mean values and ranges between the fifth and ninety-fifth percentile for 32 end-plates studied over the complete range of stimulation rates. (Reprinted with permission from Trontelj JV, Stålberg E: Single motor end-plates in myastenia gravis and LEMS at different firing rates. Muscle Nerve 1991;14:226–232.)

Lambert-Eaton Myasthenic Syndrome (LEMS)

This neuromuscular transmission disorder has been shown to be a result of an autoimmune attack against calcium channels in the presynaptic nerve terminal, resulting in impaired transmitter release. The jitter is often grossly abnormal. In stimulated SFEMG there is a dramatic reduction of jitter and blocking as the stimulation rate is increased from 1 Hz to 2 Hz up to 10 Hz to 20 Hz (48).

Reinnervation

In cases of ongoing reinnervation, the jitter value is typically increased. This is probably because of the functional immaturity of the newly formed motor-end plates, both pre- and post-synaptically. After acute nerve damage, transmission is first established in the new end-plates after about 3 weeks (depending upon the site of lesion). After about 6 months, the jitter values are normalizing, but it is usually possible to find some abnormality long after this time.

Transmission Safety in the Intramuscular Nerve Tree, Axonal Jitter, and Blocking

Transmission in the intramuscular nerve tree can be studied by means of SFEMG during electrical stimulation, by studying the axon reflex (Fig. 5–7). With different stimulation strengths, a given axon may be stimulated at two sites in different branches. The low stimulation strength activates an intramuscular nerve branch of the axon antidromically and then orthodromically, and the higher stimulation strength directly activates the proper branch to the fiber orthodromically. A difference in jitter in the two different situations should be caused by the jitter created in the non-common axon segment, which would include the nodes of Ranvier. In normal nerve, there is no extra jitter in the nodes of Ranvier.

Intramuscular axonal transmission can also be studied during voluntary activation if recordings are made from three or more muscle fibers. Two or more components in a complex recording may show concomitant jitter relative to other parts of the action potential complex. Sometimes, concomitant impulse blocking may occur. This usually is due to unreliable propagation of axonal impulses or

conduction failure in the axon to those muscle fibers from which the blocking action potentials are recorded (44) (Fig. 5–8).

As with the neuromuscular blocking encountered in myasthenia gravis, axonal blocking may increase during continuous activity and worsen with increasing activation. This may also give rise to decrement in the surface-recorded responses to repetitive stimulation. It may even respond positively to edrophonium (44); therefore, the presence of a decrement and a positive edrophonium effect is not absolute proof of a synaptic transmission defect.

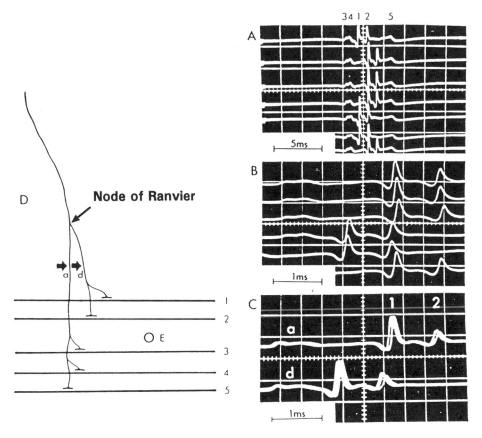

Figure 5–7. Intramuscular electrical stimulation producing a complex response of action potentials from five muscle fibers from one motor unit. Two of the muscle fibers (*1* and *2*) respond with two latencies, whereby they are always linked together. Note the different time calibrations in A and B through C. In C, seven discharges were superimposed with each of the two latencies, to show their relative constancy. D. Schematic explanation of this phenomenon based upon an axon reflex. The two fibers with dual latency are activated either directly through their own axonal branch (*d*) or, when the stimulus is subthreshhold, through the branch to the other three fibers in the recording (*a*). In this case the antidromically propagated impulse invades the branch to fibers *2* and *3*, and the response appears with a longer latency. (Reprinted with permission from Stålberg E, Trontelj JV: Demonstration of axon reflexes in human motor nerve fibers. J Neurol Neurosurg Psychiatry 1970;33:571–579.)

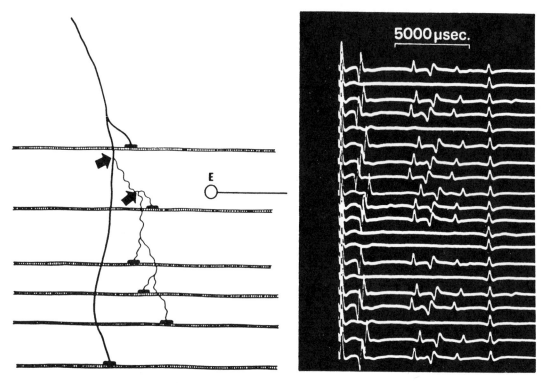

Figure 5–8. Concomitant blocking. A recording from six muscle fibers from the same motor unit. The middle four spike components intermittently block together. They also show a large common jitter in relation to the remaining two components. The block is considered to be situated in the nerve twig common to the four blocking muscle fibers (between the two arrows). The jitter of greater than 5 μsec between the 4 components indicates that this is not the case of four branches from a split muscle fiber with an abnormal motor end-plate. (Reprinted with permission from Stålberg E, Trontelj JV: Single fiber electromyography in healthy and diseased muscle. New York: Raven Press, 1994.)

Propagation Velocity of Single Muscle Fibers

Propagation velocity of the single muscle fiber action potential along the muscle fiber (29) can be measured using a multi-electrode with two arrays of recording surfaces. The time between the two recorded potentials from a muscle fiber exactly overlying two electrode surfaces is measured and the propagation velocity calculated. The normal muscle fiber propagation velocity value lies between 1.5 and 6.5 meters per second, but varies from muscle to muscle and even within a given muscle (29). Experiments on isolated muscle fibers (14) have shown that muscle fiber diameter is a major factor determining the propagation velocity. During continued activation at a firing rate of approximately 10 Hz, the propagation velocity usually decreases and is most pronounced during the first minute (29) (Fig. 5–9).

This decrease in propagation velocity explains the change in power spectrum observed with the conventional needle and surface EMG when the higher frequencies decrease and the lower frequencies increase during continuous activity. It also explains, at least in part, a decrease in the number of turns in an analysis of the EMG interference pattern during continous muscle activity.

Propagation velocity, dependent on membrane properties, also depends on the interval-to-previous discharge, called the velocity recovery function, VRF (29). In certain muscle disorders, the membrane properties are changed, which can be seen as abnormal VRF. Propagation velocity is not a parameter studied in routine EMG.

Fiber Density

Morphologic data indicate that changes from the normal "checker board pattern" of muscle fibers to a patchy distribution called fiber type grouping is an early sign of pathology. This may occur before definite changes in number of fibers within parts of the motor unit has occurred. A parameter reflecting fiber distribution called fiber density (FD) has therefore been developed. This parameter is easier to obtain than jitter and has wider applications. It reflects the distribution of muscle fibers in the motor unit and is found to be a useful complement to conventional EMG (Fig. 5–10).

METHOD

The electrode is positioned in the muscle so that a given muscle fiber action potential is obtained with its amplitude maximized. A count is made of the number of spike components (including the triggering spike) that are time-locked to the triggering action potential that has an amplitude exceeding 200 μV and a rise time shorter than 300 μs when using a low frequency limit of 500 Hz at the amplifier (many discharges must be observed to ascertain that they belong to the same motor unit) (Fig. 5–11). The sweep speed should be slow enough to cover 5 msec, or more if necessary, before and after the triggering spike. In the event that individual single fiber action potentials occur nearly simultaneously at the recording electrode, causing superimposition, the amplitude criterion for inclusion may be difficult to use. As a rule of thumb, each of the spikes giving rise to a change in signal polarity (a "notch" in the signal) should be counted. At least 20 estimations are made from different recording sites with at least three separate skin penetrations. *Note:* Occa-

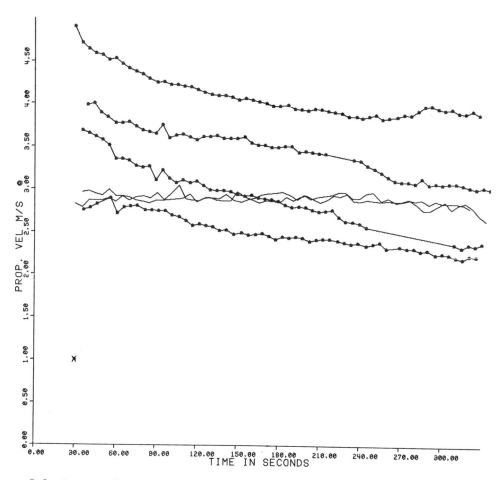

Figure 5–9. Decrease of propagation velocity in four muscle fibers during continued activity at 11, 16, 12, and 9 discharges respectively (asterisks). In a fifth fiber, tested at an innervation rate of six and 16 discharges (the two continuous lines), there is no decrease in propagation velocity.

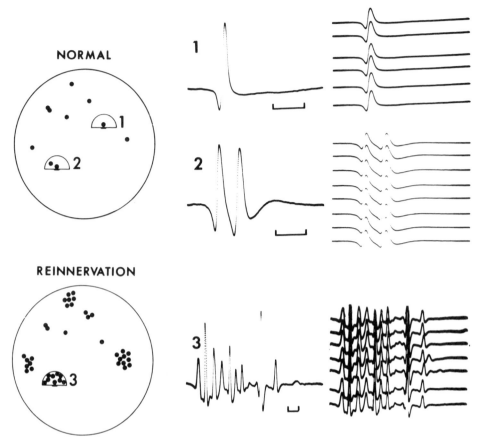

Figure 5–10. SFEMG recordings in normal and reinnervated muscle. The diagragm illustrates the number of muscle fibers of one motor unit (blacked-in). The uptake area of the recording electrode is represented as a half circle. In the normal muscle (*1* and *2*), only action potentials from one or two fibers are recorded. In reinnervation (*3*), many fibers' action potentials are recorded owing to increased fiber density in the motor unit. (Reprinted with permission from Stålberg E, Trontelj JV: Single fiber electromyography in healthy and diseased muscle. New York: Raven Press, 1994.)

sionally, positive-going, broad, jittering potentials are generated by the preceding spike component, and these should not be included in the count or used for jitter measurements.

FD Findings in Normal Muscles
The normal values vary for different muscles and, in some muscles, with age. The typical value is 1.3–1.8. Reference values for different muscles are obtained in a collaborative study (13) (see Table 5–1).

FD Values in Nerve-Muscle Disorders
In cases of abnormal motor unit organization (e.g., reinnervation), the FD values are increased, corresponding to fiber-type grouping

in the biopsy (Fig. 5–12). High values are also found in myopathies (1, 47). This most likely is due to abnormal fiber distribution owing to splitting, satellite cells, regeneration, ephatic transmission, and, sometimes, secondary neurogenic changes (1, 30).

Normal Values in SFEMG
Table 5–1 below is based on data from a multicenter study, which includes values from our own laboratories (13). Until the individual laboratory has collected its own reference values, these values can be used. Jitter values are extremely reproducible between laboratories, but FD values differ somewhat. It may be advisable to test a smaller material of controls

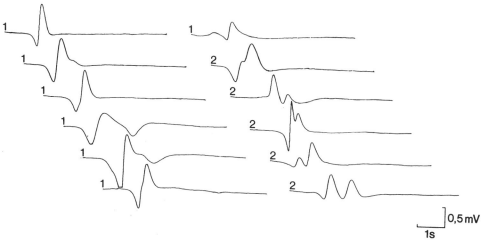

Figure 5–11. Different SFEMG recordings indicated to represent one or two fibers in FD measurements. (Reprinted with permission from Stålberg E, Trontelj JV: Single fiber electromyography in healthy and diseased muscle. New York: Raven Press, 1994.)

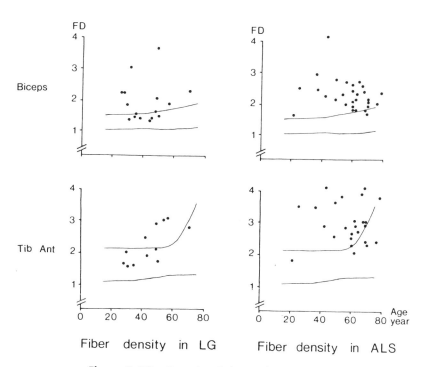

Figure 5–12. Examples of abnormal FD recordings.

for FD values in the extensor digitorum communis (EDC) muscle. If this coincides with published data, the technique is identical to that described and used for all reference values, which therefore can be adopted directly.

Jitter-Voluntary Activation

Jitter is expressed as the mean value of consecutive differences (MCD) of interpotential intervals. In a multispike recording, only MCD values between one triggering component and each other component is measured, i.e., when four spikes are present, three MCD values are obtained.

Abnormality is expressed in two ways:

1. By marking the number of recordings with jitter outside given limits for individual data. If two or more recordings exceed the limit, the finding is considered abnormal.
2. By mean MCD value for the whole study in a muscle. The distribution of individual jitter values in abnormal conditions is often skewed, with some extremely high values. Therefore, the mean MCD is calculated only from data with a jitter value less than 150 μs (unless a majority of data is abnormal and distributed near this limit).

The example of normal values for EDC from the multicenter study (13) that indicates the preference limit for mean MCD and individual jitter values is shown in Figure 5–13. For more information on muscles, the reader is referred to a comprehensive text on the subject (47).

Jitter-Axonal Stimulation

The principles given in descriptions on SFEMG electrical stimulation must be strictly adhered to in order to avoid pitfalls leading to potentially serious errors. A minimum of 20 to 30 end-plates are sampled with two or more different positions of the stimulating needle. Table 5–2 (47) shows examples of reference values. The abnormality is expressed in the same way as in the voluntary jitter study

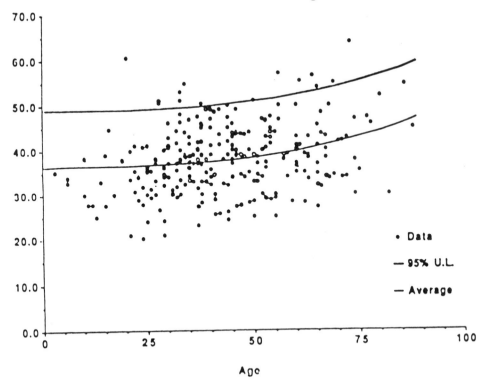

Figure 5–13. Graphs showing mean values of jitter in EDC plotted against age (A) and third-highest individual out of 20 recordings in each subject. The thick line indicates 95% confidence limit. (Reprinted with permission from Gilchrist J, Barkhaus P, Bril V, et al.: Single fiber EMG reference values: A collaborative effort. Muscle Nerve 1992;15:151–161.)

(as a number or percentage of the abnormal recordings and as the mean of all individual MCD values in the study). One out of 20 values above the upper reference limit is accepted as normal.

INDICATIONS OF SFEMG IN CLINICAL STUDIES AND IN RESEARCH

EXPERIMENTAL STUDIES OF NEUROMUSCULAR TRANSMISSION

Neuromuscular Transmission in Diseases

Diagnosis; evaluation; follow-up of neuro-
  muscular disorders
Myasthenia gravis
Lambert-Eaton myasthenic syndrome
Other myasthenic syndromes
Botulism
Other conditions with disturbed neuro-
  muscular transmission

Spatial Organisation of Motor Units in Diseases

Neurogenic disorders
Myopathies

Firing Pattern

In studies of normal and disturbed firing
  pattern

Spike Triggering

Scanning EMG
Macro EMG
Spike-triggered averaging for motor unit
  electrical or mechanical output

Propagation Velocity

Measure of fiber diameter
Membrane parameters
Fatigue

MACRO EMG

In order to obtain an overall picture of the motor unit, a special technique called Macro EMG has been developed (37).

METHOD

The recording electrode consists of a modified SFEMG electrode with the cannula insulated except for the distal 15 mm. The SFEMG recording surface is exposed 7.5 mm from the tip (the center of the bare cannula). Recording is made on two channels with the EMG equipment connected to a PC for analysis (Fig. 5–14). On one channel, the signal from the cannula (using a surface electrode as reference) is recorded and fed to an average. On the other channel, the SFEMG recording is obtained between the small surface and the cannula. The SFEMG signal serves as trigger for the averaging process. Amplifier filters are set to 5 Hz-10 KHz and 500 Hz-10 KHz for Macro and SFEMG, respectively. The electrode is inserted into the voluntarily activated muscle and a position is sought where an acceptable SFEMG potential is seen. At this moment, the averaging process begins and continues until a smooth baseline and a constant Macro MUP is obtained on the "cannula" channel. Concomitantly, fiber density of the triggering action potential is obtained.

The peak-to-peak amplitude and area of the Macro EMG signal is positively related to the number and size of muscle fibers in the entire motor unit (25). If there is atrophy of the muscle fibers, the Macro MUP should become reduced. This effect is counteracted, however, by the shrinkage of the motor unit, which reduces the distance between its fibers and the electrode, increasing the Macro MUP. When recordings from the same motor unit are repeated using a different muscle fiber as the trigger (which is separated from the first by several mm), the shape of the Macro EMG signal from one motor unit is relative constant, indicating that the recording really reflects activity in all fibers of a motor unit. (See Table 5–3.)

NORMAL FINDINGS

In normal muscle the general Macro MUP shape differs from one muscle to another (37). In the anterior tibial muscle, the potentials often have two or more separate peaks, whereas in the brachial biceps muscle, the potentials usually have a simple configuration with one or two negative peaks. There is a great scatter in individual Macro MUP amplitudes in the normal muscle. The largest Macro MUP may be up to 10 times larger than the

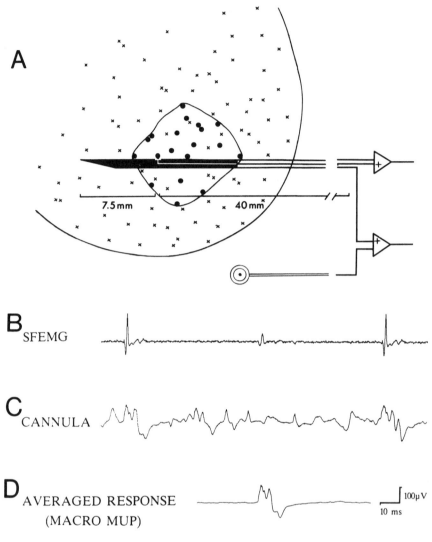

A

B SFEMG

C CANNULA

D AVERAGED RESPONSE
(MACRO MUP)

7.5 mm   40 mm

100 μV
10 ms

Figure 5–14. Recording principle of macro EMG recording.

smallest in the brachial biceps muscle for individuals under the age of 60 and up to 20 times larger in those individuals over 60 years old. Larger scatter in values can be expected if high threshold motor units are included. It is thus easy to detect the so-called size principle and to study its changes with pathology with this technique, not easily recognized with conventional EMG recordings (11). The mean Macro MUP amplitude differs fivefold for motor units recruited at 20% of maximal force as compared to those recruited at lower force, corresponding to orderly recruitment as judged from their twitches (23). This makes it important to define reference values for given ranges of contraction levels and to perform patient investigation within the same range of contraction.

Normal values given for low degree of activity, i.e., low threshold motor units, vary for different muscles. In some muscles, the values increase with age, an effect more pronounced in the anterior tibial muscle than in the brachial biceps or vastus lateralis muscles. The change with patient age reflects the enlargement of remaining motor units with the physiologic loss of neurones and reinnervation by sprouting (34, 37).

Table 5-3
Relationship Between Macro EMG Amplitude and Fiber Density

| | Macro MUP ampl | | | Fiber density | |
	Decreased	Normal	Increased	Normal	Increased
Small normal MU	+			+	
Average MU		+		+	
Large normal			+	+	
Neuropathy			+		+
Myopathy	(+)	+			+

MOTOR UNIT ESTIMATION

McComas (21) described a method for estimating the number of motor units by means of graded electrical stimulation and a surface recording of the increasing M-response amplitude. From the maximal response and the mean value of individual steps, the number of motor units was estimated. In order to ascertain the recording from just one motor unit at a time, we tried voluntary activation. An SFEMG electrode-triggered activity from one muscle fiber and surface electrode as used by McComas (21) were used for recordings. The maximal M-response used for the calculations was obtained from electrical stimulation. Brown et al. (3) have used this technique extensively and found it useful. We found that motor units in large muscles gave smaller signal amplitudes on the muscle surface and therefore developed Macro EMG, mainly for studies of motor unit size initially, not for estimating the number of motor units. Macro EMG MUPs recorded during voluntary contraction and M-response obtained from the Macro EMG electrode have been used for estimation of number of motor units (18). We have used this mainly in the study of patients with a history of polio.

FINDINGS IN MYOPATHIES

As expected, the electrical size of the motor unit reflected by the Macro MUP is decreased in myopathies as a group. In the individual case, values are often within normal limits. Large-mean-amplitude Macro MUPs have been found in some patients with FSH and limb-girdle dystrophy with slight or no clinical involvement (16) (Fig. 5-15). This finding

may indicate a compensatory hypertrophy, as seen by others (7, 21). Macro MUP parameters by themselves are thus not sensitive enough to detect early myopathic changes. The reason for the normal or near-normal amplitudes is probably the compensatory mechanisms with fiber regeneration, fiber splitting, occasional fibre hypertrophy, and general packing of fibers due owing atrophy. These changes will, however, cause an increase in the FD value. Therefore, the finding of increased FD values obtained from the SFEMG channel during the Macro EMG study, combined with normal or slightly reduced Macro MUP value, is a useful indicator of myopathy. These findings can be used to differentiate myopathy from neuropathy in questionable cases.

MACRO EMG IN REINNERVATION

During reinnervation by collateral sprouting, the most common type of compensation in neurogenic conditions, the number of muscle fibers in a given motor unit increases. In Macro EMG, this is seen as an increased amplitude of the signals. In this way, Macro EMG offers the possibility of following reinnervation quantitatively.

The individual Macro MUPs in reinnervation can have an amplitude exceeding the normal mean by a factor of 10. In the complex situation involving patients with ALS (41), the picture is variable. In some patients with rapid progression, the Macro MUPs are increased only slightly and the FD is only moderately increased. In cases of slow progression, the Macro MUPs increase much more, with individual Macro MUPs 10 to 20 times higher

TIB ANT

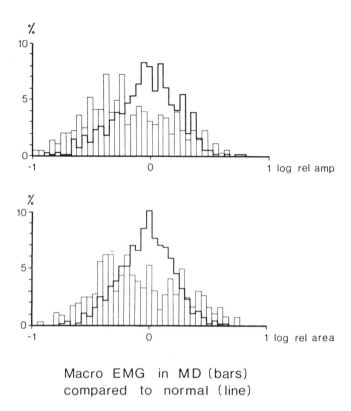

Macro EMG in MD (bars)
compared to normal (line)

Figure 5-15. Macro EMG amplitude and area values in patients with muscular dystrophies. (Reprinted with permission from Hilton-Brown P, Stålberg E: Motor unit size in muscular dystrophy; a Macro EMG and Scanning EMG study. J Neurol Neurosurg Psychiatry 1983;46:996–1005.)

than the upper normal mean. The Macro MUPs are still in parallel with the increase in FD, indicating a homogeneous and effective reinnervation. In later stages of ALS, the average Macro MUP amplitude may start to decline although the FD is still high. This has been interpreted as either fragmentation of large motor units or an effect of selective dropout of the largest motor units, leaving the smaller ones preserved.

In patients with a history of poliomyelitis, Macro EMG is usually increased dramatically, with individual values more than 20 times the normal mean value (Fig. 5–16). This reflects the preserved capacity for reinnervation in these patients, including when there is a pronounced loss of strength. The question of late effects of polio has been investigated by means of Macro EMG. In a recent study (38) of 18 patients with two examinations 4 years apart, Macro EMG and biopsy were performed in the vastus lateralis muscle. Force measurements of knee extension were performed. The results could be briefly summarized as follows: The Macro MUP amplitudes were increased at first investigation by 10 times for the stable muscles (with stable clinical situation) and 16 times for the unstable (having new weakness in that muscle) group.

Four years after the first investigation, the force was unchanged or decreased, whereas the Macro MUP amplitude has increased by 67% (p<0.01) and 35% in the stable and unstable groups, respectively. This increase could not be explained by a change in the fiber area, which was unchanged except by an increase in the number of fibers owing to reinnervation. At the stage of fully utilized reinnerva-

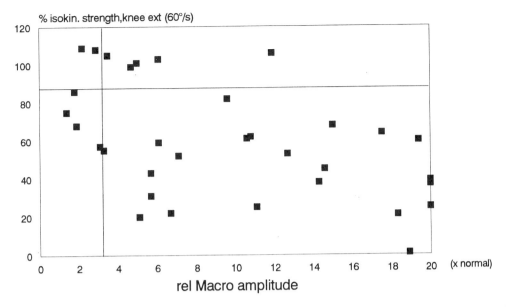

Figure 5-16. Macro EMG amplitudes (in vastus lateralis muscle) vs. strength (knee extension) in patients with history of polio. (Modified from Stålberg E, Grimby G: Dynamic EMG and biopsy changes in a 4-year follow-up study of patients with history of polio. Muscle Nerve, 1994 (in press).)

tion capacity, additional loss of motor units cannot be compensated (39). A continued loss of motor units will then present clinically as a new or accelerating decrease of strength over time.

Most EMG studies have failed to depict individual EMG parameters that may be used to diagnose or predict the so-called post-polio syndrome (PPS) (49) This is due only partly to the fact that PPS usually concerns the entire condition of the patient. Even in studies in which functional tests concern individual muscles, the EMG changes were similar in patients with unstable and stable muscle function (26). The difficulty in finding predictors for PPS is partly due to the complex relationship between the various causes for reduction of muscle strength and the compensatory processes in patients with a history of poliomyelitis.

INDICATIONS FOR MACRO EMG

Estimating motor unit size in normal
   muscle
Estimating number of motor units
Recruitment order

Neurogenic conditions

- diagnostic
- quantitative analysis of reinnervation processes

Myopathic conditions

- diagnostic (together with FD)

SCANNING EMG

In order to investigate the distribution of muscle fibers in a normal and diseased motor unit in some detail, different techniques can be used. One is by means of glycogen depletion of individual motor units. This method can hardly be applied in human muscles and only a few studies have been reported (12). In general, the fibers are scattered within the motor unit territory, although a non-random distribution pattern of muscle fibers has been suggested, with fibers arranged in a more "orderly" fashion than statistically expected (50). Electrophysiologically the territory was first studied by Buchthal et al. by means of multielectrodes containing twelve 1.5 mm long leads distributed over a distance of 25 mm (5).

With another multi-electrode technique the territory of the MU was defined by Stålberg et al. (42) using a multi-electrode with 14 different 25 μm electrodes, allowing 40 recording sites spaced 150 μm apart recording over 14 mm. The fibers were found to scatter in a manner similar to that shown by others in experimental glycogen depletion studies, i.e., without evidence of grouping.

Another technique with a higher spatial resolution has been developed to obtain a more detailed electrophysiologic cross-section of the MU; it is called Scanning EMG (31, 32). The method gives an enhanced spatial resolution of the MU compared to the multi-electrode techniques because recording is made from many more sites, spaced 50 μm. It gives a new electrophysiologic dimension to the MU structure in both normal and pathologic conditions. (15, 35). It is likely that in cases of slight change, the pathology is seen only in parts of a motor unit, which may be missed by conventional EMG sampling.

METHOD

The method has been described in related journals (32, 35). In brief, a single-fiber EMG electrode is used to trigger the activity from one MU during slight voluntary contraction, i.e., preferentially low-threshold motor units are studied. As an exploring electrode, the "scanning electrode", a concentric needle electrode is usually used, but any EMG electrode may be used (Fig. 5–17). The electrode must be in optimal condition with a sharp tip and no irregularities along the shaft in order to facilitate a smooth movement through the muscle without jumping. Small jumps may still occur and cause minor errors in terms of sudden changes in action potential shape or in territory measures, probably less than 1 mm. The scanning electrode is inserted 20 mm away from the triggering electrode, along the longitudinal axis of the muscle and perpendicular to the direction of the muscle fibers. A position is sought where one can obtain synchronous activity with that from the triggering electrode. The scanning electrode is then pushed through the triggering MU until a position is reached where no further trigger-locked spike components are detected.

Positioning of the two electrodes usually takes less than one minute. The scanning electrode is connected to a pulling stepmotor (digital linear actuator—DLA), which is controlled by a computer system. The motor is mounted in a holder with an electrode grip and a wide foot-plate. During the recording the foot-plate is handheld steadily against the skin over the muscle. The recording is cancelled if the position of the holder is visually changed in relation to the muscle. The signal recorded from the single fiber electrode triggers the oscilloscope sweep for display and also produces a TTL pulse to start the analog-to-digital (A/D) conversion process (A/D sampling frequency 20 KHz). A sweep length of 25 msec is stored each time. The signal is displayed on the computer screen. When the entire signal has been stored, the step motor is initiated to pull the concentric electrode 50 μm or in multiples thereof. The process is repeated until the scanning electrode has passed through the entire MU cross-section, up to a maximum of 20 mm. Unless the patients have pronounced tremor, they can usually cooperate well, i.e., produce a slight steady voluntary contraction during the recording procedure, which takes less than one minute. The entire procedure, i.e., positioning the electrodes and recording from one motor unit, takes less than five minutes.

3-D plots and color plots of the amplitude distribution of the MU-activity are produced by the PC. In this way, one obtains a cross-section and distribution of the MU-activity (Fig. 5–18). The following parameters may be analyzed (35):

Length of MU cross-section: The distance from first to last record with MU activity.

Number of MU fractions: The portions of motor unit activity having clearly separated peaks.

Number and length of silent portions: The silent portions occuring between the fractions.

Number of polyphasic or complex portions within the MU: The number of sections in which the activity has more than four phases or five turns.

Number and length of polyphasic or complex portion of the MU: (the sections having more than four phases or five turns). See Table 5–4.

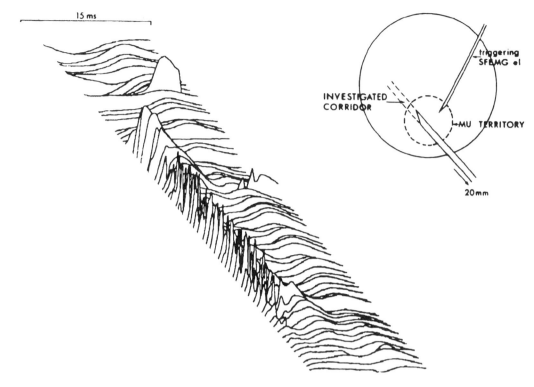

Figure 5–17. Principles of scanning EMG.

Simultaneous Macro EMG

Macro EMG can be recorded from the cannula of the scanning electrode e.g., the concentric needle passing through the MU being studied, with the electrode tip in the start position outside the MU, i.e., passing through the motor unit. As the reference electrode, either the central core (normally used as an active electrode) or a separate subcutaneous electrode can be used. This method differs slightly from conventional Macro EMG because the cannula used in scanning EMG is not partially insulated. Recording is performed before the pulling of the needle is started, as described above.

FINDINGS IN HEALTHY SUBJECTS

The Scanning EMG often shows more than one amplitude maximum. These may be separated by areas of very low amplitudes and are then called fractions (Fig. 5–18). These probably correspond to muscle fibers innervated by one major intramuscular nerve branch. If these fractions are separated in time, a recording position between them may give rise to early or late satellite components. The fractions correspond to the peaks in the Macro EMG signal.

When scanning is performed with a concentric needle electrode, a "cannula" signal is often observed. This occurs in the situation in which active muscle fibers are recorded from the cannula but not from the tip. In this way a slow, positive-going component occurs,

Table 5–4
Scanning EMG Parameters*

No clinical indications at present
Research:
    For mapping motor unit topography
    For mapping distribution of electrical activity in the muscle
    In studies of MUP shapes
    In studies of volume conduction parameters

*Reprinted with permission from Stålberg E, Dioszeghy P: Scanning EMG in normal muscle and in neuromuscular disorders. Electroenceph Clin Neurophysiol 1991;81:403–416.)

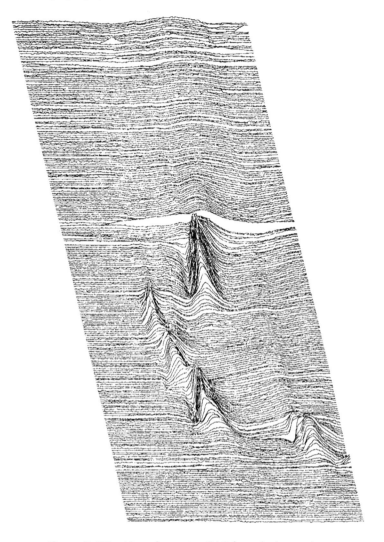

Figure 5–18. Normal scanning EMG from tibialis muscle.

which may be difficult to differentiate from the normal onset or end of the slow phase of the MUP. Scanning EMG also reveals that many motor units have at least some portion with polyphasic signals. It should be noted that a conventional EMG recording represents one trace of the scanning EMG. If a motor unit contains only few areas of polyphasic sections, there is less chance that a conventional recording is performed in that area, and therefore less chance that a polyphasic MUP is recorded. Some parameters obtained from the normal muscle are presented in Table 5–3 and more extensively in a separate report (35).

FINDINGS IN PATIENTS WITH MYOPATHY OR NEUROGENIC CONDITIONS

Some typical differences between findings in control subjects and in patients (35) are shown in Figure 5–19. The most prominent findings are summarized as follows:

> The mean length of cross section of the MU was nearly the same in all groups.
> The mean number of fractions was slightly but significantly increased in both patient groups.
> In the myopathic conditions, there were

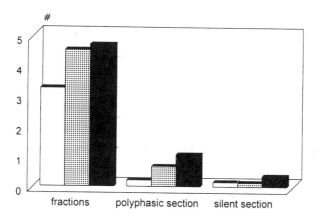

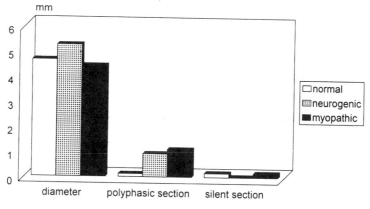

Figure 5–19. Scanning EMG results from biceps brachii normal, neurogenic, and myopathic muscles. (Reprinted with permission from Stålberg E, Dioszeghy P: Scanning EMG in normal muscle and in neuromuscular disorders. Electroencephalogr Clin Neurophysiol 1991;81:403–416.)

a larger number of recordings with silent sections than in either normal or neurogenic conditions. The most striking finding was the increase of the mean length and number of polyphasic sections in both patient groups, particularly in myopathies.

Summarizing the individual findings, we found the following: Individual scanning recordings were abnormal in some respect in 81% and 37% of all recordings in the neurogenic group and in 53% and 47% of all recordings in the myogenic group in the biceps and tibialis anterior muscles, respectively. We could not find any correlation between patient age and any of the scanning parameters interpatient groups or in the controls.

References

1. Bertorini T, Stålberg E, Yuson CP, et al.: Single fiber electromyography in neuromuscular disorders. Correlation of muscle histochemistry, single-fiber electromyography, and clinical findings. Muscle Nerve 1994;17:345–358.
2. Bischoff C, Stålberg E, Falck B: Reference values of motor unit potentials recorded with decomposition EMG. Muscle Nerve 1994;842–851.
3. Brown WF, Strong MJ, Snow R: Methods for estimating numbers of motor units in biceps-brachialis muscles and losses of motor units with aging. Muscle Nerve 1988;11:423–432.
4. Buchthal F:Diagnostic significance of the myopathic EMG. In Rowland LP, ed. Pathogensis of human muscular dystrophies; Proc 5th international conf muscular dystrophy assoc. Amsterdam-Oxford: Excerpta Medica 1977;205–218.
5. Buchthal F, Erminio F, Rosenfalck P: Motor unit terri△ry in different human muscles. Acta Physiol Scand 1959;45:72–87.
6. Dahlbäck L-O, Ekstedt J, Stålberg E: Ischemic effect on impulse tranmission to muscle fibres in man.

Electroencephalogr Clin Neurophysiol 1970;29:
579–591.

7. Dubowitz V, Brooke MH:Muscle biopsy: A modern
approach. London: WB Saunders Ltd, 1973.

8. Einarsson G, Grimby G, Stålberg E: Electromyographic and morphological functional compensation
in late poliomyelitis. Muscle Nerve 1990;13:
165–171.

9. Engel AG, Tsujihata M, Lambert EH, et al.: Experimental autoimmune myasthenia gravis: A sequential
and quantitative study of the neuromuscular junction ultrastructure and electrophysiologic correlations. J Neurophathol Experimental Neurol
1976;35:569–587.

10. Erminio F, Buchthal F, Rosenfalck P: Motor unit
territory and muscle fiber concentration in paresis
due to peripheral nerve injury and anterior cell
involvement. Neurology. 1959;9:657–671.

11. Ertas M, Stålberg E, Falck B: Can the size principle be
detected in conventional EMG recordings? Muscle
Nerve 1995;18:435–39.

12. Garnett RAF, O'Donovan MJ, Stephens JA, et al.:
Motor unit organisation of human medial gastrocnemius. J Physiol (London) 1979;287:33–43.

13. Gilchrist J, Barkhaus P, Bril V, et al.: Single fiber
EMG reference values: A collaborative effort. Muscle Nerve 1992;15:151–161.

14. Håkansson CH: Conduction velocity and amplitude
of the action potential as related to the circumference in the isolated fibre of frog muscle. Acta Physiol
Scand 1956;37:14–34.

15. Hilton-Brown P, Stålberg E: The motor unit in muscular dystrophy, a single fibre EMG, and scanning
EMG study. J Neurol Neurosurg Psychiatry
1983;46:981–995.

16. Hilton-Brown P, Stålberg E: Motor unit size in muscular dystrophy: A Macro EMG and scanning EMG
study. J Neurol Neurosurg Psychiatry 1983;46:996–
1005.

17. Karpati G, Engel WK: Type of grouping in skeletal
muscle after experimental reinnervation. Neurology
1968;18:447–455.

18. de Koning P. Functional and electrophysiological
evaluation of damaged peripheral nerve: neurotrpic
actions of org. 2766 Thesis. Utrecht 1987.

19. Kugelberg E, Edström L, Abruzzese M: Mapping
of motor units in experimentally reinnervated rat
muscle. J Neurol Neurosurg Psychiatry 1970;33:
319–329.

20. McComas AJ:Neuromuscular Function and Disorders. London: Butterworth, 1977.

21. McComas AJ, Fawcett PRW, Campbell MJ, et al.:
Electrophysiological estimation of the number of
motor units within a human muscle. J Neurol Neurosurg Psychiatry 1971;34:121–131.

22. McGill K, Dorfman L:Automatic decomposition
electromyography (ADEMG), methodologic and
technical considerations. In: Desmedt JE, ed.,
1989, 91–101.

23. Milner-Brown HS, Stein RB, Yemm R: The orderly
recruitment of human motor units during voluntary

isometric contractions. J Physiol (London) 1973;
230:359–370.

24. Nandedkar SD, Sanders DB, Stålberg E: Selectivity
of electromyographic recording electrodes. Med
Biol Engng Comp 1985;23:536–540.

25. Nandedkar S, Stålberg E: Simulation of macro EMG
motor unit potentials. Electroencephalogr Clin
Neurophysiol 1983;56:52–62.

26. Ravits J, Hallett M, Baker M, et al.: Clinical and
electromyographic studies of postpoliomyelitis muscular atrophy. Muscle Nerve 1990;13:667–674.

27. Schiller HH, Stålberg E, Schwartz MS: Regional curare for the reduction of the safety factor in human
motor end-plates studied with single fibre electromyography. J Neurol Neurosurg Psychiatry
1975;38:805–809.

28. Sonoo M, Stålberg E: The ability of MUP parameters
to discriminate between normal and neurogenic
MUPs in concentric EMG: analysis of the MUP
"thickness" and the proposal of "size index."
Electroencephalogr Clin Neurophysiol 1993;89:
291–303.

29. Stålberg E: Propagation velocity in single human
muscle fibres in situ. Acta Physiol Scand
1966;70(suppl):287:1–112 (Uppsala).

30. Stålberg E: Electrogenesis in human dystrophic muscle. In: Rowland LP, ed. Pathogensis of human muscular dystrophies; Proc 5th international conf muscular dystrophy assoc. Amsterdam-Oxford: Excerpta
Medica 1977;570–587.

31. Stålberg E: Single fiber EMG, macro EMG, and
scanning EMG. New ways of looking at the motor
unit. CRC Crit Rev Clin Neurobiol 1986;
2:125–167.

32. Stålberg E, Antoni L: Electrophysiological cross section of the motor unit. J Neurol Neurosurg Psychiatry 1980;43:469–474.

33. Stålberg E, Bischoff C, Falck B: Outliers: A way to
detect abnormality in quantitative EMG. Muscle
Nerve 1994;17:392–399.

34. Stålberg E, Borges O, Ericsson M, et al.: The quadriceps femoris muscle in 20–70-year-old subjects. Relationship between knee extension torque, electrophysiological parameters, and muscle fiber
characteristics. 1989;12:382–389.

35. Stålberg E, Dioszeghy P: Scanning EMG in normal
muscle and in neuromuscular disorders. Electroenceph Clin Neurophysiol 1991;81:403–416.

36. Stålberg E, Falck B, Sonoo M, et al.: Muli-MUP
EMG analysis—a two-year experience with a quan-
titative method in daily routine. Electroencephalogr
Clin Neurophysiol 1995;97:145–154.

37. Stålberg E, Fawcett PRW: Macro EMG changes in
healthy subjects of different ages. J Neurol Neurosurg Psychiatry 1982;45:870–878.

38. Stålberg E, Grimby G: Dynamic EMG and biopsy
changes in a 4-year follow-up study of patients with
history of polio. Muscle Nerve 1995;18:699–707.

39. Stålberg E, Hilton-Brown P, Rydin E: Capacity of
the motor neuron to alter its peripheral field. In:
Dimitrijevic M, Kakulas BA, Vrobova G, eds. Pro-

gressive neuromuscular diseases; Recent achievements in restorative neurology. Vol 2. Basel, Karger 1984;237–253.

40. Stålberg E, Sanders DB: Electrophysiological tests of neuromuscular transmission. In: Stålberg E, Young R, eds. Clinical neurophysiology. London: Butterworths, 1981.

41. Stålberg E, Sanders DB: The motor unit in ALS studied with different neurophysiological techniques. In: Rose FC, ed. Research progress in motor neurone disease. London: Pitman, 1984.

42. Stålberg E, Schwartz MS, Thiele B, et al.: The normal motor unit in man. J Neurol Sci 1976;27:291–301.

43. Stålberg E, Sonoo M, Ahrari S: Assesment of the variability in motor unit shape at consecutive discharges. Muscle Nerve 1994;17:1135–1144.

44. Stålberg E, Thiele B: Transmission block in terminal nerve twigs: A single fibre electromyographic finding in man. J Neurol Neurosurg Psychiatry 1972;35:52–59.

45. Stålberg E, Trontelj JV: Demonstration of axon reflexes in human motor nerve fibers. J Neurol Neurosurg Psychiatry 1970;33:571–579.

46. Stålberg E, Trontelj JV: Clinical neurophysiology: the motor unit in myopathy. In: Rowland LP, DiMauro S, eds. Handbook of clinical neurology, Vol 18: Myopathies. Amsterdam: Elsevier, 1992.

47. Stålberg E, Trontelj JV: Single fiber electromyography in healthy and diseased muscle. New York: Raven Press, 1994.

48. Trontelj JV, Stålberg E: Single motor end-plates in myasthenia gravis and LEMS at different firing rates. Muscle Nerve 1991;14:226–232.

49. Wiechers DO, Hubbell SL: Late changes in the motor unit after acute poliomyelitis. Muscle Nerve 1981;4:524–528.

50. Willison RG: Arrangement of muscle fibres in healthy and dystrophic muscle in man. J Neurol Neurosurg Psychiatry 1980;27:386–394.

Chapter 6

Evaluation of The Patient with Possible Radiculopathy

Albert C. Clairmont
Ernest W. Johnson

The patient who presents with leg or arm pain and is referred to the electromyographer is often suspected of having radiculopathy. In the case of a clear history of an acute precipitating event, with corroborative physical examination and imaging studies, the referral source may request electromyography (EMG) for an additional confirmation or a prognosis. In other cases, the history, physical findings, and imaging studies may be equivocal or discordant, especially regarding the exact level affected. In this case, the EMG can precisely identify the level of radiculopathy. It is important to note that the level involved per EMG does not always correspond to that suggested by imaging studies. This is because the EMG evaluates functional neurophysiology, whereas imaging studies show anatomy (5, 6, 10, 17, 19, 22). For example, the direction in which the L5-S1 disc usually protrudes involves the S1 nerve root. A far lateral protrusion may involve L5, and a medial protrusion may involve S2. Therefore, the EMG would accurately identify the nerve root affected; that may or may not correspond to the disc level identified by the imaging study.

PRACTICAL ANATOMY FOR RADICULOPATHY

Electrodiagnosis of radiculopathy requires a through knowledge of surface and peripheral neuroanatomy. All muscles acting on the limbs are plurisegmentally innervated except the rhomboids, which receive motor fibers only from C5. The rest of the limb muscles have two or more nerve roots supplying them.

Therefore, it is useful to understand that the distribution of the motor axons from the roots generally occurs proximally to distally, anteriorly to posteriorly, and medially to laterally as the roots go cephalad to caudad.

Although there is considerable overlap superficially in the lumbar paraspinals, one usually can isolate the appropriate root level by deep penetration of the paraspinal muscle bulk by the electrode. Distribution of the lumbosacral root levels occurs directly lateral to the lumbar spinous processes. There is no S2 representation in the paraspinal muscles. The S2 anterior primary rami can be studied only by exploring the gluteus maximus, the soleus, and the intrinsic muscles of the foot.

S3/S4 anterior primary rami can be investigated by exploring the external anal sphincter and the external urethral sphincter. In the cervical paraspinals, the root levels are caudal to the related spinous processes. Needle exploration of the more caudal extent of the cervical paraspinals is necessary for adequate evaluation of these muscles (Fig. 6–1).

GUIDES FOR ANATOMY IN RADICULOPATHY

In the upper limb, the only C6 motor distribution below the elbow anteriorly and medially is to the pronator teres. Anteriorly and laterally, the distribution is to the brachioradialis muscle. The only C6 motor distribution on the posterior aspect of the forearm below the elbow is to the extensor carpi radialis and supinator. There is no C7 motor distribution below the wrist. Hand intrinsics are supplied by

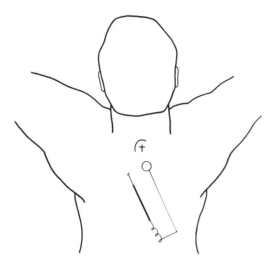

Figure 6-1. Needle electrode exploring appropriate level of cervical paraspinal muscles for C6 radiculopathy. Note the caudal extent of the position.

C8 and T1, with C8 more radialward and T1 more ulnarward.

In the lower limb, the only L4 motor distribution below the knee is to the anterior tibial muscle, and the only L5 motor distribution below the ankle is to the extensor digitorum brevis muscle.

PLANNING THE EMG

A properly performed EMG begins with an appropriately detailed history and physical examination. Pertinent positives and negatives with regard to sensory, motor, and reflex function, are noted.

Case 1

The patient is a 40-year-old mechanic who slipped on a wet, greasy floor two weeks prior to evaluation. He tried to prevent the fall by grabbing an overhead beam. This caused his neck to jerk strongly, and he felt something snap in his neck. He now presents with persistent neck pain and poorly localized right shoulder pain referred down the arm. There is numbness of the thumb. Physical examination shows some weakness of resisted external rotation of the right shoulder and abduction of the shoulder, especially through the first 30°. On resisted forward thrust of the outstretched arm, slight winging of the inferior pole of the scapula, with medial shift toward the spine, is noted. Muscle testing in other muscle groups of the upper limbs is normal. Sensory dysfunction of the thumb is equivocal, and no

other obvious sensory deficit is identified. He has an asymmetric biceps muscle stretch reflex (MSR), the right being less active.

Differential diagnosis in this patient includes cervical radiculopathy, brachial plexus stretch injury, and localized shoulder mechanism injury with pain inhibition weakness. The physician concludes that cervical radiculopathy is most likely, based on history and physical findings, and seeks corroborative evidence through electrodiagnosis. EMG examination in this patient begins with nerve conduction studies. Delayed latencies of sensory nerve action potentials (SNAPs) and slowed conduction velocities will alert one to the possibility of concurrent neuropathy. Median and radial nerve SNAPs are evaluated for differences in amplitude compared to reference values and compared side to side. In radiculopathy with axonal injury, the SNAPs may show normal latency and conduction velocity but reduced amplitude if the compromise occurs at or distal to the dorsal ganglion (Fig. 6–2). Comparison with the unaffected side should help highlight the problem. In this patient, amplitude of the right radial and median SNAP to digit I is reduced.

Flexor carpi radialis (FCR) H reflex should be done (Fig. 6–3). Unilateral delay or absence of the FCR H reflex on the affected side suggests pathology of either or both of the C6 or C7 spinal nerves. Delay of more than 1 msec side-to-side suggests slowing or blocking. Occasionally, one comes across unexpected delay or another abnormality of the FCR H reflex on the clinically uninvolved side. In such cases, imaging studies may

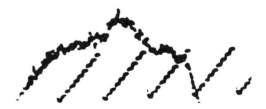

Figure 6-2. Antidromic SNAP Digit I in C6 radiculopathy. *Top trace:* Antidromic radial SNAP (Digit I). *Bottom trace:* Antidromic median SNAP (Digit I). (Caliber: Each slanted = 1 msec. Height = 10 μV. Ring recording electrodes over Digit I, 10 cm from stimulation.) Note that latencies are normal but amplitudes are reduced by over 100%.

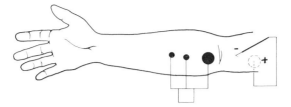

Figure 6–3. Electrode placement for H-reflex latency in flexor carpi radialis. The stimulating needle electrode (cathode) is over the median nerve. The anode is on the opposite side of the arm.

corroborate abnormal anatomy in a patient who is asymptomatic on that side (18). FCR H reflex is not affected in lesions of C5 or C8 spinal nerves.

Next, one should compare compound motor action potential (CMAP) of the weak muscle(s) with the uninvolved side. One can either directly stimulate the spinal nerve supplying the muscle with a needle electrode or stimulate the peripheral nerve supplying it. One should use surface electrodes for recording. Both amplitude and area under the negative spike are satisfactory indices of axonal loss. A meticulously performed stimulation may show a normal side-to-side difference in amplitude of about 10%. A reduction of 40% is compatible with true weakness in the clinically weak muscle group. Reduction of 50% or more suggests a less favorable prognosis for recovery of normal function, if performed after 5 days. Our patient shows a 35% reduction in amplitude of the right infraspinatus CMAP versus the left.

In this patient, median and ulnar nerve conduction studies are normal. Next, needle EMG of the affected upper limb and paraspinals is done. Whenever abnormal findings are identified, the corresponding muscle on the unaffected side must be explored. The electromyographer should sample several muscles supplied by the suspected diseased root and many muscles supplied by roots above and below that level. Table 6–1 shows the result of the needle EMG in case 1.

Summary of findings:
A 40-year-old male with a history of acute onset of neck and right upper limb pain. Physical examination reveals weakness limited to muscles with primarily a C6 root innervation. He has an asymmetric biceps muscle stretch reflex. Radial and median SNAP to digit I is reduced on the affected side, and the FCR H reflex is abnormally prolonged. Motor conduction studies show a 35% reduction in amplitude of the infraspinatus CMAP on the affected side. Needle EMG shows increased membrane irritability limited to muscles supplied by the C6 spinal nerve. There is decreased recruitment of motor units in a similar distribution, but the amplitude and duration of the MUPs are normal. Needle EMG of similar muscles on the unaffected side is unremarkable. Therefore, the diagno-

sis by EMG is acute right C6 radiculopathy. Prognosis for recovery is good.

ELECTRODIAGNOSIS OF CERVICAL RADICULOPATHY

Cervical radiculopathy is second only to lumbar radiculopathy as a cause of spinal radiculopathy. It is a common clinical problem in the person complaining of neck and arm pain. Radhakrishnan et al. (16) reported an age-adjusted incidence rate of 83.2 per 100,000 population for cervical radiculopathy in Rochester, MN. Frequency of occurrence by root level is as follows: C7 > C6 > C8 > C5.

Sensory nerve conduction studies are normal unless there is axonal loss and the lesion is at or distal to the dorsal ganglion. The FCR H reflex is often absent or delayed in lesions affecting the C6 or C7 spinal nerve. Spinal nerve stimulation can define the nature of the injury as being axonal loss or neurapraxic by stimulating the motor nerve to that muscle and noting the amplitude. When performing needle EMG of the cervical paraspinals, one should explore the more caudal extent of these muscles. In this area, the muscles are located caudal to the corresponding nerve root. Failure to explore caudally sufficiently is the most common cause of inability to find posterior ramus abnormalities in cervical radiculopathy (Fig. 6–1).

In the upper limb, the following muscles are suggested for CMAP comparison:

C5: Deltoid
C6: Infraspinatus
C7: Triceps
C8: Pronator quadratus
T1: Abductor digiti quinti

Table 6–1
Results of Needle EMG in Case 1*

Muscle (Right Upper Limb)	Root(s)	Peripheral Nerve	Membrane Irritability	No. MUAPs/ Ampl. & Duration
Rhomboid	C5	Dorsal scapular	normal	nl/nl
Supraspinatus	C5, C6	Suprascapular	increased	decr/nl
Infraspinatus	C5, C6	Suprascapular	increased	decr/nl
Pect. major (clav)	C5, C6	Medial pectoral	increased	decr/nl
Pect. min. (stern)	C7, C8, T1	Lateral pectoral	normal	nl/nl
Biceps brachii	C5, C6	Musc. cutaneous	increased	decr/nl
Serratus anterior	C5, C6, C7	Long thoracic	increased	decr/nl
Pronator teres	C6, C7	Median	increased	decr/nl
Triceps	C7, C8	Radial	normal	nl/nl
Abd. poll. brevis	C8, T1	Median	normal	nl/nl
First dorsal inter.	C8, T1	Ulnar	normal	nl/nl
Abd. digiti quinti	C8, T1	Ulnar	normal	nl/nl
Ext. indicis prop.	C7, C8	Radial	normal	nl–nl
Brachioradialis	C5, C6	Radial	increased	decr/nl
R. Cervical paraspinals	Posterior primary rami			
C2	C2		normal	
C3	C3		normal	
C4	C4		normal	
C5	C5		normal	
C6	C6		increased	
C7	C7		increased	
C8	C8		normal	
T1	T1		normal	

*MUAP: motor unit action potential; decr/nl: decreased number of MUAPs with normal amplitude and duration; nl/nl: normal. Increased membrane irritability = positive waves or fibs present.

Case 2

A 26-year-old female presents with a 6-month history of back and left lower limb pain. She experiences the most intense pain in her buttock, and describes it as deep and burning. The pain is referred to her calf. Although onset was insidious, pain has been unremitting for the past 4 months. She represents a pharmaceutical company and spends many hours driving an automobile. Additionally, her job involves frequently loading and unloading her car with product samples. She complains of numbness involving the lateral foot and lateral leg on the affected side. Climbing stairs has become very difficult for her, but she is uncertain of the reason. Physical examination reveals decreased sensory perception on the lateral foot. Left ankle jerk is slightly diminished. She can walk on her left heel but cannot perform 10 toe rises on the left. She squats and returns with some difficulty, shifting her weight to the right.

Sensory nerve conduction studies show normal superficial peroneals bilaterally. Peroneal nerve CMAP recorded from the extensor digitorum longus is normal bilaterally. Left tibial nerve CMAP stimulating at the popliteal fossa and recording from the medial gastrocnemius is 30% smaller in amplitude than the right. Initially, the H reflex is absent bilaterally. With facilitation, the right is elicited with a normal latency of 28 msec, but the left latency is prolonged by 1.5 msec. Table 6–2 shows the result of needle EMG in case 2.

Table 6–2
Results of Needle EMG in Case 2*

Muscle (Left Lower Limb)	Root(s)	Peripheral Nerve	Membrane Irritability	No. MUAPs/ Ampl. & Dur.
Adductor longus	L2, L3, L4	Obturator	normal	nl/nl
Vastus medialis	L2, L3, L4	Femoral	normal	nl/nl
Tensor fascia lata	L4, L5	Superior gluteal	normal	nl/nl
Anterior tibial	L4, L5	Deep peroneal	normal	nl/nl
Peroneus longus	L5, S1	Super. peroneal	increased	decr/incr
Ext. dig. longus	L5, S1	Deep peroneal	increased	decr/incr
Flex. dig. longus	L5, S1	Post tibial	increased	decr/incr
Medial gastroc.	S1, S2	Tibial	increased	decr/incr
Abductor hallucis	S1, S2	Tibial	increased	decr/incr
Biceps femoris	L5, S1, S2	Sciatic	increased	decr/incr
L. lumbosacral paraspinals	Posterior primary rami			
L1	L1		normal	
L2	L2		normal	
L3	L3		normal	
L4	L4		normal	
L5	L5		normal	
S1	S1		increased	

*MUAP: motor unit action potential; decr/incr: decreased number of MUAPs with increased amplitude and duration; nl/nl: normal. Increased membrane irritability = positive waves or fibs present.

Summary of findings:

A 26-year-old female with insidious onset of back and left leg pain of 6-months duration. The pain is most troublesome in the buttock. Physical examination suggests involvement of S1. Left H reflex is prolonged (1), and there is some deficit in amplitude of the corresponding medial gastrocnemius CMAP. Needle EMG shows abnormal membrane irritability only in muscles supplied by the left S1 spinal nerve. Evaluation of motor unit characteristics reveals increased amplitude and duration of motor unit potentials (MUPs) in the distribution of the affected spinal nerve. Needle EMG of the same muscles on the uninvolved side is normal. EMG diagnosis is left S1 spinal nerve compromise with ongoing degeneration and regeneration. Prognosis for eventual recovery is good.

DIAGNOSTIC VALUE OF H REFLEX IN S1 RADICULOPATHY

The H-reflex is a monosynaptic spinal reflex first described by Paul Hoffmann in 1918. It was standardized by Braddom and Johnson (1). The tibial nerve is stimulated in the popliteal fossa with needle or surface electrodes, using low voltage, 0.5 Hz stimulation, of 1-msec duration. For recording, surface electrodes are placed over the soleus muscle. The H reflex appears at 27–30 msec. (Fig. 6–4). The patient must be relaxed because mild contraction of the antagonist will inhibit the H reflex. Slight contraction of the protagonist will facilitate the reflex. Therefore, absence of the H reflex is of less importance than asymmetry of the reflex (Fig. 6–5). Latency is the most sensitive and accurate indicator in diagnosing S1 radiculopathy. Braddom and Johnson (1) calculated one standard deviation (SD) of 0.4 msec (variation side to side) and three SD of 1.2 msec. A difference in latency ≥ 1 msec lends strong support to the diagnosis of S1 radiculopathy if the history, physical

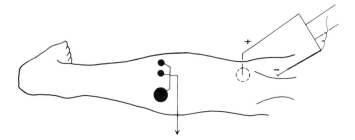

Figure 6–4. Electrode placement for H-reflex latency. The recording electrode is over the soleus, and the stimulating electrode (needle) is over the tibial nerve in the lateral popliteal space.

examination, and EMG are compatible. If the side-to-side difference is less than 1 msec but both latencies are greater than the predicted mean, one must do additional conduction studies. The value of amplitude of the H reflex remains controversial because it is dependent on many variables. A formula has been derived to predict the mean expected latency:

H-reflex Diagnostic Value

Latency of involved side is more than 1 msec greater than contralateral

Amplitude: Unproved value

Absence of H-reflex: **Less** important

Asymmetry of H-reflex: **Very** important

Figure 6–5. Diagnostic value of H-reflex latency in S1 radiculopathy.

6.14 (a constant) + 0.46 × (length in cm from medial malleolus to popliteal stimulation) + 0.1 × (age in years) = predicted mean latency.

The H reflex is useful:

- If EMG abnormalities on needle examination are limited to paraspinal muscles and the H reflex is prolonged; this suggests S1 radiculopathy. If H-reflex latencies are normal side to side, L5 radiculopathy is likely because the majority of lumbosacral radiculopathies are L5 or S1. The preponderance of L5 and S1 radiculopathies has been well documented (9, 10, 13, 23).
- If EMG abnormalities are inconclusive.
- When radicular symptoms are present for only a few days.
- If recurrent radiculopathy occurs in which paraspinal abnormalities are inconclusive.

Pease (15) and coworkers used S1 spinal nerve stimulation to elicit the H reflex. They calculated slowing of nerve conduction velocity within the S1 root by dividing the latency of the S1 spinal nerve response by the recorded ipsilateral H-reflex latency to get the S1 ratio. The S1 ratio provides a way to evaluate slowing within the spinal canal compared

to more peripheral conduction. The normal value for the S1 ratio is 0.48 msec, with 1 SD of 0.12 msec. Thus, a difference of 0.5 msec or more is diagnostically helpful. Sine (20) and colleagues have developed a technique for studying nerve conduction along proximal nerves and nerve roots. They deliver supramaximal stimuli to tibial and peroneal nerves within the popliteal space and record compound nerve action potentials (CNAPs) from an epidural needle electrode at the L4–L5 interspace. With this method, it was common to find a 25% decrement in CNAP amplitude on the clinically involved side, compared to the uninvolved side at the same level. By adjusting the pulse duration to 0.5 msec and using a current intensity predetermined by soleus-recording testing, they could obtain an H reflex to which they then applied the usual clinical criteria for interpretation.

Case 3

This 35-year-old construction worker noted acute onset of back pain while carrying a 50-pound bucket of cement 4 days prior to evaluation. He finished working, but that evening began to notice right buttock pain. The following morning, he experienced excruciating pain and found it difficult to get out of bed. Although the back pain was still present, he reports that the deep ache in his buttock was far more distressing than the back pain. In addition, he has noticed numbness of his affected leg and dorsal foot. Physical examination shows weakness of right big toe extension. He finds it difficult to walk on his heels. There is mild sensory deficit to light touch and pin prick on the dorsal right foot, the left being normal.

The electromyographer starts with needle EMG of the affected limb and related paraspinals. No abnormal membrane irritability is present in any limb muscle and a decrease in the number of motor units is noted in muscles supplied by L5 and S1. The paraspinals are remarkable for the presence of early polyphasics at L5 and S1 (Fig. 6–6). Table 6–3 shows the result of needle EMG in case 3.

Next, the electromyographer compares the CMAPs in affected and unaffected muscle and side to side. In this case, it can be helpful to use spinal nerve stimulation (Fig. 6–7). The L5 spinal nerve stimulation shows a 10% reduction in amplitude of the right extensor digitorum longus CMAP. This difference is considered significant by Chang (2), but not necessarily Colachis (3). However, Chang recorded from the anterior tibial muscle, and Colachis recorded from the extensor digitorum longus, so their findings are not directly comparable.

In the lower limb, the following muscles are suggested for CMAP comparison:

L4: Anterior tibial or vastus medialis
L5: Extensor digitorum longus
S1: Medial gastrocnemius

Performing an H reflex will help to identify the level of the lesion. In this case, the H reflex is normal bilaterally, suggesting normal neurophysi-

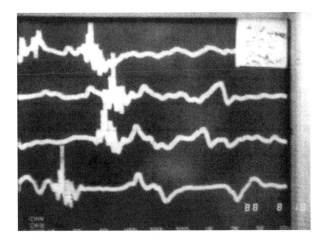

Figure 6-6. "Early" polyphasic MUP in acute radiculopathy. Monopolar needle electrode in extensor digitorum longus muscle. Duration of symptoms is 5 days. (Caliber: Line width = 10 msec/division. Line height = 200 µV/division.) (Reprinted with permission from Colachis SC, Pease WS, Johnson EW: Polyphasic motor unit action potentials in early radiculopathy: their presence and ephaptic transmission as an hypothesis. Electromyogr Clin Neurophysiol 1992;32:27–33.)

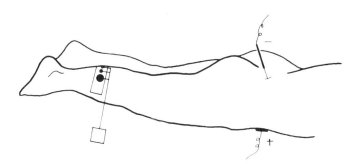

Figure 6-7. S1 spinal nerve root stimulation. Monopolar needle electrode is inserted 1 cm to 2 cm medial to the posterior superior iliac spine. Anode is placed on the anterior trunk opposite the needle.

Table 6–3
Results of Needle EMG in Case 3*

Muscle (Right Lower Limb)	Root(s)	Peripheral Nerve	Membrane Irritability	No. MUAPs/ Ampl. & Duration
Adductor longus	L2, L3, L4	Obturator	normal	nl/nl
Vastus medialis	L2, L3, L4	Femoral	normal	nl/nl
Tensor fascia lata	L4, L5	Superior gluteal	normal	decr/nl
Anterior tibial	L4, L5	Deep peroneal	normal	nl/nl
Peroneus longus	L5, S1	Super. peroneal	normal	decr/nl
Ext. hall. longus	L5, S1	Deep peroneal	normal	decr/nl
Flex. dig. longus	L5, S1	Post tibial	normal	decr/nl
Lateral gastroc.	S1, S2	Tibial	normal	nl/nl
Abductor hallucis	S1, S2	Tibial	normal	nl/nl
Biceps femoris	L5, S1, S2	Sciatic	normal	decr/nl
Gluteus medius	L4, L5, S1	Superior gluteal	normal	decr/nl
Gluteus maximus	L5, S1, S2	Inferior gluteal	normal	decr/nl
R. Lumbosacral paraspinals	Posterior primary rami			
L1	L1		normal	
L2	L2		normal	
L3	L3		normal	
L4	L4		normal	
L5	L5		early polyphasics	
S1	S1		early polyphasics	

*MUAP: motor unit action potential; decr/nl: decreased number of MUAPs with normal amplitude and duration; nl/nl: normal.

ology of S1 and thus probable right L5 spinal nerve compromise. If the H reflex is longer than predicted, one should do sensory nerve conduction studies to uncover any underlying neuropathy. In this patient, normal superficial peroneal and sural SNAPs are obtained bilaterally.

Summary of findings:
A 35-year-old patient with acute onset of back and lower limb pain. Physical findings suggest lumbosacral radiculopathy. Motor and sensory nerve conduction studies are not diagnostic. Needle EMG shows a decreased recruitment of motor units in the L5–S1 distribution. The only abnormality in the paraspinals is the presence of early polyphasic motor units (MUP) at L5 and S1 (the significance of the early polyphasic MUP will be discussed later). A normal H reflex places the lesion most likely at L5 because 95% of lumbo-sacral radiculopathies are at L5 or S1.

REVIEW OF EVALUATION OF POSSIBLE L5 RADICULOPATHY

History

The primary presenting feature of lumbar radiculopathy is pain. Onset can be acute or insidious. It usually starts in the back. A day or two later, radicular pain begins, most frequently in the buttocks. Radicular pain is almost always in the lateral buttock and then the posterior thigh, calf, or lateral shin. It is often present in the ankle or heel.

Pain is usually worst upon sitting and is especially aggravated when driving a car. There is less while standing, and least in the recumbent, side-lying position on a hard surface. See Table 6–4 for physical examination.

Table 6–4
Physical Examination

	Muscle Stretch Reflex Reduced	Weakness
L4	Quadriceps	Knee extensors
L5	Biceps femoris	Toe extensors
S1	Gastroc-soleus	Plantar flexors
C6	Biceps brachii	Ext. shoulder rotators
C7	Triceps brachii	Elbow extensors
C8	Flexor carpi radialis	Wrist flexors

ELECTRODIAGNOSIS

Place the patient prone over pillows. The electrodiagnostician should follow this sequence of steps in the examination:

1. Do a needle study of the paraspinals bilaterally, and record any spontaneous activity.
2. Do a needle study of weak limb muscles. Look for spontaneous activity and determine the recruitment interval.
3. Check for early "polyphasics" in steps 1 and 2.
4. Determine the H-reflex latency of both limbs.

5. Do a spinal nerve stimulation using surface electrodes for recording of the CMAP. Compare the area under the negative spike of the involved and uninvolved sides. Alternatively, turn the patient over and stimulate the weak muscle. Again, use surface electrodes for recording. Compare the amplitude and area if possible.
6. Do sensory nerve conduction studies to evaluate for other possible causes of neuropathy.

THE EARLY POLYPHASIC MUP

Several authors have described an abnormally high percentage of polyphasic MUPs present in the distribution of the affected nerve root early in the radiculopathy. Colachis and colleagues (4) reported 20 cases of cervical and lumbar radiculopathy in which they observed these polyphasics within 1–3 weeks of the onset of symptoms. They proposed a possible explanation (Fig. 6–8). They hypothesized that whenever a motor nerve root is inflamed, the possibility exists for ephaptic activation of a neighboring axon by an axon made active volitionally. The second axon is stimulated synchronously at the spinal nerve level with the one volitionally made active. Because of the slight variation in conduction, however, it

Early Polyphasic M.U.P

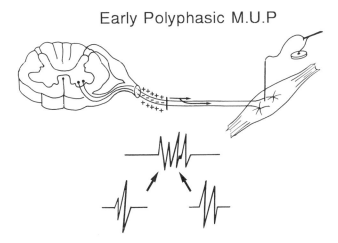

Figure 6–8. Hypothesis to explain "early" polyphasic MUP in acute radiculopathy. Ephaptic transmission between adjacent nerve axons in the region of the inflamed root results in synchronous, but not simultaneous, firing of two or more motor units. (Reprinted with permission from Colachis SC, Pease WS, Johnson EW: Polyphasic motor unit action potentials in early radiculopathy: their presence and ephaptic transmission as an hypothesis. Electromyogr Clin Neurophysiol 1992;32:27–33.)

reaches the muscle at a slightly different time, making synchronous but not simultaneous activation of their respective motor units (MUs). Thus two or three MUs appear as a single polyphasic MUP. Note that these polyphasics can occur from the onset of inflammation in the nerve root; thus the term, "early polyphasic." Clinically, one observes MUP activity that is highly polyphasic. Awareness of the early polyphasic MUP in radiculopathy provides the astute electromyographer with an additional tool with which to diagnose radiculopathy prior to the onset of fibrillation activity, which takes 7–21 days to develop.

Case 4

The patient is a 29-year-old veteran paratrooper referred from the gastroenterology service of a tertiary care center for the evaluation of visceral pain. He relates that one year ago he was involved in night-time maneuvers. He jumped and landed on a vehicle that was not supposed to be there. The veteran experienced acute back pain. Imaging studies showed a mild compression fracture of the T9 vertebra without displacement or instability. He was treated by cast application. As his back pain resolved, he began to experience poorly localized visceral pain that has become progressively more intense. He also reports numbness involving the anterior and left lateral abdominal wall. Evaluation by the gastroenterology service failed to show an organic reason for his complaints.

Physical examination reveals equivocal sensory deficit to pinprick and light touch in a distribution that corresponds somewhat with the area in which he perceives numbness. There is easily reproducible hyperesthesia in a small area of the left thoracic paraspinals at T10; otherwise the physical exam is normal. EMG of the lower six thoracic paraspinals is normal bilaterally. There are abnormal findings in the left T10 intercostal muscle and the left anterior abdominal wall muscles (AAWM), the right being normal (Table 6–5). EMG diagnosis is left T10 radiculopathy.

Thoracic radiculopathy is rare. It can occur in association with vertebral compression fractures of the dorsal spine. It can also be present at one or two levels in diabetes mellitus. Evaluating the patient with thoracic radiculopathy is difficult because there are no well-established sensory or motor nerve conduction studies for evaluating thoracic radiculopathy.

One should explore intercostally or abdominally for anterior primary distribution. Also, in the diabetic patient, it is not unusual to find abnormal membrane irritability at many levels in thoracic and lumbar paraspinal muscles, without evidence of specific radiculopathy. One examines the anterior and posterior distribution of the spinal nerve to verify radiculopathy. The most accessible muscles are the paraspinals, the intercostals, and the AAWMs. The rectus abdominis and the external abdominal obliques are supplied by the T7–T12 spinal nerves. Because of overlap, it is not possible to precisely locate the root level of innervation of a specific AAWM. Generally, the xiphoid level is supplied by T6, the umbilicus by T10, and the suprapubic region by T12. Needle EMG of the AAWM is performed with the patient laying supine. The needle electrode is inserted either perpendicularly or at a slight angle. Placement is confirmed by voluntary activation of the muscles. Any maneuver that causes activation of the muscles is satisfactory. Flexion of the neck or beginning abdominal crunch will likely produce adequate contraction. Streib (21) found that voluntary activation of the rectus abdominis was best achieved by neck flexion, and voluntary activation of the external abdominal obliques, by pelvic tilt. The electromyographer should explore with the needle electrode in the usual manner, noting abnormal insertional activity. One should then activate the selected muscle and evaluate for acute and chronic MUP changes in the usual manner.

Chronology of Electrodiagnosis in Radiculopathy

It is possible to observe several abnormalities on EMG from the onset of inflammation with accompanying pain in the nerve root (Table 6–4). If the weakness is less than 4/5 (MRC system), it is recognizable as a reduced recruitment pattern on maximal contraction. Stimulation studies and analysis of the CMAP will help one decide if the injury is neurapraxic or permanent (Fig. 6–9). If the weakness is minimal, it may be difficult to recognize the pattern as being reduced during maximal contraction. However, the electromyographer, using a minimal contraction, can observe a reduced recruitment interval. In early, mild L5 radiculopathy, Pease et al. (14) showed a recruitment interval of 70–90 msecs in the extensor digitorum longus, as compared to a normal interval of 100–120 msecs (Fig. 6–10). In unilateral radiculopathy, it is best to compare the recruitment interval of the involved muscle with the same muscle on the unaffected side.

From the onset of radiculopathy, the H-reflex latency is prolonged in S1 radiculopa-

Table 6–5
Results of Needle EMG in Case 4*

Muscle (L. Ant. Abd. Wall)	Root(s)	Peripheral Nerve	Membrane Irritability	No. MUAPs/ Ampl. & Dur.
Rectus abdominis	T7	intercostal	normal	nl/nl
Rectus abdominis	T8	intercostal	normal	nl/nl
Rectus abdominis	T9	intercostal	normal	nl/nl
Rectus abdominis	T10	intercostal	increased	decr/incr
Rectus abdominis	T11	intercostal	normal	nl/nl
Rectus abdominis	T12	subcostal	normal	nl/nl
Ext. abd. oblique	T7	intercostal	normal	nl/nl
Ext. abd. oblique	T8	intercostal	normal	nl/nl
Ext. abd. oblique	T9	intercostal	normal	nl/nl
Ext. abd. oblique	T10	intercostal	increased	decr/incr
Ext. abd. oblique	T11	intercostal	increased	decr/incr
Ext. abd. oblique	T12	subcostal	normal	nl/nl
Left intercostal	T10	intercostal	increased	decr/incr
L. Thoracic paraspinals	Post. prim. rami			
T7	T7		normal	
T8	T8		normal	
T9	T9		normal	
T10	T10		normal	
T11	T11		normal	
T12	T12		normal	

*MUAP: motor unit action potential; decr/incr: decreased number of MUAPs with increased amplitude and duration; nl/nl: normal.

thy. A latency difference of more than 1 msec from the normal limb is suggestive of S1 radiculopathy (Fig. 6–11). Similarly, in cervical radiculopathy involving C6 or C7, the H-reflex latency in FCR is prolonged. A side-to-side difference of more than 0.8 msec (18) is abnormal. F-wave latency has not proved helpful.

During the first few days after the onset of radiculopathy, spontaneous activity in the form of the early polyphasic MUP can be present (4). When present, early polyphasic MUP activity usually appears before other types of abnormal spontaneous activity. Approximately 7 to 8 days after the onset of radicular symptoms, positive sharp waves can be evoked in the appropriate paraspinal muscles. If this is the only finding in suspected lumbosacral radiculopathy, H-reflex measurement can be used to differentiate L5 from S1 disease.

By 13 to 14 days, positive waves may be present in proximal limb muscles and fibrillation potentials in the paraspinal muscles.

By 18 to 21 days, proximal and distal muscles in the distribution of the radiculopathy should show abnormalities, though not necessarily to the same degree.

If there has been substantial axonal death, reinnervation potentials that are long-duration MUPs can appear within 4 to 6 weeks. As they mature, some may appear as satellite potentials (Fig. 6–12). Months to years later, reinnervation potentials are recognized as synchronized MUPs of increased amplitude.

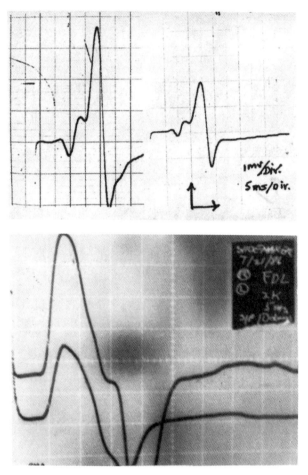

Figure 6-9. Reduced CMAP in acute radiculopathy. *Top.* Medial gastrocnemius CMAP in S radiculopathy (R); normal extremity (L). (Caliber: On photo.) *Bottom.* Extensor digitorum longus CMAP in L5 radiculopathy (*Bottom trace*); normal extremity (*Top trace*). (Caliber: Square = 5 msec, 2 mV)

Chronic Radiculopathies and Recurrent Radiculopathies

Evaluation of recurrent radiculopathies is a frequent and often difficult problem. Comparison with previous electrodiagnostic studies is most helpful. If the previous radiculopathy is severe, one would expect the muscle fibers to atrophy. Therefore, the fibrillation potentials would be small in contrast to recent denervation, when the fibrillation potentials would be larger. Kraft (12) measured the maximum peak-to-peak amplitude of fibrillation potentials in 69 patients between 7 days and 10-1/2 years after partial or complete peripheral nerve injury. He found that the mean amplitude during the first 2 months was 612 μV, progressively declining to 320 μV in the fifth

to sixth month and no greater than 100 μV after 1 year. He sectioned the sciatic nerve of guinea pigs and studied the animals for up to 17 weeks. He noticed a decline in fibrillation potential amplitude in guinea pigs, comparable to that in humans, over time. Also, by the end of the guinea pig study, Type I fibers had lost about half their initial diameter and Type II had atrophied significantly more than that.

If reinnervation has occurred, the proportion of polyphasic MUPs will have increased, with a concurrent increase in amplitude and duration. Reinnervation may occur as early as 5 to 6 weeks after injury. Single fiber EMG is useful in following the progress of reinnervation. Complex repetitive discharges may be recorded in chronic radiculopathies. These discharges result from activation of a dener-

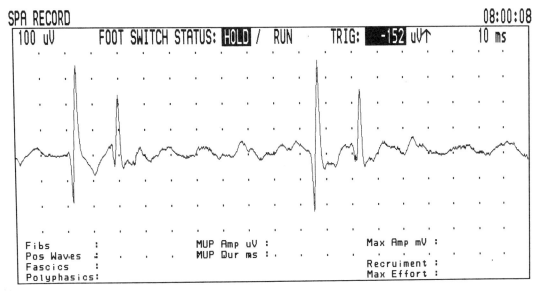

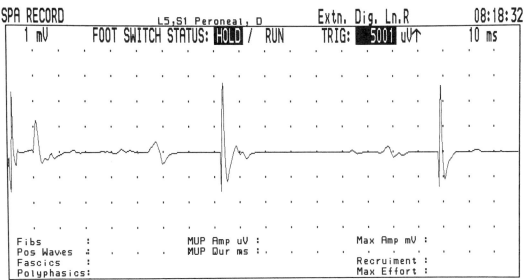

Figure 6-10. Recruitment interval (RI). *Top trace*: Normal patient. Note that the first MU is firing at 10 Hz when the second unit begins to activate. RI = 100 msec, recruitment frequency = 10 Hz. (Caliber: Each square = 10 msec, 500 μV.) *Bottom trace*: Patient with L5 radiculopathy. Note that the first MU is firing at 12.5 Hz when the second unit begins to activate. RI = 80 msec, recruitment frequency = 12.5 Hz. (Caliber: Each square = 10 msec, 1 mV. Monopolar needle electrode in extensor digitorum longus.)

vated muscle fiber that acts as a pacemaker by ephaptic transmission to neighboring dener-vated muscle fibers (Fig. 6–13).

Case 5

A 60-year-old woman presents with the history of sudden onset of right thigh pain 2 months ago. She complains of weakness of the right lower limb, and has noticed atrophy of the thigh. She gives a history of insulin-dependent diabetes mellitus that has been poorly controlled. On physical examination, there is decreased sensory perception in a glove and stocking distribution. Muscle stretch reflexes are normal in the upper limbs and left knee. The ankle jerk is diminished but symmetrical bilaterally. The right knee jerk cannot be elicited. Atrophy of the right thigh is pronounced. Muscle strength

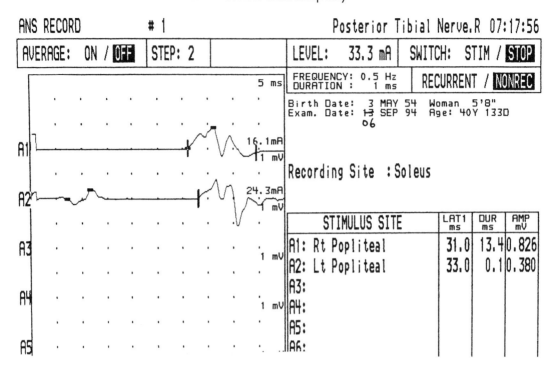

ANS RECORD	# 1	Posterior Tibial Nerve.R 07:17:56

AVERAGE: ON / **OFF** | STEP: 2 | LEVEL: 33.3 mA | SWITCH: STIM / **STOP**

5 ms

FREQUENCY: 0.5 Hz | RECURRENT / **NONREC**
DURATION : 1 ms

A1   16.1mA   1 mV

Birth Date: 3 MAY 54   Woman 5'8"
Exam. Date: ~~13~~ SEP 94   Age: 40Y 133D
       06

A2   24.3mA   mV

Recording Site : Soleus

STIMULUS SITE	LAT1 ms	DUR ms	AMP mV
A1: Rt Popliteal	31.0	13.4	0.826
A2: Lt Popliteal	33.0	0.1	0.380
A3:			
A4:			
A5:			
A6:			

A3   1 mV

A4   1 mV

A5

Figure 6–11. Prolonged H-reflex latency in S1 radiculopathy. *Top trace* (A1): Normal side. *Bottom trace* (A2): S1 radiculopathy. (Caliber: 5 msec, 1 mV; stimulate the tibial nerve at the popliteal space; surface recording over soleus.) Note the 2-msec difference between normal and abnormal sides.

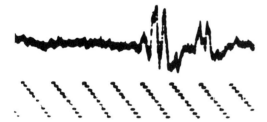

Figure 6–12. Polyphasic MUP in chronic radiculopathy. (Caliber: Each slanted line = 10 msec. Height = 200 μV. Monopolar needle electrode in infraspinatus.) Note that the satellite potential occurs 10 msec after major AP.

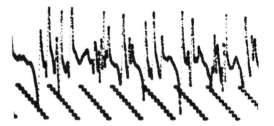

Figure 6–13. Complex repetitive discharge in posterior cervical muscles in C6 radiculopathy. (Caliber: Each slanted line = 10 msec. Height = 100 μV. Monopolar needle electrode in cervical paraspinal at C6 level.)

testing shows a 3/5 right knee extension and a 5/5 left knee extension. Resisted hip adduction gives a 4/5 on the right side and a 5/5 on the left. Right ankle dorsiflexion is a 4/5, and left ankle dorsiflexion is a 5/5. Ankle plantar flexion is 4+/5 bilaterally. Otherwise, muscle strength testing gives normal results. Imaging studies of the lumbosacral spine give normal results.

Electrodiagnostic Findings

Superficial peroneal sensory and sural SNAPs are unobtainable bilaterally. Median, ulnar, and radial nerve SNAPs are present bilaterally, but show slowed conduction velocity and decreased amplitude. Bilateral median, ulnar, tibial, and peroneal motor nerve conduction studies show slowing and some decreased CMAP amplitude. L4 spinal nerve stimulation reveals a 50% decrement of CMAP on the right. The H reflex is present and symmetrical, but abnormally prolonged.

Needle EMG shows diffuse abnormalities in the lower thoracic and lumbosacral paraspinal muscles, with more involvement localized at L3 and L4 on the right. In the lower limbs, abnormal membrane irritability is recorded diffusely in the foot intrinsics bilaterally. Pronounced, floridly abnormal mem-

Table 6–6
Results of Needle EMG in Case 5*

Muscle (Right Lower Limb)	Root(s)	Peripheral Nerve	Membrane Irritability	No. MUAPs/ Ampl. & Dur.
Iliopsoas	L2, L3	Femoral	incr ++	decr/nl
Adductor longus	L2, L3, L4	Obturator	incr +++	few/mix
Vastus medialis	L2, L3, L4	Femoral	incr ++++	few/mix
Tensor fascia lata	L4, L5	Superior glut.	incr ++	decr/mix
Anterior tibial	L4, L5	Deep per.	incr ++	decr/mix
Peroneus longus	L5, S1	Super. per.	normal	nl/nl
Ext. dig. longus	L5, S1	Deep per.	normal	nl/nl
Ext. hall. longus	L5, S1	Deep per.	normal	nl/nl
Flex. dig. longus	L5, S1	Post tibial	normal	nl/nl
Lateral gastroc.	S1, S2	Tibial	normal	nl/nl
Abductor hallucis	S1, S2	Tibial	incr (<+)	dec/occ large
1st dors. interos.	S1, S2	Sciatic	incr (<+)	dec/occ large
Gluteus maximus	L5, S1, S2	Inf. glut.	normal	nl/nl
R. lumbosacral paraspinals	Post. prim. rami			
T10–L1	T10–L1		+	
L2	L2		++	
L3	L3		++++	
L4	L4		++++	
L5	L5		++	
S1	S1		+	

*MUAP: motor unit action potential; decr/nl: decreased number of MUAPs with normal amplitude and duration; decr/mix: decreased number of MUAPs; the MUAPs are a mixture of normal and large-amplitude, long duration; few/mix: few MUAPs. They are a mixture of normal and large-amplitude, long duration; dec/occ large: slightly decreased number of MUAPs; occasionally, MUAPs of abnormally large amplitude and duration are recorded; nl/nl: normal.

brane irritability is recorded in the peripheral muscles supplied by the right L3 and L4 spinal nerves (Table 6–6). No corresponding abnormality is observed in the muscles supplied by the left L3 and L4 spinal nerves.

A patient with diabetic neuropathy can present with pain and atrophy of the thigh. Previously, this was thought to be a femoral mononeuropathy. Careful electrodiagnostic study has established this syndrome as being a multiple lumbar radiculopathy (8, 11). Dural nerve root sleeve compromise of vulnerable nerves in the diabetic patient is probably an etiologic factor. Imaging studies are usually normal. The sensory and motor conduction abnormalities result from long-standing peripheral neuropathy with both axonal and myelin damage. Similarly, diffuse, low-grade, chronic axonal loss that characteristically is worse peripherally, accounts for the

motor unit changes and increased membrane irritability in the foot intrinsics bilaterally.

Radiculopathies occur with the same frequency as other entrapment sites in individuals with generalized peripheral neuropathies and should always be considered in the diagnosis.

SUMMARY

Electrodiagnosis is an essential tool in the diagnosis and management of radiculopathy. It is helpful from the onset of radiculopathy. Measuring the recruitment interval, comparing the CMAP of the weak muscle to the patient's uninvolved side, observing early polyphasics, and measuring the H-reflex latency can give useful information before the traditional time period of 3 weeks after onset. Electrodiagnostic studies (EDX) provide information about the location and extent of the neurophysiologic dysfunction. EDX can be used as a confirmation of the loss of function suggested by imaging studies, e.g., magnetic resonance imaging (MRI). Imaging studies mostly evaluate structure and in many instances are misleading (7). The EDX examination is necessary to follow all stages of the clinical course of radiculopathy as well as to assist in determining the prognosis.

For a patient with radiculopathy, the following guidelines will help the electromyographer perform needle exploration of the fewest areas possible while still performing an adequate examination:

- Choose muscles of the suspected spinal nerve level innervated by at least two different peripheral nerves.
- Select one proximal muscle and one distal muscle at the suspected spinal nerve level; also investigate one level above and one level below.
- Explore the appropriate paraspinal level including the contralateral side.
- Examine one muscle in the contralateral uninvolved limb. This should be the same muscle as the most involved one on the affected or symptomatic limb.

References

1. Braddom RI, Johnson EW: Standardization of H reflex and diagnostic use in Sl radiculopathy. Arch Phys Med Rehabil 1974;55(4):161–166.
2. Chang CW, Lien IN: Spinal nerve stimulation in the diagnosis of lumbosacral radiculopathy. Am J Phys Med Rehabil 1990;69(6):318–322.
3. Colachis SC, Klejka JP, Shamir DY, et al.: Amplitude of M responses. Side to side comparability. Am J Phys Med Rehabil 1993;72(1):19–22.
4. Colachis SC, Pease WS, Johnson EW: Polyphasic motor unit action potentials in early radiculopathy: Their presence and ephaptic transmission as an hypothesis. Electromyogr Clin Neurophysiol 1992;32:27–33.
5. Haldeman S, Shouka M, Robboy S: Computed tomography, electrodiagnostic, and clinical findings in chronic workers' compensation patients with back and leg pain. Spine 1988;13(3):345–350.
6. Jebsen RH: Electrodiagnosis in nerve root syndromes. Northwest Medicine 1966;65(February):107–111.
7. Jensen MC, Brant-Zawadzki MN, Obuchowski N, et al.: Magnetic resonance imaging of the lumbar spine in people without back pain [see comments]. N Engl J Med 1994;331(2):69–73.
8. Johnson EW: Conservative management of cervical disc disease. In: B DS, ed. Cervical spondylosis. New York: Raven Press, 1981:145–153.
9. Johnson EW, Fletcher FR: Lumbosacral radioculopathy: A review of 100 consecutive cases. Arch Phys Med Rehabil 1981;62(7):321–323.
10. Johnson EW, Melvin JL: Value of electromyography in lumbar radiculopathy. Arch Phys Med Rehabil 1971;52(6):239–243.
11. Kimura J: Electrodiagnosis in diseases of nerve and muscle: Principles and practice. 2nd ed. Philadelphia: FA Davis Company, 1989.
12. Kraft GH: Fibrillation potential amplitude and muscle atrophy following peripheral nerve injury. Muscle Nerve 1990;13(9):814–821.
13. Lauder TD, Dillingham TR, Huston CW, et al.: Lumbosacral radiculopathy screen optimizing the number of muscles studied. Am J Phys Med Rehabil 1994;73(6):394–402.
14. Pease WS, Johnson EW, Charles M: Recruitment interval in L-5 radiculopathy: A preliminary report. Arch Phys Med Rehabil1984;65:654.
15. Pease WS, Lagattuta FP, Johnson EW: Spinal nerve stimulation in S1 radiculopathy. Am J Phys Med Rehabil 1990;69(2):77–80.
16. Radhakrishnan K, Litchy WJ, O'Fallon WM, et al.: Epidemiology of cervical radiculopathy. A population-based study from Rochester, Minnesota, 1976 through 1990. Brain 1994;117(Pt 2):325–335.
17. Saal JA, Firtch W, Saal JS, et al.: The value of somatosensory evoked potential testing for upper lumbar radiculopathy. A correlation of electrophysiologic and anatomic data. Spine 1992;17(6 Suppl):S133–137.
18. Schimsheimer RJ, de Visser BW, Kemp B, et al.: The flexor carpi radialis H-reflex in lesions of the sixth and seventh cervical nerve roots. Value of electromyography in lumbar radiculopathy. J Neurol Neurosurg Psychiatry 1985;48(5):445–449.
19. Shea PA, Woods WW, Werden DH: Electromyography in diagnosis of nerve root compression syndrome. Arch Neurol Psychiatry 1950;64(July):93–104.
20. Sine RD, Merrill D, Date E: Epidural recording of nerve conduction studies and surgical findings in radiculopathy. Arch Phys Med Rehabil 1994;75(1):17–24.
21. Streib EW, Sun SF, Paustian FF, et al.: Diabetic thoracic radiculopathy: Electrodiagnostic study. Muscle Nerve 1986;9(6):548–553.
22. Tullberg T, Svansborg E, Isacsson J, et al.: A Preoperative and postoperative study of the accuracy and value of electrodiagnosis in patients with lumbosacral disc herniation. Spine 1993;18(7):837–842.
23. Wilbourn AJ, Aminoff MJ: AAEE minimonograph#32: The electrophysiologic examination in patients with radiculopathies. Muscle Nerve 1988;11(11):1099–1114.

Chapter 7
Nerve Conduction Studies
Robert J. Weber

NERVE CONDUCTION STUDIES

Nerve conduction studies (NCS) establish the diagnosis more frequently than any of the other electrodiagnostic techniques. This is due to their high sensitivity to conduction slowing and conduction block, which are early indicators of nerve entrapment or peripheral neuropathy, the problems most frequently encountered in clinical practice. Despite their high clinical utility, conduction studies in some instances are delegated to technical assistants. This can reduce the diagnostic opportunities afforded by the sophisticated application and interpretation of these studies. New techniques such as stimulation of the spinal nerve roots continue to increase the clinical utility of NCS. In fact, direct stimulation of the spinal nerve at its origin not only extends the applicability of standard NCS techniques to the most proximal nerve segments, but also opens new assessment approaches to proximal spinal nerve problems.

The NCS appear seductively simple to perform—just shock the nerve at one point and record the signal from another. This simplicity in concept belies the underlying complexity. The study's clinical value requires the understanding and interpretation of many factors affecting the recorded signal including: the physiology of biological electrical signals; the pathophysiologic response of nerve and muscle to disease; the technical factors affecting the stimulation and recording of biological potentials; the cellular and microscopic anatomy of the neuromuscular system; and the pattern and location of injury to the neuromuscular system produced by clinical syndromes. This chapter will review the clinically

relevant aspects of each of these areas and highlight the specific elements essential to the competent clinical application of nerve conduction studies.

All neuromuscular function derives from a) the ability of specialized cells to establish an electrical potential across the cell membrane and b) the propagation of the action potential sequentially along the cell surface. In peripheral nerve cells, signal propagation results in the release of neurotransmitters at the end terminals of the cell, whereas in a muscle cell, signal propagation initiates the mechanical shortening of the cell. Neither of these "end effects" is recorded during typical NCS. Instead, we record the electrical signal generated by an intermediate aspect of the process: the motor-evoked (M) response represents the depolarization of the muscle T-system, the sensory nerve action potential (SNAP). SNAP is the volume-conducted signal of axon depolarization at the recording electrode (G1), generated as depolarization spreads along the axon. Although it is helpful to understand what generates the M response, the details of its generation can be overlooked for nerve conduction purposes. However, there are certain details associated with the generation and propagation of the depolarization wave in the nerve axon that are of practical importance in nerve conduction studies. These include the following extremely important factors:

1. The role of the bilayer axon membrane structure in potential generation;
2. The role of membrane protein structures (channel/pump) in action potential generation;

3. The role of myelin/Schwann's cells in potential propagation;
4. The relationship of axon size (diameter) to conduction velocity.

AXON POLARIZATION AND SIGNAL PROPAGATION

The emergence of a cell membrane was a key evolutionary step. It signaled the initial instance of "self" in the biological world because it partitioned the existing, undifferentiated organic chemistry of the prebiotic world into individual and ultimately autonomous segments. The regularity of present day cell membranes' bilayer structure suggests that it may have evolved from self-assembling, precursor elements. The cell membrane of the neuron serves more than the single role of enclosing and separating the "living" cytoplasmic structures from the surrounding environment, but also through the conduction of an electrical potential along its surface, the cell membrane serves another essential role, that of linking physically separated parts of complex, multicellular organisms. Although simplified, the following description of axon membrane function and signal propagation covers those aspects which are essential to electromyography. This chapter will limit its presentation to the example of the axon of the alpha motor neuron, but the principles apply to all NCS.

The axon is a cylinder consisting of a semipermeable, lipoprotein, bilayer membrane separating the intracellular from the extracellular environment. Key axonal elements such as complex proteins are assembled in the neuron cell body and then transported down the axon. That some axons extend 100,000 times their diameter, gives a rough indication of the metabolic challenge this poses. The semipermeability of the axon membrane —the ability to let some substances pass through it while blocking others—is the key to its capability to develop a transmembrane electrical potential and propagate a depolarization wave. The axon cell membrane permits the slow migration of smaller ions (e.g., the cations Na^+, C, and Ca^{++}, and the anions Cl^-, and HCO_3^-) but not the larger ions (e.g., protein anions). Thus, the axon membrane confines the negatively charged protein anions to the intracellular space, while permitting limited migration of the smaller ionic species. Even though an electric charge is created on the cell membrane (positive outside), both the intracellular and the extracellular environments must be maintained at electrical neutrality. Because protein anions cannot pass through the cell membrane, diffusion of each ion species alone cannot maintain the required electrical neutrality. Instead, an uneven concentration of those ions that can diffuse develops between the inside and the outside of the cell. This produces electrical neutrality in the two environments, but there is a difference in the concentration of specific ion "species" inside versus outside the cell. It is this local concentration gradient (i.e., difference) at the cell membrane of specific ions such as sodium that results in the electrical polarization at

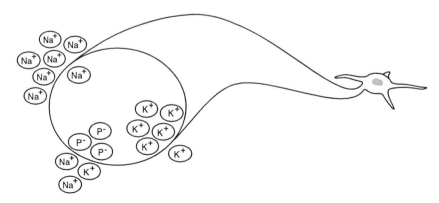

Figure 7–1. Ionic charges on axon membrane: protein anions (P⁻) cannot traverse the membrane but create attraction for oppositely charged species; Na⁺ and K⁺ ions 'see' a concentration gradient at the membrane, cluster, and produce local current potentials.

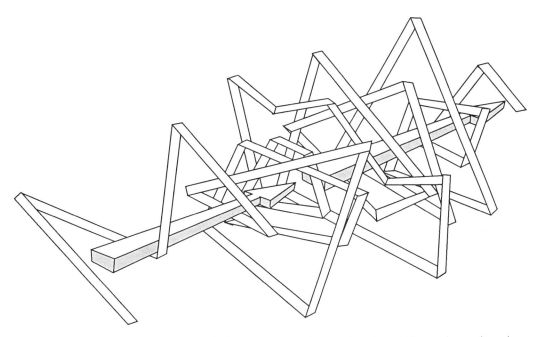

Figure 7-2. Slight changes in protein folding can open or close ion flow through the membrane channel.

the membrane (Fig. 7–1). The sodium cation "sees" a gradient across the cell membrane because of the lower intracellular concentration of Na$^+$; and, driven by the energy of this concentration gradient, would gradually diffuse through the membrane and neutralize the sodium gradient. Potassium with a high intracellular concentration mirrors this process. The "opportunity" to diffuse across the membrane gradient produces clustering of ions on the membrane and thus the membrane charge. This occurs despite the fact that the overall charge inside the cell and the charge outside the cell remain neutral. Because some of these ions clustered at the membrane will succeed in passing through it, this changed equilibrium must be maintained through the expenditure of cell energy to actively transport ions back across the membrane. Thus, the membrane sustains a static electrical charge much like that on an electronic capacitor. The Nernst equation quantitatively describes these concentration-charge relationships.

Although sustained membrane polarization is a precondition for the propagation of an electrical depolarization wave along the membrane, the system described so far is inadequate to repeatedly propagate a depolarization wave along the membrane.

Biologically useful signal conduction requires the axon membrane to: a) initiate a high-ionic current flow through an isolated membrane segment; b) pass this "active" status to adjacent membrane segments sequentially down the membrane; and c) rapidly restore the pre-discharge conditions inside the cell. These complex requirements are elegantly achieved through the operation of specialized, three-dimensional protein structures that are incorporated into the cell membrane. These proteins function as gates, rapidly opening and closing to control the concentration gradient-driven ion flow through membrane. Analogous to the way a shape change in the woven "Chinese" finger trap prevents finger movement, a slight change in protein shape sufficiently alters the channel (pore) through the protein to control ion flow (Fig. 7–2). The protein channel changes shape in response to electrical forces within the protein, which in turn alter its three-dimensional folding (conformation). The protein electrical field can be altered locally through formation of a chemical bond—typically with a synaptic neurotransmitter such as acetylcholine—or by an externally imposed electrical field. In normal nerve conduction, the electrical field needed for channel opening comes from the depolarization of the adjacent membrane. Thus, the opening (or closing) of channels can pass sequentially along the axon as a result of the electrical field influence of neighboring membrane areas (Fig. 7–3). In NCS, the depolarization wave is initiated by an external electrical field imposed by the electromyographer through the use of an electronic nerve stimulator, whereas in nature, the depolarization wave results from neurotransmitter action.

Once the protein channel (gate) opens, there is a rapid, transmembrane flow of the ions positioned along the membrane, driven by the transmembrane concentration gradient. This flow neutralizes (and somewhat over-compensates for) the local gradient, and flow then ceases. The local intracellular environment is now electrically and ionically disturbed and must be restored to the previous condition, —both for stability of the cell and in order to permit reuse of the membrane depolarization wave for signal transmission. This is accomplished through energy expenditure by cell membrane proteins that are able to attach to and actively transport these "excess" ions out of the cell. The "sodium pump" is the best known of these proteins. It is able to attach and transport sodium ions out of the cell against the exterior concentration gradient and is the principal mechanism for restoring and maintaining the membrane in the charged state.

In summary, the static charge on the axon cell membrane results from physical characteristics of the membrane. The membrane maintains a separation between the intracellular and extracellular environments. This separation produces a high concentration of protein anions inside the cell and produces a concentration gradient across the cell membrane for a number of ionic species. The gradient results in the clustering of charged ions on the cell surface, producing a static, transmembrane potential of up to 90 millivolts. Although this process is mostly passive, the initiation of rapid current flow through the membrane and the ability to transmit this flow sequentially along the membrane (depolarization wave propagation) requires active "machinery." Three-dimensional proteins in the cell membrane contain gated channels that open in response to chemical or electrical influences, initiating the rapid, transmembrane ionic flows necessary to generate an action current. This ionic current flow in turn opens adjacent membrane channels through the effect of its generated electrical field. The propagating depolarization wave is thus passed along from channel to channel in much the same way a row of stacked dominos falls: each

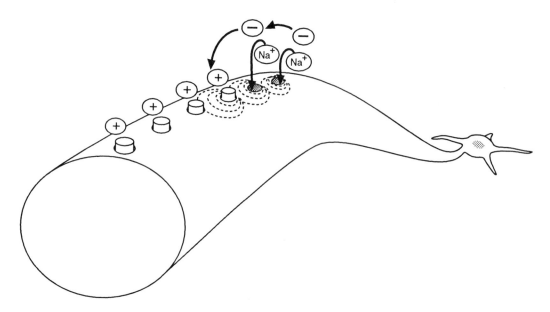

Figure 7–3. Membrane channels open and close as the result of the electrical field created by ion flow through adjacent channels.

from the influence of its neighbor. Once this propagation wave passes, the intracellular milieu is restored by the active transport of ions (principally sodium), across the membrane through the action of the "membrane pump" proteins.

CONDUCTION VELOCITY

The time required for conduction along an axon is related to the time required for a membrane channel opening following adequate stimulus and that time required for ions to reach a sufficient flow rate through the channel to create an effective local electrical field. Once this new electromagnetic field is created, it acts on its neighbor (propagates) at the speed of light (which for practical purposes is instantaneous). Thus, the time it takes to conduct a signal along a nerve axon is proportional to the sum of the opening and flow time for each membrane channel multiplied by the number of channels involved. It follows that the greater the distance between membrane proteins, the lower the conduction time and the faster the nerve conduction velocity will be. The Distance between the protein channels is limited by the distance over which the ionic electrical field can act to open a neighboring channel. It turns out that in the system we have described so far (an unmyelinated nerve), this distance is proportional to the square root of the diameter of the axon. Although conduction velocity in this nerve model increases as the axon size increases, the square root relationship imposes some practical limits on how fast an unmyelinated nerve is able to conduct a signal without becoming prohibitively large. As organisms become larger and more complex, fast nerve conduction becomes essential if the organism is to be able to respond rapidly to its environment or to perform complex behaviors. The limitation imposed by this "square root of axon diameter" relationship is obvious when you consider that if a one-micron, unmyelinated axon conducts at approximately one meter per second, scaling that axon up to conduct at 100 meters per second would require an axon approximately the size of a man's arm ($1 \mu m \times 100^2$). Whereas this system works admirably in the squid (squid giant axons have thrilled physiologists for de-

cades) and in the human autonomic nervous system where conduction velocity is not critical, the small-diameter unmyelinated nerve fibers cannot accommodate the requirements necessary for either rapid mobility or complex cognitive processing in man. Because the distance between depolarization points on the nerve is transversed at the speed of light, the obvious strategy is to increase the spacing between these active areas. The development of nerve myelination has accomplished this task in a manner analogous to that in which microwaves are used to transmit telephone signals across the country: towers receive the signal from a distant tower and, amplify and retransmit it to another tower along the route. The Schwann's cell envelopes the axon in concentric myelin sheaths, dividing the axon into regularly spaced segments of myelin. The small gaps between the myelin are the nodes of Ranvier. Myelin is a waxy, insulating substance, and in the myelinated nerve the cell membrane proteins are concentrated at the nodes of Ranvier, and the myelinated segments between are barren (9). This intensifies the electrical field generated at the active node and permits the strengthened electrical field to jump (saltatory conduction) from one node of Ranvier to the next. This significantly increases the space between depolarization points compared with that of an unmyelinated nerve, reduces their number, and significantly increases conduction velocity. Thus, the nodes of Ranvier become the equivalent of the microwave relay transmission tower. In this system, conduction velocity, i.e., the distance between nodes, is also related to the size of the axon; however, with myelination the conduction velocity relationship is directly related to the diameter of the axon rather than to its square root. Thus, there is a linear relationship between an increase in axon size and velocity; and, axons of practical size (10 to 20 microns) can generate conduction velocities (40–100 msec) adequate for the effective signaling. To review:

I. The physical structures of the cell membrane:
    A. Confines protein anions to the cell interior;
    B. Controls the flow of smaller

ions through the semipermeable membrane;

    C. Contains special channel/ion pump proteins that connect the intra-cellular and extracellular space.

II. Despite the fact that there is electrical neutrality within the cell and electrical neutrality outside of the cell, the axon membrane contains a static charge of approximately 90 mV with a positive on the exterior. This results from the transmembrane concentration gradients of various ions.

III. The axon membrane proteins, acting under the influence of an electrical field, can change their shape, which permits the rapid flow of charged ions through the membrane. This flow, in turn, generates an electrical field.

IV. Axonal membrane proteins adjacent to an active channel will respond to the electrical field created by that channel in a like manner, thus propagating a depolarization wave.

V. Axonal membrane proteins can use the chemical energy of the cell to actively transport ions across the membrane. This mechanism can maintain or restore the transmembrane electrical potential after its depolarization.

VI. Schwann's cell myelin produces highly insulated axon segments that alternate along the axon with bare nodes of Ranvier. The membrane proteins are concentrated at the nodes of Ranvier. This intensifies their electrical field, increases the distance over which the Schwann's cell can activate channels, and thus decreases conduction time (increases conduction velocity) along the axon.

These are the key physiologic and anatomical factors that influence conduction along the axon membrane. Interference with the operation of any of these elements will result in change in function detectable by clinical electrodiagnostic studies.

PATHOPHYSIOLOGY

As testimony to the sophisticated nature of nerve function and the crudeness of our un-derstanding, we are able to detect only three altered states of nerve function. These are the slowing of conduction, the blocking of conduction (neurapraxia), and the loss of conduction through axonal death (axonotmesis). The myriad subtle modifications in the cellular chemistry that lead to these events lie beyond both our understanding and assessment. Although the terms neurapraxia and axonotmesis appear frequently, they can generate confusion because the neura/axono prefixes suggest reference to the whole nerve or the axon, respectively. In practice, either is used to indicate single axon or whole nerve involvement. More fundamentally confusing is the fact that they refer to end effects rather than to the underlying, pathophysiological cause of nerve dysfunction (i.e., they are product, not process). This tends to obscure the fact that there are multiple causes for each of the three nerve conduction status changes we can observe clinically. The fundamental causes as well as the observed conduction change itself, should be considered in the interpretation of NCS.

Because the conduction time along a nerve depends on the number of discreet depolarization points (channels) that must be activated. It follows that conduction time will increase (conduction velocity slow) if more depolariza-

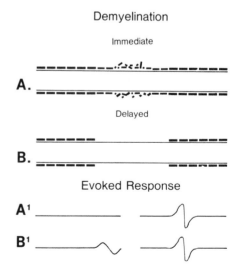

Figure 7–4. Demyelination pictured immediately following the onset of injury (*A*, *A*¹) and some weeks later (*B*, *B*¹) after myelin debris has been removed. The evoked responses with stimulation proximal to and distal to the lesion are demonstrated at *A*¹ and *B*¹ at the bottom.

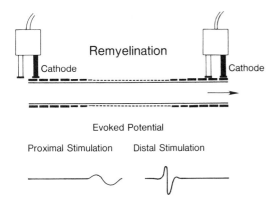

Figure 7-5. Remyelinated axon; note the decreased internodal distance and decreased thickness of myelin. The evoked potential with stimulation above and below the lesion that would be obtained from a nerve with all axons remyelinated is seen at the bottom. Conduction is slowed, and the response is temporally dispersed across the lesion.

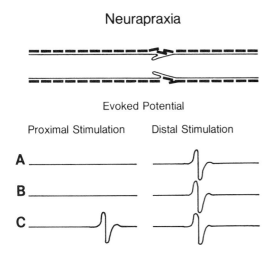

Figure 7-6. *A, B,* and *C* show the evoked responses from stimulation proximally and distally to the lesion: *A,* immediately post-injury; *B,* 7 days post-injury; *C,* some weeks following injury after neurapraxia has resolved.

tion points are required. This situation occurs in three pathophysiologic instances: in demyelination, in which (after an interval) function resumes as in an unmyelinated axon (Fig. 7–4) (see conduction block); in re-myelination, in which segments are shorter because the re-myelinated Schwann cell size is reduced; and in reinnervation, in which both the axon diameter is smaller and smaller Schwann's cells produce shorter segments (Fig. 7–5). In practice, variations on these extremes are usually

seen: spotty demyelination with demyelinated segments intermixed with normal; demyelination mixed with partial or light re-myelinization; light/partial re-myelination mixed with normal segments. When a long segment of myelin loss is present, the conduction velocity will be in the below-20-msec range. Faster velocities suggest that either the demyelination is confined to a short segment that is "diluted out" by the adjacent normal segment or some mixed or segmental type of pathophysiology exists. When re-myelination is successful over a longer segment, nerve conduction velocity will often remain just below normal values; unfortunately, this situation is electrodiagnostically indistinguishable from a nerve injury in which the larger diameter axons have been lost. Thus, only change over time can distinguish continuing, chronic injury from limited injury but maximum recovery after decompression of nerve entrapment.

Conduction block, i.e., neurapraxia often occurs at discreet points along the axon. Usual causes include local trauma, acute focal or multifocal demyelination, e.g., autoimmunity, post-viral syndrome, or focal vascular insults of the nerve. By definition, a neurapraxic axon remains alive despite the inability to transmit a signal along its entire length. The normal segments of the axon above and below the block still conduct a signal when appropriately stimulated. Investigators have attributed conduction block to mechanical distortion of the axon (1) (Fig. 7–6) and to an impedance mismatch (59, 60) in the membrane between the myelinated and demyelinated section. The absence of cell membrane proteins beneath the myelinated segments provides a convincing mechanism for conduction block in demyelination (9) because conduction through the recently demyelinated segment would be blocked when the segment length exceeds the distance over which the electrical field of the last intact node of Ranvier is able to act. Thus, an acutely demyelinated axon segment would first exhibit conduction block and then resume conducting in the slow, unmyelinated manner once the membrane proteins had been inserted along the course of the demyelinated membrane. None of these mechanisms explain the very transient conduction blocks of large diameter fibers that occur with brief nerve compression. These blocks resolve completely and rapidly, suggesting that they result from a focal, intracellular energy failure related to interference with vascular or cytoplasmic flow.

Many processes can produce axon death (axonotmesis). When the neuron itself dies, there is no possibility of nerve regeneration; however, when only a portion of the axon has been disrupted, the surviving portion may die back to an intact node, stabilize, and then attempt regeneration. Wallerian degeneration occurs following these injuries, and is the process of cellular reorganization accompanying dissolution of the disrupted neural segment. Axons are dependent on the neuron cell body to generate the major subcellular structures needed for their function. These structures are mechanically transported down the axon as part of the axoplasmic flow. Enough of these materials are present, however, for the axon to function for several days without resupply. An axon cleanly separated from the rest of the neural cell will continue to conduct an action potential wave when externally stimulated for

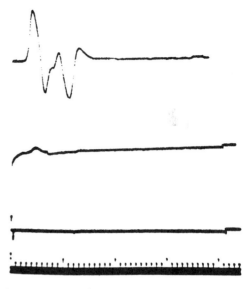

Figure 7–8. Evoked potential recorded from the thenar eminence with median nerve stimulation at the wrist in an individual with surgically demonstrated complete section of the median nerve following a stab wound in the upper. *Top* response was recorded 4 days post-injury, the *middle*, 7 days post-injury, and the *bottom* response, 10 days post-injury. The time base is in msec/ divisions, and the amplitude of the time base is 1 mV.

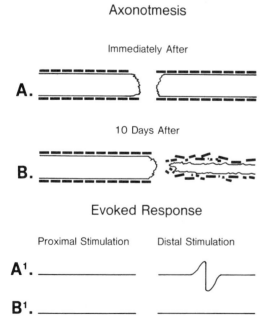

Figure 7–7. Axonotmetic lesion with axon changes demonstrated A, immediately after injury and B, 10 days after injury. The evoked responses obtained by stimulation proximally and distally to the lesion at the corresponding times (A¹ and B¹) are demonstrated at the bottom.

3 to 7 days following this injury (Figs. 7–7, 7–8). During this period, response of the separated axon to external stimulation will appear normal, making it impossible to distinguish between mere neurapraxia and the early stages of axonotmesis (Wallerian degeneration). At the end of this period, axon conduction abruptly fails, that is, there is not a gradual decline but rather a precipitous one. Once conduction fails, a physical dissolution of the axon segment beyond the injury begins. Because of this delay between injury and the failure of conduction, electrodiagnostic distinction between axonotmesis and neurapraxia can be made only by studying the nerve function after a delay ranging from 3 to 7 days after the injury (Figs. 7–7, 7–8). Although early electrodiagnostic studies are useful after an injury to determine if some function is preserved (or that the injury is progressing), they cannot determine the viability of the segment distal to the injury, nor determine if the nerve remains in continuity when there is complete conduction block.

Whereas discrete axons often exhibit only

one pathophysiologic change (conduction slowing, conduction block, axonotmesis), an "injured" nerve composed as it is of thousands of individual axons is likely to demonstrate a mixture of these features. All three abnormalities may be found within a short segment or they may occur separately along a single nerve. Even individual axons may exhibit different pathophysiological responses at different locations along their course. This complicates the interpretation of conduction studies and highlights the importance of integrating clinical as well as electrodiagnostic information when formulating the diagnosis.

THE RECORDED RESPONSE AND TEMPORAL DISPERSION

The compound motor action potential (CMAP) and the SNAP are easily recognized by their familiar shapes (see Figs. 7–14 and 7–21 later in this chapter). Except for minor amplitude differences, they vary little from nerve to nerve. The recorded signal consists of the summated negative and the positive voltage contributions from each axon conducting in the nerve. The normal shape of recorded responses derives from the fact that there is a "normal" distribution of axon velocities in human nerves, which produces the typical summation pattern. Figure 7–9 illustrates this summation of individual axon responses into an extended response, i.e., a temporally dispersed response. If each axon conducted at the same velocity, then the duration of the summated evoked response would be the same as that of a single axon, and the size of both the negative and the positive components of the recorded response would be directly proportional to the number of axons, i.e., additive (summation of area more closely relates to this than does summated amplitude). Conversely, if each axon in a nerve conducted at a significantly different velocity than each of the others (so that there was no overlap of their evoked signals), then the compound signal would be a 'saw-tooth' with each deflection equal to that produced by one individual axon. In the real world, axons exhibit a relatively narrow range of conduction velocities. Although the signals do not arrive simultaneously from all of the axons, the variation of

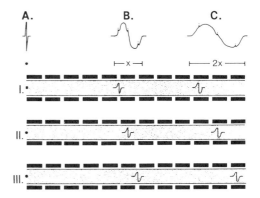

Figure 7–9. Temporal dispersion. Three axons of various conduction speeds, I (fastest) to III (slowest), are illustrated. The summated response of the signals from each of these axons is shown (*A* through *C*) at distances along the nerve. Conduction begins at the left and proceeds to the right. At point *A*, the signals in each axon arrive almost simultaneously, producing a very compact recorded response. At point *B*, the signals are less well synchronized, producing a smaller amplitude and longer duration response. This spreading is increased by the time the signals arrive at point *C*. The greater the number of axons contributing to the signal, the smoother is the curve of the recorded evoked response.

their arrival time is well grouped, and there is significant overlap of the axon signals. Thus, in a normal situation, the arrival of a positive deflection generated by one axon may overlap that of a negative deflection generated by another, and they will completely or partially cancel each other. This phenomenon is known as phase cancellation, and it is the reason there is not a direct, one-to-one, relationship between the size (either amplitude or area) of an evoked response and the number of axons activated (Fig. 7–10). The typical sensory or motor response that we record during nerve conduction studies gains its recognizable shape as a result of the axon potentials summating (additive and cancellation) in a pattern determined by the typical mix of conduction velocities in normal human nerves. Because each nerve has a similar mix, each recorded response is similar. Were the normal velocity mix different, normal evoked potentials would also have a significantly different shape. This changing of the axon velocity distribution is precisely what occurs in pathology with significant alteration of the recorded response (see Fig. 7–47 later in this chapter). Comput-

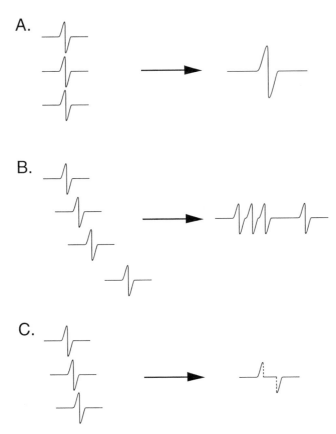

Figure 7–10. Summation and phase cancellation. *A. Simultaneous signal arrival (all axons at same velocity) amplitude area a summation of signals while duration same as single axon. B. No overlap (all axons distinct velocities); duration of envelope is difference between fastest and slowest axon. C. Phase cancellation: negative-positive components of axons of slightly different velocities cancel.*

ers have made it relatively easy to model the way the evoked potential shape varies as the distribution and range of conduction velocities of individual axons changes. Such studies demonstrate that in a typical nerve, up to 50% of the size of the evoked potential can be lost merely by altering the conduction velocity mix of axons within the nerve, i.e., absent any conduction block. Thus, we must alter the traditional interpretation of nerve conduction studies that a "significant" (often 10% or 15%) drop in the size of the evoked potential across a point of injury indicates (i.e., requires) the presence of conduction block. The amplitude/area loss in NCS across lesions, particularly if it is less than 50% of the normal response, can result entirely from conduction slowing of some axons within the nerve, resulting in increased phase cancellation. Clinically, it is likely that a combination of conduc-

tion block and phase cancellation will exist. Needle EMG examination can be helpful in this situation because blocked axons cannot contribute to the voluntary recruitment pattern, whereas axons that are merely slowed will still be recruitable. Therefore, the finding of the preservation of good voluntary recruitment in the face of a significant drop in the size of the evoked potential across the lesion would favor conduction slowing (phase cancellation) as the primary cause; conduction block would be favored as the cause if the voluntary recruitment is severely reduced. Conduction slowing might also increase temporal dispersion of the recorded signal more than would a predominantly neurapraxic injury.

The effect of the arrival of the signal of axons at different times during recording of the evoked response is termed the temporal dispersion of the response. It affects not only the amplitude and area of the recorded response as explained above, but also can produce additional phases in the response (baseline crossings) and extend its duration. Temporal dispersion is a normal aspect of NCS because axons range in both size and conduction velocity. Signals recorded from nerves are briefer than the M responses because they contain only axon depolarization waves. Those recorded over muscle are of longer duration owing to the extended action potential time of the muscle membranes. Normally, nerve responses (SNAP) will last less than 2 msec, whereas motor responses (CMAP) will be less than 5 msec in duration (negative peak). Recorded responses requiring longer than this indicate slowing and spreading of the range of conduction velocities of axons within the nerve and indicate increased or abnormal temporal dispersion (Fig. 7–11).

INTRANEURAL ANATOMY AND LESION LOCALIZATION

The physical arrangement of axons within nerves protects against the complete loss of specific motor functions in cases of partial nerve lesions. It is also central to the electro-

myographer's ability to localize the point of injury along the course of the nerve. In a typical telephone or fiber optic cable, groups of fibers are bundled and remain together throughout the length of the cable. The telephone lines from XYZ company travel together in one of these small bundles. If someone cuts that portion of the cable, the XYZ company will lose the use of all of its telephones. Similarly, neurons are grouped by function both in the brain and in the spinal cord, and focal lesions there often cause discrete motor loss. If motor axons were grouped in nerves analogous to the arrangement in telephone cables, partial injury might affect only one muscle while leaving others unaffected (Fig. 7–12). That arrangement also would make it difficult to locate the site of injury because there would be no difference in the observed effect of partial injury whether it occurred proximally or distally in the nerve. Fortunately, the body employs a scheme of continually mixing axons between the different fascicles within the nerve, thus altering which axons travel together and their location within the nerve (Fig. 7–13). In this arrangement, a partial nerve injury tends to spare some axons to every muscle supplied by the nerve distal to the injury rather than to com-

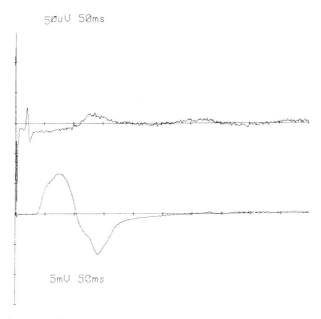

50uV 50ms

5mV 50ms

Figure 7–11. Typical motor and sensory response. Both shape and duration of response depend on the presence of "normal" distribution of axon conduction velocities in the nerve. 50 msec duration of sweep.

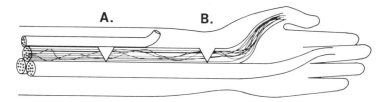

Figure 7-12. Hypothetical nerve in which all axons stay in a single fascicle until they exit the nerve. Note that a lesion at *A* or *B* would appear identical on EMG examination both on both distal examination and on examination of the mid-forearm branch.

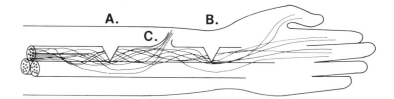

Figure 7-13. Typical nerve illustrating the movement of axons from one fascicle to another during their course. Here lesions at *A* and *B* may be easily distinguished electromyographically by the fact that lesion *A* produces changes in the distribution *C*, whereas the lesion at *B* does not.

pletely wipe out specific functions. In addition, the fact that the full distribution of the nerve below the lesion shares the abnormality makes it possible to determine the site of the lesion by analyzing the distribution of abnormalities seen. Intraneural anatomy thus serves both to reduce the functional impact of partial nerve injuries and to assist the clinician in locating the lesion.

DEFINING REFERENCE VALUES IN NCS

Reference NCS values usually are determined by performing a standardized testing method on a group of individuals that are free of neurologic symptoms and that have a distribution of age, sex, and other features representative of the general population. "Normal" is typically defined statistically as the mean value plus or minus two standard deviations (SDs). Although this approach is helpful, problems such as non-parametric distributions of population characteristics in the "reference" group can result in skewed statistics. More often, the difficulty is that the subject has a unique characteristic that significantly influences conduction values but that differs from that of the reference group. Although different from the

reference group median, this characteristic is not an indication of nerve pathology. Examples of this type of characteristic are extreme limb length, height, or extremes of age. Even when unique factors are not present, difficulty can arise from the wide range of values normal to the population. The breadth of this reference population range is dramatic when compared to the limited variation in values found in different nerves in a single individual. A review of a typical reference nerve conduction value reveals that the range of normal variation is ($\pm$ two SDs) which is approximately 25% of the mean conduction velocity. This compares to typical side-to-side variation in a single subject of several percentage points and to day-to-day variation of repeat testing of less than 10%. When judged against a population-based, set of normal NCS values, an individual whose usual conduction value is at the fast end of the range would have to experience as much as a 40% conduction velocity slowing before "falling-out" of, i.e., dropping below the reference range. In certain circumstances, the sensitivity of NCS can be increased without an undue increase in the rate of false positives if the tested individual also serves as the control. This approach is appropriate for cases of focal injury or entrapment. It runs into obvious difficulties when one attempts to apply it in the face of a generalized neuropathic process such as diabetic neuropathy in which both of the nerves would be affected. This approach is exemplified by a side-to-side comparison of the median and by median-to-ulnar nerve comparisons for carpal tunnel syndrome. With intrasubject comparison, the percentage change in NCS required to detect abnormality is much less than that necessary when using a population-based reference value.

EVOKED POTENTIAL RECORDING

Evoked potentials are recorded using a G1 (recording) and a G2 (reference) electrodes attached to the separate grids of the differential amplifier. The signal that appears simultaneously at the two electrodes is canceled by the differential amplifier. This makes the placement of the two electrodes in relation to the generator source (nerve or muscle) and to each other important. Surface (silver cup) electrodes are usually used because they record a summated signal that permits quantitative analysis of the evoked potential. For motor conduction studies, G1 is placed over the motor point of the muscle belly, and G2 is placed distally over the tendon or another electrically silent area. The initial deflection of motor responses should be sharply negative, and the signal should be a smooth, biphasic curve (Fig. 7–14). A signal that shows initial

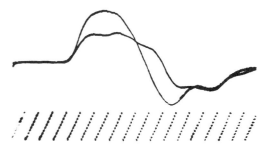

Figure 7–15. Superimposed are evoked potentials recorded at the median thenar motor point and a more medial site over motor point of three muscles. The larger amplitude response is from the single muscle. The separate components of the smaller response result from recording responses from three separate median-innervated muscles.

positive deflection (see Fig. 7–23 later in this chapter) is volume conducted, i.e., initiated at a distance from G1. The source must be more clearly defined by changing the electrode placement or using needle recording to confirm the generator. Whereas a distorted response may originate from the desired muscle, it may also be from a "distant" muscle that was accidentally cross-stimulated. Polyphasic or complex signals may be seen as a result of the unintentionally simultaneous recording of two muscles or from the effects of pathology on the nerve being studied (Fig. 7–15).

In sensory conduction studies, both the G1 and the G2 electrodes are placed directly along the course of the nerve with the G1 electrode located closest to the stimulator. Ground electrode placement can reduce shock artifact and usually is best between the stimulating and the G1 electrodes. The impedance of dry skin is high and may produce an excessive shock artifact. The use of a standard electrode paste or gel is usually sufficient to overcome this difficulty, but occasionally light abrasion of the skin may be necessary to obtain a satisfactory recording. This is particularly helpful for short segment sensory conduction studies.

The separation between the G1 and G2 electrodes affects the measured latency and the amplitude of the recorded evoked potential. In sensory studies, the optimal distance is usually 3 cm to 4 cm. This separation can be standardized by embedding the two electrodes in a plastic bar. An alternate technique

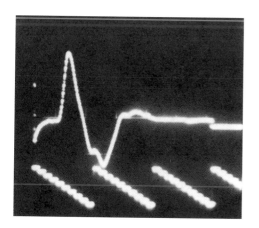

Figure 7–14. Motor nerve evoked potential with recording electrode over motor point of a single muscle. Note initial negative deflection.

of recording is to place the G1 electrode directly over the nerve with the G2 electrode approximately 3 cm away from the recording electrode and perpendicular to the course of the nerve (35). This "monopolar" recording results in a lower-amplitude signal but one less subject to change from small G1 movement (Fig. 7–16). The sensitivity of the response to electrode separation and placement results from the wave length characteristics of the nerve signal and the phase cancellation effects. Maximum amplitude results when the electrode separation is equal to one fourth the wavelength of the nerve signal (57) (Fig. 7–17).

Needle electrodes offer advantages in certain circumstances because they enable the investigator to isolate the stimulation to a specific nerve or the response to a specific muscle. When placed intramuscularly, the needle electrode disproportionately records the muscle fiber spike potentials from motor units located very close to the needle tip. The negative rise time of the potential for a fiber located near the needle tip is fast, and very large ampli-

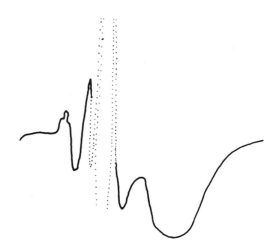

Figure 7–18. Evoked motor response recorded using a needle electrode in the muscle. Note that the initial deflection is of low amplitude (full screen deflection represents 6 millivolts), indicating that the needle tip is not directly against fibers depolarized by the fastest conducting axons.

tudes are seen (Fig. 7–18). Needle electrodes are most useful for confirming that the evoked potential that is recorded originates in the muscle under investigation and is not a volume-conducted signal from nearby. Because the large-amplitude spike response recorded through an intramuscular needle electrode originates from the motor units at the needle tip, recording conduction velocities with this technique require care in identifying the earliest deflection and can be erratic in highly denervated muscles. In that case the amplitude observed is NOT diagnostically useful because small needle movements can alter it considerably.

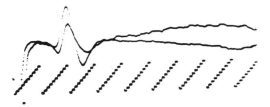

Figure 7–16. Sensory evoked response obtained using standard recording electrode placement of the reference electrode (large amplitude response) and off-nerve placement (monopolar technique) of the reference electrode (small amplitude response).

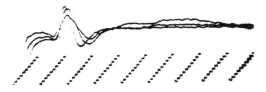

Figure 7–17. Three sensory evoked responses recorded with increasing separation of the reference from the recording electrode along the nerve axis. Separation is 3 cm (largest amplitude, shortest duration), 6 cm, and 8 cm (smallest amplitude, longest duration), respectively. Optimum separation is related to the wave length of the signal.

GENERAL FACTORS AFFECTING NERVE CONDUCTION

In addition to the "normal" variation among individuals, three nonpathologic factors in addition to the "normal" variation among individuals significantly affect NCS: nerve temperature; subject age; and subject height. Temperature is the most challenging of these in day-to-day application because either a cold environment, vasoconstriction, or evaporative cooling from sweating can quickly lower the temperature of superficial, peripheral nerves.

There is a direct relationship between nerve temperature and conduction velocity. Henriksen reported a drop in conduction velocity of approximately 2.4 msec for every 1°C of temperature decreased in the forearm (measured by a needle thermistor at a depth of 2 cm) (22). Johnson, using intramuscular temperature, found a decrease of 5% per 1°C (28). Haller found a linear correlation in normal subjects among skin, subcutaneous, and intramuscular temperatures of the calf with various induced temperatures (21). He suggested that the skin temperature be measured 15 cm proximal to the medial malleolus and that an arithmetic correction for conduction velocity then be made to an equivalent of 32° C.

Arithmetic correction for temperature is effective for small variations from normal, but may have drawbacks beyond this range. The correlation in normal subjects among surface, subcutaneous, and deep temperatures and their relation to conduction velocity has been shown to exist, but it is uncertain whether these relationships hold in all pathologic circumstances. Temperature affects the size of evoked potentials in NCS. This occurs on top of the considerable range in normal amplitude reported for both sensory and motor conduction studies. Direct nerve and muscle factors and technical factors such as skin/electrode impedance, depth of the nerve placement of recording electrodes, and stimulation technique also contribute to amplitude variation. Given this variation, amplitude is diagnostically less useful than is velocity. Comparison of amplitudes side-to-side and along the course of the nerve (above and below entrapment points), plus observation of amplitude change occurring over time after injury is more helpful than the absolute value of the recorded amplitude.

Temperature significantly affects the size of recorded potentials (24). The amplitude and duration of evoked potentials (and therefore the area under the negative spike) decrease with increasing nerve temperature throughout the normal physiologic temperature range. This finding is counter intuitive; because higher temperatures cause conduction velocity to increase, we might well expect that velocity increases would cause a better summation of the evoked response and thus a larger recorded amplitude. The paradoxical, observed change may be due to a disproportionate change in the rate of conduction of the various sizes of axons or to the summated effect of the reduction of individual axon depolarization durations (4). At the cellular level, lower temperature is known to slow both ion diffusion and protein conformational changes. (The effect of slowed conformation changes in the membrane protein channels should be mentioned.) Whatever the fundamental cause, the net result is that cooling reduces the magnitude of phase cancellation and thus increases the amplitude of the recorded sensory response (Fig. 7–19).

Because nerve temperature affects both the recorded nerve conduction velocity and the amplitude in clinically important ways, and because no amplitude "correction" for temperature is available, it is essential that limb temperature be controlled during NCS. In addition, recording the temperature from a standard location at each examination provides an excellent reference point for serial studies in individuals patients. This extra step may not be necessary to demonstrate that entrapment, e.g., carpal tunnel syndrome, is not present when the latency recorded is normal. However, the information may prove invaluable for comparison some years later, when one reexamines the patient for signs of an early peripheral neuropathy.

Age significantly affects nerve conduction at the extremes of youth and maturity. At birth, motor conduction velocities are approximately one half of the velocities of a normal adult. Values reach the low end of the normal range for the adult population by the age of 2 years old, and are in the mid-normal range by the age of 4 years old (Fig. 7–20) (3). Because conduction velocity correlates with gestational age, historically it was used to determine the degree of prematurity in newborns, i.e., to separate prematurity from low weight for gestational-age infants (45).

Population-based studies indicate that ageing related neuronal loss and nerve conduction slowing can be statistically demonstrated by the fourth decade of life (16). This slowing is small and is obscured by the wide range of the normal values for the population. It results

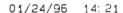

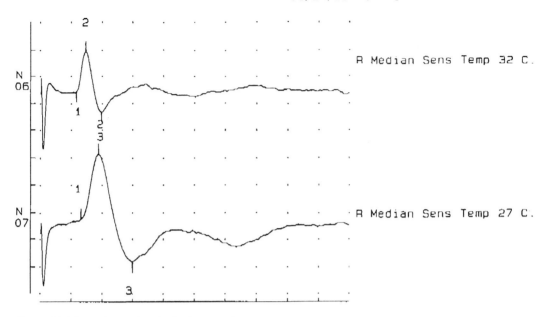

01/24/96 14:21

R Median Sens Temp 32 C.

R Median Sens Temp 27 C.

Figure 7–19. Palm-stimulated orthodromic median sensory response. Note that the amplitude increases with cooling.

from the gradual loss of larger-sized neurons that accompanies aging. Norris found that conduction velocity decreased 1.5% percent per decade after age 60. This slowing is seen throughout the body (proportionate slowing); however, some authors have reported that disproportionate, i.e., unevenly distributed, slowing can occur at common entrapment points. (41). Although this slowing is gradual on a population basis, our experience has been that some seniors beyond age 70 can show accelerated affects. These individuals may show other signs of neuronal loss. Separate reference values based on age are required for both young and old.

Height is inversely correlated with nerve conduction velocity. Distal conduction slowing is normal in very tall subjects (8). This may be due to greater axonal tapering and lighter myelination in the "extended" segment. Tall individuals may be subject to greater large-axon loss with aging because of a higher metabolic stress related to supplying the more distant axon. Thus, aging and distal cooling may exaggerate this finding. In elderly and in very tall individuals, it is important to test a sufficient number of nerves to determine if the slowing recorded at an entrapment

point is merely an accentuation of general peripheral slowing or isolated entrapment. It is important to temper the diagnosis of general peripheral neuropathy in these individuals. Motor unit reorganization on needle EMG and other pathophysiologic changes should be sought to confirm the diagnosis. Mathematical correction or the use of a separate reference data set should be used whenever one encounters extremes of age or height.

Other biological factors such as gender (28) are also known to affect NCS values. However, these factors are not quantitatively sufficient to require individual correction.

Technical factors may produce clinically important changes in the recorded response. Amplifier filters can drastically change recorded responses—amplitude, latency, and duration— by eliminating signal components. This alteration in the recorded frequency component is the electrical equivalent of changing the axon velocity distribution of the nerve. Filtering out the high frequencies of the SNAP delays the peak latency enough to affect clinical values (Fig. 7–21), whereas the loss of low frequencies impacts the M amplitude (Fig. 7–22). Obvious but underappreci-

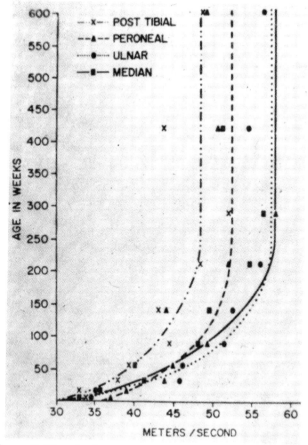

Figure 7-20. Conduction velocity as a function of age in children.

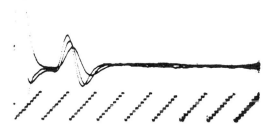

Figure 7-21. Sensory evoked response recorded from identical stimulation and recording electrode placements with shifts in the high frequency filter settings. The largest amplitude response with shortest latency was obtained with the high frequency cut at 3.2 kHz. Settings at 1.6 and 0.8 kHz produced the intermediate and low amplitude responses, respectively. Note the clinically significant shift in the recorded peak latency. (Caliber: Each slanted line = 1 msec. Height = 20 μV.)

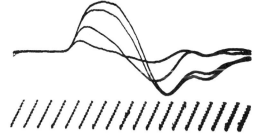

Figure 7-22. Motor evoked responses obtained with low frequency filter cutoffs of 16, 32, 160, and 500 Hz (largest to smallest amplitude response). Note that there is no shift in the latency of the initial deflection but that the accuracy of identification of the deflection becomes more difficult as amplitude decreases. (Caliber: Each slanted line = 1 msec. Height = 2 mV.)

ated is the effect of amplification on the recorded response. Misreading of the amplification scale is more likely with transient analog displays, than with digital instru-

ments with persistent displays. The degree of amplification affects the visual perception of latency, an effect minimized by using standard amplification settings (Fig. 7-23).

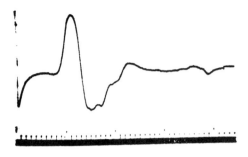

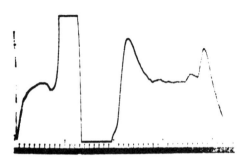

Figure 7-23. Median evoked response in a patient with carpal tunnel syndrome recorded at amplifier settings of 1 mV (*above*) and 100 μV (*below*) per division (division equals height of time base). Estimates of latency can be affected by the amplification.

NERVE STIMULATION

Each NCS requires an external stimulation designed to initiate depolarization simultaneously in all of the normal axons, in order to produce a complete, easily recordable response. Whereas a magnetic pulse or a mechanical tap can be used, typically stimulation is with an electrical discharge between two surface electrodes (bipolar stimulation). This produces an electromagnetic field intense enough to open axon membrane channels and initiate a depolarization wave. The electrodes are oriented along the nerve with the cathode in the direction of the intended conduction. In a perfectly conducting medium, stimulation would produce a uniform electromagnetic force in a hemispheric pattern around the electrodes. The irregularity of the body tissue planes, conductivity, and impedance all work to distort the stimulating signal. This distortion can introduce some uncertainty into judging the point of initial nerve activation of deep nerves. By convention, a supramaximal stimu-

lus 10% percent above the level necessary to produce the largest observed amplitude of the recorded response is used. Depolarization of the nerve proceeds in both directions along the nerve following stimulation.

Theoretical assessment of the electrical field produced by bipolar surface stimulation indicates that it is shaped as a downward-directed cone with an angle of approximately 70⁰ (Fig. 7-24) (13). Depolarization of the nerve (or nerves) can begin anywhere within the volume of this cone. Distortion of the shape and intensity of the field is produced in the patient by connective tissue planes, bones, etc. The deeper the nerve is located, and the greater the stimulation intensity used, the larger the volume of the cone and the more uncertain the exact point on the nerve at which depolarization begins. This is due to both to the increase in volume covered by the field, and to the increased distortion of the field by the greater tissue irregularity encountered.

This small uncertainty as to the point of initial depolarization of the nerve creates a measurement error in the length of the nerve segment used in the conduction study (doubled when two stimulation points are required), and contributes to both expanding the normal value range of normal and increasing the variation seen upon repeat testing. Using excessive stimulus intensities increases the size of the stimulation field and thus increases error in NCS.

Overstimulation also increases the chance that the stimulus will activate nearby nerves (Fig. 7-24D). Unintended and unrecognized stimulation of additional nerves is a major cause of error in conduction studies. Overstimulation should be considered (in addition to injury and anatomic variation) whenever there is a change in the configuration of the evoked potential between two points of stimulation along the nerve.

A needle cathode is often more effective for stimulation of a deep, difficult-to-isolate nerve (Fig. 7-24E). A standard monopolar EMG needle works well, paired with a surface disc anode. Inserting the needle tip to a point near the nerve bypasses the high skin impedance. Thus, a low-voltage, short-duration stimulus (50 μsec) is adequate. Needle electrodes seldom cause bleeding (easily con-

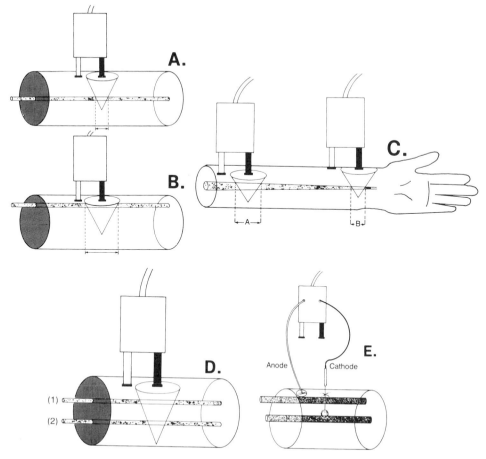

Figure 7–24. *A.* When the intensity of the stimulation field is just adequate to produce nerve depolarization, the initial depolarization point is more likely to be directly below the cathode. *B.* Very large stimulation intensities increase the uncertainty of this location and increase the changes of stimulation of nearby nerves. *C.* The cone approximates the volume of tissue in which the electrical field produced by the cathode is sufficient to initiate nerve depolarization. Initial depolarization may begin anywhere along the nerve within this volume. *D.* The high intensity stimulation required to produce depolarization of nerve (*2*) causes depolarization of the adjacent nerve (*1*). This often occurs when attempting to stimulate a deep-lying nerve from the surface. *E.* A needle electrode can be used to produce a small, localized stimulation field (*sphere*). Needle stimulation can ensure stimulation of a specific nerve (while excluding others) or permit stimulation of deep-lying nerves. The lower intensity of the stimulation is better tolerated by the patients.

trolled with pressure), and they do not risk causing infection owing to their small size (inoculum) and minimal trauma. Theoretical analysis indicates that there is no risk of electrically generated thermal injury to the nerve from this technique because of low heat generation and excellent dispersion by the tissue.

From a practical perspective, with each stimulation the electromyographer should attempt to activate all target nerve axons so that total nerve function is recorded; one should avoid unintended stimulation of nearby nerves and minimize patient discomfort. These goals

are interrelated by their dependence on the electrical voltage and duration of the stimulus.

The proper physical application of the stimulus is the most important aspect of technique. Standard stimulation points for clinical studies are chosen both for their clinical relevance and because they are points where the nerve is relatively accessible. Firm pressure used to seat the electrodes between the adjacent structures permits stimulation with less current but should not directly induce pain. Experience reduces the number of stimuli needed for a study by providing an educated guess about the stimulus intensity required. Typically, a stimulation of 0.1 msec and 150–250 volts with a constant voltage stimulator is sufficient. Longer durations (0.2–0.5 msec) are more effective with large sensory axons. Electrical coupling gels and light skin abrasion reduce skin impedance and thus the stimulation intensity required.

CONDUCTION LATENCY

Latency is the time required for a conduction signal to reach a recording electrode following stimulation at a single point on the nerve. Latency rather than velocity is usually used to assess the terminal nerve segments when a second stimulation point needed to establish point-to-point conduction velocity is not available because of "space" restrictions. Motor latencies are obtained by stimulating near the terminal end of the nerve and recording the compound motor action potential. The time that is required for this distal conduction, i.e., motor latency, has several components:

1. Latency of activation: the time between the initiation of the electrical discharge of the stimulator and the actual beginning of saltatory conduction along the axon; it represents the initial channel opening and ion flow time.
2. Fast, saltatory conduction along the large, myelinated axon (Fig. 7–25, A–B).
3. Slower conduction along the smaller diameter myelinated axons as they taper distally (Fig. 7–25, C–D).

4. Still slower conduction along the even smaller diameter axon as it branches distally (Fig. 7–25, D–E).
5. Very slow conduction along the non-myelinated, terminal twigs of the axon (Fig. 7–25, E–F).
6. Chemical transmission (diffusion) of the signal across the myoneural junction—approximately 0.2 to 0.5 msec (Fig. 7–25, F–G).
7. Muscle depolarization (Fig. 7–25, G).

Residual latency is the difference between the observed latency and the calculated time required to conduct along the same terminal segment distance using the conduction velocity of the large myelinated fibers obtained with standard nerve conduction studies. For example: if the median nerve forearm conduction velocity is 50 msec and the distal segment used for the motor latency is 8 cm, then the calculated time for conduction along this segment would be 0.08 m · 50 msec = 0.0016 sec or 1.6 msec. If the actual measured latency is 3.5 msec, then 3.5 msec − 1.6 msec = 1.9 msec, which is the residual latency.

In sensory latencies, the evoked potential recorded is directly generated by the nerve, and the latency (i.e., conduction time) required consists only of these factors: (a) the latency of activation; (b) a saltatory conduction along the myelinated axon; and (c) slower saltatory conduction as the axon diameter tapers distally and cools (Fig. 7–26).

Because sensory latency consists only of "nerve factors," it can be arithmetically converted into a conduction velocity. Most authors ignore the latency of activation in this

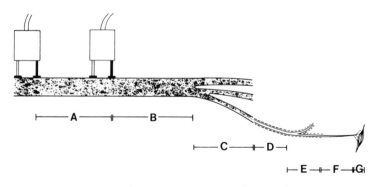

Figure 7–25. Conduction "environments" of a typical motor axon.

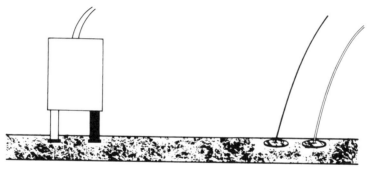

Figure 7–26. Conduction along a sensory axon showing stimulation and recording electrodes. Note the contrast between this rather uniform conducting medium and that illustrated for the motor axon in Figure 7–25.

F - Wave

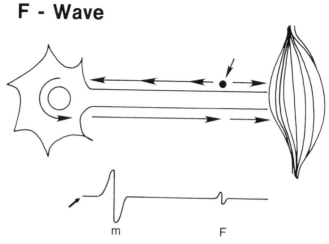

m   F

Figure 7–27. F response. The course of the depolarization following stimulation (*dot*) is shown by the arrows. Initially, depolarization travels both directly to the muscle fiber, producing the Mm response, and retrograde up the axon to the neuron, where it is repropagated in a small percentage of neurons, then back down the axon to produce the delayed F response.

process. Because motor latencies include the disparate factors that make up the residual latency, they cannot be arithmetically converted into nerve conduction velocities.

SPECIAL CONDUCTION TECHNIQUES

H and F Wave use in Proximal Conduction Studies

NCS are traditionally performed by stimulating the nerve at two separate locations and comparing evoked potentials recorded at a third point. From this, the conduction velocity of the segment can be calculated, and changes in the size and shape of the evoked response caused by abnormality in the tested segment can be quantified. This approach is difficult in very proximal lesions, e.g., Guillain-Barré syndrome, root or plexus injuries, thoracic outlet syndrome, and intragluteal sciatic nerve injuries because we are not able to use standard surface stimulation proximal to these lesions. Either direct spinal root stimulation techniques or the use of late waves enables us to evaluate these lesions. Although each of those techniques have limitations, they are better than alternatives that assess only the distal effects of these proximal injuries.

The F wave results from the recurrent discharge of a small percentage (1–5%) of the alpha motor neurons that are antidromically activated during peripheral nerve stimulation. Therefore, both the afferent and the efferent arcs of this late wave must follow the same alpha motor neuron axons and the response passes through the proximal nerve segment twice (Fig. 7–27). Those anterior horn cells that re-discharge vary from stimulation to

stimulation; thus, the latency, shape, and amplitude of the F response vary slightly from stimulation to stimulation (14, 39). If a number of stimulations are recorded and the shortest latency selected, a consistent value, representing the fastest conduction motor fibers, is obtained.

The F wave is not suppressed by high intensity or frequency stimulation. Its amplitude is smaller than that of the H wave, usually less than 500 μV. With small-amplitude F-waves, the initial deflection is hard to identify and care must be taken to ensure that the shortest latency (earliest takeoff) of the wave is used. Recording multiple responses is essential to establish the latency; at least 10 responses should be recorded for each analysis (Fig. 7–28). There should be no voluntary motor activity in the background during F-wave recording.

The F wave occurs in all motor nerves and often remains present in the face of severe disease. Weber developed the following formula for predicting the F wave in the ulnar nerve (59):

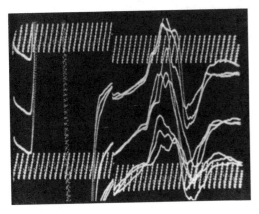

Figure 7–28. Recording of ulnar F responses obtained in nine sequential stimulations of the nerve. (Caliber: Each slanted line = 1 msec. Height = 200 μV.)

031 × (the distance in centimeters from the spine of C7 to the tip of the ulnar styloid) + (the constant 11.05) − (0.123 × the forearm velocity of the ulnar nerve).

Figure 7–29. Multiple regression technique-derived F-wave formula.

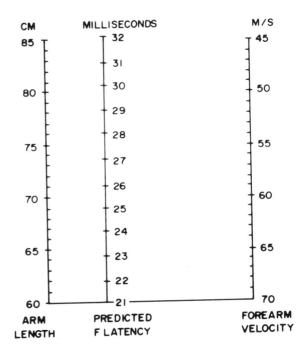

NOMOGRAM FOR PREDICTING ULNAR F WAVE LATENCY

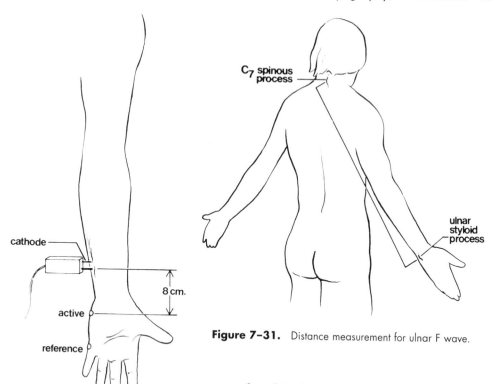

Figure 7–31. Distance measurement for ulnar F wave.

Figure 7–30. Stimulation and recording technique for obtaining the F wave in the ulnar nerve. Note that the cathode is placed proximally to the anode.

Normal latency should not exceed the predicted value by more than 2.5 msec (mean + 2 SDs). The nomogram gives the upper limit value (Fig. 7–29). Side-to-side variation on the ulnar nerve should not exceed 1 msec (mean + 2 SDs), and side-to-side comparisons in other nerves remain within this general range. For this technique, the ulnar nerve is stimulated at the wrist just as for the usual ulnar motor latency, except that the anode and the cathode positions are reversed (Fig. 7–30). Stimulation at the wrist avoids the necessity of recording an F wave on the upslope of the M wave, which results from proximal stimulation (unless special collision techniques are used). For testing and for distance measurement, the arm is positioned with the elbow extended and the shoulder abducted approximately 20° (Fig. 7–31).

Because the ulnar forearm velocity is part of the formula to predict latency, the wide range of normal nerve conduction velocities found in the population is eliminated. Thus, the velocity narrows the range of the predicted F value. It also negates the effect of distal slowing from proximal entrapment. Therefore, these predicted values should be used for entrapments only, not for investigation of generalized neuropathy.

The H wave is generated by a monosynaptic spinal reflex. The afferent axons are I-a afferent fibers of the muscle spindle and the efferents are axons of the alpha motor neuron (Fig. 7–32). In infants, the H-wave is found in many nerves, but in adults it occurs in only a few. The tibial H-wave latency for an individual can be predicted from the following formula, which was developed by Braddom (5): (0.46 × the length in centimeters from the mid-popliteal crease to the tip of the medial malleolus) + (one-tenth of the patient's age) + (the constant, 9.14). This value may also be obtained from a nomogram. The normal variation from the predicted value is rather large (4.8 msec), but it can be reduced in unilateral problems by comparing of the symptomatic to the nonsymptomatic side. In this instance, the sides should vary by no more than 1.2 msec.

The H wave can usually be elicited by stimulating at an intensity below that which is

H - Wave

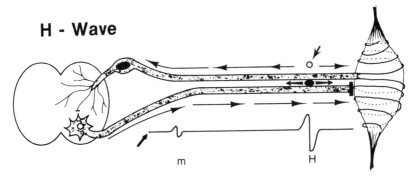

Figure 7–32. The H response is obtained by stimulation of the afferent sensory fiber (*top*), resulting in orthodromic conduction to the spinal cord. There, synaptic stimulation of the alpha motor neuron occurs, resulting in the evoked H response in the muscles. A few motor axons are often directly stimulated, producing the rudimentary M response illustrated.

necessary to evoke muscle contraction (M response) because the larger-diameter I-a afferent axons are more easily stimulated. It is suppressed by supramaximal stimulation intensities and by stimulation frequencies greater than 1 Hertz. Therefore, it can be distinguished from the F wave through the use of a slowly increasing stimulation intensity. When this technique is used, the H wave will appear before or near the threshold stimulation intensity for eliciting the M response, increase in amplitude to several mV, and finally diminish and disappear as the intensity of the stimulation increases (the F wave will then be seen) (40).

Although these techniques offer a method of confirming distal conduction abnormalities (particularly useful in ulnar lesions at the elbow), they should not be routinely relied upon to replace direct stimulation studies for segments of the nerve that are easily accessible. Central "relay" components complicate the use of either of these techniques for peripheral conduction velocity determination. Whereas the F wave can be employed to check proximal conduction in most nerves, the H wave has a more limited scope in adults, where it's usually confined to the tibial, median, and femoral nerves.

SPINAL NERVE STIMULATION

The ability to directly stimulate spinal nerves makes it possible to assess conduction across the most proximal peripheral nerve segments. Johnson has long advocated root stimulation with monopolar needle electrodes. This approach is now routine for C8 spinal nerve stimulation, but, it can be as effective for other roots as well. Not only can peripherally directed conduction be assessed, but root or cauda equina function also has been assessed through reflex responses. Stimulation from the surface can be accomplished with high-voltage electrical and magnetic stimulators. Studies assessing the location of the initial depolarization by these techniques have been reported. The majority view is that depolarization begins near the spinal foramen; however, there can be considerable variation. Nevertheless, this variability is likely to be less than the conduction uncertainty encountered at other proximally located stimulation sites such as in the supraclavicular space. Although small uncertainties of the site of initial activation have practical implications for evaluation of the nerve root itself, it should have little appreciable impact when assessing major plexus entrapments or injuries. We favor needle stimulation of the root because it causes less patient discomfort than high voltage stimulation and is more reliably accomplished for deep-lying roots than is magnetic stimulation.

Spinal nerve stimulation provides both a direct measurement of the conduction velocity and information about the distribution of velocities (temporal dispersion) of all axons composing the root. This is a significant advantage over use of the F wave and H wave. Its relative limitation is that change in the size and shape of the evoked potential generated by the root stimulation cannot be directly compared with an evoked response generated distal to the suspected lesion. This is an obvious consequence of the peripheral nerve containing axons from more than a single nerve root. Because the number of axons that a particular nerve root contributes to a given peripheral nerve varies, the "normal" response generated in a specific muscle by spinal nerve stimulation is also highly variable. Nonetheless, considerable information can be obtained from the shape and temporal dispersion of the response, and in discrepancies between conduction velocities calculated from spinal nerves, and from peripheral nerve stimulation.

C8 is the most frequently stimulated spinal nerve. The procedure is safe and relatively painless, particularly if stimulation can be restricted to several trials. A standard monopolar, Teflon-coated EMG needle is used as a cathode with a large surface electrode applied near the midline serving as the anode. Stimulation can often be obtained with a stimulus duration of 0.10 milliseconds and an intensity of less than 100 V. Somewhat higher intensities available with commercial EMG stimulators can be employed without danger of tissue injury related to electrical or thermal effects. To stimulate C8, the needle should be inserted approximately one inch lateral to the inferior border of the C7 dorsal spine, angled 30° to 45° degrees toward the midline, and advanced through the paraspinal muscle until it strikes the transverse process (Fig. 7–33). If the first attempt at stimulation is not successful, the needle can be slightly repositioned until a good response is obtained.

The CMAP action potential can be recorded from any of the innervated muscles. With C8, the abductor digiti V is usually chosen because the lower plexus, ulnar components are most often at interest in proximal entrapment syndromes. Normal velocity is 68 ± 3 msec (lower normal limit is normal, 62 msec). Distance is measured from the point of needle insertion to the standard point of stimulation at the wrist to obtain the distal ulnar latency. The arm is positioned as for the F wave study. Using a similar technique but recording from the median nerve over the thenar eminence, the normal conduction velocity is 70 ± 2.7 msec (lower limit of normal is 65 msec). The mean latency difference with C8 stimulation between the median nerve and the ulnar nerve is 0.0 ± 0.86 msec (maximum

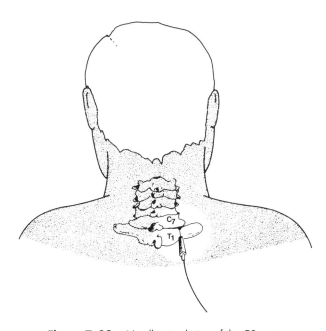

Figure 7–33. Needle stimulation of the C8 root.

variation = 1.7 m/second) (58). If the spinal nerve stimulation response is abnormal, it is important that all peripheral segments be tested in order to localize the point of abnormality. The spinal stimulation, F and H wave techniques offer a means of confirming observed abnormalities in peripheral conduction across particularly challenging areas, such as the ulnar groove, because peripheral slowing should also be detectable by these techniques.

Stimulation of each of the cervical roots up through C5 can be performed in a manner analogous to that for C8. In the lumbar region (37), the root also is approached from a lateral position at approximately a 30° to 45° angle. For S1, the point of entry is medial to the posterior superior iliac spine and approximately 1.5 to 2.0 inches lateral to the midline. A longer needle electrode may be required. A sacral root to the sphincter can be stimulated by a needle at the foramens (51). Although the technique is well tolerated, it is helpful to prepare the individuals by explaining what to expect, letting them know when the stimulus is coming, and providing some counterirritant pressure on the back in the area of the stimulation to reduce its sensory impact.

COMMON NERVE CONDUCTION ERRORS

Computerized electrodiagnostic equipment makes it increasingly easy to "capture" a nerve response. Unfortunately, there is no guarantee that the signal recorded is the one that was sought or that it was not distorted by technical problems. The increasing automation of the process keeps the electromyographer from "seeing" the clues that something is amiss. It is a useful exercise to periodically review the sources of error in order to maintain an index of caution:

1. Recording a volume-conducted signal (sometimes generated by a volume-conducted stimulus to an untargeted nerve). Often a slight, initial positive response is the only clue to a problem. It results from initial depolarization occurring away from G1. It is surprising how closely an ulnar volume-conducted response, recorded over the thenar muscles, resembles the expected median response if the median response is absent in a patient with severe carpal tunnel syndrome.

2. Mistaking a general slowing of conduction for focal entrapment. Nerves can be unevenly involved in an early neuropathy; one should be certain the others are normal before deciding that the "tested" one is entrapped.

3. Be careful to monitor temperature throughout the course of the examination. Evaporative cooling and vasoconstriction can quickly drop temperatures. It is easy to miss the effects of cool nerves, age, and height when testing using very short sensory segments.

4. Technical mistakes happen! Sooner or later you will reverse the cathode and anode, use an improper filter or amplifier setting, or mismeasure or stimulate the wrong nerve. If the signal or value does not "look right," take the time to exclude technical error.

5. Deviating from standard NCS techniques can be a problem with short segment studies in which normal ranges are quite tight.

6. Watch for anatomic variation. The challenge of the Martin-Gruber anastomosis is not the "wildly" fast median nerve velocity recorded in carpal tunnel syndrome, but the amplitude change in the ulnar-evoked potential it produces in normal subjects.

7. Internal inconsistency. Ignoring inconsistencies in the findings deprives one of the best check on one's work. Patients rarely have inexplicable, inconsistent findings; neither should your reports.

REPORTING VALUES: A NUMBERS GAME

The use of computers has also increased the tendency to report results of NCS to an ever higher number of decimal places. Whereas NCS reported to two or three decimal places seem more precise, they are, in fact, deceptive. The accuracy of any NCS value is limited by the precision with which its least reliable component can be known. Although the time component can be accurately "recorded" by the computer to several decimal places, the significance of the value is restricted by the uncertainty in the distance the signal has traveled. Measurement of this distance is restricted mechanically and by the inherent uncertainty as to the point of initial depolarization along the nerve. Clinical studies will vary by up to 5% between trials and up to 10% if repeated after an interval of several days. In these circumstances, the number of significant digits reported is also limited by these uncertainties. Therefore, velocity values are "accurate" at whole msec levels with a first decimal place value inherently uncertain, i.e., for 50 msec a variation of 1 msec represents a 2% variation, which exceeds the 5% measurement accuracy underlying the test. Similarly, a latency variation of 0.1 msec represents a 5.5% variation for a normal 8-cm median sensory (mean median nerve reference value 1.8 msec) conduction study. While each study has its own technical aspects affecting accuracy/reproducibility, the general guideline of reporting in full numbers for conduction velocities and in increments of 0.1 msec for latencies remains valid.

SPECIFIC NERVE EXAMINATIONS

Phrenic Nerve

Phrenic nerve motor function originates from the fourth cervical root, with contributions from C3 and C5. It is the sole motor supply for the diaphragm. The right and left phrenic nerves follow different courses to the diaphragm, the right nerve being shorter and more vertical. Loss of diaphragmatic function is a catastrophic event, occurring most frequently with spinal cord injury, peripheral nervous system disease, and trauma. Electrodiagnostic studies are often crucial in determining both the prognosis and the appropriate treatment.

STANDARD MOTOR CONDUCTION TECHNIQUE

The phrenic nerve is easily stimulated using a standard bipolar surface stimulator pressed

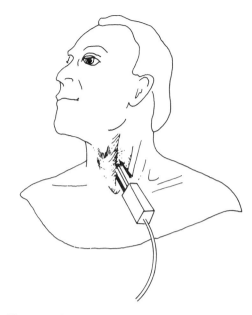

Figure 7–34. Stimulation technique for the phrenic nerve.

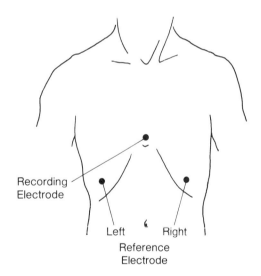

Figure 7–35. Evoked potential recording technique from the diaphragm for phrenic nerve stimulation.

deeply along the lateral edge of the sternocleidomastoid in the supraclavicular space (Fig. 7–34). MacLean has noted the benefits of stimulation in this location using a needle electrode, which he reports to be both safe and more effective in isolating the stimulus to the phrenic nerve (38). G1 is placed over the xiphoid, and G2 is placed in the eighth intercostal space at the costochondral junction

(Fig. 7–35). This location helps isolate the diaphragmatic response from those that occur through inadvertent brachial plexus stimulation. The normal latency on the right is 7.4 ± 0.73 msec; on the left, it is 7.5 ± 0.97 msec (38). The highest normal latency seen was 8.6 msec, although some authors have reported slightly higher values, up to 9.4 msec (2). Amplitudes range widely and are lower than might be anticipated; adult amplitudes range 0.2 to 2.0 mV and neonatal amplitudes are frequently less than 0.2 mV. There is no superficial sensory component of this nerve.

Suprascapular Nerve

The suprascapular nerve (C5, C6) enters the suprascapular fossa through the suprascapular foramen (Fig. 7–36). This U-shaped, bony notch is bridged by the superior transverse scapular ligament, converting it into an enclosed foramen. The nerve forms two branches. The first one passes to the supraspinatus muscle, branching to the glenohumeral and acromioclavicular joints. The second passes around the lateral margin of the scapular spine, supplying the infraspinatus muscle, the scapula, and the glenohumeral joint.

Nerve compromise may be due to: isolated "neuritis"; compression by the transverse scapular ligament; relatively minor, repeated trauma to a metabolically compromised nerve; or the stretching of the nerve during an extreme motion of the scapula (forced scapular protraction). The infrascapular branch can be stretched or compressed as it passes around the scapular spine.

Supraspinatus weakness disrupts normal glenohumeral motion by decreasing stabilization of the humeral head, and paralysis may prevent initiation of shoulder abduction. Patients may substitute for this weakness by dipping the shoulder and flexing the trunk toward the side of the injury, because the resulting pendular arm motion helps initiate abduction. Infraspinatus weakness decreases external rotator strength, but is not usually functionally limiting.

The suprascapular nerve provides no cutaneous innervation. Suprascapular nerve en-

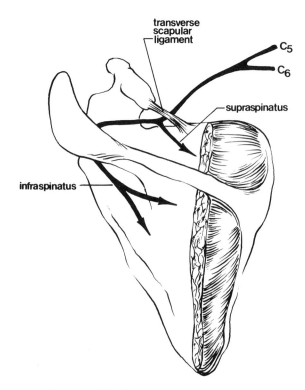

Figure 7-36. Suprascapular nerve anatomy.

trapment may present as shoulder pain, sometimes with limitation of movement, and be mistaken for pericapsulitis of the shoulder.

Suprascapular nerve injury may result in a prolongation of the motor latency to or loss of the evoked response in the supraspinatus and/or infraspinatus muscle. Needle EMG examination should be performed to confirm the diagnosis. Positive waves, fibrillation potentials, motor unit loss, etc., should be confined to the appropriate muscles. Careful exploration of the C5, C6 paraspinals must always be included because C5 radiculopathy can mimic suprascapular nerve entrapment. Investigation of the infraspinatus muscle is essential when the supraspinatus is normal and shoulder pain is the major complaint.

MOTOR CONDUCTION TECHNIQUES

Because of its short length and the inaccessibility of the distal portion of the nerve for stimulation, standard studies utilize only a motor latency determination. One stimulates the nerve in the supraclavicular fossa using a standard bipolar surface stimulator that is pressed deeply into the space behind the clavicular head of the sternocleidomastoid just above the clavicle (Fig. 7–37). The cathode is situated lateral to the anode. The study is uncomfortable for the patient and should be organized to minimize the number of stimulations.

Surface electrodes are adequate for recording in individuals with normal findings, but a needle electrode may be required with patients with abnormal findings to ensure that the recorded signal originates from the desired muscle (see the section on recording technique) (Fig. 7–38). Kraft reported normal latency to the supraspinatus of 2.7 ± 0.5 msec (upper limit of normal is 3.7 msec) and to the infraspinatus of 3.3 ± 0.5 msec (upper limit of normal is 4.3 msec) (31) (Fig. 7–39). There is no superficial sensory component of this nerve.

Axillary Nerve

The axillary nerve (C5, C6) forms an anterior branch that supplies the deltoid and overlying skin and a posterior branch that supplies the teres minor and the posterior portion of the

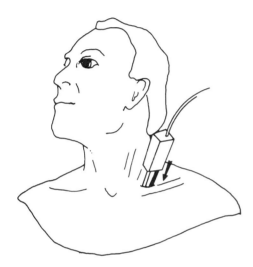

Figure 7-37. Technique of supraclavicular stimulation of the upper brachial plexus used in various upper extremity nerve conduction studies.

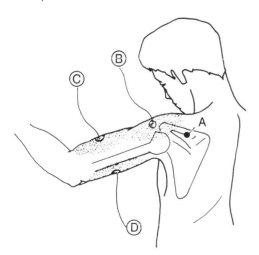

Figure 7-38. Motor recording points illustrated for various upper extremity nerve conduction studies. A. Supraspinatus. B. Axillary. C. Musculocutaneous. D. Radial.

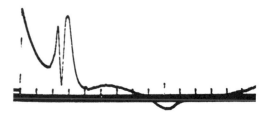

Figure 7-39. Motor response recorded with needle electrode in the supraspinatus muscle with suprascapular nerve stimulation. (Caliber: Each slanted line = 2 msec. Height = 200 μV.)

deltoid. Its sensory continuation pierces the deep fascia along the lower part of the posterior deltoid border and continues as the upper lateral cutaneous nerve of the arm. It supplies an oval-shaped area over the lateral aspect of the upper arm.

The axillary nerve is infrequently injured. Gunshot wounds, shoulder dislocations, and errant intramuscular injections account for most injuries. Loss of the teres minor is not functionally significant; however, denervation of the deltoid limits shoulder abduction. Although some authors disagree, abduction can occur in the absence of a functioning deltoid, particularly in very muscular individuals. Sensory loss can occur independent of motor loss.

MOTOR CONDUCTION TECHNIQUE

Stimulation is the same as for the suprascapular nerve (Fig. 7–37). Recording is done with surface electrodes: G1 over the most prominent portion of the middle deltoid, and G2 over the junction of the deltoid tendon and the humerus (Fig. 7–38). The mean latency is 3.9 ± 0.5 msec, with a normal range of 2.8 to 5.0 msec (31).

Direct recording of a sensory response from the axillary nerve is not practical; however, somatosensory evoked potential recording is possible.

Musculocutaneous Nerve—Lateral Cutaneous Nerve of the Forearm

The musculocutaneous nerve (C5, C6) supplies the biceps, coracobrachialis, and brachialis minor muscles and provides sensation to the lateral aspect of the forearm through its terminal branch, the lateral cutaneous nerve of the forearm. The latter proceeds obliquely across the arm and emerges through the deep fascia several centimeters above the elbow crease. There, it lies in close relationship to the antecubital veins—usually medial and deep to their confluence. At that point the nerve divides into posterior and anterior branches, which then proceed along the forearm, providing cutaneous sensation to the volar and dorsal aspects of the radial side of the forearm (see Fig. 7–41 later in this chapter).

In some individuals, the nerve also supplies sensation to the radial side of the hand.

The proximal portion of the musculocutaneous nerve is infrequently entrapped or injured. Gunshot wounds are the most frequent cause of proximal injury and usually damage both the nerve and the lateral cord of the plexus. Injury occasionally occurs in shoulder dislocation, violent compressive injuries to the anterior portion of the shoulder, or stretch injuries of the arm. Compression during surgery has been reported, as has spontaneous palsy occurring in weight lifters. In weight lifters, compression probably takes place during the nerve's passage through the coracobrachialis or the biceps muscle (6).

Injury to the terminal sensory portion, the lateral cutaneous nerve of the forearm, is more frequent. That nerve may be tethered as it passes through deep fascia and at the point where it forms its two terminal branches. The nerve is occasionally injured during phlebotomy in the antecubital space. Most frequently, injury occurs during cardiac catheterization in association with canalization of the vein.

Because there is much overlap among sensory nerves supplying the forearm and hand, injury to this nerve may produce only a small area of numbness or dysesthesia. Paralysis of the motor portion leads to loss of strength for elbow flexion; however, but the pronator teres and other forearm muscles are still able to carry out effective elbow flexion, albeit with more pronation than supination.

MOTOR CONDUCTION TECHNIQUE

The musculocutaneous nerve is stimulated in the supraclavicular fossa at the lateral attachment of the sternocleidomastoid to the clavicle (Fig. 7–37). The recording electrode is placed just distal to the midpoint of the biceps over the area of its greatest mass, and the reference electrode is placed at the elbow (Fig. 7–38). The mean normal latency is 4.5 ± 0.6 msec, with a normal range of 3.3 to 5.7 msec (31) (Fig. 7–40).

SENSORY CONDUCTION TECHNIQUE

Lateral Cutaneous Nerve of the Forearm
Sensory studies can be performed using surface stimulation and recording. With the anti-

dromic technique reported by Spindler, the nerve is stimulated in the antecubital space just lateral to the biceps tendon, with the recording electrode 12 cm distal along the course of the nerve (Fig. 7–41). Latency mea-

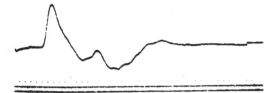

Figure 7–40. Motor evoked response recorded from the biceps with musculocutaneous nerve stimulation. Height of the time base equals 1 meter. 1-msec division.

sured to the negative peak is 2.3 ± 0.1 msec (upper limit of normal is 2.5 msec), and the mean amplitude is 24 ± 7.2 μV. Side-to-side comparison of latencies gave a mean plus 2 SD of 0.30 msec, whereas the mean plus 2 SD comparison side-to-side comparison of the ratio of the smaller over the larger amplitude was 0.73 (49).

Long Thoracic Nerve (of Bell)

The long thoracic nerve (C5, C6, C7) supplies only the serratus anterior muscle, giving branches to each muscle's slip as it passes vertically down the chest wall. It is anchored proximally at the scalenus medius and on each slip

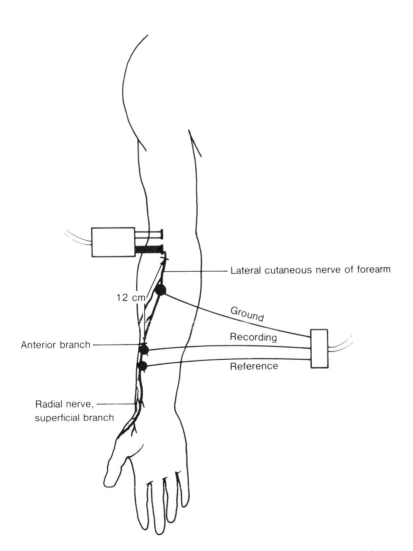

Lateral cutaneous nerve of forearm

12 cm

Ground

Recording

Anterior branch

Reference

Radial nerve, superficial branch

Figure 7–41. Sensory conduction technique illustrated for the lateral cutaneous nerve of the forearm (musculocutaneous nerve).

of the serratus. This anchoring increases its susceptibility to stretch injury from either contralateral bending of the neck or depression of the ipsilateral shoulder. Palsies may result from use of a heavy knapsack, which depresses the shoulders, or from inappropriate positioning during surgery. The nerve is most frequently damaged during competitive wrestling.

The serratus assists the trapezius in elevation of the shoulder and pulls the medial border of the scapula against the chest wall during elevation of the arm. Paralysis results in winging of the scapula, i.e., separation from the thoracic wall. This separation is demonstrated by having the patient place the extended arms directly in front and pressing forward against a wall with the hand. This causes the medial aspect of the scapula to prominently wing out from the thoracic wall.

MOTOR CONDUCTION TECHNIQUE

The long thoracic nerve can be stimulated in the supraclavicular space using a surface stimulator. The technique is similar to that used for the other proximal portions of the plexus (Fig. 7–37). Recording is done from the serratus muscle slips at the midaxillary line using needle or surface electrodes. Kaplan reported a mean latency of 3.9 ± 0.6 msec (upper limit of normal is 5.1 msec) using surface recording electrodes (30). Side-to-side comparison of the evoked potential and latency and needle EMG examination should be included in the evaluation. Needle exploration of the muscle may be more useful than conduction studies for following the progress of recovery. This nerve has no superficial sensory component.

Radial Nerve

The radial nerve (C5 through T1) is more likely to be damaged by trauma or acute compression and is less frequently involved in chronic entrapment syndromes than are other distal upper extremity nerves. Crutch palsy can occur from external pressure on the nerve in the axilla. The radial nerve is the nerve most frequently damaged with arm fractures, occurring in perhaps 10% of mid-humeral shaft fractures (spiral groove). It is also in-

jured, if less frequently, with fractures of the proximal third of the radius (posterior interosseus branch) (Fig. 7–42). With humeral fractures or open trauma, surgical repair of the nerve is required if its continuity is interrupted. Although EDX studies cannot prove that the nerve is severed, the demonstration of preserved voluntary function on needle EMG or the presence of an evoked potential from stimulation after the time necessary for Wallerian degeneration does prove continuity and that surgery can be deferred.

The nerve is vulnerable to compression as it runs from the lateral epicondyle to the supinator muscle (radial tunnel). In this area, it passes the radiohumeral joint, where it may be tethered by connective tissue and thus more

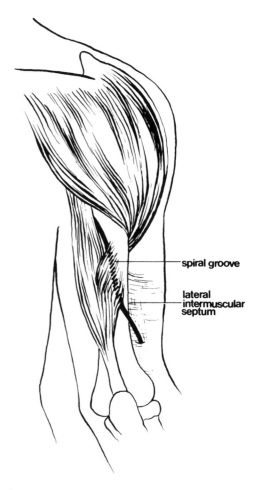

spiral groove

lateral intermuscular septum

Figure 7–42. Radial nerve course through the spiral groove. The immobility of the nerve in this location makes it vulnerable to injury during upper arm trauma and fractures.

easily injured. It also may be compressed by the tendon of the overlying extensor carpi radialis brevis (Fig. 7–43).

Because the radial nerve divides into its two major branches (superficial and posterior interosseus) in the tunnel, either the entire nerve or either of its separate branches can be entrapped there. The purely sensory superficial branch can be damaged near the wrist by handcuffs or watchbands (17, 43).

Posterior Interosseus Nerve Syndrome

This purely motor posterior interosseus nerve arises in the radial tunnel from the division of the radial nerve. Injury has been reported from direct trauma, compression by ganglia or vascular anomaly, and rheumatoid synovitis. The nerve seems to be most vulnerable to repeated trauma from firm wrist extension where it passes through the supinator muscle at the fibrous arcade of Frohse. Additionally, full pronation of the forearm may exert pressure on the nerve at the sharp, tendinous edge of the extensor carpi radialis brevis muscle. Paresis following Frisbee throwing has been reported (18), as has tennis elbow-based neuropathy (44).

In posterior interosseus syndrome, the patient has difficulty extending the fingers and thumb and frequently complains of a dull, aching pain, i.e., lateral epicondylitis. The radial wrist extensors are normal, and there is no

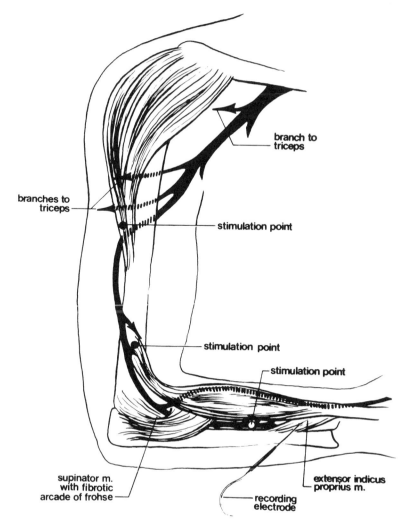

Figure 7–43. Radial nerve with major motor distributions, stimulation points, and recording points marked.

superficial sensory loss. Needle EMG may be positive in several of the supplied muscles: extensor digitorum, extensor digiti minimi, extensor carpi ulnaris, abductor pollicis longus, extensor pollicis longus, extensor pollicis brevis, and extensor indicus proprius. Each should be explored.

Sleep palsies have two forms: the "Saturday night palsy," in which the individual sleeps with the arm draped over or pressed against the hard edge of a piece of furniture, and the "sleep palsy," in which the weight of another individual's head compresses the nerve against the patient's arm. In either instance, the individual experiencing the radial nerve injury is often in a deeper-than-normal sleep induced by the use of alcohol or a sedative.

Wrist and finger extension is compromised, but the triceps is spared; therefore, triceps involvement indicates a more proximal lesion. Occasionally the brachioradialis and, less often, the extensor carpi radialis longus muscles may be spared. Sensory loss (hypesthesia and hypalgesia) is seldom prominent in radial nerve palsy because the area of exclusive radial nerve sensory innervation is often confined to the dorsum of the thumb.

Nerve conduction across the lesion may be slowed or it may be partially or completely blocked. Forearm conduction usually remains normal. Special care is necessary to avoid confusion caused by the volume-conduction spread of the stimulus to adjoining nerves; one should watch to see which muscles are responding or use a needle recording electrode to confirm the signal source. Needle EMG following sleep palsy may be markedly abnormal; despite this, prognosis for recovery (generally within 2 months) is excellent if a radial evoked response can be obtained with stimulation at the elbow 7 days after the injury or if there continues to be some voluntary motor units present in the extensor muscles on the initial needle EMG (21). Recovery from intra-axillar compression, humeral fractures, intermuscular injections, etc., is less satisfactory than those associated with the sleep palsies, and residual weakness is frequent.

MOTOR CONDUCTION TECHNIQUE

The radial nerve has less-well-defined landmarks to identify stimulation points, and the muscles used for recording are less isolated than for many other nerves. Radial motor conduction studies are therefore less reproducible or precise than those of the median and ulnar nerves. Stimulation points include the supraclavicular space, axilla; the point posterior to the deltoid insertion at the beginning of the spiral groove; the area between the brachioradialis and biceps; and in the mid-forearm (Figs. 7–42 and 7–43). The last site requires needle electrode stimulation. Recording has been reported from the triceps, anconeus, brachioradialis, extensor communis, and extensor indicis proprius muscles. The latter are the most practical for general use, although certain clinical problems may dictate the use of another recording site.

When investigating the proximal portion of the nerve, surface recording from the extensor indicis is usually satisfactory; however, needle recording may be necessary when studying the segment from just above the elbow to the mid-forearm. Four stimulation points for standard study are the supraclavicular space; the area lateral to the triceps; the groove between the brachioradialis and the biceps just above the elbow crease; and approximately 3–4 cm proximal to the recording electrode in the mid-forearm. The first three points can be stimulated using a hand-held surface stimulator pressed deeply between the muscles, whereas the distal point requires needle electrode stimulation (Figs. 7–43, 7–44). The arm is positioned in 10° abduction with, the elbow flexed 10–15°, and the forearm pronated.

Normal conduction velocity for the proximal segment is 72 msec ± 6.3 msec (lower limit of normal is 60 msec). For the distal segment, the normal value is 61.6 ± 5.9 msec (lower limit of normal is 50 msec) (25).

Conduction to the triceps has been reported by Gassel using Erb's point stimulation and surface recording (Fig. 7–38D). Normal motor latency is dependent on the distance to the recording electrode, because the motor endplates are spread out along the muscle. Distance was measured with the arm at the side using obstetric calipers; which better approximates the nerve length (21). At 21.5 cm, the latency is 4.5 SD = 0.42 msec (upper limit of normal is 5.3 msec); and at 31.5 cm and,

5.3 msec, the SD = 0.5 (upper limit of normal is 6.3 msec) (20). Motor amplitudes greater than 2 mV are expected with this NCS.

To investigate the mid-arm segment in cases of trauma or the sleep palsies, it is helpful to stimulate proximally just posterior to the insertion of the deltoid, rather than at Erb's point, thus avoiding stimulation of other plexus elements. Normal velocities are essen-tially the same as described above, with the proximal segment conduction velocity ap-proximately 10% faster than that of the distal segment. Loss of this velocity relationship is suggestive of nerve entrapment.

To investigate entrapments in the radial or supinator tunnels, the distal radial segment is tested using needle recording and stimulating electrodes. In sleep palsies and fractures, vol-untary motor function is often absent, and evoked potential analysis is used to determine prognosis; i.e., preservation of a response after 5 days provides a good prognosis.

SENSORY CONDUCTION TECHNIQUE

The superficial radial nerve derived from ra-dial nerve bifurcation in the radial tunnel, is used for radial sensory conduction studies. With the orthodromic technique, one stimu-lates the digital branches on the dorsum of the thumb. Recording is done 14 cm proximally along the nerve using surface electrodes (Fig. 7–45). The forearm is positioned in neutral, and the recording electrodes are placed over the crest of the radius. A hand-held surface stimulator should be used, rather than ring electrodes, to reduce the overflow of stimula-tion to the median nerve branches that supply the palmar surface of the thumb. Because of this potential for median nerve stimulation, Trojaberg preferred to stimulate the nerve at the wrist for conduction studies of the more proximal segments of the nerve (50). Anti-dromic techniques have been described for the distal segment that use stimulation at the wrist and recording with ring electrodes at the

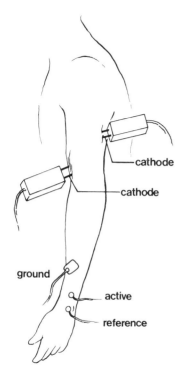

Figure 7–44. Standard stimulation and recording lo-cations for radial nerve motor conduction studies. G-1 over extensor indicus proprius, G-2 over tendon.

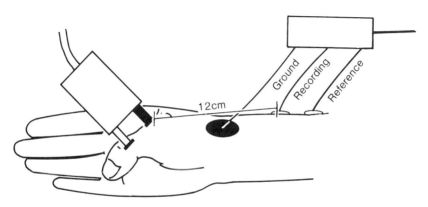

Figure 7–45. Standard stimulation and recording locations for orthodromic sensory conduction studies of the radial nerve. Note that individual digital nerve branches may be stimulated.

thumb. Normal values are essentially the same as those for the orthodromic technique.

Computer averaging is usually necessary to obtain conduction values for segments proximal to the wrist. Using a surface stimulator at the wrist, recording can be done by means of surface electrodes placed in the groove between the biceps and brachioradialis, posterior to the insertion of the deltoid, or in the axilla.

The orthodromic distal latency is 3.3 ± 0.4 msec (the upper limits of normal is 4.1 msec; the amplitude range is 15–35 μV). Using needle stimulation and, measuring from the initial deflection, proximal conduction values (Trojaberg) are wrist to elbow, 66 ± 8.0 msec (the lower limits of normal is 50 msec); and elbow to the axilla, 67 ± 6.5 msec (the lower limits of normal is 54 msec) (50).

Ulnar Nerve

NCS of the ulnar nerve (C7, C8, T1) is among the most technically challenging. The nerve's length and mobility, coupled with the number of potential points of entrapment, make testing difficult, while similarity of symptoms from ulnar entrapment and from other sources further complicates diagnosis. Proximal entrapment occurs in thoracic outlet syndrome (which is discussed elsewhere in this chapter), in Pancoast's tumor, by axillary lymph nodes, in vascular aneurysms, and from deformed clavicles, cervical ribs, and other anatomic structures. These can be investigated with F waves, C8 root stimulation, and somatosensory evoked potentials (Fig. 7–46). The ulnar nerve is seldom injured in the upper arm, but may occasionally be entrapped as it passes through the intermuscular septum or the arcade of Struthers.

Compromise at the elbow is most frequent and occurs from two basic problems: a) constriction by fibrous bands; or b) pressure or trauma to the nerve in the ulnar groove. The contribution to nerve injury of subluxation in the ulnar groove to nerve injury is unknown. Fibrous bands occur proximal to the groove and can produce nerve injury through constriction and by repeated trauma as the nerve is pulled to and fro. The point of nerve injury can often be localized by moving the stimulator sequentially at 1-cm to 2-cm intervals

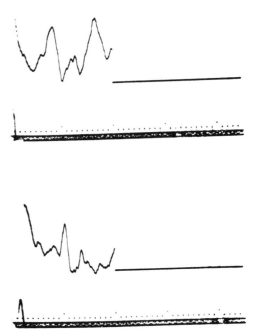

Figure 7–46. Evoked nerve potential in the ulnar nerve recorded at supraclavicular point using a signal average: (the technique for somatosensory evoked potentials). Upper response latency is 8.5 msec, whereas that obtained from the opposite side is pictured on the bottom and is delayed to 10.5 msec. (Caliber: 1 msec, 10 μV.)

along the nerve to look for an abrupt change in the evoked potential.

Direct compression at the elbow is often associated with weight loss or prolonged bed rest. It may result from arm positioning during anesthesia or during unconsciousness. Injury from acute compression is more easily demonstrated than that from chronic compression. In the latter, some fast-conducting fibers may

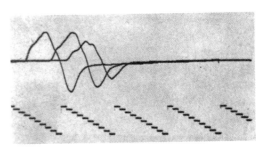

Figure 7–47. Hypothenar motor evoked responses from ulnar nerve stimulation at the wrist, below the elbow, and above the elbow. Note the loss of amplitude and area of the evoked response with conduction across the elbow. (Caliber: each slanted line = 10 msec, Height = 5 mV.)

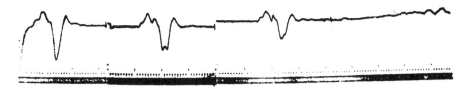

Figure 7–48. Ulnar nerve conduction series in severe, chronic ulnar nerve entrapment at the elbow. Evoked potentials obtained from left to right with stimulation at the wrist, below elbow, and above elbow. Note that all responses are small and velocities slowed owing to loss of many of the large-diameter axons. In this instance, it is difficult to determine if the entrapment at the elbow is ongoing or resolved, in view of the lack of dramatic change in conduction in this segment. This picture often confronts the electromyographer in patients with longstanding ulnar injuries both before and after surgical decompression. The height of the time base equals 1 mV, and the intervals are 1 msec. Forearm conduction velocity equals 34 msec, and across the elbow is 30 msec.

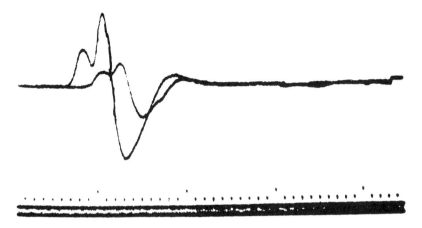

Figure 7–49. Evoked response with ulnar nerve stimulation below and above elbow. Note loss of response and slowing across elbow. (Caliber: same as in Figure 7–48.)

remain, preserving a normal maximum conduction velocity. Evoked potential analysis, sensory conduction, and needle electromyography may be needed to identify mild, chronic injury changes (Figs. 7–47, 7–48, and 7–49).

Observing the status of various branches, some help in the localization of abnormalities comes from observing the status of various branches: the flexor carpi ulnaris may be supplied above, in, or below the ulnar groove. Thus, when the flexor carpi ulnar is involved, it indicates ulnar injury at or above the elbow, but normal findings in this muscle do not preclude injury at the elbow. Forearm ulnar lesions are difficult to localize because of the absence of nerve branches in the forearm and because of the occurrence in 15%–20% of people of a Martin-Gruber anastomosis (Martin-Gruber) from the median to the ulnar nerve in the upper forearm (Fig. 7–50). When this anastomosis is present, the evoked poten-

tial obtained by stimulating the ulnar nerve below the level of the anastomosis is larger than that obtained from stimulating the nerve above the anastomosis—in direct proportion to the number of axons that join the ulnar from the median nerve (Figs. 7–51 and 7–52). Thus, sequential stimulation along the course of the ulnar nerve from distal to proximal would produce a point of sudden drop in the amplitude and area of the evoked response similar to that which would be seen in the presence of a partial ulnar palsy. The ulnar nerve enters the forearm between the two heads of the flexor carpi ulnaris (cubital tunnel) and may be entrapped there. The ulnar nerve gives off its dorsal cutaneous branch (in the hand) approximately 6 cm above the ulnar styloid, and preservation of sensation (and normal conduction) in this branch indicates a more distal problem. The next, more distal branch is the palmar sensory branch. This

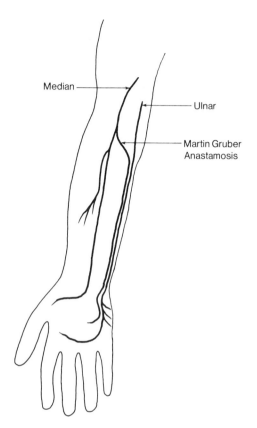

Figure 7–50. Communication in the forearm between the median and ulnar nerve: the Martin-Gruber anastomosis.

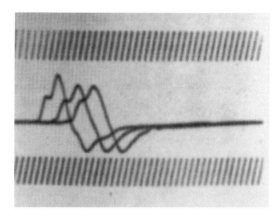

Figure 7–51. Evoked response recorded with stimulation of the ulnar nerve at the wrist, below the elbow, and above the elbow in an individual with the Martin-Gruber anastomosis. This response must be distinguished from the changes seen in ulnar entrapment.

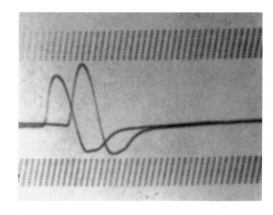

Figure 7–52. Paradoxical response to median nerve stimulation in same patient as in Figure 7–51. Proximal stimulation here produces larger evoked potential. Note also the initial positive deflection with elbow stimulation. (Caliber: each slanted line = 1 msec. Height = 5 mV.)

arises several centimeters proximal to the wrist crease and supplies sensory innervation to the ulnar aspect of the palm. It serves as another marker of the point of nerve injury.

The ulnar nerve has already split into its terminal branches when it enters Guyon's canal: the superficial branch (sensation to the little and ring fingers and palm; motor innervation to the palmaris brevis muscle), and the deep branch (motor innervation to the remaining ulnar-innervated muscles). The deep branch lies on the bony roof of the canal and separates into its terminal motor branches before exiting the canal. It is more susceptible to compression because of its position on the bony surface and its sharp turn around the hamate. Individual terminal branches can be injured in the distal canal. Handlebar palsy from bicycling compresses the nerve in the canal and may produce either painless weakness of the interossei or numbness, or both,

demonstrating that unequal compromise of the two principal branches can occur at any point from the beginning of the canal distalward.

The deep branch gives off motor twigs to the hypothenar muscles and then exits the canal. It must pass over the pisohamate ligament and under the fibrous arch from which the abductor and opponens digiti V originate. It turns sharply around the hook of the hamate and proceeds as the deep palmar branch, supplying the ulnar interossei, the two ulnar lumbricals, and the adductor pollicis brevis. These points are potential sites of entrapment (Fig. 7–53).

Unfortunately, from the standpoint of localizing lesions along the course of the deep branch, it divides into its terminal motor fascicles quite proximally in Guyon's canal. Thus, proximal, partial injuries of the deep branch may involve all or only some of the distal fascicles and can produce falsely localizing distributions of abnormalities. Thus, it is not possible to localize the injury based on the specific distribution of abnormalities in the deep palmar branch, except that it is distal to the separation from the sensory component.

Conduction studies to the abductor V and to the adductor pollicis brevis are helpful, but needle exploration of both these muscles and several of the dorsal interossei should also be routinely done in suspected ulnar lesions. Sampling of many muscles is necessary in distal lesions, both because of the possibility of specific branch injury or entrapment and because of the prevalence of anatomic variation in the nerve supply of the hand.

MOTOR CONDUCTION TECHNIQUE

Numerous cadaver studies have shown that arm position greatly affects the actual versus the surface-measured length of ulnar nerve segments. This is reflected in the wide variation in calculated conduction velocities among reported serial studies of normal subjects depending on the arm position used in each study. A technique in which the shoulder is abducted approximately 45°, and externally rotated; the elbow is acutely flexed so that the angle between the arm and forearm is less than 70°; and the forearm is supinated gives surface-measured distances closest to the actual nerve segment lengths. For recording, G1 is placed at the midpoint between the proximal

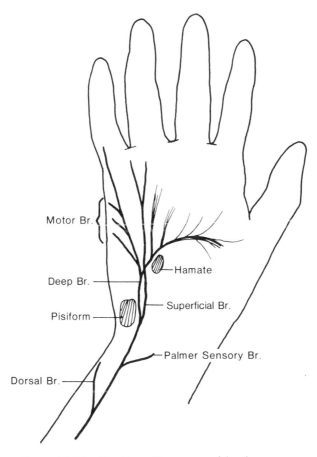

Figure 7–53. Distal branching pattern of the ulnar nerve.

wrist crease and the metacarpal phalangeal joint over the abductor digiti V, and the reference electrode G2 is placed on the little finger. Distal stimulation is 8 cm proximal to the recording electrode—lateral to and under the flexor carpi ulnaris tendon. Proximal stimulation points are just distal to the ulnar groove at the elbow, at a point approximately 12 cm proximal to this at the junction of the mid- and distal third of the arm, and in the supraclavicular space (Fig. 7–54). The mean value for the distal latency is 3.2 ± 0.5 msec (the upper limits of normal is 4.2 msec). The mean value for the forearm segment (below the elbow to the wrist) is 61.8 ± 5 msec (the lower limits of normal is 53 msec). The mean value for the across-elbow segment is 62.7 ± 5.5 msec (the lower limits of normal is 52 msec) (12). The amplitude range is 2–10 mV with no meaningful difference in mean amplitudes means with stimulation above or below the elbow.

Checkles noted that individuals show considerable variation when he compared these across-elbow to those below-elbow segment conduction velocities (12). The 95% confidence interval for normal was a slowing of up to 7% in the across-elbow segment compared to that of the forearm segment of the nerve. Thus, a small amount of slowing is acceptable in the across-elbow segment when using this technique. This compares to the finding of up to 45% slowing in normal individuals when this conduction comparison is made by testing with the elbow fully extended. (26, 48). This reinforces the importance of using evoked response analysis in addition to velocity changes in electrodiagnosis. Thus, a slowing of greater than 10% across the elbow when tested in the 70° flexed position is significant, particularly when accompanied by an arm amplitude decrease.

Jebsen reported a mean value of 62.8 ± 6 msec for conduction between the supraclavicular and above-elbow stimulation points (26). Calipers were used to measure this distance, and the lower limit of normal obtained by this technique was 51 msec.

Investigation of entrapment of the deep palmar branch of the ulnar nerve can be accomplished by recording over the adductor pollicis brevis in the dorsal web space. The mean latency for this response, stimulated as above, was found by Johnson and Melvin of

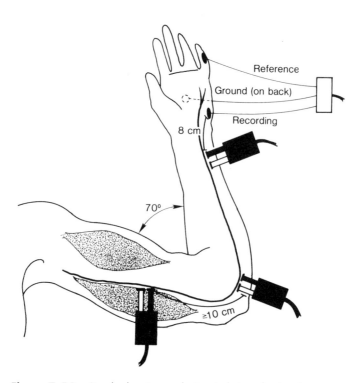

Figure 7–54. Standard motor conduction technique for the ulnar nerve.

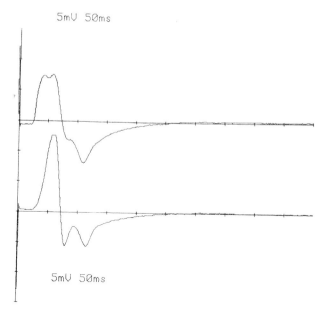

Figure 7–55. Ulnar motor recordings: hypothenars (above), dorsal web space (below).

Ohio State University (unpublished data) to be 3.34 ± 0.6 msec (Fig. 7–55) (upper limit of normal is 4.6 msec).

SENSORY CONDUCTION TECHNIQUE

Both orthodromic and antidromic techniques have been reported for the ulnar nerve. Checkles used an antidromic technique with arm positioning similar to that described for the motor conduction studies above (10). The mean conduction velocity of the forearm segment was 61.9 msec, and, for the across-elbow segment, 64.0 msec (10). All of the problems of positioning mentioned for the motor studies hold true for the sensory study. After analyzing their data, Checkles et al. felt the most reliable means of determining abnormal conduction at the elbow (with 95% confidence) was the use of an absolute conduction velocity in the across-elbow segments of not less than 50 msec.

With the ready availability of electronic averaging equipment and better amplifiers, orthodromic techniques have become more popular. Stimulating the digital nerves on the little and ring fingers (using ring electrodes, with the cathode proximal and recording 14 cm proximally, Melvin et al. (38) found a mean latency value to the peak of 3.0 ± 0.20 msec

(upper limit of normal is 3.4 msec) (Fig. 7–56). They also recorded proximally at the elbow and found a mean conduction velocity of 57.0 ± 5.0 msec (lower limit of normal is 47 msec). Amplitudes are sensitive to both recording and stimulating electrode placement and values of 7.0 μV are expected. The use of shorter segments may improve sensitivity in entrapments by avoiding dilution of slowing by long normal segments. The common digital nerve can be stimulated between the fourth and fifth metacarpals with a bipolar surface stimulator at the palmar crease (cathode proximal) (Fig. 7–57). Recording is at a point 8 cm proximal along the course of the nerve, and the mean latency is 1.86 ± 0.16 msec (upper limit of normal is 2.2 msec, at greater than 30°C). The difference between this and the analogous median conduction study is 0.02 ± 0.18 msec, with a maximum acceptable difference of 0.38 msec (mean plus 2 SD) (Fig. 7–58) (Weber, SUNY, unpublished data). Amplitudes with these techniques again range widely, but are considerably greater than those for longer segment studies; values are generally greater than 20 μV and often above 100 μV.

The superficial ulnar branch and the dorsal cutaneous branch can be tested and compared. Palmar stimulation was as above, but the re-

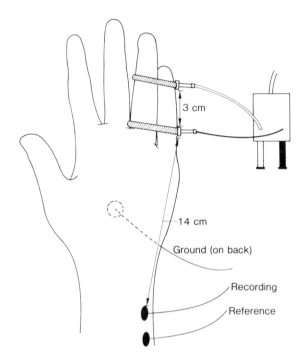

Figure 7–56. Standard orthodromic ulnar stimulation technique using ring electrodes over the fingers (cathode proximal).

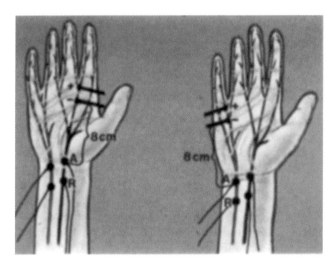

Figure 7–57. Palmar stimulation technique of the ulnar nerve (*right*). This technique has the advantage of producing a large amplitude evoked response that is easy to detect without the use of a signal average. Occasionally a shock artifact will obscure very short latency responses. This cause can be confirmed by increasing the separation between the cathode and recording electrodes. Low-intensity stimulation will decrease the shock artifact. The analogous technique for the median nerve is also illustrated.

cording point was 12 cm proximal along the course of the nerve (Fig. 7–59). This same recording point was then used for the dorsal cutaneous branch. A flexible tape was used to measure distally 12 cm along the course of the nerve onto the dorsal area of the hand between the ring and little fingers. There, stimulation was performed in a method analogous to that described within the palm (Fig. 7–60). In both cases, low-intensity stimulation

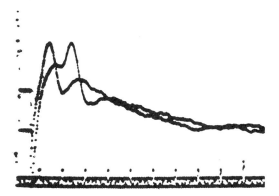

Figure 7-58. Sensory evoked potentials recorded from the ulnar nerve and from the median nerve using the palmar stimulation technique. Note the short latencies and large amplitudes of the evoked responses. Median response is delayed because of carpal tunnel syndrome. (Caliber: 1 msec, 10 μV.)

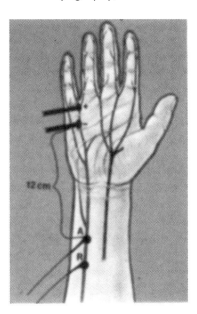

Figure 7-59. Technique for recording the sensory response from the volar branches of the ulnar nerve for comparison with that of the dorsal branch. Note that the same recording point is used for both studies. A. active electrode. R. cathode.

is used in order to avoid volume-conduction spread of the stimulus. With this technique, the mean latency from stimulation of the palm was 2.4 ± 0.2 msec (upper limit of normal is 2.7 msec), whereas that from the dorsal cutaneous branch was 2.2 ± 0.2 msec (upper limit of normal is 2.6 msec). The difference between the two mean latencies in the same hand is 0.2 ± 0.3 msec, i.e., the acceptable variation between the superficial and dorsal sensory branches was 0.5 msec (mean plus 2 SD) (58).

Median Nerve

The median nerve (C6, C7, C8, T1) is formed by the union of the medial and lateral cords of the brachial plexus. It descends into the arm, lying lateral to the brachial artery, and crosses in front of the artery at about the point of insertion of the coracobrachialis muscle. The nerve continues into the forearm between the two heads of the pronator teres and under the fibrous, arching origin of the flexor digitorum sublimis (Fig. 7–61). In this area, it gives rise to the anterior interosseus branch that supplies the flexor pollicis longus, pronator quadratus, and the index and long finger slips of the flexor digitorum profundus. Entrapment here can involve either the anterior interosseous branch alone or both it and the median nerve supply to the hand. The remaining portion of the median nerve, destined to innervate the hand, then passes between

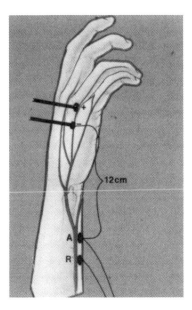

Figure 7-60. Technique for recording the sensory response from the dorsal branch of the ulnar nerve. A. active electrode; R. cathode.

the flexor digitorum superficialis and the profundus, being it is adherent to the superficialis. Approximately 5 cm proximal to the flexor retinaculum, the nerve becomes superficial,

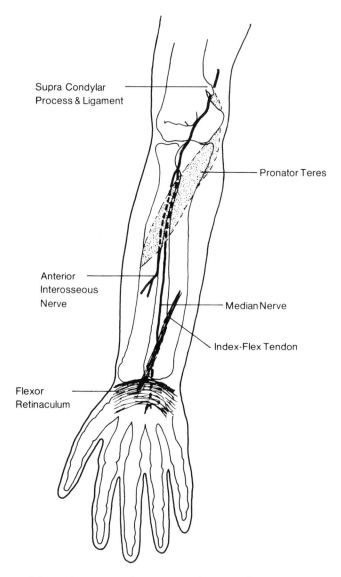

Figure 7-61. Course of the median nerve in the arm. Note the potential entrapment points at the supracondylar process and in the forearm.

lying just medial to the tendon of the flexor carpi radialis at the wrist.

Median nerve entrapment at the wrist—carpal tunnel syndrome—is discussed in Chapter 8. There are, however, a number of other causes of median neuropathy. In the upper arm, injury can occur by the same mechanisms that affect the radial nerve, i.e., sleep palsies, rifle slings, crutch compression, or trauma.

Just above the elbow, an infrequent anatomical variation provides a potential point of entrapment. About 5% of individuals have a supracondylar process that extends medially from the humerus 5 cm above the condyle. The median nerve passes over this process posteriorly to anteriorly before passing into the pronator canal. In 1% of individuals (20% of those with a supracondylar processes), a supracondylar ligament converts this condyle into a forearm, which encloses the nerve. Injury can occur through either compression or repetitive trauma, and symptoms can be identical to those of pronator canal entrapment. Detection depends on routinely stimulating the median nerve proximal to the entrapment point and then separating it from a possible pronator syndrome by inching the stimulation along the nerve to localize the injury point.

The median nerve may be compromised as it enters the forearm between the heads of the pronator teres and passes under the edge of the retinaculum of the flexor sublimis (i.e., pronator syndrome). The pronator teres muscle innervation originates proximal to this point, and is spared in the pronator syndrome. The anterior interosseous nerve has separated by this point and its involvement is inconsistent (see the section on anterior interosseus syndrome). Its involvement results in weakness of the long thumb flexor, the flexor profundus slips to the index and long fingers, and the pronator quadratus.

The median nerve supply to the hand may be injured by compression before entering the carpal canal by compression as it emerges from under the edge of the flexor digitorum sublimis (Fig. 7–61). This so-called pseudo-carpal tunnel syndrome is clinically indistinguishable from the true carpal tunnel syndrome (CTS) because injury at this point involves the same elements that would be involved in the carpal canal.

Although potentially causing a wider symptom distribution, proximal median entrapment produces symptoms similar to those of carpal tunnel syndrome (CTS). Even entrapment of the anterior interosseus nerve, which lacks a cutaneous sensory supply to the hand, can produce a vague aching discomfort referred to the hand similar to CTS. Investigation of the full course of the median nerve is appropriate when carpal tunnel-like symptoms are present in order to rule out each of the potential sources of entrapment.

STANDARD MOTOR CONDUCTION TECHNIQUE

The strong clinical interest generated by CTS has perhaps made median nerve conduction values the best documented. The nerve is easily accessible, and the thenar eminence offers an excellent evoked response recording point. The recording electrode is placed over the motor point of the abductor pollicis brevis, and the reference is placed on the distal thumb. The distal stimulation point is 8 cm

proximal to the recording electrode measured along the approximate course of the nerve (Fig. 7–62). The normal distal latency is 3.7 ± 3.0 msec (the upper limits of normal is 4.2 msec) (42); the amplitude range is 5.0–25.0 mV; the forearm velocity is 57 msec with a range of 50–67 msec; the amplitude range is 5–23 mV. Additional studies of median motor conduction using stimulation at the neck (supraclavicular point) (N), 10 cm proximal to the elbow (AE), at the elbow (E), and 5 cm distal to the elbow (BE) and the wrist (W) provide the following values (27):

	Mean	Lower Limit
N-AE	62.9 msec	50.9 msec
N-E	61.8 msec	50.8 msec
E-W	58.6 msec	51.0 msec
BE-W	55.1 msec	44.7 msec

The test is performed with the arm abducted approximately 10^0 at the shoulder and the elbow fully extended. All distance measurements are made with a steel tape, except for the exception of the supraclavicular fossa, which is best measured with calipers. The distribution of values in segment comparisons was not distributed in the usual pattern, which indicates that a longer-than-expected tolerance in the range of acceptable values must be accepted. For clinical screening purposes, the above-elbow-to-wrist segment is the most useful, because it includes the supracondylar ligament, the pronator canal, and the pseudo-carpal tunnel syndrome entrapment points. When this segment's findings are abnormal, shorter segments must be studied in order to isolate the point of entrapment.

The Martin-Gruber anastomosis is described more fully in the sections covering the ulnar nerve and the carpal tunnel syndrome (Fig. 7–50). This diversion of median nerve fibers to the ulnar nerve in the forearm can cause confusion when investigating a suspected forearm median nerve problem because it causes the evoked motor response recorded from the hand to significantly vary in size and shape between proximal and distal stimulation. A larger response is generated from stimulation at the elbow in individuals with the anastomosis because all median nerve axons to the hand are activated at that point,

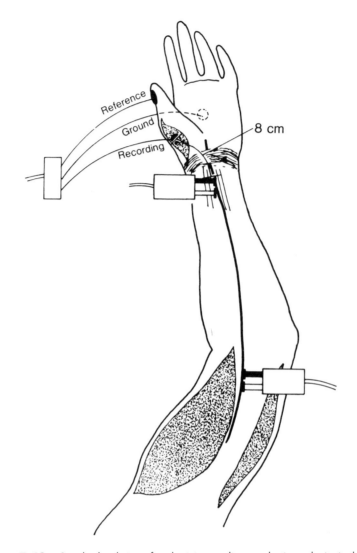

Figure 7-62. Standard technique for obtaining median conduction velocity in the forearm.

regardless of whether they travel with the median or the ulnar nerve. Proximal stimulation may produce a response with an initial, small positive deflection from the initial recording of a volume-conducted component originating from a muscle located away from the usual thenar site and supplied by the ulnar running axons.

SENSORY CONDUCTION TECHNIQUE

The distal techniques of median sensory conduction are described in more detail in the section on carpal tunnel syndrome. Forearm conduction velocity can be obtained using either orthodromic or antidromic techniques.

The standard antidromic technique consists of recording with ring electrodes from the index and long finger digital branches and stimulating the nerve at a point over the wrist 14 cm proximal to the recording electrode and then proximally at the elbow. Using this technique, the mean conduction velocity in the forearm, measured to the peak, is 56.9 ± 4.5 msec (the lower limits of normal is 48 msec), amplitude range 10–90 μV; the 14-cm distal latency is 3.2 ± 0.2 msec, range 2.9–3.7; the amplitude range is 7–75 μV (42). Using computer averaging techniques, proximal orthodromic segment conduction velocities can be measured by stimulating the nerve at the hand or wrist and recording along the nerve course, at Erb's point, or at the spinal cord. Somatosensory evoked potentials derived from median nerve stimulation have been well defined and may offer an excellent technique for assessing proximal median nerve sensory function.

Anterior Interosseus Nerve

This nerve arises from the posterior aspect of the median nerve as it passes between the two heads of the pronator teres. It runs with the interosseus artery, along the anterior aspect of the interosseus membrane, deep to and supplying the flexor pollicis longus, the flexor digitorum profundus (two lateral leads), and the pronator quadratus (Fig. 7–61).

The most frequent cause of anterior interosseus nerve syndrome is repeated forceful use of the forearm muscles. It is occasionally seen bilaterally following floor-scrubbing using a hand brush. In some individuals, fibrous constricting bands have been reported to cause a true compressive entrapment. Anterior interosseous compression also can occur from compression during unconsciousness.

Patients note vague aching in the forearm, developing either gradually or suddenly. Weakness, if present, is usually noticed during pinch grip. Physical examination reveals weakness of the flexor pollicis longus and other muscles supplied. Individual motor branches rather than the entire nerve may be comprised. Sensory examination is normal.

Needle electromyography provides the best initial approach to diagnosis because all the terminal branches can be tested. It should be used in conjunction with the standard studies of the median and ulnar nerves to detect proximal pathology in our experience. The flexor pollicis longus is the individual branch most likely to be abnormal.

MOTOR CONDUCTION TECHNIQUE

To assess conduction, the median nerve is stimulated at the elbow, and the response from the pronator quadratus recorded using a needle electrode. The electrode is inserted proximal and just volar to the ulnar styloid, parallel to the plane of the radius and ulnar, with the forearm supinated (Fig. 7–63). The latency is 5.3 ± 0.5 msec (upper limit of normal is 6.3 msec). Surface recording of the pronator quadratus from the dorsum, 3 cm proximal to the ulnar styloid, with a distance of 17–28 cm, resulted in with a latency range of 2.8 to 4.4 msec and an amplitude range of 2.2–5.0 mV (40).

Lateral Cutaneous Nerve of the Thigh

The lateral cutaneous nerve of the thigh is a purely sensory nerve (L2, L3) that provides sensation to the lateral one-third of the thigh. It passes around the pelvis and emerges into the thigh beneath or through the inguinal ligament approximately 1 cm medial to the anterior superior iliac spine. It forms branches that travel some distance distally (Fig. 7–64) before penetrating the fascia lata to become subcutaneous.

Entrapment is most frequent at the inguinal ligament. Obesity, underlying metabolic or toxic neuropathies, direct trauma, and indirect trauma by corsets, belts, or braces are known causes of nerve injury, but often no clear etiology is found. Another potential site of entrapment is the point of penetration of the distal branches through the fascia lata. The nerve also can be injured by intrapelvic masses or inflammation, e.g., appendicitis, which causes identical sensory symptoms on the thigh.

Entrapment, produces burning pain and numbness known as meralgia paresthetica over the lateral thigh known as meralgia paresthetica. Sitting may exacerbate the symptoms. Complete anesthesia in the area is rare. The presence of actual thigh weakness is inconsistent with this diagnosis, because the lateral cutaneous nerve is a purely sensory nerve.

SENSORY CONDUCTION TECHNIQUE

The nerve is evaluated antidromically by stimulating the anterior branch. A needle electrode is most effective for stimulation. It is inserted approximately 1 cm medially and distally to the anterior iliac spine. Depth depends on patient size. Surface recording is obtained 12 cm distal to the ligament (Fig. 7–64). Nor-

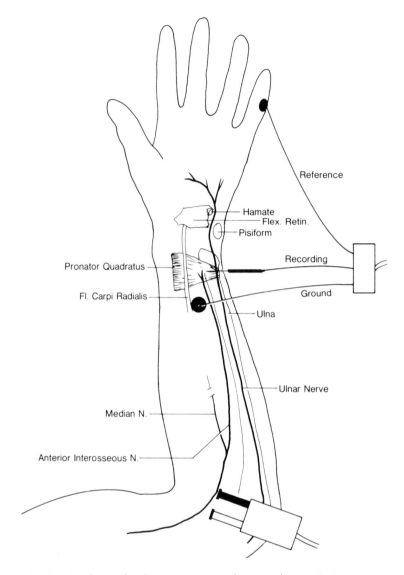

Figure 7–63. A technique for obtaining motor conduction in the anterior interosseous nerve.

mal latency is 2.6 ± 0.2 msec, giving an upper limit of less than 3.1 msec; and there should be little change in the latency across the ligament (7) (Fig. 7–65). Amplitude ranges from 10 to 25 μV. Strip electrodes placed perpendicular to the course of the nerve are helpful for recording. Placing recording electrodes more distally on the lateral thigh may avoid the interfering motor artifact of the tensor fascia lata.

Mild, chronic entrapments may produce a prolongation of the latency, but in most instances of true meralgia, no evoked potential is recordable. Because there is anatomic variation in nerve location, the asymptomatic extremity should be examined when the potential is absent on the patient's symptomatic side to confirm technique.

Femoral Nerve

The femoral nerve (L2, L3, L4) passes through the psoas major and supplies the iliacus and pectineus muscles before passing beneath the inguinal ligament. In the thigh, the anterior branch supplies the sartorius and gives off the intermediate and median cutaneous branches to the thigh. The posterior

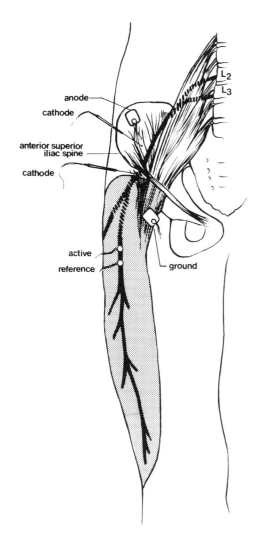

Figure 7-64. Anatomy and stimulation technique for the lateral cutaneous nerve of the thigh.

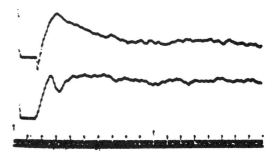

Figure 7-65. Evoked sensory response recorded antidromically from each side in the lateral cutaneous nerve of the thigh. Time base divisions are 1 msec; and the height = is equivalent to 10 μV. The lower response is from the asymptomatic side. Note the slight prolongation of the latency on the symptomatic side (*top*).

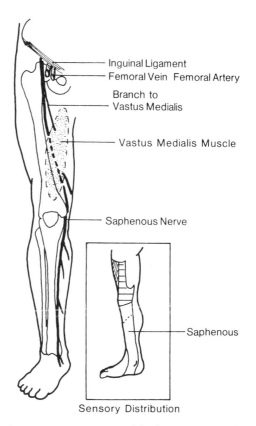

Figure 7-66. Anatomy of the femoral nerve and its distal sensory continuation of the saphenous nerve.

branch forms the saphenous (sensory) nerve and also supplies the quadriceps and knee joint (Fig. 7–66).

Femoral neuropathy has many causes, including: diabetes, polyarteritis nodosa, trauma from hip fracture, pressure during the birth process, hemorrhage into the psoas muscle secondary to anticoagulation therapy, alcohol abuse, self-retaining surgical retractor blades, or prolonged dorsal lithotomy positioning. Surgical tourniquets can produce injury, and as many as 40% of total hip procedures may result in some femoral injury. Symptoms include medial leg and thigh sensory changes, knee instability, or frank quadriceps weakness.

Severe hip flexor weakness is rare because these muscles also receive branches directly from the spinal roots. The patellar reflex may be decreased or absent.

MOTOR CONDUCTION TECHNIQUE

Three stimulation points are commonly used: just above the inguinal ligament, just below the ligament, and at a distal point along Hunter's canal. Recording is from the medialis because it receives the most direct branch of the femoral nerve. Above the inguinal ligament, the nerve lies lateral to the pulsation of the femoral artery and can be easily stimulated with a needle electrode if surface stimulation proves inadequate (Fig. 7–67). Needle stimulation may be necessary in Hunter's canal; and this stimulation point is often omitted.

Johnson et al. found a mean latency from the above-inguinal ligament stimulation point of 7.1 ± 0.7 msec (upper limit of normal is 8.5 msec) and a mean latency of 6.0 ± 0.07 msec (upper limit of normal is 7.4 msec) from the below-inguinal ligament stimulation point (29). The velocity of the distal segments was 66.7 ± 7.4 msec; however, in 25% of their controls, the evoked response was not well enough defined at all points of stimulation to determine a conduction velocity. It is often more practical to use the latency rather than pursue a conduction velocity.

Johnson reported a mean latency difference of 1.1 ± 0.4 msec (upper limit of normal is 1.9 msec) across the clinically important inguinal ligament segment. Evoked potential morphology changes across the ligament should be

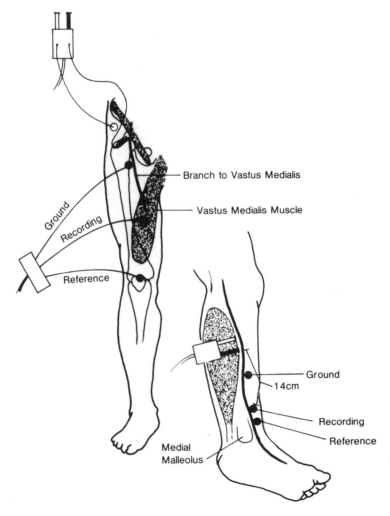

Figure 7–67. Stimulation and recording technique for motor conduction in the femoral nerve (note needle stimulation at the inguinal ligament). Lower insert shows technique for recording sensory evoked response antidromically in the saphenous nerve.

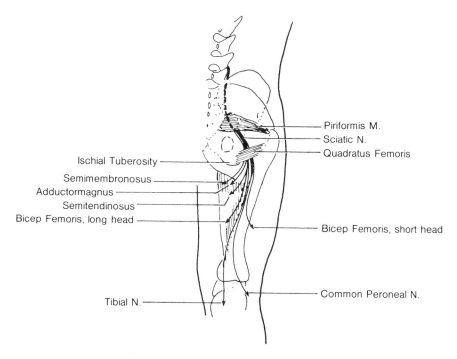

Figure 7-68. Anatomy of the sciatic nerve in the gluteal region.

minimal. The distance across the inguinal ligament was 5.5 ± 1.6 cm, and the distance from above the inguinal ligament to G1 was 35.4 ± 1.9 cm (29). Individual motor branches may be tested using needle recording electrodes to isolate the evoked potential. Because diabetic lumbar radiculopathy can mimic femoral neuropathy, needle examination of the paraspinals should always be performed.

Many femoral nerve problems are actually proximal to the inguinal ligament. Whereas late waves, needle EMG, or somatosensory evoked potential (SSEP) may be helpful, L3 and L4 spinal root stimulation offers the best assessment opportunity. It provides both a direct measure of velocity and a somewhat quantitative evaluation of axon function. (See the section on: spinal nerve root stimulation.)

STANDARD SENSORY CONDUCTION TECHNIQUE: SAPHENOUS NERVE

The saphenous nerve (L3, L4) provides sensation for the medial aspect of the knee, leg, and foot, and injury produces an aching or burning sensation in its area. It may be entrapped as it penetrates the roof of the adductor canal or injured by compression or inade-

quate support of the leg during surgery. It is injured frequently during vein stripping because of its vulnerable location near the saphenous vein.

For antidromic studies, G2 is placed just anterior to the medial malleolus in the space between the malleolus and the tibialis anterior tendon, and G1 is placed 3 cm proximal to this, also just below the anterior tibialis tendon. The nerve is stimulated 14 cm proximal to the G1 electrode using a standard bipolar surface stimulator (Fig. 7-67), which is pressed firmly under the medial edge of the tibia, separating the gastric soleus from the bone. The response is measured to the peak of the evoked potential. Wainapel reported a normal latency of 3.6 ± 0.4 msec, with an amplitude of 9.0 ± 2.3 µV (54).

Sciatic Nerve

The sciatic nerve consists of two separate but closely bound divisions throughout its length. The lateral division supplies the short head of the biceps before becoming the peroneal nerve. The medial division supplies the remaining other hamstrings (Fig. 7-68), before separating as the tibial nerve. Sciatic injury from buttocks compression often occurs during coma or narcosis. Transient symptoms from sitting on a hard seat or wallet are daily experiences for many thin individuals. Compression from tightness of the piriformis muscle remains controversial. Marked injury is seen in femoral shaft fractures and other thigh trauma; however, most femoral injury (lateral division) occurs from misdirected intramuscular injections.

MOTOR CONDUCTION TECHNIQUE

Thigh-level sciatic injuries can be assessed using conventional NCS techniques. A needle electrode is required for proximal stimulation because the nerve lies quite deep, located approximately one-third of the way between the ischial tuberosity and the femoral trochanter. The distal stimulation point is in the popliteal fossa (needle or surface stimulation), and recording is from the abductor digiti minimi (lateral division) (Fig. 7–69). Yap reported a normal conduction velocity for the thigh segment of 51.3 ± 4.4 msec, with a lower limit of normal of 42 msec (60). Responses can be recorded from any sciatic-innervated muscle; however, the normal conduction velocity differs for each muscle, e.g., medial gastrocnemius, 53.8 ± 3.3 msec; lower limit, 49.1 msec. Injury proximal to the ischium (wallet or narcosis-associated compression, injection palsy, etc.) shows only indirect changes, such as mild, generalized conduction slowing from large axon loss, by this technique.

Spinal root stimulation is the most effective means of evaluating function proximal to the ischium. Both L5 and S1 levels should be studied. Late wave abnormalities, i.e., H and F wave changes can be present in injection palsy or other proximal injuries. Both the tibial (H and F wave) and the peroneal (F wave) branches should be tested because single division injury is common (see the section on H and F waves section). Direct conduction studies must be performed if the late wave studies are abnormal, in order to localize the level of injury.

Sensory Conduction Technique

Sciatic sensory status can be studied with SSEP.

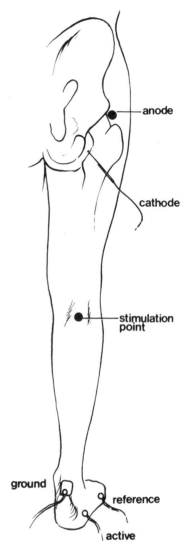

Figure 7–69. Stimulation technique for motor conduction studies in the sciatic nerve.

Peroneal Nerve

The sciatic divisions separate at the apex of the popliteal fossa, creating the tibial and peroneal nerves. The peroneal nerve is vulnerable to compression as it spirals around the caudolateral margin of the fibular head before dividing into its two branches, the deep and the superficial peroneal nerves (Figs. 7–70, 7–71, and 7–72). "Crossed leg palsy" results from compression of the nerve between the ipsilateral fibular head and the contralateral patella and femoral condyle when the legs are casually crossed while sitting. Recent weight loss, diabetics, and sedatives increase susceptibility to compression. Trauma, cast pressure, or prolonged, unaccustomed squatting or kneeling can also cause compromise. Inversion ankle sprains may produce stretch injuries to the peroneal nerve, and should be suspected in individuals with a history of repeated ankle sprains. Popliteal space masses and accessory ossicles can also produce nerve injury. The absence of involvement of the popliteal sensory branches in these entrapments help to clinically localize lesions (Figs. 7–70). Symptoms include painless foot drop, dorsiflexion or eversion weakness, and decreased sensation on the dorsum of the foot. (Fig. 7–72).

Although EMG abnormalities should be confined to the peroneal nerve territory, the association of peroneal palsy with neuropathy may produce more widely distributed changes. Trauma can be confined to a single nerve branch; thus, conduction to the nerve

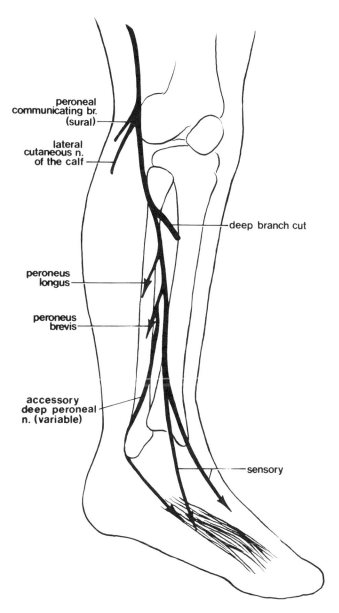

Figure 7–70.   Superficial branch of the peroneal nerve.

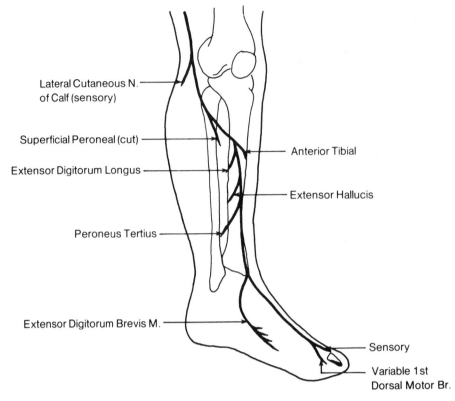

Lateral Cutaneous N. of Calf (sensory)

Superficial Peroneal (cut)

Extensor Digitorum Longus

Peroneus Tertius

Extensor Digitorum Brevis M.

Anterior Tibial

Extensor Hallucis

Sensory

Variable 1st Dorsal Motor Br.

Figure 7-71. Deep branch of the peroneal nerve. Following major injury, surface conduction studies may not be sensitive enough to detect limited residual function.

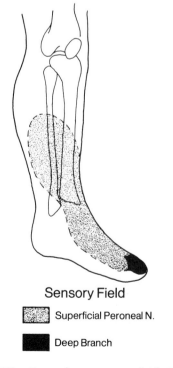

Sensory Field

Superficial Peroneal N.

Deep Branch

Figure 7-72. Peroneal nerve sensory distribution.

and needle EMG should routinely be performed for at least the main branches.

MOTOR CONDUCTION TECHNIQUE

The common peroneal nerve is stimulated in the popliteal fossa and at the lower limit of the fibular head (Fig. 7–73). Distal stimulation of the deep branch is at the border of the anterior tibialis tendon and at the posterior border of the lateral malleolus when an accessory peroneal nerve (APN) is present. Calculation provides conduction velocities for the fibular head segment and for the leg segment distal to the fibular head. The extensor digitorum brevis is composed of separate muscle slips, which in some individuals (22%) may be supplied by both the deep peroneal nerve branch and by a separate APN (22%) that originates from the superficial peroneal nerve (32). The APN passes behind the lateral malleolus, and its presence can be recognized by the unusual finding of a smaller evoked response when stimulating at the ankle rather

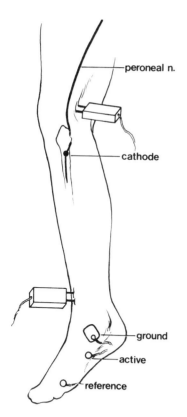

Figure 7-73. Standard motor conduction study technique for the peroneal nerve.

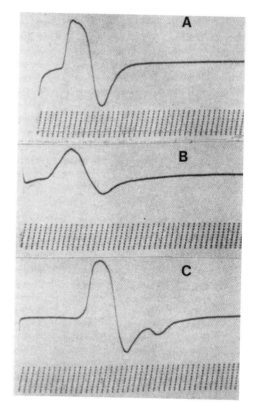

Figure 7-74. Accessory peroneal nerve: motor evoked response recorded from the extensor digitorum brevis with peroneal nerve stimulation at *C,* knee; *B,* behind lateral malleolus; and *A,* standard distal location anterior ankle. The drop in the evoked potential size with distal stimulation is the clue to presence of anomalous innervation.

than proximally (Fig. 7–74). These additional axons can be tested by stimulating behind the lateral malleolus.

Peroneal palsy from compression or entrapment at the fibular head produces slowing and/or blocking of conduction in the relatively short segment of the nerve just around the fibular head. Normal peroneal conduction velocity is 49.9 ± 5.9 msec, (lower limit of normal is 38 msec) and the velocity of the proximal segment should be equal to or greater than that of the leg segment (11). Neurapraxia and evoked potential dispersion are often prominent in mild injury. Motor amplitude range is broad, but minimum values of greater than 2 mV are generally reported. The nerve is susceptible to the effects of generalized neuropathy, which may imitate local entrapment (Figs. 7–75, 7–76, 7–77, and 7–78).

Both the deep and the superficial branches should be tested. When no clear response is detected with surface recording electrodes,

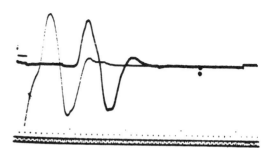

Figure 7-75. Evoked responses obtained by stimulation of the peroneal nerve at the ankle and above the fibular head in an 82-year-old man in good health. The slight amplitude loss is the result of increased temporal dispersion associated with aging. The proximal response (*right*) changes little above and below the fibular head. Minor changes between stimulation points are common in older people, and care should be taken to avoid overinterpretation of such minor changes. (Caliber: 1 msec. Negative spike = 2.5 mV.)

needle recording electrodes should be used, and needle EMG exploration should be undertaken to achieve better sensitivity of the examination (56).

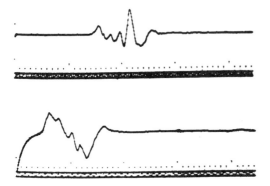

Figure 7-76. Motor evoked responses from the peroneal nerve in an 83-year-old adult-onset diabetic patient. (The time base = 1 msec; and height = 500 μV.) Such dispersion and changes in the form of the evoked potential between stimulation points are more related to the underlying disease than to any superimposed entrapment. Conservative interpretation of results regarding entrapment may be best when a longstanding peripheral neuropathy coexists. The peroneal evoked response using the extensor digitorum brevis as the recording point may be polyphasic and dispersed because of the presence of multiple muscle slips.

SENSORY CONDUCTION TECHNIQUE

The superficial sensory branch on the dorsum of the foot can be assessed antidromically. DiBenedetto has described an antidromic technique for the superficial branch involving stimulation using bipolar stimulation 2 cm medial and 5 cm proximal to the lateral malleolus and recording over the dorsum of the foot with 1 cm by 3 cm silver straps (15). Light abrasion of the skin may be required, and in 2%–3% of normal individuals, no response is seen. Measurement is to the first negative deflection. M conduction velocity for individuals below the age of 15 years old is 53.1 ± 5.2 msec (lower limit of normal is 43 msec); and for those over the age of 15, the mean velocity is 47.3 ± 3.4 msec (lower limit of normal is 40 msec). The mean amplitude is 13 μV (15). In a group of patients with neuropathy, response was absent more often in the superficial peroneal than in the sural nerve (68% versus 32%). The absence of response is, of course, more difficult to interpret than is the finding of a delayed response, as technical error must be considered. Thus, the better-established sural or tibial nerve conduction

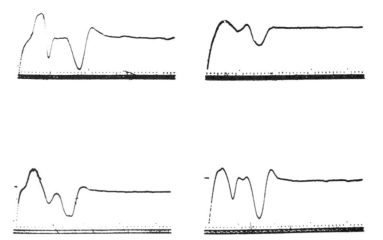

Figure 7-77. Evoked potentials recorded from the peroneal nerve with distal stimulation from the involved side (upper two tracings) and the uninvolved side (lower two tracings) 3 days (left tracings) and 7 days (right tracings) following the onset of an acute peroneal palsy. Recording was from the midpoint of the anterior tibialis muscle. (Time base = 1 msec; height = 2 mV.) Note the excellent reproduction of the waveform in the uninvolved side 4 days apart, indicating the reliability of evoked response comparisons. The significant loss of amplitude in the upper right tracing and the decreased evoked potential area decrease, when compared to the upper left tracing, are proportional to the percentage of motor axons that have undergone Wallerian degeneration. Had the patient not been seen at 3 days after the injury, late comparison between the two sides would have given essentially identical information concerning the proportion of axons lost.

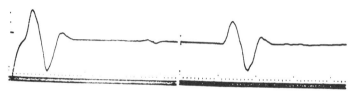

Figure 7–78. Evoked response change in a 73-year-old adult-onset diabetic man. Note the temporal dispersion and decreased amplitude of the motor evoked potential from proximal stimulation. The peroneal nerve, because of its length, is affected early in neuropathies, and the possibility of an underlying neuropathy should always be considered when small changes in the evoked potential are present between two stimulation points in this nerve. (Caliber: same as in Figure 7–77.)

studies would appear to be more reliable for screening.

Tibial Nerve

The tibial nerve (L4, L5, S1, S2) originates at the "separation" of the sciatic nerve at the apex of the popliteal fossa. It is quite superficial in the middle of the popliteal fossa (lateral to the popliteal vessels) and in the distal third of the calf. It forms the medial and lateral plantar nerves as it passes through the tarsal tunnel below the medial malleolus (see the section on tarsal tunnel syndrome).

The tibial nerve above the tarsal canal is relatively free from entrapments. It can be injured in the popliteal space by cysts, masses, or physical compression. In the leg, it is vulnerable to direct trauma and to ischemia during vascular compartment syndromes.

MOTOR CONDUCTION TECHNIQUE

The usual approach is to stimulate the nerve in the mid-popliteal space using a standard bipolar surface stimulator (29). The distal stimulation point is just above the tarsal tunnel, along the lower tibial border at the upper edge of the medial malleolus. G1 is placed over the motor point of the abductor hallucis, approximately 1 cm posterior to and below the navicular tubercle (Fig. 7–79). Normal conduction velocity is 49.8 ± 6.0 msec (lower limit of normal is 38 msec), and the motor latency to the abductor hallucis is 4.8 ± 0.8 msec (upper limit of normal is 6.4 msec). Using the same stimulation technique, the motor conduction for the lateral plantar branch is obtained by recording from the abductor digiti quinti motor point. This is lo-

cated directly below the lateral malleolus at the sole-regular skin junction (Fig. 7–79). The latency is 5.8 ± 0.84 msec, with an upper limit of normal of 7.5 msec. Motor amplitudes greater than 2 mV are expected.

SENSORY CONDUCTION TECHNIQUE

See tarsal tunnel syndrome for a discussion of distal sensory studies. Sensory conduction can be obtained for the leg segment using computer averaging techniques. Somatosensory studies provide an alternative means of assessing sensory conduction.

Tarsal Tunnel Syndrome (TTS)

The tarsal tunnel covers a broad portion of the ankle, bounded medially and posteriorly by the flexor retinaculum, anteriorly by the medial malleolus, and laterally by the tarsals. It contains the tibial nerve vessels and the tendons of the posterior tibialis, flexor digitorum longus, and flexor hallucis longus covered by the flexor retinaculum (lancinate ligament). It might better be termed a course of passage for these structures rather than a tunnel in view of its loose structure. Unlike the transverse carpal ligament, the flexor retinaculum is composed of multiple, deep fibrous septa to which the nerve may be attached and that blend with the periosteum (Fig. 7–80). Anchoring of the nerve increases its susceptibility to traction or compression and is enhanced by post-trauma scar formation. Nerve entrapment here has been attributed to fibrosis following ankle fracture, compression by a ganglion or varix of the posterior tibial vein, tendon sheath cysts, valgus deformity of the ankle, and compression by an accessory or

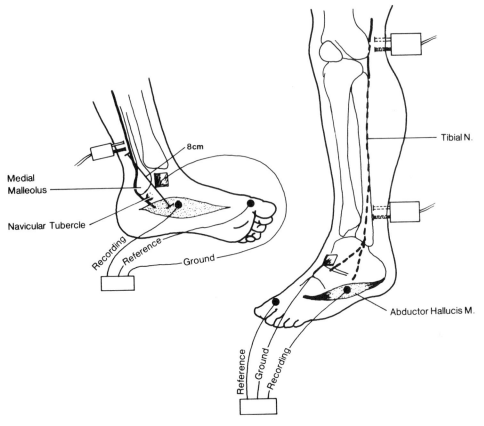

Figure 7–79. Motor conduction technique for the tibial nerve.

hypertrophied abductor hallucis muscle. TTS is also said to be associated with sudden weight gain or fluid retention. In the majority of surgically explored cases, however, no underlying cause has been identified.

The tibial nerve divides into medial and lateral plantar branches just after entering the tunnel. It also gives off the calcaneal branch, which provides cutaneous and deep sensation to the medial heel area. The medial plantar nerve supplies the abductor hallucis, the flexor digitorum brevis, the flexor hallucis brevis, and the first lumbrical. The lateral plantar nerve has both a superficial (third plantar, fourth dorsal interosseous) and a deep (two or three lateral lumbricals, remaining interossei, adductor hallucis) branch. Branches can be individually entrapped in their separate compartments or in any combination.

In contrast to the carpal tunnel syndrome, TTS affects females only sightly more often than males. The typical symptoms are inter-mittent burning pain and tingling in the foot that often worsens with prolonged standing. The symptoms may be most prominent at night and seem to be proportional to the amount of standing or walking done during the day. Sensory change distribution depends on which branches are involved. Sensation on the dorsum of the foot should be normal, with the exception of the distal phalanges of the toes. Tapping over the nerve may produce tingling in the foot (Tinel sign), and tenderness, proximal and distal to the site of compression (the Valleix phenomenon), may be present. Symptoms may be provoked by holding the ankle in forced inversion or applying a venous tourniquet on the calves.

TARSAL TUNNEL MIXED NERVE CONDUCTION

The medial and lateral plantar nerves—mixed nerve terminal branches of the tibial nerve—

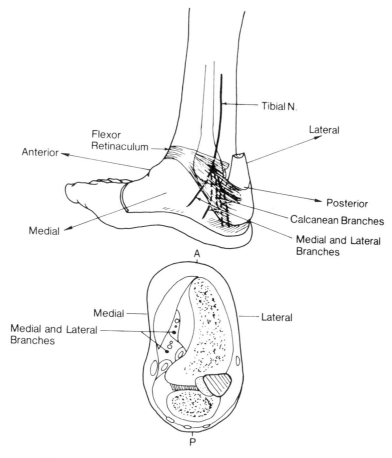

Figure 7–80. The tarsal tunnel and course of the tibial nerve.

provide a reliable means of assessing the tarsal tunnel. Saeed and Gatens were able to obtain clear responses at 14 cm in all normal subjects, representing a wide age range (46). The robustness of the technique makes it the preferred technique in suspected tarsal tunnel syndrome. Recording is along the tibial nerve just proximal to the transverse retinaculum. Stimulation is at 14 cm as illustrated near the first or fifth metatarsal base (Fig. 7–81). Reference values are: medial branch 3.16 msec mean, range 2.6–3.7, amplitude range 10–30 μV; lateral branch 3.15 msec mean, range 2.7–3.7, amplitude range 8–220 μV. It is interesting to note that there was a significant loss of recordable signals at greater distances and a significant delay in latency at ages greater than 69 years. The mean in the older group of 4.0 msec actually exceeds the 3.7 msec upper limit of normal for the study. This reinforces the importance of caution in interpretation of NCS at both the extreme periphery and in patients of advanced age.

MOTOR CONDUCTION TECHNIQUE

The tibial nerve is stimulated at the superior border of the medial malleolus, above the flexor retinaculum and motor latencies to the abductor hallucis (medial plantar) and abductor digiti quinti pedis (lateral plantar) muscles, and recorded with surface electrodes (Fig. 7–79). Because both motor branches are stimulated, it is sometimes difficult to obtain a well-defined initial deflection for latency measurement for each branch. Needle electrodes may be helpful in isolating the responses. Latency should not exceed 6.1 msec for the medial plantar and 6.7 msec for the lateral plantar branch. More than a 1.0 msec difference between the branch latencies suggests branch compromise. Minimum amplitude is 2 mV.

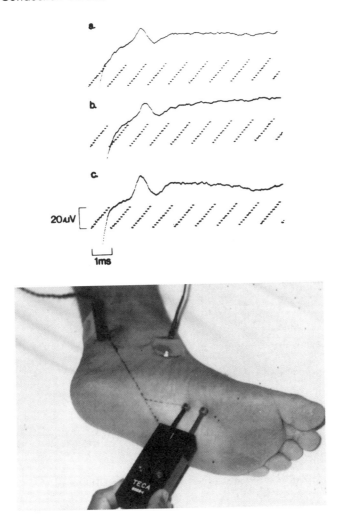

Figure 7–81. *A.* Compound nerve AP stimulating medial plantar nerve. *B.* Compound nerve AP stimulating lateral plantar nerve. *C.* Antidromic sural nerve sensory AP (14 cm). *Bottom:* Medial plantar nerve stimulation. (Courtesy of P. Gatens, M.D.)

SENSORY CONDUCTION TECHNIQUE

Sensory conduction is more sensitive to compression and can be recorded more precisely than can motor studies. Although computer averaging may be required to observe the response, the technique is simple to perform. Care must be exercised in distinguishing between tarsal tunnel syndrome, early peripheral neuropathy, and aging changes. The tibial sensory nerve is more sensitive than the sural nerve to the effects of peripheral neuropathy. Bilateral absence of the response (or symmetrical changes of any kind) is more likely due to peripheral neuropathy or aging than to nerve entrapment.

Tibial sensory studies are performed orthodromically, recording the response from behind and just proximal to the medial malleolus from surface electrodes (Fig. 7–82). Studies of the medial and lateral branches are done using ring electrodes on the great and little toes respectively. A signal average is required because normal amplitudes range from 0.5 μV upward (Fig. 7–83). Normal values are medial branch—35.2 $\pm$ 3.6 msec with a lower limit of 28 msec—and lateral branch—31.7 $\pm$ 4.4 msec, with a lower limit of 23 msec (42). Other techniques, including stimulation at intervals along the nerve branches, have been reported. Because of the sensitivity of the nerve conduc-

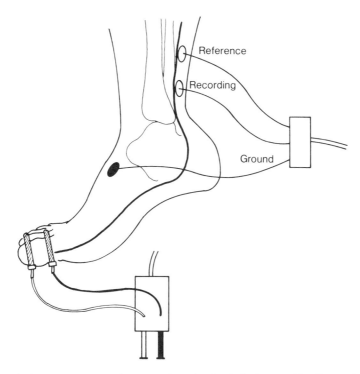

Figure 7–82. Orthodromic sensory conduction study in the distal tibial nerve. The illustrated technique employs the medial branch, whereas the analogous study may be performed on the lateral branch by placing the ring electrodes around the small toe.

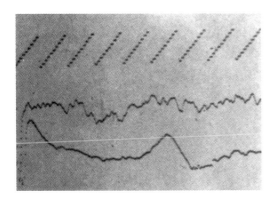

Figure 7–83. Averaged tibial orthodromic sensory response (*lower*) and real time response using technique illustrated in Figure 7–31.

tion values to aging, foot temperature, and to neuropathy, each electromyographer should establish standard values for the equipment and technique while simultaneously gaining practical experience in use of the techniques.

Sural Nerve

The purely sensory sural (L5, S1, S2) nerves forms at mid calf from the joining of a tibial and a peroneal component. It can be stimulated once easily when it emerges through the deep fascia. It then runs subcutaneously, passing behind the lateral malleolus and along the lateral foot until it terminates on the lateral aspect of the small toe. It supplies sensation to the posterolateral aspect of the lower third of the leg and the dorsolateral aspect of the foot (Fig. 7–84).

The sural nerve is relatively free of entrapments, and therefore it is frequently used to assess the general physiologic status of the peripheral nervous system. Entrapment can occur as the nerve passes through the deep fascia near its origin or by fibrous adhesions from ankle fractures at the medial malleolus. Boot top compression has been reported. Symptoms consist of numbness, burning, or dysesthesia in the appropriate distribution.

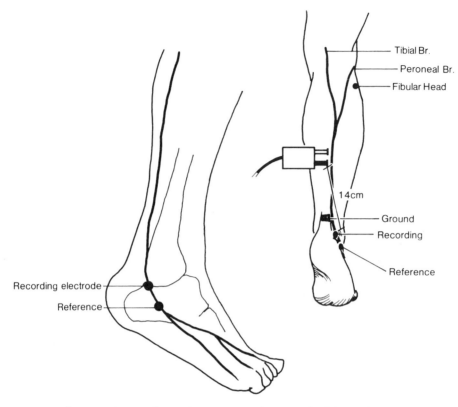

Figure 7-84. Technique for sensory conduction study of the sural nerve.

SENSORY CONDUCTION TECHNIQUE

Antidromic conduction studies are performed using surface stimulation and recording (Fig. 7–84). The G1 and G2 electrodes are placed 3–4 cm apart along the course of the nerve as it passes posterior and inferior to the lateral malleolus. It is best to maintain the ankle at approximately 90° (the neutral position) during the study. The nerve can be stimulated along its course using a standard bipolar surface stimulator. A sweep speed of 2 msec/cm and an amplification of 20 μV/cm for recording are used. Best results are obtained at 14 or 17 cm. At shorter distances, separating the evoked response from the shock artifact may be a problem, and at longer distances, the nerve may be too deeply located to stimulate.

The mean latency value at 14 cm is 3.5 ± 0.25 msec (Fig. 7–85), giving an upper limit of normal of 4.0 msec and an, amplitude range of 5–30 mV. Particular attention should be directed to ensuring that the foot temperature is above 29°C, measured at the recording point. The mean amplitude of the evoked response is 23.7 ± 3.8 μV (47). Although techni-

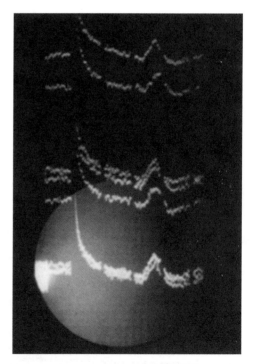

Figure 7-85. Sural sensory response. Time base height = 20 μV *(lower = time base height)*. Trace is interrupted at 1-msec intervals. Stimulus applied after 1-msec delay.

cal problems may affect amplitude values, an amplitude below $10\ \mu V$ peak-to-peak suggests the presence of peripheral neuropathy. This impression should be confirmed through the use of multiple conduction studies, e.g., other sural, tibial sensory, and peroneal sensory studies.

References

1. Aguayo A: Neuropathy due to compression and entrapment. In: Dyck P, Thomas P, Lambert E, eds. Peripheral Neuropathy. Philadelphia: WB Saunders, 1975.
2. Awad EA: Electrodiagnostic evaluation of phrenic nerve and diaphragm in high quadriplegia. Abstract, AAPM&R 40th Annual Assembly, 1978.
3. Baer RD, Johnson EW: Motor nerve conduction velocities in normal children. Arch Phys Med Rehabil 1965;46:698–704.
4. Bolton CF: Factors affecting the amplitude of the human sensory compound action potentials. AAEE Minimonograph (#17, October 1981.)
5. Braddom RL, Johnson EW: Standardization of H reflex and diagnostic use in S-1 radiculopathy. Arch Phys Med Rehabil 1974;55:161.
6. Braddom RL, Wolfe C: Musculocutaneous nerve injury after heavy exercise. Arch Phys Med Rehabil 1978;59(6):290–293.
7. Butler ET, Johnson EW, Kay Z: Normal conduction velocity in the lateral femoral cutaneous nerve. Arch Phys Med Rehabil 1974;55:31–31.
8. Campbell WW Jr, Ward LC, Swift TR: Nerve conduction velocity varies inversely with height. Muscle & Nerve 1981;4(6):520–523.
9. Catterall WA: The molecular basis of neuronal excitability. Science 1984;223:653–661.
10. Checkles NS, Balmaseda M: Standardization of ulnar sensory fiber conduction velocity. Abstract, AAPM&R 38th Annual Assembly, 1976.
11. Checkles NS, Bailey JA, Johnson EW: Tape and caliper surface measurements in determination of peroneal nerve conduction velocity. Arch Phys Med Rehabil 1969;50:214–218.
12. Checkles NS, Russakov AD, Piero DL: Ulnar nerve conduction velocity-effect of elbow position on measurement. Arch Phys Med Rehabil 1971;52:362–365.
13. Cockrell JL, Levine SP, Miller HF: Prediction of the excitation site resulting from surface electrical stimulation of a myelinated nerve. Abstract, AAPM&R 41st Annual Assembly, 1979.
14. Dawson G, Merton P: "Recurrent" discharges from motoneurons. Abstract, XX International Congress on Physiology. Bruges, Belgium, 1956.
15. DiBenedetto M: Sensory nerve conduction in lower extremities. Arch Phys Med Rehabil 1970;51:253–258.
16. Dorfman LJ, Bosley TM: Age-related changes in peripheral and central nerve conduction in man. Neurology 1979;29:38–44.
17. Dorfman L, Jayaramar: Handcuff neuropathy. JAMA 1978;239:957.
18. Fraim CJ: Unusual cause of nerve entrapment. Letters to the Editor. JAMA 1979;242:2557.
19. Gassel MM: A test of nerve conduction to muscle of the shoulder girdle as an aid in the diagnosis of proximal neurogenic and muscular disease. J Neurol Neurosurg Psychiatry 1964;27:200–205.
20. Gassel MM, Diamantopoulous E: Pattern of conduction times in the distribution of the radial nerve. Neurology 1964;14:222–231.
21. Haller EM, DeLisa JA, Brozovich FV: Nerve conduction velocity: relationship to skin, subcutaneous and intermuscular temperatures. Arch Phys Med Rehabil 1980;61:199–203.
22. Henriksen JD: Conduction velocity of motor nerves in normal subjects and patients with neuromuscular disorders. M.S. Thesis, University of Minnesota, Minneapolis, 1956.
23. Hulley WC, Wilbourn AJ, McGinty K: Sensory nerve action potential amplitudes: Alterations with temperature. Abstract, AAEE 24th Annual Meeting, 1977.
24. Izzo KL, Sridhara CR, Sharma R: Side, age, and sex influences on lower extremity sensory nerve conduction studies. Abstract, AAEE 27th Annual Meeting, 1980.
25. Jebsen RH: Motor conduction velocity in the proximal and distal segments of the radial nerve. Arch Phys Med Rehabil 1966;47:597–601.
26. Jebsen RH: Motor conduction velocities in the median and ulnar nerves. Arch Phys Med Rehabil 1967;48:185–194.
27. Johnson EW, Olsen KJ: Clinical value of motor nerve conduction velocity determination. JAMA 1960;172:1–6.
28. Johnson EW, Ortiz PR: Electrodiagnosis of tarsal tunnel syndrome. Arch Phys Med Rehabil 1966;47:776.
29. Johnson EW, Wood PK, Powers JJ: Femoral nerve conduction studies. Arch Phys Med Rehabil 1968;49:528–532.
30. Kaplan PE: Electrodiagnostic confirmation of long thoracic nerve palsy. J Neurol Neurosurg Psychiatry 1980;43:50–52.
31. Kraft GH: Axillary, musculocutaneous and suprascapular nerve latency studies. Arch Phys Med Rehabil 1972;53:383–387.
32. Lambert EH: The accessory peroneal nerve. Neurology 1969;19:1169–1176.
33. Licht S: History. In: Johnson EW, ed. Practical electromyography. Baltimore: Williams & Wilkins, 1980.
34. MacLean IC: Nerve root stimulation to evaluate conduction across the lumbosacral plexus. Abstract, AAPM&R 41st Annual Assembly, 1979.
35. MacLean IC, Mattioni TA: Phrenic nerve conduction studies: A new technique and its application in quadriplegic patients with high spinal cord injury. Arch Phys Med Rehabil 1981;62:70–73.
36. Magladery JW, McDougal DB: Electrophysiological studies of nerve and reflex activity in normal man. Bull Johns Hopkins Hosp 1950;86:265.

37. Magladery J, Porter W, Parka A, et al.: Electrophysiological studies of nerve and reflex activity in normal man. IV. Two-neuron reflex and identification of certain action potentials from spinal roots and cord. Bull Johns Hopkins Hosp 1951;88:499.

38. Melvin JL, Harris DH, Johnson EW: Sensory and motor conduction velocities in the ulnar and median nerves. Arch Phys Med Rehabil 1966;47:511–519.

39. Melvin JL, Schuchmann JA, Lanese RR: Diagnostic specificity of motor and sensory nerve conduction variables in carpal tunnel syndrome. Arch Phys Med Rehabil 1973;54:69–74.

40. Mysiw WJ, Colachis SC: Electrophysiologic study of the anterior interosseous nerve. Am J Phys Med Rehabil 1988;67:50–54.

41. Norris AH, Shock NW, Wagman IH: Age changes in the maximal conduction velocity of motor fibers in human ulnar nerves. J Appl Physiol 1953;5:589.

42. Oh SJ, Sarala PK, Cuba T, et al. Tarsal tunnel syndrome: Electrophysiologic study. Ann Neurol 1979;5:327–330.

43. Rask MR: Watchband superficial radial neurapraxia. JAMA 1979;421:2702.

44. Roles NC, Maudsley RH: Radial tunnel syndrome. Resistant tennis elbow as a nerve entrapment. J Bone Joint Surg (Br) 1972;54B:499–508.

45. Ruppert ES, Johnson EW: Motor nerve conduction velocities in low birth weight infants. Pediatrics 1968;42:255.

46. Saeed MA, Gatens PF: Compound nerve action potentials of the medial and lateral plantar nerves through the tarsal tunnel. Arch Phys Med Rehabil 1982;63:304–307.

47. Schuchmann JA: Sural nerve conduction and a standardized technique. Arch Phys Med Rehabil 1977;58:166.

48. Spiegel MH, Johnson EW: Conduction velocity in the proximal and distal segments of motor fibers in the ulnar nerve of human beings. Arch Phys Med Rehabil 1962;43:57–61.

49. Spindler HA, Felsentahl G: Sensory conduction in the musculocutaneous nerve. Arch Phys Med Rehabil 1978;59:20–21.

50. Trojaberg W, Windruup EH: Motor and sensory conduction to different segments of the radial nerve in normal subjects. J Neurol Neurosurg Psychiatry 32:354–359.

51. Turk MA, Weber RJ: EMG assessment of bladder function and rehabilitation potential. Abstract, 8th International Congress of PM&R, Stockholm, Sweden, 1980.

52. Turk ,MA, Burkhart JA, Traetow D, et al. An alternate method of estimating peroneal motor nerve conduction velocity. Abstract, AAEE 23rd Annual Session, 1976.

53. Varghese G, Dulalas R, Rogoff JB: Influence of interelectrode distance on antidromic sensory potentials. Electromyogr & Clin Neurophysiol 1983;23(4):297–301.

54. Wainapel SF, Kim DJ, Ebel A: Conduction studies of the saphenous nerve in healthy subjects. Arch Phys Med Rehabil 1978;59:316–319.

55. Waxman SG: Conduction in myelinated, unmyelinated, and demyelinated fibers. Arch Neurol 1977;34:585–589.

56. Waxman SG, Brill MH: Conduction through demyelinated plaques in multiple sclerosis: Computer simulation of facilitation by shortening the nodes. J Neurol Neurosurg Psychiatry 1978;41:408–417.

57. Weber RJ, van den Hoven R, Kukla RD: Dorsal vs. Palmar branch ulnar nerve sensory conduction: sensitive discriminator of ulnar entrapment. Arch Phys Med Rehabil 1980;61:475.

58. Weber RJ, Bowers D: Determination of the anatomical distribution of the C-8 nerve root by percutaneous root stimulation. Muscle & Nerve 1980;3:441.

59. Weber RJ, Piero DL: F wave evaluation of thoracic outlet syndrome: A multiple regression derived F wave latency predicting technique. Arch Phys Med Rehabil 1978;59:464.

60. Yap CB, Hirota T: Sciatic nerve motor conduction velocity study. J Neurol Neurosurg Psychiatry 1967;30:233–239.

Chapter 8

Carpal Tunnel Syndrome

William J. Hennessey
Ernest W. Johnson

In his 1854 lecture on surgical pathology, Sir James Paget described the first known documented case of carpal tunnel syndrome (CTS). An old fracture had caused compression of the median nerve at the wrist (40). In 1933, Learmonth described the first surgical release of the median nerve owing to post-traumatic osteoarthritis (35). In 1938, Moersch provided the first description of spontaneous median nerve compression and is credited with coining the term "carpal tunnel syndrome" (39). Phalen published a series of articles on CTS from 1950 to 1970 that have created a heightened awareness of this common clinical entity in the medical community (44–46).

CTS is a group of signs and symptoms secondary to dysfunction of the median nerve within the carpal tunnel. Subtle abnormalities of median nerve function can be identified with the technologically advanced electromyographic instruments currently available to the electrodiagnostician. Today, CTS is the most common entrapment neuropathy referred to the electrodiagnostician for evaluation. Electrodiagnostic studies are a reliable tool in assessing median nerve dysfunction (22). Interpretation of the electrodiagnostic data has important implications for the diagnosis, prognosis, and treatment of CTS.

ANATOMY OF THE CARPAL TUNNEL

The carpal tunnel is defined by the transverse carpal ligament and the carpal bones (16). The transverse carpal ligament is attached medially to the pisiform bone and the hamulus of the hamate, and laterally to the scaphoid tuberosity and the crest of the trapezium. The floor

of the carpal tunnel is comprised of the lunate and capitate bones.

The flexor retinaculum is comprised of the transverse carpal ligament and the palmar carpal ligament. The transverse carpal ligament forms the roof of the carpal tunnel. The palmar carpal ligament is attached to the styloid processes of the ulna and radius, and it is made up of thickened antebrachial fascia lying over the tendons of the flexor muscles. It merges distally with the proximal transverse carpal ligament. The transverse carpal ligament forms part of the roof of Guyon's canal, and the palmar carpal ligament forms the floor of Guyon's canal. This relationship of the flexor retinaculum to the carpal tunnel and to Guyon's canal occasionally leads to co-existing ulnar deficits with CTS (2,5,51,52).

The median nerve and 10 tendons pass through the carpal tunnel, including the four tendons of the flexor digitorum profundus, the four tendons of the flexor digitorum superficialis, the flexor pollicus longus tendon, and the tendon of the flexor carpi radialis, which runs through the groove of the trapezium to insert upon the base of the second metacarpal bone. At the level of the carpal tunnel, the median nerve is immediately surrounded by the transverse carpal ligament anteriorly, the radial portion of the flexor digitorum superficialis tendons medially and posteriorly, and the flexor pollicus longus tendon laterally (Fig. 8–1).

RISK FACTORS FOR CTS

CTS is three to four times more common in women and is thought to be due in part to occupation (33,46,48,49). CTS has been

195

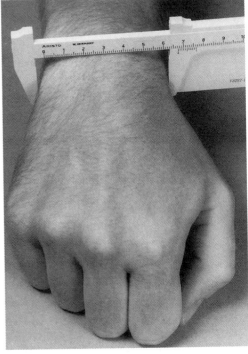

Median Nerve

Transverse Carpal Ligament

Flexor Digitorum Superficialis m.
(tendons)

Flexor Carpi Radialis m.
(tendon)

Flexor Pollicis Longus m.
(tendon)

Flexor Digitorum Profundus m.
(tendons)

Figure 8-1. Cross-sectional view of the carpal tunnel and its contents at the level of the first row of carpal bones.

shown to be common in such occupations that have been filled predominantly by women.

A square wrist dimension is another known risk factor for the development of CTS (14, 24). Johnson and colleagues determined that the more square the wrist, the longer the median sensory distal latency (24). The wrist dimensions were measured with a standard engineering caliper at the level of the distal wrist flexor crease (Fig. 8–2). As the wrist thickness (A-P measurement) to width (M-L measurement) ratio approached 0.7, CTS was much more common (Fig. 8–2).

A familial association can contribute to the development of CTS. Radecki reported that 27% of patients referred for electrodiagnostic evaluation who had a family history of CTS were diagnosed with CTS (48).

CTS occurs more frequently in the dominant hand (49). If it is present bilaterally, symptoms are usually more severe on the dominant-hand side. This is due to the increased repetitive usage of the wrist flexors and extensors on the dominant side. Some authors feel that the kinesiology of the wrist flexor tendons play a major role in the development of CTS (46, 54).

CTS occurs frequently in middle-aged people, mostly between the ages of 30 and 60 years (46, 49). Patients with disease processes, such as diabetes mellitus or Guillain-Barre syndrome, are more vulnerable to nerve entrapment syndromes (23). Patients with conditions such as gout or rheumatoid arthritis, or those who are pregnant, can develop localized

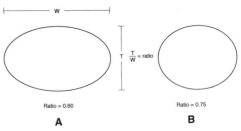

$\frac{T}{W}$ = ratio

Ratio = 0.60   Ratio = 0.75

A   B

Figure 8-2. *Top.* Measurement technique of wrist dimension at the distal flexor wrist crease with a standard engineering caliper. *Bottom. A.* "Rectangular" wrist with low risk for CTS. *B.* "Square" wrist with higher risk for CTS.

wrist swelling that is contributory to the development of CTS (23,37,46,53). Pregnancy-related CTS usually occurs during the third trimester and often resolves after delivery (37). Women whose CTS resolved after delivery are at a greater risk for its recurrence later in life. Except for pregnancy, many of the conditions mentioned above develop during the middle-aged years when CTS is most prevalent, thus increasing the risk for CTS. In summary, risk factors for the development of CTS include the female gender, square-shaped wrists, a family history of CTS, repetitive wrist movements, "middle-age", and the presence of certain other co-existing conditions.

CLINICAL DIAGNOSIS OF CTS

By definition, CTS is a clinical diagnosis because a syndrome is an aggregate of signs and symptoms associated with any morbid process. Symptoms of CTS include numbness and tingling in the median nerve distribution of the thumb, index finger, long finger, and radial half of the ring finger (28, 46). The palm is not involved because its sensory innervation is by the palmar cutaneous branch of the median nerve, which does not travel through the carpal tunnel. Patients also frequently complain of pain in the wrist at nighttime or after frequent use of the hands or fingers.

In more advanced cases, patients may complain about thumb or index finger weakness and occasionally report dropping items (which could be due to the motor or sensory impairment). Less frequently, patients might complain only about forearm, elbow, or shoulder pain. Pain can be referred to any location in the upper limb because the median nerve has fibers from the C6 to T1 nerve root levels.

Physical examination findings supportive of the diagnosis of CTS include hypesthesia in the median nerve distribution, impaired two-point discrimination, Tinel's sign, Phalen's sign, and thenar weakness with or without noticeable atrophy (Fig. 8–3). A positive Tinel's sign occurs by gently tapping over the median nerve within the carpal tunnel and inducing paresthesias (not pain) distally in the median nerve distribution (59, 62). "Gentle" has never been defined but implies avoiding a hard tap that could induce paresthesias distally

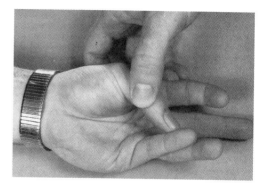

Figure 8–3. Abductor pollicus brevis muscle strength evaluation. The patient is asked to place the touch pads of the thumb and little finger together. The examiner then applies pressure over the thumb interphalangeal joint and directs a force toward the second metacarpophalangeal joint while the patient is instructed to keep the touch pads together. Although it is impossible to isolate the abductor pollicus brevis muscle, this manuever is the most reliable technique.

along any nerve pathway. Tinel's sign can help localize the median nerve injury to the level of the carpal tunnel because paresthesias will only be induced when tapping over the injured nerve site.

A positive Phalen's sign occurs by holding the wrists in complete flexion for 30 to 60 seconds and inducing or exaggerating paresthesias (not pain) in the median nerve distribution in the hand. Phalen's sign induces ischemia within the entrapped median nerve, which already has compromised blood flow prior to the wrist flexion test (57). Phalen noted the wrist flexion test was negative in the presence of advanced sensory loss.

Both Tinel's sign and Phalen's sign have had been extremely variable in sensitivity and specificity, thus limiting their clinical utility (12, 34). Thenar atrophy and weakness are usually only present in advanced cases of CTS. Sensory complaints noted by history often cannot be confirmed by examination early in cases of CTS. Physical signs are frequently absent in early CTS. In these cases, the diagnosis should be suspected on the basis of presenting symptoms and risk factors and confirmed by electrodiagnostic evaluation of the median nerve (12).

ELECTRODIAGNOSIS OF CTS

CTS is a group of signs and symptoms resulting from dysfunction of the median nerve within the carpal tunnel. Median nerve dysfunction can be confirmed by performing nerve conduction study techniques that have been demonstrated to be extraordinarily sensitive. In some cases, nerve conduction studies are able to detect subtle nerve dysfunction before symptoms develop. Electrodiagnostic evaluation of the median nerve across the carpal tunnel is indicated for the following reasons:

1. To confirm the diagnosis in cases in which no physical deficits are noted and CTS is suspected;
2. To identify CTS in the presence of a peripheral neuropathy;
3. To rule out other pathology, most commonly a sensory peripheral neuropathy, C6 or C7 radiculopathy, or a more proximal entrapment of the median nerve;
4. To follow up after a failed response to conservative treatment or carpal tunnel release for clinically diagnosed carpal tunnel syndrome without electrodiagnostic evaluation;
5. To establish the severity of median nerve compromise;
6. To determine prognosis.

As with all entrapment neuropathies, the nerve MUST be examined proximal and distal to the suspected site of entrapment in order to establish the point of entrapment and the degree of nerve compromise.

A brief review of the four types of nerve damage is as follows:

1. **Conduction block (neurapraxia):** The segmental block of axonal conduction owing to a focal region of demyelination. The nerve conducts normally above and below the lesion but not across it. Weakness occurs with conduction block of motor fibers.

   The compound muscle action potential (CMAP) and sensory nerve action potential (SNAP) are either decreased in amplitude or absent with stimulation proximal to the wrist and have normal amplitudes with stimulation of the median nerve in the midpalm.

2. **Conduction slowing:** The conduction of an action potential through a partially demyelinated region can be slowed but not blocked completely. This occurs if there is widening of the nodal area rather than destruction of the entire internodal segment of myelin. In this situation, more time is required to propagate the action potential through the widened nodal region. Conduction slowing alone does not necessarily produce symptoms (weakness or paresthesias). However, conduction block leads to motor or sensory impairment.

   The latencies and durations of the CMAPs and SNAPs are prolonged with stimulation proximal to the carpal tunnel and are normal with midpalmar stimulation in patients with carpal tunnel syndrome accompanied by conduction slowing of median nerve fibers. The increased duration of an action potential is also referred to as temporal dispersion.

3. **Axonotmesis:** The loss of continuity of the nerve axons and myelin sheath but retained continuity of the connective tissue sheath. Myelin is dependent upon its axon; if the axon degenerates, so will the myelin sheath.

   Axonotmesis results in death of axons, and the CMAP and SNAP are decreased with stimulation proximal and distal to the carpal tunnel. It is important to wait 5 days to differentiate neurapraxia from axonal death because the axons can remain excitable for up to 5 days during wallerian degeneration, and both cause the same degree of weakness.

4. **Neurotmesis:** The disruption of the axon, myelin sheath, and neural connective tissue. The severity of the injury depends upon the degree of connective tissue involvement (endoneurium → perineurium → epineurium).

   Nerve conduction study findings are similar to those of axonotmesis except that there is less than a full recovery because of retrograde neuronal degeneration, scar tissue, and misdirection of growing axons into foreign tubes. Neurotmesis and axonotmesis cannot be distinguished by a single routine nerve conduction study. The degree of functional nerve recovery over time helps distinguish these two entities.

All four types of nerve injury can occur in different nerve fibers within the same nerve. The action potential generated via routine nerve conduction study is representative of the various types of nerve injury occurring in all of the different nerve fibers of the nerve being examined (i.e., conduction block, conduction slowing, axonotmesis, and neurotmesis).

MEDIAN SENSORY AND MOTOR DISTAL LATENCY DETERMINATIONS

Numerous studies have published reference values for median motor and sensory distal latency determinations. Reference values must be collected using standard techniques, adequate sample sizes, and temperature controls (9, 20). The median motor distal latency is determined with an 8-cm technique, and the median sensory distal latency is determined with a 14-cm antidromic technique (Fig. 8–4) (9,20,26,38). Sensory studies are usually more sensitive than motor studies for the electrodiagnosis of CTS (2,22,29,58). However, motor nerve fiber dysfunction can be the only median

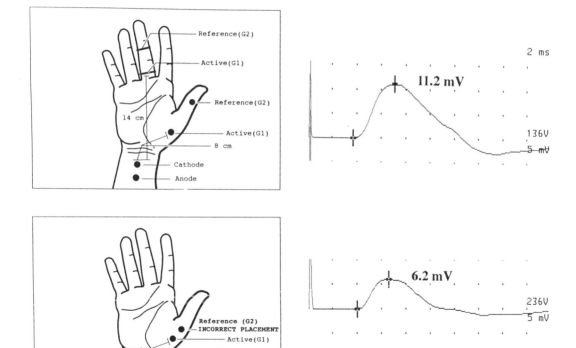

Figure 8–4. *Top left.* Standard median nerve 8-cm motor and 14-cm antidromic sensory techniques for recording potentials. The G2 electrode for recording the median CMAP should be over an electrically silent area, such as the interphalangeal joint of the thumb. If G2 is placed over the thenar muscles, the amplitude and duration will decrease. *Top right.* Median CMAP at 8 cm with G1 over the abductor pollicis brevis motor point and G2 over the thumb interphalangeal joint (an electrically silent area). *Bottom left.* Standard median nerve 8-cm motor technique for recording potentials except G2 is improperly placed over the thenar muscles. *Bottom right.* Median CMAP at 8 cm with G1 over the abductor pollicus brevis motor point and G2 only 2 cm distal to G1 and still over the thenar muscles as depicted in the picture to the left of this potential. Note the decrease in CMAP amplitude and duration compared to the above potential as a result of failure to place G2 over an electrically silent area.

Table 8–1
Normal Reference Values for Distal Latency

Sample size	Temp (°C)	Distance	Median fibers	Distal latency (msec)
44	32.4	8 cm	motor	3.2 (0.4)[t20]
120	31.0	14 cm	sensory	3.0 (0.4)[*26]
155 (elderly)	34.0	8 cm	motor	3.6 (0.6)[t9]
155 (elderly)	34.0	14 cm	sensory	2.9 (0.4)[t9]

*measured to the negative peak of the action potential.
[t]measured to the onset of the action potential.

nerve abnormality in acute CTS (13). Median motor nerve conduction parameters are important for prognosis and localization of the lesion when a median SNAP is unobtainable. Suggested reference values are shown in Table 8–1.

The use of a single reference value as "the upper limit of normal" is discouraged. A young patient with risk factors, history, and physical examination supportive of CTS might have a sensory distal latency value of 3.6 msec, which is approaching the mean plus two standard deviations (3.8 msec). Although 3.6 msec still could be considered "normal," it can also be considered supportive of median nerve dysfunction owing to CTS, especially if the negative spike duration is increased with nerve stimulation proximal to the carpal tunnel (Fig. 8–5). The electrodiagnostic data must be viewed in light of the clinical presentation and relative to the other nerve conduction values obtained for that individual.

Temporal dispersion can be the first electrodiagnostic sign of median nerve dysfunction. The negative spike of the SNAP is usually 1.0 msec in duration in healthy middle-aged adults (Fig. 8–5) (63). This duration frequently increased up to 2.5 msec in elderly healthy adults 60 to 95 years of age (21). Duration analysis in isolation of other conduction parameters may be less useful in elderly patients because of the variable durations of the negative spikes of the action potentials.

Awareness of the influence of temperature on nerve conduction is essential for accurate interpretation of electrodiagnostic data. For each decrease of 1°C, the patient's distal latency increases 0.2 msec, the nerve conduction velocity decreases 2 msec, the duration increases, and the amplitude increases (1, 8, 19).

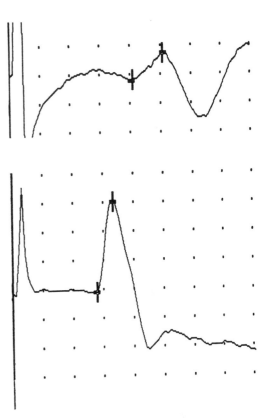

Figure 8–5. *Top.* Median SNAP at 14 cm is prolonged at 5.0 msec measured to the negative peak and with abnormal amount of temporal dispersion (2.0-msec duration). *Bottom.* Normal median SNAP with a peak latency of 3.3 msec and a duration of 1.0 msec. (Caliber: Horizontal graticule = 1.0 msec; vertical graticule = 10 mV. Filter: 20 Hz to 2 KHz)

A cool hand could lead to misinterpretation of data as supportive of CTS if the electrodiagnostician is not aware of the influence of temperature on nerve conduction parameters (Fig. 8–6). The touch pad of the digit being tested should be at least 31°C. The hand does not necessarily need to be warmed up prior

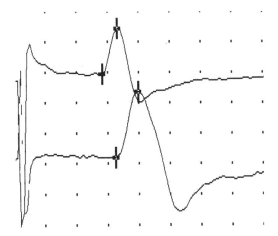

Figure 8–6. *Top.* Median SNAP from digit 3 at 14 cm measures 3.3 msec to negative peak with touch pad of digit at 32° C. *Bottom.* Same individual with touch pad of tested digit at 28° C with distal latency to negative peak measurement of 4.0 msec. Note the increase of distal latency, amplitude, and duration of bottom response from the cool hand. (Caliber: Horizontal graticule = 1.0 msec; vertical graticule = 20 mV. Filter: 20 Hz to 2 KHz)

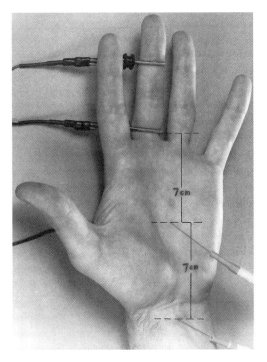

Figure 8–7. *Left.* Antidromic 14-cm and 7-cm median sensory nerve conduction technique with monopolar needle stimulation.

MEDIAN SENSORY 14-cm AND 7-cm TECHNIQUE

Evaluation of the median nerve sensory fibers at the wrist (14 cm) and at the midpalmar site (7 cm) with antidromic recording of the SNAP at the long finger (digit 3) is a sensitive test for evaluating median nerve dysfunction (Fig. 8–7) (63). This test adds specificity to the electrodiagnostic evaluation of CTS compared to a distal latency determination at 14 cm. It allows evaluation of the proximal 7-cm segment for CTS and the distal 7-cm segment for peripheral neuropathy (Figs. 8–8, 8–9, 8–10) (63). The long finger is chosen for recording potentials because its nerve conduction parameters are most often abnormal in CTS as compared to those of the other fingers (36).

In the original study describing this technique, the distal 7-cm latency measured was 52% of the total response time (63). The proximal 7 cm is considered prolonged and supportive of CTS if it measures greater than half

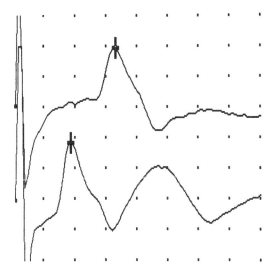

Figure 8–8. *Top.* Median SNAP at 14 cm. *Bottom.* Median SNAP at 7 cm. These potentials were recorded in a healthy adult subject. Note that the palmar response amplitude is 25% larger and also slightly more than 50% of the 14 cm distal latency. These are typical "normal" responses. Note the motor artifact depicted to the right of the SNAP of the bottom recording. The characteristic long duration of the motor artifact enables the electrodiagnostician to distinguish the artifact from the SNAP. (Caliber: Horizontal graticule = 1.0 msec; vertical graticule = 10 mV. Filter: 20 Hz to 2 Khz)

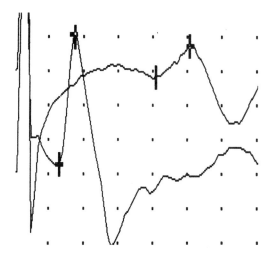

Figure 8–9. *Top.* Median SNAP from digit 3 at 14 cm measures 5.1 msec. *Bottom.* Median SNAP at 7 cm in midpalm. Note the much larger amplitude in the bottom recording. This is consistent with neurapraxia (conduction block) across the carpal tunnel. The proximal 7-cm segment conduction time is greater than the distal 7-cm segment, which also supports a diagnosis of CTS. The increased duration (1.7 msec) of the top response (carpal tunnel segment) is also abnormal. (Caliber: Horizontal graticule = 1.0 msec; vertical graticule = 10 mV. Filter: 20 Hz to 2 KHz)

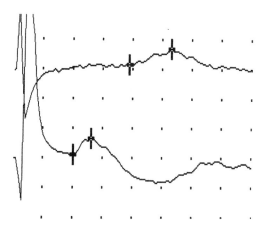

Figure 8–10. *Top.* Median SNAP from digit 3 at 14 cm. *Bottom.* Median SNAP at 7 cm in midpalm. Note that both response times are prolonged and have an increased duration. This supports a diagnosis of CTS and a peripheral neuropathy. This tracing was obtained from a patient with CTS and diabetic peripheral neuropathy. Examination of other perpheral nerves, particularly the sural nerves, was necessary to confirm the peripheral neuropathy. (Caliber: Horizontal graticule = 1.0 msec; vertical graticule = 10 mV. Filter: 20 Hz to 2 KHz)

of the total 14-cm distal latency (Fig. 8–9). There are cases in which the 14-cm distal latency might be 3.6 msec but the proximal 7-cm segment latency time is greater than half of the 14-cm latency time. The temporal dispersion noted in the proximal segment in these cases is also helpful for detecting focal demyelination in early CTS (Fig. 8–9).

This technique can be performed with monopolar needle electrode stimulation or bipolar surface stimulation. The needle electrode technique delivers a supramaximal stimulation with a shorter duration (0.05 msec) and thus with less discomfort. Needle electrode stimulation also reduces the shock artifact.

Assessment of the degree of conduction block or axonotmesis of sensory fibers is possible with the 14- and 7-cm technique. The palm-to-wrist ratio for amplitudes has been shown to vary from 75% to 236% with a mean palmar response 28% greater than the wrist response (63). The palmar response would be expected to be larger because the SNAP amplitude increases as the distance between the stimulation site and the recording site shortens (Fig. 8–11). This is due to physiologic temporal dispersion with phase cancellation of fast and slow conducting axons within the SNAP (see Chapter 4) (32). The amplitude of the SNAP also decreases as the distance between the two ring electrodes decreases. This also is due to phase cancellation (see Chapter 4). The ring electrodes should be 4 cm apart. An understanding of the amplitude changes owing to ring electrode placement and stimulating site distance from electrodes is imperative for appropriate SNAP amplitude analysis (Fig. 8–11).

MEDIAN MOTOR NERVE MIDPALMAR STIMULATION

Palmar stimulation of the recurrent motor branch of the median nerve must be a routine part of the median motor nerve study in suspected cases of CTS; this provides prognostic and diagnostic information. This technique is necessary to localize the lesion in cases in which the median SNAP cannot be obtained because of advanced sensory deficits or in cases

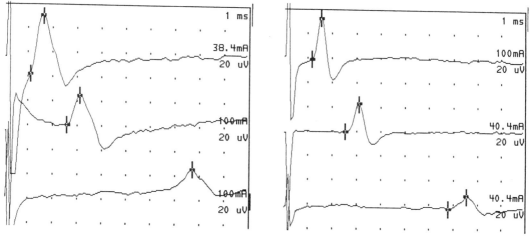

Figure 8–11. Demonstration of normal *decrease* in median SNAP amplitude with *increase* of distance between G1 and stimulation site. Amplitude *decrease* can also occur with placement of ring electrodes less than 4 cm apart on tested digit. *Left.* Antidromic SNAP to long finger at midpalm (top), 14 cm (middle), and at elbow (bottom) with ring electrodes 4 cm apart. *Right.* Antidromic SNAP to long finger at midpalm (top), 14 cm (middle), and at elbow (bottom) with ring electrodes 1 cm apart. (Caliber: Horizontal graticule = 1.0 msec; vertical graticule = 20 mV. Filter: 20 Hz to 2 KHz)

of acute CTS (duration of a few weeks) in which motor fibers occasionally are preferentially affected (13). Because some instances of acute CTS will have only conduction block and minimal slowing of median motor nerve fibers, this technique can be the only way to demonstrate CTS in these instances. CMAP reference values have varied to include values as low as a few millivolts (mV) to as high as 20 mV as normal. With such variation, the only way to determine if the wrist stimulation CMAP amplitude is normal is to examine the median nerve CMAP proximal and distal to the carpal tunnel to determine if there is any nerve compromise.

The median motor nerve fibers are stimulated with a standard 8-cm orthodromic technique with a recording of the CMAP over the abductor pollicus brevis muscle. The palmar stimulation site is located where the tip of the flexed ring finger contacts the thenar crease (the "life line" of the palm) as shown in Figure 8–12.

Although this technique can be performed with a bipolar surface stimulator, the use of a monopolar needle electrode for stimulation is recommended (Fig. 8–13). A surface stimulation could make nerve depolarization technically more difficult due to the thickness of

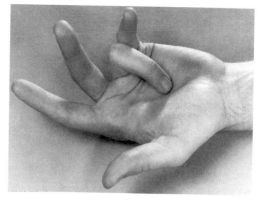

Figure 8–12. Stimulation site for midpalmar study of the recurrent motor branch of the median nerve.

the palm skin. A needle stimulation, with the needle electrode just penetrating the corneum, will provide effective stimulation with shorter duration (0.05 msec). Amplitude analysis in this setting is more reliable because supramaximal stimulation is more easily accomplished.

In a study by Pease and colleagues, healthy subjects had a mean increase in amplitude of 0.6 millivolts (range up to 2.0 mV) with midpalmar stimulation compared to wrist stimulation (42). In contrast, patients with varying severity of CTS had a mean increase of 2.2

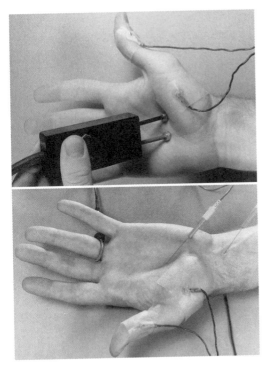

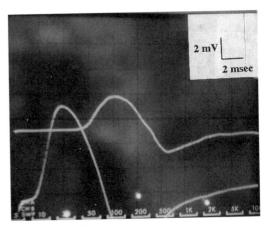

Figure 8–14. *Top.* Median motor nerve CMAP at 8 cm. *Bottom.* Recurrent median motor nerve CMAP distal to the carpal tunnel. These responses are from a patient's acute case of CTS as noted by the neurapraxic response (conduction block) with the CMAP distal to the carpal tunnel nearly twice as large as that obtained with wrist stimulation of the median nerve. The increased duration (temporal dispersion) of the CMAP from wrist stimulation indicates that there is also conduction slowing of the median nerve under the palmar carpal ligament. (Caliber: Horizontal graticule = 2.0 msec; vertical graticule = 5 mV. Filter: 2 Hz to 10 KHz)

Figure 8–13. *Top.* Stimulation technique of the recurrent motor branch of the median nerve using a bipolar surface stimulator. The cathode and anode are oriented in a direct line with the pathway of the recurrent motor nerve in order to reduce shock artifact. *Bottom.* Monopolar needle electrode montage for evaluation of the median motor nerve fibers across the carpal tunnel. The ring electrode on the ring finger serves as the anode and the needle electrode serves as the cathode. The CMAP is recorded from the abductor pollicis brevis muscle.

mV with midpalmar stimulation (Fig. 8–14) (44). This demonstrates the usefulness of this technique in identifying conduction block. Excellent functional recovery should occur in CTS largely with conduction block of median motor nerve fibers.

The electrodiagnostician must be aware of a possible source of error with midpalmar stimulation of the motor nerve. The shape of the CMAP must be the same at wrist and midpalmar stimulation. Stimulation in the midpalm can lead to depolarization of ulnar motor fibers to the deep head of the flexor pollicis brevis (especially with surface electrode stimulation). This could lead to misinterpretation of electrodiagnostic data (Fig. 8–15).

If a patient has identical wrist and mid-

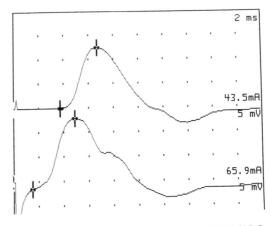

Figure 8–15. *Top.* Median motor nerve CMAP (12.0 mV) from 8 cm wrist stimulation technique. *Bottom.* Median and ulnar nerve CMAP (14.2 mV) from midpalmar stimulation. Although there is a 14% increase in size of the midpalmar CMAP, there is no sign of neurapraxia. The shape of the midpalmar CMAP is changed because of depolarization of the ulnar nerve innervated thenar muscles. This can occur with supramaximal stimulation. The electrodiagnostician must be aware of this possible source of error. The shape of the wrist and midpalmar CMAP waveforms *must be similar* prior to interpretation of the data. (Caliber: Horizontal graticule = 2.0 msec; vertical graticule = 5 mV. Filter: 2 Hz to 10 KHz)

palmar amplitudes on the side with CTS, the other median nerve should be examined. A midpalmar stimulation motor amplitude of 6 mV on the symptomatic side compared to an amplitude of 12 mV on the asymptomatic side is useful information with evidence of axonotmesis on the symptomatic side. Median motor CMAPs from side to side are highly correlated and usually have less than a 5% difference (20).

The side-to-side analysis is simple if the amplitudes are different. However, CTS can occur bilaterally(4, 56). If amplitudes are identical on the right and left sides and with wrist and midpalmar stimulation on the affected side, it is difficult to assess if axonotmesis of motor fibers is present. In these cases where both upper limbs in an individual are affected with CTS, ipsilateral median abductor pollicus brevis CMAP amplitude and ulnar-innervated abductor digiti minimi CMAP amplitude comparison is recommended. Ipsilateral hypothenar CMAP amplitudes usually differ from thenar CMAP amplitudes by less than 1.0 mV (20).

MEDIAN MOTOR NERVE CONDUCTION VELOCITY

The median motor nerve conduction velocity and mixed (motor/sensory) nerve conduction velocity in the forearm is frequently noted to be abnormally reduced with values commonly ranging from 40 m/s to 50 m/s in CTS (2, 43, 60). The reason for this remains unknown. It is hypothesized that because the fast conducting large diameter motor axons are more

adversely affected than the small diameter fibers, the motor conduction velocity may reflect only the function of the smaller diameter fibers that conduct more slowly (43). In addition to distal wallerian degeneration, nerve compression may cause retrograde axonal degeneration as proximal to the motor neuron cell body. The sensory nerve conduction velocity has not been shown to be reduced in CTS (2, 60).

The motor nerve conduction velocity is also helpful for assessing CTS in the presence of a Martin-Gruber anastomosis (17, 18).

MARTIN-GRUBER ANASTOMOSIS AND CTS

A Martin-Gruber anastomosis is defined as a median to ulnar nerve fiber communication that only involves motor fibers and occurs in the forearm. The C8 or T1 motor nerve fibers initially communicate from the lower trunk to the middle or upper trunk or from the ulnar motor nerve to the median motor nerve in the arm. In the forearm, these C8 or T1 motor nerve fibers rejoin the ulnar nerve (Fig. 8–16). Martin-Gruber anastomoses infrequently arise from the anterior interosseous nerve< which also has C8 and T1 motor nerve fibers (55).

The Martin-Gruber anastomosis has reportedly been present in 17% to 25% of subjects (17, 31). It has been reported as being bilateral in 68% of subjects (7). This anomaly is probably inherited as an autosomal dominant trait (31). Median motor nerve determinations can be confusing unless the electrodi-

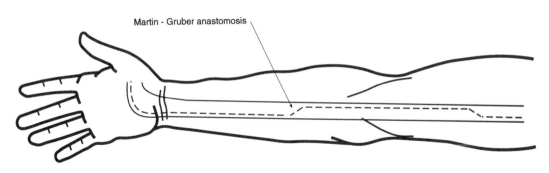

Figure 8–16. Example of a Martin-Gruber anastomosis with return of C8 and/or T1 motor fibers to the ulnar nerve in the forearm.

Wrist Stimulation

Elbow Stimulation

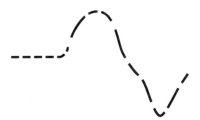

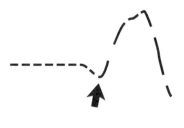

Elbow Latency (6.0 msec) - Wrist Latency (4.0 msec) = Forearm Latency (2.0 msec)

$$\frac{\text{Forearm Measurement (200 mm)}}{\text{Forearm Latency (2.0 msec)}} = 100 \text{ m/sec}$$

Figure 8–17. Martin-Gruber anastomosis with CTS electrodiagnostic findings. Note the positive deflection obtained only with stimulation of the median nerve at the elbow (arrow), the larger amplitude with stimulation of the median nerve at the elbow, and the falsely fast nerve conduction velocity of the forearm segment.

agnostician is aware of the Martin-Gruber anastomosis and its influence on nerve conduction variables.

Stimulation of the median nerve in the antecubital fossa also stimulates those ulnar motor fibers traveling with the median nerve, whereas stimulating the median nerve at the wrist does not. This anastomosis can be verified by stimulation of the median nerve in the antecubital space and recording the CMAP over the thenar muscles.

Three clues to the presence of a Martin-Gruber anastomosis associated with CTS on electrodiagnostic testing include the following (Fig. 8–17):

1. An initial positive deflection of the CMAP is obtained when stimulating the median nerve at the elbow. This positive deflection is not present when stimulating the median nerve at the wrist. It is a result of the action potential generated from ulnar-innervated thenar muscle fibers (probably the deep head of the flexor pollicus brevis) whose motor point is not under (but near) the recording electrode (Fig. 8–17). The positive deflection occurs before the median CMAP because the ul-

nar fibers are not entrapped at the level of the carpal tunnel.

2. A larger CMAP is obtained when stimulating the median nerve at the elbow (Fig 8–17). This is because the CMAP is the result of median and ulnar motor thenar muscle (presumably the deep head of the flexor pollicus brevis) depolarization. The wrist stimulation does not activate the ulnar nerve fibers that were stimulated from the median nerve at the elbow; thus, a smaller amplitude results. This finding is present in individuals with a Martin-Gruber anastomosis whether or not they have CTS.

3. An artificially fast median motor nerve conduction velocity (NCV) is calculated. The NCV can be as fast as 100 m/s to 150 m/s (Fig. 8–17). The NCV is fast because only the median motor nerve fibers in the carpal tunnel are stimulated at the wrist, resulting in a prolonged latency, whereas the proximal latency represents the normal conduction time of the ulnar nerve fibers escaping the carpal tunnel. Thus, the difference between the normal proximal latency and the prolonged distal la-

tency is small and contributes to a falsely fast NCV.

WITHIN-HAND NERVE-TO-NERVE COMPARISONS

Numerous efforts have been made to improve the sensitivity and specificity for the electrodiagnosis of CTS. The concept of comparison of distal latencies has developed over the past few decades to increase the electrodiagnostic sensitivity of CTS, especially in cases in which routine distal latency measurements are within normal limits (2,4,21,25,27,41,56,61). These techniques have several advantages. They allow the subject to serve as his or her own control and avoid the use of the contralateral limb, which may also have CTS. Within-hand nerve comparisons can be performed quickly when dually innervated digits (thumb and ring finger) are chosen for study. This testing also helps assess if a peripheral neuropathy is present because other sensory nerves are examined.

Within-hand comparisons have been reported to have an electrodiagnostic sensitivity approaching 90% (41, 56). These studies were performed on middle-aged subjects and thus their data serves the vast majority of patients. Recently, it has been determined that comparison values used for middle-aged subjects are not valid in elderly subjects greater than 60 years of age (21). In elderly patients, nerve-to-nerve comparison values can vary so much that the usefulness of these techniques may be less valuable. For elderly subjects, examination of the median nerve proximal and distal to the carpal tunnel is thus even more essential.

MEDIAN AND RADIAL SENSORY LATENCIES TO THE THUMB

Johnson and colleagues have studied the median and radial sensory nerve fibers with a 10-cm antidromic technique (27). Ring electrodes were placed over the thumb and the superficial branch of the radial nerve was stimulated 10 cm from the proximal electrode (G1) on the dorsolateral surface of the wrist. With the same recording electrodes, the median nerve

was stimulated 10 cm from the proximal electrode (G1) ulnar to the flexor carpi radialis tendon. The median nerve 10-cm measurement was made from the G1 electrode to the middle of the distal flexor wrist crease and then proximally along a line between the flexor carpi radialis tendon and the palmaris longus tendon.

In their study, Johnson and colleagues determined the difference between these two SNAPs measured to the negative peak to be 0.4 msec or less in 78 healthy subjects (27). In 20 patients with CTS, this difference was 1.0 msec or greater (Figs. 8–18 and 8–19).

Although current studies indicate that radial and ulnar sensory comparisons to the median nerve have equal electrodiagnostic sensitivities, the radial nerve comparison is conceivably a better choice and is recommended as an initial screening test for CTS. The radial nerve is felt to be better for comparison because of the following reasons:

1. It is less frequently involved with entrapment syndromes compared to the ulnar nerve.
2. Ulnar nerve deficits are occasionally associated with carpal tunnel syndrome. This is explained by the ulnar nerve's relationship to the carpal tunnel. The flexor retinaculum serves as the roof (transverse carpal ligament) and as the

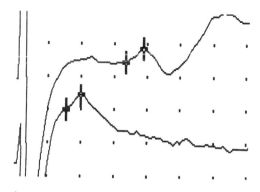

Figure 8–18. Median to radial SNAP comparison to digit I at 10 cm. The top tracing with a median SNAP peak distal latency of 3.9 msec compared to the bottom tracing of the radial SNAP measured to the peak at 2.0 msec supports a diagnosis of CTS. (Caliber: Horizontal graticule = 1.0 msec; vertical graticule = 10 mV. Filter: 20 Hz to 2 KHz)

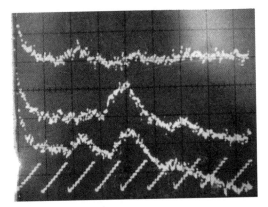

Figure 8–19. The Bactrian sign. This sign is the result of simultaneous stimulation of the median and radial sensory nerve fibers by using a bipolar surface stimulator midway between the two standard stimulation sites for these nerves. The delayed median nerve response provides the second hump of the camel's back. *Top.* Radial nerve response. *Middle.* Median nerve response. *Bottom.* Radial-median sensory nerve response (Bactrian sign). (Caliber: Slanted line = 1 msec. Each dot along slanted line = 0.1 msec. Vertical line = 20 mV. Filter: 2 Hz to 10 KHz)

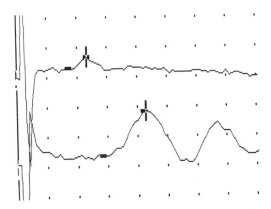

Figure 8–20. *Top.* Antidromic radial SNAP from the thumb at 10 cm (no motor artifact). *Bottom.* Antidromic median SNAP from the ring finger at 14 cm followed by motor artifact. Note how similar these two potentials appear and how one might be misinterpretted as the other. The motor artifact is usually denoted by its longer duration. However, this SNAP looks remarkably similar to the motor artifact owing to its falsely prolonged duration because it was obtained from a cool hand. For another example of motor artifact, see Figure 8–8.

(Caliber: Horizontal graticule = 1.0 msec; vertical graticule = 20 mV. Filter: 20 Hz to 2 Khz)

floor (palmar carpal ligament) of Guyon's canal (2,5,51,52).

3. There is no interfering motor artifact when studying the radial sensory nerve (Fig. 8–20) (27).

4. A superficial radial sensory nerve deficit can also cause a numb thumb.

5. The radial sensory nerve distal latency is not affected by advancing age (up to 95 years) (20).

6. A C6 radiculopathy can be detected by viewing a reduced radial SNAP or median SNAP. Some radiculopathies can occur at or distal to the dorsal root ganglion (i.e., they are actually "nerve-opathies"). This can result in a diminished SNAP, especially in middle- to older-aged patients with foramenal encroachment at the lower cervical vertebrae secondary to degenerative discs and osteoarthritic spurring.

MEDIAN AND ULNAR SENSORY LATENCIES TO THE RING FINGER

Johnson and colleagues studied the median and ulnar sensory nerve fibers with a 14-cm antidromic technique (25). Recording ring electrodes were placed 4.0 cm apart over the ring finger. The median nerve stimulation was performed ulnar to the flexor carpi radialis tendon and the ulnar nerve was stimulated posterior to the flexor carpi ulnaris tendon.

In their study, Johnson and colleagues determined the difference between these two SNAPs measured to the negative peak to be 0.3 msec or less in 37 healthy subjects (25). In 18 patients with CTS, this difference was 1.0 msec or greater (Fig. 8–21).

Although this technique is not recommended for the routine electrodiagnosis of CTS, it is useful to determine if coexisting ulnar deficits are present or to help to quickly determine if a sensory peripheral neuropathy and CTS are present.

MISCELLANEOUS ELECTRODIAGNOSTIC TECHNIQUES FOR CTS

Stevens has described an 8-cm compound nerve action potential (CNAP) comparison of the median and ulnar nerve fiber distal latencies measured from palm to wrist (56). The median nerve is stimulated in the midpalm

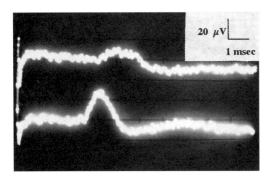

Figure 8-21. Antidromic 14-cm ring finger median and ulnar SNAP comparison in a patient with CTS. *Top.* Antidromic median SNAP from digit four measuring 4.0 msec to the negative peak. The prolonged duration (temporal dispersion) of this response also serves as a useful clue to the presence of median nerve dysfunction. *Bottom.* Antidromic ulnar SNAP from digit four measuring 3.5 msec to the negative peak. The electrodiagnostician may suspect CTS with a difference greater than 0.3 msec.

in the second metacarpal interspace, and the ulnar nerve is stimulated in the midpalm in the fourth metacarpal interspace. The CNAP (orthodromic sensory/antidromic motor potential) is recorded with a bar electrode with the recording and reference disks 3 cm apart. The bar electrodes were placed just ulnar to the flexor carpi radialis tendon for the median nerve and just radial to the flexor carpi ulnaris tendon for the ulnar nerve (Fig. 8–22). The upper limit of normal for the median CNAP was 2.2 msec in 202 tested "normal" hands. A difference of greater than 0.2 msec between the median and ulnar nerve CNAPs measured to the negative peak was supportive of CTS.

The CNAP comparison is a sensitive technique and is an option available to the electrodiagnostician. The CNAP latency can be in the normal range, however, if either the

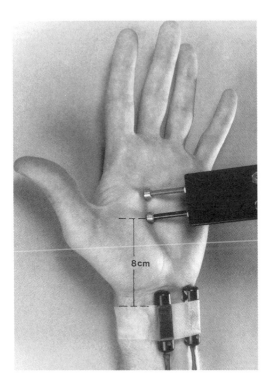

Figure 8-22. Median and ulnar 8-cm CNAP study montage. The cathode and anode are directed in line with the pathway of the median nerve. The bipolar surface stimulator is placed in the midpalm (cathode is proximal) in the second metacarpal interspace for the median nerve and in the fourth metacarpal interspace for the ulnar nerve.

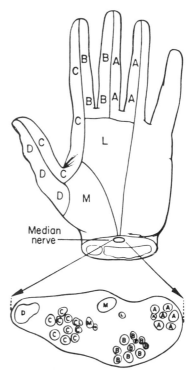

Figure 8-23. Topography of the median nerve at the level of the radial styloid. A. Funiculi correspond to sensory fibers to area A. B. Funiculi correspond to sensory fibers to area B. C. Funiculi correspond to sensory fibers to area C. D. Funiculi correspond to motor fibers to the thenar muscles. L. Funiculi correspond to motor fibers to the first and second lumbricals. (Reprinted with permission from Livingstone C: In: Sunderland S, ed. Nerve and nerve injuries, 2nd ed., 1978.)

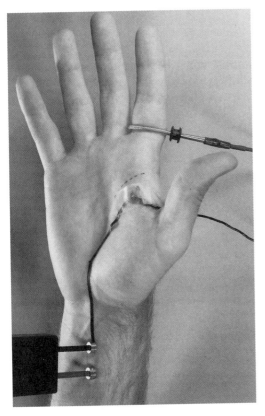

Figure 8–24. First lumbrical motor study montage. The reference (G2) ring electrode is over the base of the index finger. The active (G1) electrode is 1 cm proximal to the midpalmar crease and to the radial side of the long flexor tendon. Surface stimulation is at 12 cm following the course of the median nerve.

motor or sensory fibers are spared in selected cases of CTS. The CNAP comparison is also more time consuming than the ring finger comparison technique. The ring finger (median/ulnar) comparison technique and thumb (median/radial) comparison technique have also been shown to be comparable to the CNAP comparison for the electrodiagnosis of CTS (41, 47, 61). The ring finger technique also lacks the prognostic information available with motor/sensory wrist and midpalm methods.

Evaluation of the first lumbrical CMAP is an additional motor nerve conduction technique that could be useful for individuals suspected of CTS who have normal latencies and amplitudes to the abductor pollicis brevis (10). Three of 36 patients (8%) who had an abnormal sensory study but normal motor la-

tencies to the abductor policus brevis were found to have abnormal lumbrical latencies (10). These abnormal latencies can occur with selective nerve fiber involvement in CTS (Fig. 8–23).

The first lumbrical motor study technique is demonstrated in Figure 8–24. The first lumbrical latency at 12 cm and the abductor pollicus brevis latency at 8 cm had an upper limit of normal measuring 4.2 msec. The mean lumbrical amplitude was 2 mV with a range of 600 μV to 8 mV. A typical first lumbrical response is shown in Figure 8–25.

Kimura has published what has become known as the "inching technique" (although increments were measured in centimeters) for the electrodiagnosis of CTS (30). He examined 12 total sites (five proximal to the distal flexor wrist crease, one at the wrist crease, and six sites distal to the wrist crease) and determined that a latency change greater than

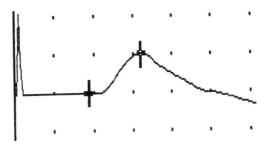

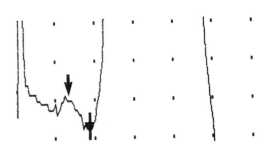

Figure 8–25. *Top.* A "normal" first lumbrical CMAP obtained with a 12-cm technique. (Caliber: Horizontal graticule = 2 msec; vertical graticule = 2 mV.) *Bottom.* A view of the top recorded potential at a gain setting of 500 uV/division. The lumbrical CMAP often might be only 1.0 mV or 2.0 mV and the premotor potential that the arrow is pointing to should not be misinterpreted as the lumbrical CMAP. The premotor potential is a result of the depolarization of the sensory branches of the median nerve. (Filter: 2 Hz to 10 KHz)

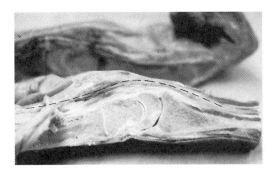

Figure 8-26. Longitudinal section through the long finger of the right hand. The dashed line represents the course of the median nerve. Note its varying depth, which can make it difficult to stimulate the median nerve fibers directly beneath the bipolar surface stimulator, particularly in the carpal tunnel segment of the palm.

0.2 msec from one location to the next was supportive of median nerve entrapment at that site.

The inching technique is prone to error when using surface stimulation. Supramaximal stimulation of median nerve fibers, particularly in the thick skin of the palm, can lead to depolarization of nerve fibers proximal and distal to the cathode of the bipolar surface stimulator. The course of the median nerve is superficial at the wrist, deep in the carpal tunnel segment of the palm, and superficial again in the distal palm (Fig. 8–26).

Provocative maneuvers have also been attempted in order to increase the sensitivity of the electrodiagnosis of median nerve dysfunction. Performance of complete wrist flexion for several minutes followed by testing has been shown in some cases to prolong the distal latency to abnormal limits (50). It has not been shown to increase the senstivity of detecting median nerve abnormalities compared to most other techniques discussed in this chapter.

ACUTE CTS IN INDUSTRY

CTS is probably the most common cumulative trauma disorder with about one half of the cases reported being occupationally related (6). Prompt recognition of this entity can result in proper treatment for the patient and save the employee and employer time and money. Repetitive motions of the wrists in the workplace can result in the development of CTS in as short a time as 2 weeks, particularly

in people with risk factors for CTS (13, 15). The acute syndrome is manifested by a conduction block of sensory, motor, or both fiber types within the carpal tunnel (Figs. 8–9 and 8–14). The changes in amplitude across the carpal tunnel can be markedly different in comparison to the distal latencies, which may be only slightly prolonged or even within normal limits (13). Alternatively, acute CTS can result in changes that are predominantly related to conduction slowing without much change in amplitudes noted. The severity of the symptoms did not correlate with the severity of the electrodiagnostic abnormalities (13).

TREATMENT OF CTS

Conservative treatment of CTS includes wearing a wrist splint that holds the wrist in a neutral position (Fig. 8–27) (3). Patients are advised to wear the splint at least every night during the sleeping hours until symptoms resolve or lessen to a stable degree (usually in 4 to 8 weeks).

A steroid injection within the carpal tunnel can provide symptomatic relief of pain, often well beyond the expected pharmacologic effect of the steroid (11). One half of a cc (20 mg) of triamcinolone hexacetonide is recommended because it is the least-water-soluable steroid. Anesthetics, such as lidocaine, should not be used in order to avoid accidental injection into the median nerve after the area becomes numb. The injection is performed ulnar to the palmaris longus tendon and a few millimeters beyond the distal wrist crease with

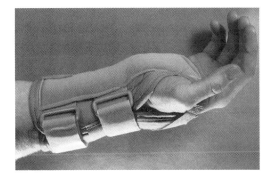

Figure 8-27. A carpal tunnel splint with the wrist properly placed in a neutral position for the optimal treatment of CTS. Many over-the-counter splints have the wrist improperly positioned at 10° to 20° of extension.

a 25-gauge needle angled at about 35° and pointed distally toward the carpal tunnel. Alternatively, nonsteroidal anti-inflammatory medication can be precribed for patients with CTS.

A reduction in activities associated with repetitive wrist movements can also facilitate recovery from median nerve symptoms. Coexisting disease processes such as diabetes mellitus or gout should also be medically controlled.

Carpal tunnel release surgery should be reserved for patients who fail to respond to conservative treatment, who have persistent pain or weakness, and who have electrodiagnostically confirmed dysfunction of the median nerve within the carpal tunnel as the etiology of their symptoms.

SUMMARY

Electrodiagnostic evaluation of the median nerve for CTS is an extension of the history and physical exam. A high clinical suspicion of CTS should prompt the electrodiagnostician to perform only one or two confirmatory tests. Diagnostic uncertainty or "normal findings" after a few electrodiagnostic techniques in a clinically suspected CTS should prompt the electrodiagnostician to further test the patient. *In all cases, both the sensory and motor fibers of the median nerve should be examined proximal and distal to the carpal tunnel in order to localize the median nerve dysfunction to the level of the carpal tunnel and determine the degree of nerve compromise.*

Recommended steps for electrodiagnostic evaluation of the median nerve in suspected cases of CTS should include the following:

1. Compare antidromic median and radial SNAP peak latencies at the thumb. A difference greater than 0.4 msec is suggestive of CTS.
2. Compare antidromic median SNAP peak latencies at 14 cm and 7 cm, recorded from the long finger. If the 14 cm latency is greater than twice the distal 7 cm latency, it is supportive of CTS. Also compare the wrist and midpalmar amplitudes and durations for the extent of nerve compromise.
3. Compare the median nerve CMAP amplitudes recorded from the abductor pollicus brevis muscle with wrist and midpalmar stimulation. Determine the degree of conduction block (neurapraxia). An increase greater than 10% with midpalmar stimulation is supportive of conduction block.
4. Perform median motor nerve conduction velocity. A falsely fast nerve conduction velocity and an initial positive deflection of the CMAP on elbow stimulation is supportive of CTS with a Martin-Gruber anastomosis.
5. If CTS is confirmed with electrodiagnostic evaluation, screen the contralateral upper limb with an antidromic median to radial SNAP comparison at the thumb.
6. Antidromic median-to-ulnar nerve SNAP comparisons should be performed if there is a suspected coexisting peripheral neuropathy.
7. Needle EMG electrode examination of muscles in the upper limb is not recommended for the electrodiagnosis of CTS. This should be performed only if another disease process, such as a radiculopathy, is suspected.

Case Studies

Patient number one is a 35-year-old, right-hand-dominant male with a 4-week history of right wrist pain shooting into his hand. He never paid attention to determine from which digits the pain radiated. Six weeks ago he started working on a widget assembly line.

A median-to-radial sensory screen to the thumb revealed a difference of 0.5 msec (see Table 8–2). This was a borderline abnormality. The median sensory 14-cm and 7-cm technique revealed a normal latency across the carpal tunnel segment. The median motor study revealed a significant degree of neurapraxia of median motor fibers within the carpal tunnel. The NCV of 110 m/s indicated the presence of a Martin-Gruber anastomosis with CTS.

This case demonstrates the need to examine both the median motor and sensory fibers. Median sensory studies are more sensitive for the electrodiagnosis of CTS in most cases. However, this patient developed an industrial-related, acute case of CTS involving primarily the median motor nerve fibers. Examination of the median nerve proximal and dis-

Table 8-2
Nerve Conduction Values for Patient 1

Nerve	Distance	Digit	DL (msec)	Amplitude	NCV (m/s)
median sensory	10 cm	thumb	3.0	30 μV	
radial sensory	10 cm	thumb	2.5	20 μV	
median sensory	14 cm	long finger	3.4	30 μV	
median sensory	14 cm	long finger	1.6	40 μV	
median motor	8 cm	APB	3.8	7.0 mV	110.0
median motor	mid palm	APB		12.0 mV	

DL = distal latency
NCV = nerve conduction velocity

Table 8-3
Nerve Conduction Values for Patient 2

Nerve	Distance	Digit	DL (msec)	Amplitude	NCV (m/s)
median sensory	10 cm	thumb	3.7	20 μV	
radial sensory	10 cm	thumb	2.9	12 μV	
median sensory	14 cm	long finger	3.9	20 μV	
median sensory	14 cm	long finger	1.8	25 μV	
median motor	8 cm	APB	3.6	7.0 mV	50.0
median motor	mid palm	APB		10.0 mV	

tal to the carpal tunnel revealed that this was a neurapraxic injury. This has an excellent prognosis with prompt initiation of treatment.

Patient number two is a 51-year-old, right-hand-dominant woman with a medical history of well-controlled type II diabetes mellitus who presented with numbness and tingling in the right hand. Results of an electrodiagnostic evaluation of her right upper limb are presented in Table 8–3.

A median-to-radial sensory screen to the thumb revealed a difference of 0.8 msec. This was suspicious for CTS. Both latencies were a little more prolonged than might be expected, which might be owing to the patient's diabetes. Therefore, a median sensory study to the long finger was performed proximal and distal to the carpal tunnel. This revealed a prolonged time of 2.0 msec across the carpal tunnel. This was diagnostic of CTS. The distal 7-cm latency of 1.8 msec as well as the 10-cm radial and 14-cm median latencies suggested that a mild diabetic peripheral neuropathy might be present. A median motor study was performed proximal and distal to the carpal tunnel and revealed a 3.0 mV increase in amplitude, indicative of a neurapraxic injury to the median motor fibers within the carpal tunnel.

The electrodiagnostic evaluation of a patient for CTS with a possible underlying perpheral neuropathy can be challenging. Examination of only the

distal latency to the long finger at 14 cm and to the abductor pollicus brevis (APB) at 8 cm could have resulted in a "normal" study with regard to a CTS evaluation and might have led to a diagnosis of only peripheral neuropathy. The ulnar sensory nerve and both sural nerves should be studied next for a diabetic neuropathy evaluation. This case emphasizes the need to examine the median nerve fibers proximal and distal to the carpal tunnel in order to distinguish CTS from an underlying peripheral neuropathy.

References

1. Bolton CF, Sawa GM, Carter K: The effects of temperature on human compound action potentials. J Neurol Neurosurg Psychiatry 1981;44:407–414.
2. Buchthal F, Rosenfalk A, Trojaborg W: Electrophysiologic findings in entrapment of the median nerve at the wrist and elbow. J Neurol Neurosurg Psychiatry 1974;37:340–360.
3. Burke DT, Burke MM, Stewart GW, et al.: Splinting for carpal tunnel syndrome: In search of the optimum angle. Arch Phys Med Rehabil 1994;75:1241–1244.
4. Cassvan AA, Ralescu S, Shapiro E, et al.: Median and radial sensory latencies to digit I as compared with other screening tests in carpal tunnel syndrome. Am J Phys Med 1988;67:221–224.

5. Cassvan A, Rosenberg A, Rivera LF: Ulnar nerve involvement in carpal tunnel syndrome. Arch Phys Med Rehabil 1986;67:290–292.

6. Centers for Disease Control: Occupational diseases survaillance: carpal tunnel syndrome. JAMA 1989; 77:889.

7. Crutchfield CA, Gutmann L: Hereditary aspects of median- ulnar nerve communications. J Neurol Neurosurg Psychiatry 1980;43:53–55.

8. Denys EH: AAEE minimonograph #14: the influence of temperature in clinical neurophysiology. Muscle Nerve 1991;14:795–811.

9. Falco FJE, Hennessey WJ, Braddom RL, et al.: Standardized nerve conduction studies in the upper limb of the healthy elderly. Am J Phys Med Rehabil 1992;71:263–271.

10. Fitz WR, Mysiw WJ, Johnson EW: First lumbrical latency and amplitude. Control values and findings in carpal tunnel syndrome. Am J Phys Med Rehabil 1990;69:198–201.

11. Gelberman R, Aronson D, Weisman M: Carpal tunnel syndrome: results of a prospective trial of steroid injection and splinting. J Bone Joint Surg 1980; 62A:1181–1184.

12. Golding DN, Rose DM, Selvarajah K: Clinical tests for carpal tunnel syndrome: An evaluation. Br J Rheumatol 1986;25:388–390.

13. Gordon C, Bowyer BL, Johnson EW: Electrodiagnostic characteristics of acute carpal tunnel syndrome. Arch Phys Med Rehabil 1987;68:545–548.

14. Gordon C, Johnson EW, Gaten PF, et al.: Wrist ratio correlation with carpal tunnel syndrome in industry. Am J Phys Med Rehabil 1988;67:270–272.

15. Gordon C, Lubbers LM, McCosker SP: Carpal tunnel syndrome. Phys Med Rehabil: State Art Rev. 1992;6:223–232.

16. Gray H: Muscles and fasciae of the hand. In: Goss CM, ed. Gray's anatomy. Philadelphia: Lea & Febiger, 1973;29:473.

17. Guttmann L: Median-ulnar nerve communications and carpal tunnel syndrome. J Neurol Neurosurg Psychiatry 1977;40:982–986.

18. Guttmann L, Gutierrez A, Riggs JE: The contribution of median-ulnar communications in the diagnosis of mild carpal tunnel syndrome. Muscle Nerve 1986;9:319–321.

19. Halar EM, DeLisa JA, Soine TL: Nerve conduction studies in upper extremities: Skin temperature corrections. Arch Phys Med Rehabil 1985;66:605–609.

20. Hennessey WJ, Falco FJE, Braddom RL: Median and ulnar nerve conduction studies: Normative data for young adults. Arch Phys Med Rehabil 1994; 75:259–264.

21. Hennessey WJ, Falco FJE, Braddom RL, et al.: The influence of age on distal latency comparisons in carpal tunnel syndrome. Muscle Nerve 1994;17: 1215–1217.

22. Jablecki CK, et al.: Literature review of the usefulness of nerve conduction studies and electromyography for the evaluation of patients with carpal tunnel syndrome. Muscle Nerve 1993;16;1392–1414.

23. Johnson EW: Sixteenth Annual AAEM; Edward H. Lambert Lecture. Electrodiagnostic aspects of diabetic neuropathies: Entrapments. Muscle Nerve 1993;16:127–134.

24. Johnson EW, Gatens T, Poindexter D, et al.: Wrist dimensions: Correlation with median sensory latencies. Arch Phys Med Rehabil 1983;64:556–557.

25. Johnson EW, Kukla RD, Wongsam PE, et al.: Sensory latencies to the ring finger: Normal values and relation to carpal tunnel syndrome. Arch Phys Med Rehabil 1981;62:206–208.

26. Johnson EW, Melvin JL: Sensory conduction studies of median and ulnar nerves. Arch Phys Med Rehabil 1967;48:25–30.

27. Johnson EW, Sipski M, Lammertse T: Median and radial sensory latencies to digit I: Normal values and usefulness in carpal tunnel syndrome. Arch Phys Med Rehabil 1987;68:140–141.

28. Johnson EW, Wells RM, Duran RJ: Diagnosis of carpal tunnel syndrome. Arch Phys Med Rehabil 1962;43:414–419.

29. Kemble F: Electrodiagnosis of carpal tunnel syndrome. J Neurol Neurosurg Psychiatry 1968;31: 23–27.

30. Kimura J: The carpal tunnel syndrome: Localization of conduction abnormalities within the distal segment of the median nerve. Brain 1979;102:619–635.

31. Kimura J, Murphy MJ, Varda DJ: Electrophysiological study of anomalous innervation of intrinsic hand muscles. Arch Neurol 1976;33:842–844.

32. Kimura J, et al.: Relation between size of compound sensory or muscle action potentials and length of nerve segment. Neurology 1986;36:647–652.

33. Kopell HP, Goodgold J: Clinical and electrodiagnostic features of carpal tunnel syndrome. Arch Phys Med Rehabil 1968;49:371–375.

34. Kuschner SH, Ebramzadeh E, Johnson D, et al.: Tinel's sign and Phalen's test in carpal tunnel syndrome. Orthopedics 1992;15:1297–1302.

35. Learmonth J: The principle of decompression in the treatment of certain diseases of peripheral nerves. Surg Clin North Am 1933;13:905–913.

36. Macdonnel RAL, Schwartz MS, Swash M: Carpal tunnel syndrome: Which finger should be tested? An analysis of sensory conduction in digital branches of the median nerve. Muscle Nerve 1990;13: 601–606.

37. Melvin JL, Burnett CN, Johnson EW: Median nerve conduction in pregnancy. Arch Phys Med Rehabil 1969;50:75–80.

38. Melvin JL, Schuchmann JA, Lanese RR: Diagnostic specificity of motor and sensory nerve conduction variables in the carpal tunnel syndrome. Arch Phys Med Rehabil 1973;54:69–74.

39. Moersch FP: Median thenar neuritis. Proc Surg Meetings Mayo Clin 1938;13:220–222.

40. Paget J: Lectures on surgical pathology. Philadelphia: Lindsay and Blakiston, 1854.

41. Pease WS, Cannell CD, Johnson EW: Median to radial latency difference test in mild carpal tunnel. Muscle Nerve 1989;12:905–909.

42. Pease WS, Cunningham ML, Walsh WE, et al.: Determining neurapraxia in carpal tunnel syndrome. Am J Phys Med Rehabil 1988;69:117–119.

43. Pease WS, Lee HH, Johnson EW: Forearm nerve conduction velocity in carpal tunnel syndrome. Electromyogr Clin Neurophysiol 1990;30:299–302.

44. Phalen GS: Spontaneous compression of the median nerve at the wrist. JAMA 1951;145:1128–1132.

45. Phalen GS: The carpal tunnel syndrome: 17 years' experience in diagnosis and treatment of 654 hands. J Bone Joint Surg 1966;48:211–228.

46. Phalen GS: Reflections on 21 years' experience with the carpal tunnel syndrome. JAMA 1970;212:1365–1367.

47. Preston DC, et al: The median-ulnar latency difference studies are comparable in mild carpal tunnel syndrome. Muscle Nerve 1994;17:1469–1471.

48. Radecki P: The familial occurrence of carpal tunnel syndrome. Muscle Nerve 1994;17:325–330.

49. Reinstein L: Hand dominance in carpal tunnel syndrome. Arch Phys Med Rehabil 1981;62:202–203.

50. Schwartz MS, Gordon JA, Swash M: Slowed nerve conduction with wrist flexion in carpal tunnel syndrome. Ann Neurol 1980;8:69–71.

51. Sedal L, McLeod JC, Walsh JC: Ulnar nerve lesions associated with carpal tunnel syndrome. J Neurol Neurosurg Psychiatry 1973;36:118–123.

52. Silver MA, Gelberman RH, Gellman H, et al.: Carpal tunnel syndrome: Associated abnormalities in ulnar nerve function and the effect of carpal tunnel release on these abnormalities. J Hand Surg 1985;10A:710–713.

53. Slater RR, Bynum DK: Diagnosis and treatment of carpal tunnel syndrome. Orthop Rev 1993:1095–1105.

54. Smith EM, Sonstegard DA, Anderson WH: Carpal tunnel syndrome: Contribution of flexor tendons. Arch Phys Med Rehabil 1977;58:379–385.

55. Spinner M: The median nerve. In: Injuries to the major branches of peripheral nerves of the forearm. Spinner M, ed. Philadelphia: WB Saunders, 1978;2:210–211.

56. Stevens JC: AAEE minimonograph #26: The electrodiagnosis of carpal tunnel syndrome. Muscle Nerve 1987;10:99–113.

57. Sunderland S: Nerve lesion in carpal tunnel syndrome. J Neurol Neurosurg Psychiatry 1976;39:615–626.

58. Thomas JE, Lambert EH, Cseuz KA: Electrodiagnostic aspects of carpal tunnel syndrome. Arch Neurol 1967;16:635–641.

59. Tinel J: Presse Med 1915;47:388.

60. Uchida Y, Sugioka Y: Electrodiagnosis of retrograde changes in carpal tunnel syndrome. Electromyogr Clin Neurophysiol 1993;33:55–58.

61. Uncinci A, Lange DJ, Soliven B, et al.: Ring finger testing: The most sensitive technique to detect mild carpal tunnel syndrome. Muscle Nerve 1987;10:647.

62. Wilkins RH, Brody IA: Neurological classics: Tinel's sign. Arch Neurol 1971;24:573–575.

63. Wongsam PE, Johnson EW, Weinerman JD: Carpal tunnel syndrome: Use of palmar stimulation of sensory fibers. Arch Phys Med Rehabil 1983;64:16–19.

Chapter 9

Late Responses: The H, F, and A Waves

W. Jerry Mysiw

H REFLEX

The H reflex was initially described by Hoffman in 1918 (47), but its clinical value did not become apparent until the 1950s with the studies of Magladery and McDougal (74). Since that time, the H reflex has become a clinically important tool in the diagnosis of radiculopathy and peripheral neuropathy. Ongoing studies continue to define the importance of the H reflex in both understanding the physiology of abnormal muscle tone and using the H reflex as a quantifiable parameter useful in the management of spasticity. The next section will first review the physiologic basis of the H reflex and then discuss how this phenomena can be clinically applied.

Physiology

The H reflex represents the consequence of a submaximal electrical stimulation of I_a sensory fibers; this impulse then enters the dorsal horn of the spinal cord where it synapses with alpha motor neurons, ultimately resulting in a compound muscle action potential that is recorded as the H wave (47, 74). Although electrophysiologic evidence largely supports the observation that the H reflex is monosynaptic (75), evidence exists that questions the veracity of this observation (17). Nevertheless, the H reflex clearly results from orthodromic conduction along both the I_a sensory nerve and the alpha motor neuron that comprise this reflex.

The H reflex is most reliably recorded from the soleus after stimulation of the tibial nerve. Stimulation of the median nerve usually produces an H reflex that is recordable over the flexor carpi radialis muscle, but its onset la-

tency is often obscured by the preceding M wave. Stimulation of the femoral nerve less commonly produces an H reflex that is recordable over the quadriceps muscles. H reflexes are otherwise recorded over additional muscles in the newborn-to-one-year-of-age period (9, 11), with central nervous system disorders producing an upper motor neuron lesion (76, 117); with the addition of facilitation techniques, such as with Jendrassik's maneuver; or, more significantly, with forceful agonist muscle contractions (15, 41, 96).

H reflexes have also been recorded over the pronator teres, flexor digitorum sublimis, brachioradialis, extensor carpi radialis longus, extensor digitorum communis, extensor indices, extensor pollicus longus-brevis, anterior tibialis, and peroneal longus muscle when these facilitation techniques are utilized. Thus, H reflexes have been recorded in muscles supplied by C5, C6, C7, C8, L2, L3, L4, L5, S1, and S2 nerve roots, implying that H reflexes are ubiquitous in adults with a normal neurologic system when facilitation techniques are utilized (129).

The H reflex is characterized by a comparatively stable onset latency but a more variable amplitude. The amplitude of the H reflex is largest when associated with a submaximal compound muscle action potential (CMAP). With additional increases in stimulation intensity, the amplitude of the H-reflex response decreases while the CMAP, or M wave, amplitude conversely increases (Fig. 9–1) (12, 13, 51). The H reflex is usually absent when the amplitude of the M response has been maximized. It has been estimated that 24% to 100% of the motoneuron pool that partici-

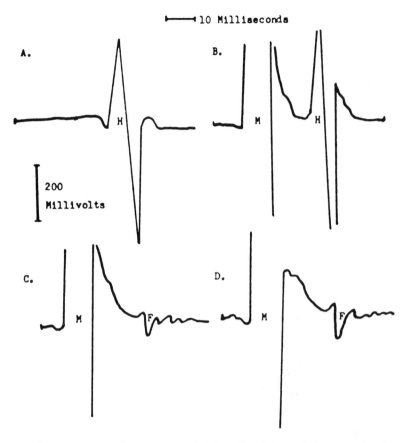

Figure 9-1. H reflex, M wave, and F wave recorded from the abductor hallucis muscle after stimulation of the tibial nerve. *A through D* represents the consequence of increasing stimulation intensity from submaximal and supramaximal. Initially, only the H reflex is observed (*A*), then the M wave with H reflex (*B*). At supramaximal intensity, the H reflex is replaced with an F wave.

pates in the formation of the M wave may also contribute to the formation of the H reflex (113, 115).

The decrease in H-reflex amplitude and the simultaneous increase in the CMAP amplitude, with subsequent increase in stimulation intensity, was initially believed to result from the collision of H-reflex impulses with the antidromic conduction of impulses arising from the alpha motor neurons (74). The validity of this assumption is predicated on a substantially greater conduction velocity for the I_a sensory nerve compared to the alpha motor neuron, thereby allowing the afferent sensory impulse to reach the spinal cord, synapse with the alpha motor neuron, and then collide with the antidromically conducted impulse within the alpha motor neuron. However, data have failed to substantiate the conduction velocity of the I_a sensory nerve being sufficiently faster

than the alpha motor neuron to account for this theory. Specifically, human studies have documented mean conduction velocities of 55.1 m/s in cutaneous afferent nerves, 57.6 m/s in muscle afferent nerves, and motor conduction velocities of 52.4 m/s (110). Thus, this small variation in conduction velocity is insufficient to account for a central delay of 4 msec to 5 msec that results from the combination of the 0.5 to 1.0 msec consumed by a single synapse and the 3-msec to 4-msec rise time of the excitatory postsynaptic potentials generated from the afferent activation of alpha motor neurons (16,17,70,71,72,74,106). For a collision to occur within the alpha motor neuron, the conduction velocity of the I_a sensory afferent segment of the reflex would need to be substantially faster than the antidromically conducting impulse in the alpha motor neuron to overcome the 4-msec to 5-msec central delay. However, as previously stated, the disparity between the conduction velocity of the I_a sensory afferent and the alpha motor neurons are not sufficient to support this collision hypothesis. Finally, the observation that H reflexes are present with higher stimulation intensity, in conjunction with facilitation via forceful muscle contraction, provides further evidence that collision does not account for the loss of the H reflex during stimulation with higher intensity. It is, therefore, more likely that the inhibition of the H reflex with supramaximal stimulation intensity results from the alpha motor neuron being in a refractory state, from the antidromic impulse conducting within the alpha motor neuron, or from Renshaw cell-mediated inhibition (125, 126).

Several distinctions exist between the H reflex and the F wave that allows one to distinguish between these two late responses (Table 9–1). First, the H reflexes are largely limited to the soleus and the flexi carpi radialis muscles, whereas facilitation techniques are often required in an otherwise intact adult neurologic system to produce H reflexes in additional muscle groups. Conversely, the F wave is ubiquitous in that it can be elicited from any muscle after proper stimulation of the respective motor nerve (55).

A second distinction between the H reflex and F wave is the stability of the H reflex and the inherent variability of the F response. Repetitive stimulation utilizing consistent stimulation parameters and technique produces H reflexes that are identical in shape and latency. On the other hand, repetitive stimulation utilizing consistent stimulation parameters and technique appropriate for F wave studies demonstrates responses that are variable in latency, amplitude, shape, and persistence (55). The stability of the H reflexes with consistent stimulation techniques and parameters reflects the physiologic consequence of stimulating the same motor neuron pool, whereas the variable F-wave responses reflect the inconsistent recurrent activation of the alpha motor neuron pool (55).

As previously mentioned, the onset latency of the H reflex is more stable than that of the F wave, but, conversely, H-reflex and F-wave latencies recorded from individual single muscle fibers demonstrate greater variability from the H reflex compared to the F wave. This observation is presumed to reflect greater variability in the synaptic delay of the H reflex at the anterior horn cell, whereas the turnaround time for recurrent discharges resulting in an F wave is comparatively stable (50,51,56,111). The variability of the central synapse of the H reflex is supported by single fiber EMG studies. For example, the mean jitter or MCD (mean of consecutive differences) of the H reflex has been estimated at less than 140 μsec in both the flexi carpi radialis and the soleus muscles, whereas the mean MCD for M responses in both of these muscles is less than 40 μsec. It is believed, therefore, that the M

Table 9–1
Comparison of Features Distinguishing H Reflexes and F Waves

	F wave	H reflex
Physiology	motor neuron "backfiring"	monosynaptic reflex
afferent	alpha motor neuron	I_a sensory
efferent	alpha motor neuron	alpha motor neuron
distribution	ubiquitous	soleus; flexor carpi radialis
facilitation	increased amplitude	increased amplitude; greater distribution of muscles
Technique		
stimulation	supramaximal	submaximal
Waveform		
latency	variable	stable
amplitude	variable	stable
shape	variable	stable
persistence	variable	stable
jitter	<H	>F

jitter contributes comparatively little to the overall H reflex jitter and that the majority of the jitter noted in the H reflex is indicative of the variability of the central synapse (50, 111).

A number of studies have begun to explore the clinical relevance of H-reflex jitter. For example, H-reflex jitter studies have documented increasing jitter with age; a direct correlation between H-reflex jitter and H-reflex latency; and a dramatic increase in jitter during sleep. In addition, H-reflex jitter has been shown to approximate 300 μsec in motor neuron disease (50, 111). Therefore, this technique offers another intriguing way to understand the interplay between the central and peripheral nervous systems. However, for now the considerable variability in H-reflex jitter and the relative paucity of clinical studies exploring the utility of this technique renders the H-reflex jitter to be of uncertain clinical significance.

Although the latency of the H reflex is stable with a given set of stimulation parameters, it is possible to affect the H-reflex latency with either facilitory or inhibitory techniques. For example, it has been found that facilitory techniques such as Jendrassik's maneuver shorten the central delay of the soleus H reflex; however, the extent of impact on central delay appears variable (1, 2). The impact of facilitory and inhibitory conditioning stimuli on the central delay of the H reflex is more consistent. Specifically, facilitory techniques may shorten the central delay by approximately 0.4 msec, whereas inhibitory conditioning may lengthen the central delay approximately 0.9 msec (1, 2). Again, this technique appears to have potential value in assessing the excitability of the motoneuron pool, but the clinical significance of this observation remains uncertain.

Change in H-reflex amplitude is thought to reflect the excitability of the motor neuron pool subsequent to segmental and supraspinal influences (56). A significant body of information exists about the influence of body position and muscle contraction on subsequent H-reflex gain. For example, passive stepping and pedaling movements of the lower limb produce ipsilateral H-reflex inhibition, with maximum inhibition occurring at the most flexed position (19). The same set of experiments also suggests that the rate of passive stretch is exponentially related to the H-reflex gain. The implication, then, is that the inhibition of H-reflex gain under these circumstances is related to segmental influences (19).

The soleus H-reflex amplitude is known to attenuate during quiet standing, relative to the amplitude recorded with the subject in a prone position (63). Supraspinal influences on H-reflex amplitude are also supported by the observation that the H-reflex gain is attenuated during the swing phase of gait. It is known that soleus H-reflex amplitude is augmented with background EMG(46); specifically, ankle plantar flexion will increase H-reflex amplitude, whereas ankle dorsal flexion attenuates the reflex gain (40). Changes in H-reflex amplitude with ambulation have been correlated with anterior tibialis muscle activity. However, activation of antagonist muscles alone does not account for this phenomenon, as soleus H-reflex gain has been shown to attenuate during the swing phase of gait in the absence of anterior tibialis muscle contraction (30).

In addition to the reciprocal inhibition of the H-reflex amplitude with activation of antagonist muscles, contralateral movement affects H-reflex amplitude. For example, contralateral median nerve stimulation enhances the degree of reciprocal inhibition, whereas contralateral radial nerve stimulation reduces the reciprocal inhibition exerted by the extensor muscles on the flexor carpi radialis H reflex (107).

A number of paired stimulation techniques have been developed to evaluate the excitability of the motor neuron pool. A subthreshold conditioning stimulus has been shown to produce a facilitory affect on the subsequent test stimulus at intervals of approximately 25 msec; a period of inhibition then develops that persists for approximately 500 msec (Fig. 9–2) (56, 114). Within this time frame, a relative period of facilitation appears to occur between 50 msec and 200 msec. This initial facilitation is thought to represent the consequence of excitatory postsynaptic potentials, whereas the inhibition is likely the consequence of presynaptic inhibition of afferents (56, 114). The impact of conditioning stimuli on the H reflex is not yet fully understood; newer studies continue to explore this relationship and its physi-

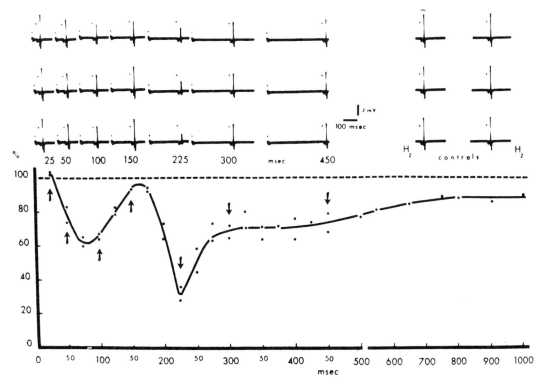

Figure 9-2. This study by Taborikova and Sax[k157] explored the effect of a conditioning stimulus on the H reflex. The conditioning stimulus intensity was below threshold for evoking an H wave whereas the test stimulus intensity was below the intensity necessary to evoke an M wave. To the right are the mean amplitude of three H reflexes in control subjects. To the left is the mean amplitude of three H reflexes generated at conditioning-test intervals of 25, 50, 100, 150, 225, 300, and 450 msec. (Reprinted with permission from Kimura J, ed. Electrodiagnosis in diseases of nerve and muscle: Principles and practice. Philadelphia: FA Davis, 1989.)

ologic relevance. For example, contralateral H-reflex conditioning results in facilitation of the soleus H reflex at conditioning-test intervals of 100 or more msec (62). Paired shock techniques have also been used to evaluate the effect of cutaneous stimulation on the soleus H reflex; at interstimulus intervals of approximately 100 msec, selective cutaneous stimulation produces a significant decrease in H-reflex amplitude.

Vestibular influences have been noted on the H reflex. Specifically, lateral tilting results in both inhibition of the ipsilateral soleus H reflex and facilitation of the contralateral soleus H reflex (3). Similarly, it has been noted that backward tilting of the head/body results in an increase in the excitability of Renshaw cells projecting to soleus motor neurons, thereby inhibiting the H reflex (82).

More recently, transcranial stimulation of the motor cortex has been utilized to study corticospinal control of spinal inhibitory mechanisms in humans. It has been documented that cortical stimulation induces a short latency inhibition of H reflexes in the soleus (49). More specifically, data generated from transcranial stimulation imply that the corticospinal tract can inhibit soleus motoneurons through multiple spinal mechanisms.

The fact that the H reflex is influenced by suprasegmental input has rendered it attractive in evaluating the physiologic basis for disorders of muscle tone (95, 96). It has been demonstrated that H reflex latencies are significantly shorter and reflex amplitudes are significantly greater (H/M ratios) in spastic hemiplegic subjects compared to control subjects (67). The H/M ratio-increase with spasticity appears to correlate with tendon reflex changes to a greater extent than the degree of muscle tone (64). The presence of clonus appears to coincide with elevations of both the

H/M ratio and late facilitation of the soleus H-reflex recovery curve (64). In addition, the magnitude of vibratory inhibition of the H reflex decreases with increasing hypertonia (64).

The impact of tendon vibration on the H-reflex amplitude after spinal cord injury (SCI) is dependent on the maturity of the neurologic lesion. Specifically, tendon vibration causes a significant attenuation of H-reflex amplitude in acute SCI (less than 2 weeks post-injury) and has relatively little effect in chronic SCI subjects (greater than one year post-injury) (18). These data are presumed to reflect a decline over time in the level of presynaptic inhibition contributing to the enhancement of spinal reflexes.

Paired stimulation to the median nerve in a hemiplegic limb demonstrates an absolute potentiation of the H-reflex amplitude with delays between 100 msec and 400 msec and a peak at 200 msec (95, 96). This response does not appear to correlate with tone or reflexes. Reciprocal inhibition of H reflexes reveals three periods of inhibition: the first occurs from -1.0 msec to 1.0 msec of delay between radial and median nerve stimulation; the second peaks at 10 msec of delay; and the third peaks at 100 msec of delay. Each period of delay-producing inhibition is believed to be subsequent to various mechanisms. Specifically, the first period of delay is thought to result from disynaptic reciprocal inhibition. The second period of inhibition is believed to be the consequence of presynaptic inhibition, whereas the third period of inhibition may be related to either presynaptic inhibition or other polysynaptic-mediated mechanisms (95).

Specific electrophysiologic techniques are being explored for their utility in the assessment of pathophysiologic mechanisms of spasticity. For example, the F wave has been advocated as an assessment for alpha-motoneuron activity. Achilles tendon to H-reflex maximal amplitude ratio has been used to assess gamma-motoneuron activity. The maximal H-reflex amplitude before and after vibrating the Achilles tendon has been advocated as an adequate technique for the assessment of presynaptic inhibition (85, 88). However, it is important to understand that the theoretical aspects of these data remain unclear. Work is ongoing to explain the impact of various central nervous lesions on muscle tone and to develop reproducible electrophysiologic techniques capable of providing clinically relevant physiologic insight.

CLINICAL APPLICATIONS

Because the H reflex represents the physiologic consequence of an interaction between the peripheral and central nervous systems, it is an intriguing technique for evaluating specific aspects of both sensory and motor function. Attempts have been made to correlate the clinical efficacy of spinal manipulation (91), massage therapy (90), and analgesia from transcutaneous electrical nerve stimulation (5, 44) with subsequent changes in H-reflex amplitude. Researchers have additionally used the H reflex in an effort to characterize the physiologic mechanisms of spasticity and to utilize this information in the pharmacologic management of spasticity (86, 87, 92). These assessments are primarily predicated on changes in H-reflex amplitude or the H-maximum amplitude/M-maximum amplitude ratio. However, extreme caution is warranted in interpreting the clinical significance of H-reflex amplitude variability because of the considerable number of factors that influence H-reflex amplitude. Studies intended to draw clinical implications from changes in H-reflex amplitude are compelled to account for variables such as facilitory contractions of agonist muscles or inhibitory contractions of its antagonist muscles (40). Similarly, activation of agonist muscles in the contralateral limb have been shown to facilitate H-reflex amplitude, whereas antagonist muscle activation in the contralateral limb results in inhibition and a subsequent decline in H-reflex amplitude (107). Cutaneous activation also bears consideration in interpreting H-reflex amplitude changes, as both inhibitory and facilitatory effects have been observed (127). Body position should be considered; it should be consistent in studies attempting to draw clinical significance from amplitude variability of the H-reflex, because trunk position affects H-reflex amplitude, and hip, knee, and ankle flexion all decrease H-reflex amplitude (3, 14, 19).

Consistent with the data that a large number of factors affect H-reflex amplitude is the observation that in the clinical setting, the upper limit of normal for side-to-side H-reflex amplitude difference in the soleus muscle is 400%, whereas the normal side-to-side H-reflex amplitude in the flexor carpi radialis variability approaches 300% (33). The mere presence of H reflexes in muscle groups not typically associated with the reflex may serve as an early indication of subtle neurologic system disease if that H-reflex is elicited without the use of facilitatory techniques. For example, the presence of H reflexes in the anterior tibialis muscle has been reported as unusually high in the children of patients with Huntington's disease (24, 53). In addition, H reflexes have been documented in the anterior tibialis muscle of patients with phenylketonuria and may be utilized for documenting early central nervous system manifestations of the disease (38).

The primary clinical utility of the H reflex stems from the ability to assess conduction along the proximal segment of sensory fibers and the entire length of motor fibers within a mixed peripheral nerve. Consequently, the H reflex has been documented as abnormal in various types of polyneuropathies and represents an important adjunct in the early detection of peripheral neuropathy (61, 66, 79). The H reflex also offers a unique ability to show the proximal integrity of the peripheral nerve; hence, the H reflex has been documented as abnormal in plexopathies, piriformis syndrome (36), and nerve root injury (10,36,54,77,93,129).

The primary clinical value of the H reflex is in the detection of an S1 radiculopathy and, to a lesser extent, a C6 or C7 radiculopathy (Fig. 9–3) (51, 108, 109). Subsequently, the H reflex has been referred to as the electromyographic counterpart to the ankle reflex. However, the physiologies of the two reflexes are not entirely the same, as the H reflex bypasses the muscle spindle. In addition, either the H reflex or the ankle reflex may be absent with subsequent sparing of the counterpart. A unilateral absence of an H reflex or the side-to-side prolongation of the H-reflex by as little as 1.0 msec in the tibial nerve and 0.8 msec in the median nerve is highly suggestive of

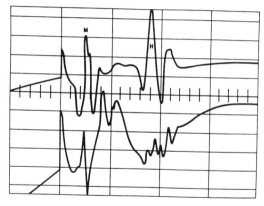

Figure 9–3. H reflex recorded over the soleus in a patient with a unilateral S1 radiculopathy. The H reflex from the unaffected side revealed a latency of 29.8 msec (*top trace*), whereas the H reflex from the affected side showed a latency that was comparatively prolonged at 32.1 msec (*bottom trace*).

an S1 or a C6/C7 radiculopathy, respectively. Unilateral H-reflex abnormalities in the absence of other electromyographic evidence for radiculopathy may be interpreted as early evidence of a nerve root injury. However, other etiologies for focal injuries to the peripheral nerve should be considered. On the other hand, H reflexes may be normal in proven radiculopathies, presumably because of incomplete nerve root involvement with sparing of sufficient fibers to produce a normal latency (10). Finally, the unilateral absence of an H reflex must be interpreted cautiously in an individual with a pre-existing S1 or C6/C7 nerve root injury as the reflex may not reappear despite the resolution of the radiculopathy (see Chapter 6) (51).

Technical Considerations

Proper electrode placement for recording the H reflex involves placing the recording and reference electrodes over the appropriate muscles. Several specific patterns of electrode placement have been advocated for recording the soleus H reflex. One approach advocates placing the active electrode at the point where a line between the tibial nerve in the popliteal crease and the tibial nerve at the uppermost portion of the medial malleolus is bisected (Fig. 9–4). The reference electrode is placed over the Achilles tendon (13, 51). A second electrode distribution often used to record the

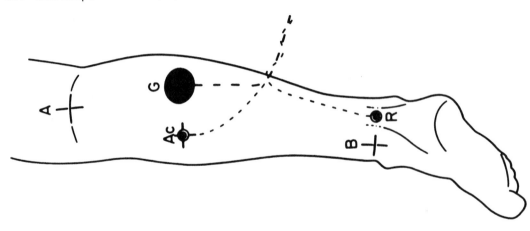

Figure 9–4. Electrode placement for H-reflex studies. The active electrode (Ac) is placed at the midpoint between the popliteal crease (A) and the tibial nerve at the superior border of the medial malleolus. The reference electrode (R) is placed over the Achilles tendon and the ground (G) is lateral to the active electrode. Stimulation is at the tibial nerve (A).

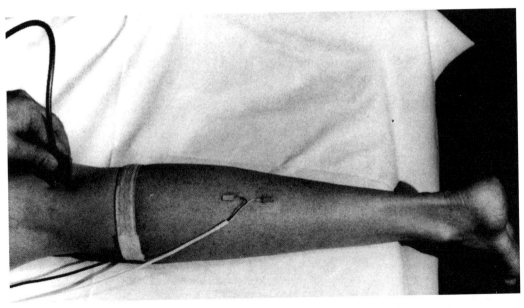

Figure 9–5. A second electrode placement technique for recording the H reflex. The active electrode is in the midline of the calf, 2 cm distal to the insertion of the gastrocnemius muscle. The reference electrode is 3 cm distal to the active electrode. (Reprinted with permission from Kimura J: Electrodiagnosis in diseases of nerve and muscle: Principles and practice. Philadelphia: FA Davis, 1989.)

H reflex from the soleus involves placing the active electrode 2 cm distal to the insertion of the gastrocnemius and the reference electrode approximately 3 cm distal to the active electrode (Fig. 9–5) (56). A third electrode array advocates placing the active electrode over the medial soleus distal to the insertion of the gastrocnemius, with the reference and ground electrodes arranged lateral to the active elec-

trode. Considerable variation in H-reflex waveform is noted with the different electrode placement techniques (80). Additionally, consistency in electrode placement is warranted as more distal electrode placement increases H-reflex latency (80). Finally, the electrode placement for recording the H reflex over the flexor carpi radialis involves placing the recording electrode over the prominence of the muscle at approximately one-third the distance from the medial epicondyle to the radial styloid. The reference is placed distally over the brachioradialis tendon. In all H-reflex studies, the stimulating cathode is placed proximally to the anode over the peripheral nerve.

Instrument parameters include a sweep speed of 10 msec/cm for the lower limb and 5 msec/cm in the upper limb. Amplifier gain is typically adequate at 0.5–1.0 mV/cm. Filter settings used in motor nerve conduction studies are appropriate for the H reflex with a high-pass filter of 2 Hz and a low-pass filter of 10 kHz. The H reflex is most effectively elicited with stimulation parameters that include an impulse of submaximal intensity and a long duration that is firing at slow stimulation rates. Specifically, it is recommended that initially a subthreshold stimulation intensity be used that is subsequently slowly increased until the amplitude of the H reflex has maximized as the M response is becoming apparent. The potential for confusing an H reflex with an F response is diminished when the observed late response amplitude decreases in the presence of increasing M-wave amplitude. Hence, a late response appearing with variable latency and waveform that is smaller in amplitude than the concurrent M wave should be considered an F wave and not confused with the H reflex. Adjusting the stimulation intensity in an effort to obtain an H reflex of maximal amplitude may require decreasing the stimulation intensity to levels that are subthreshold for eliciting the M response.

The optimal stimulation duration is approximately 0.5 to 1.0 msec (26). This recommendation is based on the observation that long-duration stimulation impulses selectively stimulate sensory fibers at threshold, whereas short-duration impulses of less than 200 μsec selectively stimulate motor fibers (124). Similarly, the H reflex is suppressed with rapid stimulation rates; therefore, stimulation frequencies of 0.2 Hz to 0.5 Hz are advocated (26).

Normal Values

The normal lower limb H-wave latency typically falls within a range of 28 msec to 33

msec. In the upper limb, the latency of the H reflex recorded from the flexor carpi radialis is typically less than 22 msec (56). H-reflex latency has been documented to correlate with age and height. Two strategies have been developed to predict H-reflex latency in the lower limb while correcting for the influences of age and height. One technique uses a regression equation in which the predicted H-reflex latency in milliseconds equals 9.14 + 0.46 (leg length in centimeters from the stimulation site to the top of the medial malleolus) + 0.1 (age in years) (12, 13, 51). Similarly, a nomogram based upon this equation may be used to predict the H-wave latency; specifically, the predicted H-reflex latency is determined by a line connecting the patient's age and leg length (Fig. 9–6) (12, 13, 51). The predicted H-reflex latency and the normal range of H-reflex latencies are important variables in the diagnosis of peripheral neuropathy or bilateral nerve root injury.

Perhaps the most valuable clinical application of the H reflex is in the diagnosis of unilateral radiculopathy. With unilateral radiculo-

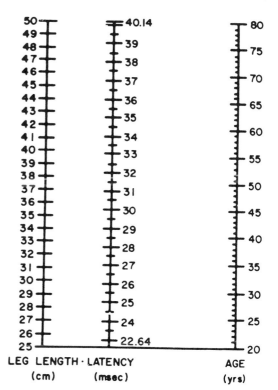

Figure 9–6. Nomogram for predicting H-reflex latency based on leg length and age.

pathy, comparison of side-to-side H-reflex latencies provides meaningful diagnostic information. Reported normal upper limit of side-to-side variability of H-reflex latencies has ranged between the upper limits of 1.0 msec to 1.8 ms (13, 26, 31). Hence, each laboratory is encouraged to develop its own normal range, as the precision of this technique has important clinical implications. Less information is known about the normal side-to-side variability of H-reflex latency in the upper limb; in the upper limb, the upper limit of side-to-side variability has been estimated at 0.8 msec to 1.0 msec (89).

Other Considerations

A less conventional technique for obtaining the S1 H reflex involves S1 spinal nerve stimulation (52, 99). This technique uses a needle as the cathode, which is inserted at the S1 level, 1 centimeter medial to the posterior, superior iliac spine. The anode is placed over the anterior abdomen. Recording and reference electrodes are placed in a standard fashion. Under these circumstances, the normal side-to-side variability of H-reflex latency is less than 0.8 msec. This technique presumably offers the advantage of greater precision by bypassing most of the afferent arm of the S1 H-reflex.

F WAVE

The first description of the F wave is credited to Magladary and McDougal in 1950 (74). The F wave was initially presumed to represent the consequences of yet another reflex, however, the preservation of the F wave in both human and animal models, in whom afferent impulses were removed by a posterior root sectioning, suggested that the F-wave is generated by a mechanism other than a reflex (42,81,83,84,119). Single-fiber EMG studies have additionally supported the observations that the F-wave is not generated through reflexive mechanisms. Specifically, single-fiber EMG studies have documented that F waves occur only in motor units in which stimulation produces both antidromic and subsequent orthodromic conduction (120). Finally, the comparatively minimal jitter documented

with F waves does not support the presence of a central synapse (121). It is, therefore, assumed that the F wave represents the activation of a motor neuron with subsequent orthodromic and antidromic conduction. The antidromically conducted impulse then sequentially depolarizes the axon hillock, the anterior horn soma, and the dendrites (26). This sequence of events presumes that electrical activity within the dendrites again depolarizes the axon hillock, generating an impulse that is conducted to the periphery.

Physiology

Approximately 1% – 2% of all motor neurons within a peripheral nerve participate in the generation of an F-wave response after a given single electrical impulse (26). F-to-M ratios in normal subjects approach a maximum of 5% (33). Sequential stimulation reveals that 10%–20% of generated F waves are identical or repeated responses (33, 103). These three issues have generated considerable speculation as to the responsible interactions between the peripheral and central nervous systems generating the observed F wave. In part, the observed responses have been explained as a preferential bias for larger motor neurons to participate in the production of an F wave. This bias for larger motor neurons has been explained as the consequence of one of three physiologic phenomena. First is the belief that Renshaw cell inhibition is less effective with larger motor neurons (28, 29, 45). Second, it has been speculated that the slower conduction of smaller alpha motor neurons renders that population more susceptible to collision with faster-conducting afferent impulses (45, 68). Finally, its been speculated that the depolarization characteristics of larger motor neurons render them more likely to backfire and activate an axon hillock that is no longer in a refractory state (7,105). However, contradictory data exists to support the observation that motor neurons of all sizes produce F waves with similar probability (23). These data, generated from individual intramuscular microstimulation of motor axons, suggest that larger motor neurons are preferentially responsible for the recurrence of identical waveforms (repeater F wave) (23).

Despite this persistent controversy, the fact that the central nervous system influences the characteristics of observed F-wave responses is incontrovertible. Specific examples include the F-wave characteristics recorded in subjects with upper motor neuron disorders. For example, in acute hemiplegia, F-response persistence, duration, and amplitude are decreased compared to the contralateral uninvolved limb. In chronic hemiplegia, persistence, duration, and maximum amplitude all normalize and are comparable to the contralateral side (25). It appears that the changes observed in chronic hemiplegia do not result in an appreciable change in the maximum amplitude of observed F waves; instead, the number of F responses with larger amplitude increases, resulting in a larger mean amplitude. These data suggest that F-wave characteristics are indicative of alpha-motoneuron excitability. Finally, interventions aimed at decreasing spasticity have documented normalization of F-response characteristics (86, 87, 92).

Other central nervous system influences on F-wave characteristics that warrant consideration during routine clinical studies include the observation that weak voluntary contraction of the muscle where the F-wave is being recorded results in F responses with larger amplitude (122). The importance of posture appears less important to subsequent F-wave characteristics compared to that previously described with the H reflex. At best, the data are conflicting about the importance of posture on F-wave characteristics (104). Sleeping during the recording of F-wave responses provides another example of the importance of the CNS on the characteristics of recorded F-wave responses; specifically, recording F waves during sleep results in a prolongation of the F-wave minimum latency and a decrease in both the persistence and size of the recorded F waves (48).

Clinical Applications

The CNS influences on F-response characteristics have been studied in an effort to understand the mechanism of spasticity and to evaluate the efficacy of subsequent interventions. A number of pharmacologic interventions for spasticity have documented improvement in F-wave characteristics,(86, 87, 92), but there has been little effort to correlate this improvement with clinical benefits, rendering the usefulness of F-response characteristics in the management of spasticity to be unproven.

The clinical utility of F responses has been substantiated in disorders of the peripheral nerve. The F response, for example, is essential for diagnosing and staging polyneuropathies (69). The importance of the F wave in the electrophysiologic evaluation for polyneuropathy is underscored by the recommendation that upper and lower limb F-wave determination should be included in all diagnostic polyneuropathy protocols. This recommendation is based on the observation that F-wave latencies have been repeatedly documented as abnormal when other measures of motor conduction appear unremarkable (26). The consensus statement from the San Antonio Conference on Diabetic Neuropathy has additionally recommended that all research protocols using electrodiagnostic techniques to monitor the progression of neuropathy should include upper and lower extremity F-response latencies (4).

F-wave abnormalities may be the first electrophysical evidence of acute Guillain-Barre syndrome, with a diagnostic sensitivity that exceeds 90%. Electrophysiologic studies performed an average of 8 days after the onset of neurologic symptoms have documented that lower limb F waves are abnormal in approximately 66% of subjects and upper limb F waves are abnormal in 56% of subjects (123). The F-wave abnormalities typically reported in Guillain-Barre syndrome include a prolongation of latency and chronodispersion, a decrease in persistence or a total absence of the F wave, and a decrease in F-wave amplitude (37, 55). However, the severity of F-wave abnormalities does not correlate with clinical outcome (22, 55).

Axonal neuropathic processes result in less obvious F-wave abnormalities than those noted with demyelinating disorders. However, F-wave studies are significantly more sensitive than conventional motor conduction studies in detecting evidence of axonal polyneuropathy (22,66,69,101). Hence, the F wave is an integral part in the evaluation of disorders such as amyotrophic lateral sclerosis

(ALS). For example, in mild cases of ALS, F-response latencies tend to to be normal; however, in more advanced cases in which there is significant reduction in the compound muscle action potential amplitude, F-response latencies are slowed, approaching 125% of the upper limit of normal (22). F-wave values that exceed 125% of normal should then imply that there is another mechanism of injury to the peripheral nerve that is in addition to the ALS.

The diagnostic significance of F-wave studies in the presence of focal compression injuries of peripheral nerves is dependent upon the accessibility of the injured nerve segment to other electrophysiologic techniques. In carpal tunnel syndrome, F-waves have demonstrated high sensitivity but low specificity, rendering this technique unimportant compared to other electrophysiologic approaches that are both sensitive and specific (65). The importance of the F wave is greater in more proximal focal injuries to the peripheral nerve, such as thoracic outlet syndrome. F-wave latencies have been documented as prolonged in patients with thoracic outlet syndrome, but with true neurogenic thoracic outlet syndrome, abnormal F-wave characteristics are preceded by abnormalities in the electromyographic portion of the examination (98, 131).

F waves have been utilized in an effort to diagnose suspected injuries at the nerve root level. Studies have documented that F-wave characteristics may be abnormal in the presence of suspected nerve root injury when electromyographic findings have remained normal (10). In the presence of cervical spondylosis, for example, the number of repeater F-waves increases significantly, whereas other F-wave characteristics, such as persistence and shape, remain unaffected (101). However, the majority of data suggest that the F-wave is not sufficiently sensitive or specific in the diagnosis of nerve root injury (130). Several theories have been advanced to explain this technique's lack of sensitivity compared to electromyographic testing. Most problematic is that F waves are elicited in peripheral nerves containing motor fibers from multiple nerve roots. Hence, recording the minimal F-wave latency in the presence of a single nerve root injury is likely to result in normal F-wave studies because of the unimpeded conduction along the uninjured nerve roots. The second consideration is that the focal injury to the nerve root may be mild so that it is undetectable when recording over the entire length of the peripheral nerve. Little data are available exploring the diagnostic utility of using other F-wave characteristics, such as persistence, duration, chronodispersion, etc., to enhance the diagnostic sensitivity of F waves in disorders of the nerve root. Dynamic maneuvers such as ambulation in cases of suspected neurogenic claudication have documented post-exercise changes in F-wave characteristics such as a decreased persistence or increased latency (70).

Technical Considerations

F-wave techniques do not differ substantially from standard motor nerve conduction studies. The recording electrode is placed over the motor points of the tested muscle, and the reference electrode is placed over the muscle tendon. Typical instrument parameters include a sweep speed of 5 ms/cm and a gain of 200 μV/cm. Filter settings utilized in motor nerve conduction studies are appropriate for the F wave with a high-pass filter of 2 Hz and a low-pass filter of 10 kHz.

Stimulus parameters must remain consistent within a given electrophysiologic laboratory as stimulus parameters have considerable impact on subsequent recorded F-wave characteristics. At issue is the relative importance of the stimulation intensity, the duration of the stimulating impulse, the rate of stimulation, and the total number of F-wave responses necessary for meaningful analysis. Stimulation intensity should be supramaximal; increasing stimulation intensity beyond 125% supramaximal to 150% supramaximal appears to cause no significant variations in recorded F-wave characteristics (21). Similarly, increasing the stimulation duration from 0.1 msec to 0.2 msec produces no appreciable change in recorded F-wave characteristics. However, stimulation rate is an important variable that must be controlled. One study, comparing the impact of stimulation rates ranging between 0.2 Hz and 2 Hz, documented greater F-wave amplitudes and persistence at the higher stimulation rates (32). Another study, comparing F-wave characteristics at stimulation rates ranging between 0.5 Hz and 3.0 Hz, documented a similar increase in amplitude and persistence of recorded F-wave responses, but additionally documented a decrease in minimum latency (21). These data support the observation that normal values established for a given laboratory must adhere to consistent stimulation parameters in subsequent clinical studies.

The minimum number of stimulations or recorded F waves required for an adequate clinical evaluation remains controversial. At balance is the issue of patient comfort versus the number of stimulations necessary to maximize the sensitivity of the technique. According to one study, the probability of obtaining the minimal F-wave latency within the first 10 of 100 stimulations was only 30%. Sixty stimuli were required to achieve a 95% probability of observing the minimum latency responses (8, 78). Another study showed that only one to 10 stimuli are required to obtain the minimum latency within one millisecond of that found by analyzing 100 responses (35). The same study showed that an estimate of persistence after 10 stimuli is within 90% of the persistence documented after 100 stimuli. Approximately 30 stimuli are necessary to fall within 97% of the persistence documented with 100 stimuli. A larger number of stimuli appear to be necessary to adequately study chronodispersion and amplitude.

Normal Values

The majority of studies utilizing F waves report only the minimum F-wave latency. In the upper limb, the minimum latency is typically less than 35 msec. In the lower limb, the F-wave minimum latency is typically less than 60 msec. Side-to-side differences in the minimum latency appear important; this difference should not exceed 2 msec in the upper limb and 4 msec in the lower limb (33, 56).

In an effort to maximize the information obtained from F-wave studies, other F-wave characteristics have been standardized. The chronodispersion represents the difference in time between the slowest and fastest conducting F-waves after a series of stimulations. In both the upper and lower limbs, the chronodispersion does not exceed 7.5 msec (94). The mean amplitude for a population of F waves, expressed as the F/M ratio, may range from 1% to 5% (33). Persistence, which represents the ratio of the number of recorded F responses to the number of stimulations applied, may be as low as 50% in a normal population; more typically, persistence approaches 80%–90% (102). Finally, the reappearance of individual motor units within a series of F waves is believed to be indicative of the selectivity of motor neuron populations available for F-waves. In normal subjects, the number of repeater F waves typically does not exceed 5% (103).

A number of studies have been dedicated to increasing the diagnostic yield of F-wave latencies. For example, it has been documented that F-wave latencies are affected by age, height, and limb length (34, 53, 102); consequently, nomograms have been developed that correct for these variables (Fig. 9–7) (128). The relative advantage of reporting a mean F-wave latency as opposed to a minimum F-wave latency has also been studied. These studies suggest that calculating a mean

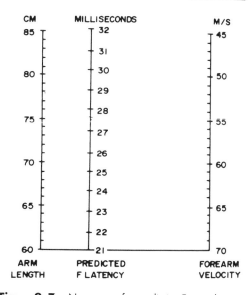

Figure 9–7. Nomogram for predicting F-wave latency in the ulnar nerve. The arm length is calculated from the C_7 spinous process to the ulnar styloid. The observed minimum latency should not exceed the predicted latency by more than 2.5 msec.

F wave decreases the coefficient of variation. The coefficient of variation for the mean F wave has been estimated at 7.6%, whereas the coefficient variation for the minimum F-wave latency was 8.6% (35, 116). Occasionally, reporting median F-wave latencies is advocated as F-wave latencies are not always normally distributed (103).

F-wave Conduction Velocity

Additional attempts to enhance the clinical value of the F wave have included converting the F-wave latency to a conduction velocity. This F-wave conduction velocity can be calculated by knowing the distance between the stimulus site and the C7 spinous process for upper limb studies and the T12 spinous process for lower limb studies (57, 59). The F-wave conduction velocity equals $[(D \times 2)(mm)] \div [(F-M-1)(msec)]$, in which D represents the distance from the stimulus site to the appropriate spinous process; F represents the minimum latency; and M represents distal motor latencies. In the upper limb, the F-wave conduction velocity has been estimated at approximately 65 ± 5 m/s. In the lower limb, the F-wave conduction velocity has been estimated at approximately 50 ± 4 m/s. These values then correlate rather closely with motor nerve conduction velocities. Conversion of F-wave latency to conduction velocities permits analysis of F tacheodispersion. Tacheodispersion represents a variation of chronodispersion: tacheodispersion represents the range of F-wave conduction velocities, whereas chronodispersion represents the range of F-wave latencies within a population of F waves. This technique has been suggested as a more sensitive means of detecting disorders that affect peripheral nerve conduction (20).

F-wave Ratio

The F-wave ratio has been studied as an alternative to the F-wave conduction velocity. The F-wave ratio offers the advantage that distance measurements are not required, thereby minimizing a potential source of error. The F-wave ratio is based on the assumption that stimulating an F-wave at either the elbow or the knee results in similar conduction times along both the above-joint and below-joint

segments; hence, the F-wave ratio should approach a unity. Actually, the F-wave ratio in the upper limb is approximately 1 ± 0.1; in the lower limb, the F-wave ratio is approximately 1.1 ± 0.1. The equation used to determine the F ratio equals $[(F-M-1)(msec)] \div [(M \times 2)(msec)]$, in which F represents the minimum F latency; M represents the distal motor latency; and 1 is an estimate of the central turnaround time of the F wave (56, 58).

Other Considerations

The F wave represents a standard electrophysiologic technique that in many ways is inadequately utilized. In most circumstances, only the minimum F latency is recorded after 10 stimulations, ignoring all other potential information discernible from looking at chronodispersion, amplitude, duration, persistence, and the number of repeater waves. This is somewhat understandable in a clinical setting, as there is a paucity of data available regarding the impact of pathologic disorders on these F-response characteristics. Additionally, increasing the number of stimulations and recording a greater number of F-wave characteristics has the disadvantage of increasing both patient discomfort and the required time for the study. Additional studies will be required to determine if attention must be directed to all F-wave characteristics to maximize the diagnostic sensitivity of this technique. One must determine if these F-wave characteristics are important only for serially documenting changes over time, subsequent to intervention studies.

A WAVE

The A wave is an example of a late or intermediate response that is rarely observed during the course of F-wave studies of primarily the hand and foot (39). The A wave is believed to represent the physiologic consequence of an incomplete peripheral nerve injury, with subsequent collateral sprouting from the nerve to the muscles at a more proximal location to the stimulation site. Several features of the A wave distinguish this waveform from the F wave. First, unlike the F wave, the A wave maintains a constant latency and shape; second, the A wave is encountered after a stimula-

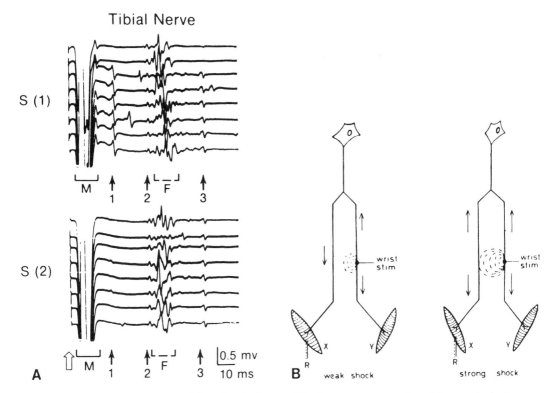

Figure 9–8. *A.* A waves recorded from the tibial nerve. The A waves at arrows 1 and 2 precede the F wave, whereas the A wave at arrow 3 follows the F wave. Stronger shocks at *S(2)* eliminated the earlier A waves noted at *S(1)*. *B.* Diagramatic representation of an A wave generated by a submaximal stimulation; however, at supramaximal stimulation, collision precludes the A wave. (Reprinted with permission from Kimura J: Electrodiagnosis in diseases of nerve and muscle: Principles and practice. Philadelphia: FA Davis, 1989.)

tion of submaximal intensity. These observations are explained by the following sequence of events. First, a submaximal impulse results in both antidromic and orthodromic activation of the peripheral nerve. The antidromic impulse conducts proximally, reaches the point of collateral sprouting, and then proceeds to conduct both proximally and distally. The impulse that precedes proximally may generate an F-wave, whereas the portion of the impulse that precedes distally generates the A wave (Fig. 9–8) (43, 56). Stimulation at supramaximal intensity typically results in a loss of the A wave as activation of the entire peripheral nerve results in a collision of the impulse along the collateral sprout. A waves can be observed after supramaximal stimulation intensity, but the mechanism for this is uncertain (56).

The A wave typically is of a shorter latency than the F wave, but on occasion the collateral sprout is immature and poorly myelinated; the resulting slowed conduction along this segment may result in an A wave with a latency that is longer than that of the F wave. As was noted in F waves, more proximal stimulation results in a decrease in the A-wave latency. However, as collateral sprouting does not always occur at the point of injury, this technique may not allow for accurate localization of the site of peripheral injury (56).

The A wave is noted in a variety of disorders affecting the peripheral nerve; these include pressure injuries to the peripheral nerve, peripheral neuropathies, amyotrophic lateral sclerosis, and root injuries (56). However, because the A wave can be observed in normal subjects, its clinical significance is limited (112).

References

1. Abbruzese M, Reni L, Favale E: Changes in central delay of soleus H reflex after facilitory or inhibitory conditioning in humans. J Neurophysiol 1991; 65(6):1598–1605.

2. Abbruzese M, Reni L, Favale E: Interindividual variability of central delay changes in the soleus H-reflex pathway. Muscle Nerve 1992;15(1):21–26.

3. Aiello I, Rosati G, Sau GF, et al.: Modulation of soleus H reflex by lateral tilting in man. Muscle Nerve 1992; 15:479–481.

4. American Diabetes Association: Report and recommendations of the San Antonio conference on diabetic neuropathy. Muscle Nerve 1988;661–667.

5. Arsenault AB, Belanger AY, Durand MJ, et a.: Effects of TENS and topical skin anesthesia on soleus H-reflex and the concomitant influence of skin/muscle temperature. Arch Phys Med Rehabil 1993; 74(1): 48–53.

6. Ashby P, LaBelle K: Effects of extensor and flexor group I afferent volleys on the excitability of individual soleus motoneurons in man. J Neurol Neurosurg Psychiatry 1977; 40:910–919.

7. Barakan TH, Dowman CBB, Eccles JC: Electric potentials generated by antidromic volleys in quadricep and hamstring motoneurones. J Neurophysiol 1949; 12:393–424.

8. Barron SA, Mazliah J, Bental E: The minimum F-response latency: The results from 10,000 stimuli of normal ulnar nerves. Electromyogr Clin Neurophysiol 1987;27:499–501.

9. Blom S, Haybarth KE, Skoglund S: Post-tetanic potentiation of H-reflexes in humans and infants. Exp Neurol 1964; 198–211.

10. Bobinac-Georgijevski A, Sokolovic-Matejcic B, Graberski M: The H- or F-wave latencies in medial gastrocnemius in the electrodiagnostic study of sciatica with suspected S_1 radiculopathy. Neurol Croatica 1991; 40(2):85–91.

11. Borg J: Axonal refractory period of single short toe extensor motor units in man. J Neurol Neurosurg Psychiatry 1980; 43(10):917–924.

12. Braddom RL, Johnson EW: H reflex: Review and classification with suggested clinical uses. Arch Phys Med Rehabil 1974; 55:412–417.

13. Braddom RL, Johnson EW:. Standardization of H reflex and diagnostic use in S_1 radiculopathy. Arch Phys Med Rehabil 1974;55:161–66.

14. Brooke JD, Cheng J, Misiaszek JE, Lafferty K: Amplitude modulation of the soleus H reflex in the human during active and passive stepping movements. J Neurophysiol 1995;73(1):102–111.

15. Burke D, Adams RW, Skuse NF: The effects of voluntary contraction on the H reflex of human limb muscles. Brain 1989;112:417–433.

16. Burke D, Gandevia SC, McKeon B: Monosynaptic and oligosynaptic contributions to human ankle jerk and H reflex. J Neurophysiol 1984;52:435–448.

17. Burke D, Gandevia SC, McKeon B: The afferent volleys responsible for spinal proprioceptive reflexes in man. J Physiol 1983;339:535–552.

18. Calancie B, Broton JG, Klose KJ, et al.: Evidence that alterations in presynaptic inhibition contribute to segmental hypo- and hyperexcitability after spinal cord injury in man. Electroencephalogr Clin Neurophysiol 1993;89:177–186.

19. Cheng J, Brooke JD, Misiaszek JE, et al.: The relationship between the kinematics of passive movement, the stretch of extensor muscles of the leg, and the change induced in the gain of the soleus H-reflex in humans. Brain Res 1995;672(1–2):89–96.

20. Chroni E, Panayiotopoulos CP: F tacheodispersion. J Neurol Neurosurg Psychiatry 1993;56(10):1103–1108.

21. Clinchot DM, Colachis SC, Kaplansky BD, et al.: Effects of stimulus parameters on characteristics of the F-response in normal subjects. Am J Phys Med Rehabil 1994;73:313–318.

22. Cornblath DR, Mellits ED, Griffin JW, et al.: Motor conduction studies in Guillain-Barre syndrome: Description and prognostic value. Ann Neurol 1988; 23(4):354–359.

23. Dengler R, Kossev A, Wohlfahrt K, et al.: F waves and motor unit size. Muscle Nerve 1992;15:1138–1142.

24. Deuschl G, Lucking CH, Schenk E: Hand muscle reflexes following electrical stimulation in choreatic movement disorders. J Neurol Neurosurg Psychiatry 1989;52(6):755–762.

25. Drory VE, Neufeld MY, Korczyn AD: F-wave characteristics following acute and chronic upper motor neuron lesions. Electromyogr Clin Neurophysiol 1993;33(7):441–446.

26. Dumitru D, ed. Electrodiagnostic medicine. Philadelphia: Hanley Belfus, 1995;191–206.

27. Dyck PJ, Karnes JL, Douke J, et al.: Clinical and neuropathological criteria for the diagnosis and staging of diabetic polyneuropathy. Brain 1985;108(4): 861–880.

28. Eccles JC: The central action of antidromic impulses in motor nerve fibers. Pflugers Arch 1955;260: 385–415.

29. Eccles JC, Eccles RM, Iggo A, et al.: Distribution of recurrent inhibition among motoneurones. J Physiol 1961;159:479–499.

30. Edamura M, Yang JF, Stein RB: Factors that determine the magnitude and time course of human H-reflexes in locomotion. J Neuroscience 1991;11(2): 420–427.

31. Falco FJE, Hennessey WJ, Goldberg G, et al.: H-reflex latency in the healthy elderly. Muscle Nerve 1994;17:161–167.

32. Fierro B, Raimondo D, Modica A: F-wave study at different stimulation rates. Electromyogr Clin Neurophysiol 1991;31(6):357–360.

33. Fisher M: AAEM minimograph #13: H reflexes and F waves: Physiologic and clinical indications. Muscle Nerve 1992;15:1223–1233.

34. Fisher MA: F response latency determination. Muscle Nerve 1982;5:730–734.

35. Fisher MA, Hoffen B, Hultman C: Normative F wave values and the number of recorded F waves. Muscle Nerve 1994;17(10):1185–1189.

36. Fishman LM, Zybert PA: Electrophysiologic evidence of piriformis syndrome. Arch Phys Med Rehabil 1992;73(4):359–364.

37. Fraser JL, Olney RK: The relative diagnostic sensitivity of different F-wave parameters in various polyneuropathies. Muscle Nerve 1992;15(8):912–918.

38. French JH, Clark DB, Butler HG, et al.:Phenylketonuria: Some observations on reflex activity. J Pediatr 1961;58:17–22.

39. Fullerton PM, Gelliatt RW: Axon reflexes in human motor nerve fibres. J Neurol Neurosurg Psychiatry 1965;28:1–11.

40. Funase K, Imavaka K, Nishihira Y, et al.: Threshold of the soleus muscle H-reflex is less sensitive to the change in excitability of the motoneuron pool during plantarflexion or dorsiflexion in humans. Eur J Appl Physiol 1994;69(1):21–25.

41. Garcia HA, Fisher MA, Gilai A: H-reflex analysis of segmental reflex excitability in flexor and extensor muscles. Neurology 1979;29:984–991.

42. Gassel MM, Wiesendanger M: Recurrent and reflex discharges in plantar muscles of the cat. Acta Physiol Scand 1965; 65:138–142.

43. Gilchrist JM: The axon reflex as ephaptic transmission: An hypothesis. Electromyogr Clin Neurophysiol 1988;28:209–213.

44. Goulet C, Arsenault AB, Levin MF, et al.: Absence of consistent effects of repetitive transcutaneous electrical stimulation on soleus H-reflex in normal subjects. Arch Phys Med Rehabil 1994;75(10):1132–1136.

45. Guiloff RJ, Moderres-Sadeghi H: Preferential generation of recurrent responses by groups of motor neurons in man. Brain 1991;114:1171–1181.

46. Hayashi R, Tako T, Yanagisawa N: Comparison of amplitude of human soleus H-reflex during sitting and standing. Neuroscience Research 1992;13(3):227–233.

47. Hoffman P: Uber die beziehungen der sehnen reflexe zur wilkurlichen bewegung und zum tonus. Z Biol 1918;68:351–370.

48. Ichikawa T, Yokota T: F wave change by decreased motoneuronal excitability: A sleep study. Bull Tokyo Med Dent Univ 1994;41(1):15–22.

49. Iles JF, Pisini JV: Cortical modulation of transmission in spinal reflex pathways of man. J Physiol 1992; 455:425–446.

50. Jabre JF, Stålberg EV: Single fiber EMG study of the flexor carpi radialis H reflex. Muscle Nerve 1989;12:523–527.

51. Johnson EW, ed. Practical electromyography. Baltimore: Williams & Wilkens 1980:46–52, 94–109, 217–221.

52. Johnson EW, Pease W, Gatens P, et al.: Combination of "H" reflex and S_1 spinal nerve stimulation in S_1 radiculopathy. Arch Phys Med Rehabil 1985; 66:546.

53. Johnson EW, Radecki P, Paulson G: Huntington disease: Early identification by H reflex testing. Arch Phys Med Rehabil 1977;58:162.

54. Katirji B, Wilbourn AJ: High sciatic lesion mimicking peroneal neuropathy at the fibular head. J Neurol Sci 1994;121(2):172–175.

55. Kiers L, Clouston P, Zuniga G, et al.: Quantitative studies of F-responses in Guillain-Barre syndrome and chronic inflammatory demyelinating polyneuropathy. Electroencephalogr Clin Neurophysiol 1994;93(4):255–264.

56. Kimura J, ed. Electrodiagnosis in diseases of nerve and muscle: Principles and practice. Philadelphia: FA Davis, 1989:332–374.

57. Kimura J: F-wave velocity in the central segment of the median and ulnar nerves: a study in normal subjects and in patients with Charcot-Marie-Tooth disease. Neurology 1974;24:539–546.

58. Kimura J: Proximal versus distal slowing of motor nerve conduction velocity in the Guillain-Barre syndrome. Ann Neurol 1978;3:344–350.

59. Kimura J, Bosch P, Lindsay GM: F-wave conduction velocity in the central segment of the peroneal and tibial nervos. Arch Phys Med Rehabil 1975;56:492–497.

60. Kimura J, Yanagisawa H, Yamada T, et al.: Is the F wave elicited in a select group of motorneurons? Muscle Nerve 1984;7:392–399.

61. Knoll O, Dierker E: Detection of uremic neuropathy by reflex response latency. J Neurol Sci 1980; 47(2):305–12.

62. Koceja DM, Kamen G: Contralateral influences on triceps surae motoneuron excitability. Electroencephalogr Clin Neurophysiol 1992; 85:177–182.

63. Koceja DM, Trimble MH, Earles DR: Inhibition of the soleus H-reflex in standing man. Brain Research 1993;629(1):155–158.

64. Koelman JH, Bour LJ, Hilgevoord AA, et al.: Soleus H-reflex tests and clinical signs of the upper motor neuron syndrome. J Neurol Neurosurg Psychiatry 1993;56(7):776–781.

65. Kuntzer T: Carpal tunnel syndrome in 100 patients: Sensitivity, specificity of multi-neurophysiological procedures, and estimation of axonal loss of motor, sensory and sympathetic median nerve fibers. J Neurol Sci 1994; 127(2):221–229.

66. Lachman T, Shahani BT, Young RR: Late responses as aids to diagnosis in peripheral neuropathy. J Neurol Neurosurg Psychiatry 1980;43(2):156–162.

67. Levin MF, Hui-Chan C: Are H and stretch reflexes in hemiparesis reproducible and correlated with spasticity? J Neurol 1993;240:63–71.

68. Lloyd DPC: Neuron patterns controlling transmission of ipsilateral hind limb reflexes in cat. J Neurophysiol 1943; 6:293–315.

69. Logigian EL, Kelly JJ Jr, Adelman LS: Nerve conduction and biopsy correlation in over 100 consecutive patients with suspected polyneuropathy. Muscle Nerve 1994;17(9):1010–1020.

70. London SF, England JD: Dynamic F waves in neurogenic claudication. Muscle Nerve 1991;14(5):457–461.

71. Lorente de No R. Limits of variation of the synaptic delay of motorneurons. J Neurophysiol 1938;1:187–194.

72. Lorente de No R: The synaptic delay of the motoneurons. Amer J Physiol 1935;111:272–282.

73. MacLeod WN: Repeater F waves: A comparison of sensitivity with sensory antidromic wrist-to-palm latency and distal latency in the diagnosis of carpal tunnel syndrome. Neurology 1987; 37:773–778.

74. Magladery JW, McDougal JB: Electrophysiological studies of nerve and reflex activity in normal man.

I. Identification of certain reflexes in the electromyogram and the conduction velocity of peripheral nerve fibers. Bull Johns Hopkins Hosp 1950; 86:265–290.

75. Magladery JW, Porter WE, Park AM: . Electrophysiological studies of nerve and reflex activity in normal man. IV. The two-neurone reflex and identification of certain action potentials from spinal roots and cord. Bull Johns Hopkins Hosp 1951; 88:499–519.

76. Magladery JW, Teasdall RD.: Stretch reflexes in patients with spinal cord lesions. Bull Johns Hopkins Hosp 1958;103:236–41.

77. Marin R, Dillingham TR, Chang A, et al.: Extensor digitorum brevis reflex in normals and patients with radiculopathies. Muscle Nerve 1995; 18(1):52–59.

78. Marra TR: F wave measurements: A comparison of various recording techniques in health and peripheral nerve disease. Electromyogr Clin Neurophysiol 1987;27:33–37.

79. Marya RK, Chandran AP, Maini BK, et al.: Role of H-reflex latency studies in the diagnosis of subclinical diabetic neuropathy. Indian J Physiol Pharmacol 1986;30(2):133–138.

80. Maryniak O, Yaworski R: H-reflex: Optimum location of recording electrodes. Arch Phys Med Rehabil 1987;68:798–802.

81. Mayer RF, Feldman RG: Observations on the nature of the F wave in man. Neurology 1967;17:147–156.

82. Mazzocchio R, Rossi A, Rothwell JC: Depression of Renshaw recurrent inhibition by activation of corticospinal fibres in human upper and lower limb. J Physiol 1994;487–498.

83. McLeod JG, Wray S: An experimental study of the F wave in the baboon. J Neurol Neurosurg Psychiatry 1966;29:196–200.

84. Miglietta OE: The F-response after transverse myelotomy. In: Desmedt JE, ed. New developments in clinical neurophysiology. Basel:Karger, 1973;323–327.

85. Milanov I: Examination of the segmental pathophysiological mechanisms of spasticity. Electromyogr Clin Neurophysiol 1994;34:73–79.

86. Milanov I: Mechanisms of tetrazepam action on spasticity. Acta Neurol Belg 1992;92(1):5–15.

87. Milanov I, Georgiev D: Mechanisms of trizanidine action on spasticity. Acta Neurol Scand 1994; 89(4):274–279.

88. Milanov IG: A comparison of methods to assess the excitability of lower motoneurones. Canadian J Neurological Sciences 1992;19(1):64–68.

89. Miller TA, Newall AR, Jackson DA: H-reflexes in the upper extremity and the effects of voluntary contraction. Electromyogr Clin Neurophysiol 1995;35(2):121–128.

90. Morelli M, Seaborne DE, Sullivan SJ: H-reflex modulation during manual muscle massage of human triceps surae. Arch Phys Med Rehabil 1991; 72(11):915–919.

91. Murphy BA, Dawson NJ, Slack: Sacroiliac joint manipulation decreases the H-reflex. Electromyogr Clin Neurophysiol 1995;35(2):87–94.

92. Nance PW: A comparison of clonidine, cyproheptadine and baclofen in spastic spinal cord injured patients. J Am Paraplegic Society 1994;17(3):150–156.

93. Ongerboer de Visser BW, Schimsteimer RJ, Hart AA: The H reflex of the flexor carpi radialis muscle; A study in controls and radiation-induced brachial plexus lesions. J Neurol Neurosurg Psychiatry 1984;47(10):1090–1101.

94. Panayiotopoulos CP: F chronodispersion: A new electrophysiologic method. Muscle Nerve 1979; 2:68–72.

95. Panizza M, Balbi P, Russo G, et al.: H-reflex recovery curve and reciprocal inhibition of H-reflex of the upper limbs in patients with spasticity secondary to stroke. Am J Phys Med Rehabil 1995;74:357–363.

96. Panizza M, Lelli S, Nilsson J, et al.: H-reflex recovery curve and reciprocal inhibition of H-reflex in different kinds of dystonia. Neurology 1990;40:1152–1158.

97. Panizza M, Nilsson J, Hallett M: Optimal stimulus duration for the H reflex. Muscle Nerve 1989; 12(7):576–579.

98. Passero S, Paradiso C, Giannini F, et al.: Diagnosis of thoracic outlet syndrome. Relative value of electrophysiological studies. Acta Neurol Scand 1994; 90(3):179–185.

99. Pease WS, Lagattuta FP, Johnson EW: Spinal nerve stimulation in S_1 radiculopathy. Am J Phys Med Rehabil 1990;69(2):77–80.

100. Peioglou-Harmoussi S, Fawcett PRW, Howel D, et al.: F- response behavior in a control population. J Neurol Neurosurg Psychiatry 1985;48:1152–1158.

101. Peioglou-Harmoussi S, Fawcett PR, Howel D, et al.: F- response frequency in motor neuron disease and cervical spondylosis. J Neurol Neurosurg Psychiatry 1987;50(5):593–599.

102. Peioglou-Harmoussi S, Fawcett PRW, Howel D, et al.: F- responses: A study of frequency, shape and amplitude characteristics in healthy control subjects. J Neurol Neurosurg Psychiatry 1985;48:1159–1164.

103. Petajan JH: F waves in neurogenic atrophy. Muscle Nerve 1985;8:690–696.

104. Raudino F: Effects of positional changes on F wave. Electromyogr Clin Neurophysiol 1994;34(5): 285–287.

105. Renshaw B: Influence of discharge of motoneurons upon excitation of neighboring motoneurons. J Neurophysiol 1941;4:167–183.

106. Renshaw B: Activity in the simplest spinal reflex pathways. J Neurophysiol 1940;3:373–387.

107. Sabatino M, Sardo P, Ferraro G, et al.: Bilateral reciprocal organisation in man: Focus on IA interneurone. J Neurol Transmission-General Section 1994;96(1):31–39.

108. Sabbahi MA, Khalil M: Segmental H-reflex studies in upper and lower limbs of patients with radiculopathy. Arch Phys Med Rehabil 1990;71(3):223–227.

109. Schuchman JA: H-reflex latency in radiculopathy. Arch Phys Med Rehabil 1978;59(4):185–187.

110. Shefner JM, Logigan EF: Conduction velocity in motor, cutaneous-afferent, and muscle-afferent fibers within the same mixed nerve. Muscle Nerve 1994;17(7):773–778.

111. Soliven B, Maselli RA: Single motor unit H-reflex in motor neuron disorders. Muscle Nerve 1992; 15(6):656–660.

112. Stålberg E, Trontelj JV: Demonstration of axon reflexes in human motor nerve fibres. J Neurol Neurosurg Psychiatry 1970;33:571–579.

113. Taborikova H: Fraction of the motoneuroneurone pool activated in the monosynaptic H-reflexes in man. Nature 1965;209:206–207.

114. Taborikova H, Sax DS: Conditioning of H-reflexes by a preceding subthreshold H-reflex stimulus. Brain 1969;92:203–212.

115. Taborikova H, Sax DS: Motoneurone pool and the H-reflex. J Neurol Neurosurg Psychiatry 1968; 31:354–361.

116. Taniguchi MH, Hayes J, Rodriguez AD: Reliability determination of F mean response latency. Arch Phys Med Rehabil 1993;74(11):1139–1143.

117. Teasdall RD, Park AM, Languth HW, et al.: Electrophysiological studies of reflex activity in patients with lesions of the nervous system. Bull Johns Hopkins Hosp 1952;91:245–256.

118. Thomas JE, Lambert EH: Ulnar nerve conduction velocity and H-reflex in infants and children. J Appl Physiol 1960;15:1–9.

119. Thorne J: Central responses to electrical activation of the peripheral nerves supplying the intrinsic hand muscles. J Neurol Neurosurg Psychiatry 1965; 28:482–495.

120. Trontelj JV: A study of the F response by single fiber electromyography. In: Desmedt JE, ed. New developments in electromyography and clinical neurophysiology. Basel: Karger, 1973;318–322.

121. Trontelj JV: A study of the H-reflex by single fibre EMG. J Neurol Neurosurg Psychiatry 1973;36: 951–959.

122. Upton ARM, McComas AJ, Sica REP: Potentiation of "late" responses evoked in muscles during effort. J Neurol Neurosurg Psychiatry 1971;34:699–711.

123. Vajsar J, Taylor MJ, MacMillan LJ, et al.: Somatosensory evoked potentials and nerve conduction studies in patients with Guillain-Barre syndrome. Brain Development 1992;14(5):315–318.

124. Veale JL, Mark RF, Rees S: Differential sensitivity of motor and sensory fibres in human ulnar nerve. J Neurol Neurosurg Psychiatry 1973;36:75–86.

125. Veale JL, Rees S: Renshaw cell activity in man. J Neurol Neurosurg Psychiatry 1973;36:674–683.

126. Veale JL, Rees S, Mark RF: Renshaw cell activity in normal and spastic man. In: Desmedt JE, ed. New developments in electromyography and clinical neurophysiology. Basel:Karger, 1973;3:523–537.

127. Walk D, Fisher MA: Effects of cutaneous stimulation on ipsilateral and contralateral motoneuron excitability: An analysis using H reflexes and F waves. Electromyogr Clin Neurophysiol 1993;33(5):259–264.

128. Weber R, Piero D: F-wave evaluation of thoracic outlet syndrome: A multiple regression derived F-wave latency predicting technique. Arch Phys Med Rehabil 1978;59:464–469.

129. White JC: The ubiquity of contraction enhanced H-reflexes: Normative data and use in the diagnosis of radiculopathies. Electroenceph Clin Neurophysiol 1991;81:433–442.

130. Wilbourn AJ, Aminoff MJ: AAEE minimongraph #32: The electrophysiologic examination in patients with radiculopathies. Rochester: American Association of Electromyography and Electrodiagnosis, 1988.

131. Wulff CH, Gilliatt RW: F waves in patients with hand wasting caused by a cervical rib and band. Muscle Nerve 1979;2:452–457.

Chapter 10

Entrapment Neuropathies and Other Focal Neuropathies

Lawrence R. Robinson

GENERAL APPROACHES TO THE STUDY OF ENTRAPMENTS

There are a number of general considerations when evaluating any patient with suspected entrapment or focal neuropathy. This section discusses the patient's history and physical examination, the timing of electrodiagnostic changes, pathophysiology, and principles of localization, as well as initial electrodiagnostic approaches.

PATIENT HISTORY

A directed history is critical to performing the electrodiagnostic medical consultation. It is required for generating an appropriate list of differential diagnoses and planning the electrophysiologic examination. Many times, the electrodiagnostic medical consultant has more experience in the diagnosis of focal neuropathies and other neuromuscular conditions than the patient's referring physician and thus may think of new possible diagnoses based upon the patient's history.

A number of the history's components are especially pertinent to the evaluation. Knowing the quality and precise distribution of symptoms, combined with an intimate knowledge of peripheral nervous system anatomy, will usually be very helpful in developing a sensible differential diagnosis. Finding out whether symptoms are intermittent or constant will suggest a likelihood of finding abnormalities on the electrophysiologic examination; constant symptoms are more likely to be associated with electrophysiologic abnor-

malities. Although symptoms of entrapment neuropathies are usually initially reported in one or two limbs, one should also ask about other limbs to rule out a more generalized process. The patient with hand numbness, for example, could have entrapment neuropathy in the upper limbs; however, if the lower limbs are also involved, then one might perform a wider search for a peripheral polyneuropathy. When patients report the sudden onset of symptoms upon awakening, it should prompt extensive questioning about where and how the patient slept and if he or she was intoxicated or otherwise medicated. If there is a recent history of surgery or trauma, a detailed history may help point to those areas of the peripheral nervous system that might have been placed at risk.

Although an extensive search of the past medical history is not always productive in the evaluation for possible entrapment neuropathies, several questions should always be asked. One should routinely ask about any medications the patient is on. This brings up not only other prior pertinent diagnoses that may not have been mentioned (e.g., diabetes mellitus), but also possible exposure to neurotoxic agents or anticoagulants. One should elicit any history of systemic disease that might contribute to the chief complaint, such as a history of diabetes mellitus, extensive alcohol intake, or rheumatologic disease. Also, one should know whether or not the presenting symptoms have occurred in the past so that one is prepared for the finding of old electrophysiologic changes. A history of prior trauma may be pertinent, as in the case of tardy ulnar palsy. The patient's vocational history may play a role in the diagnosis, as many occupations increase the risk of developing focal entrapment neuropathies.

The family history becomes pertinent when one is considering congenital diseases. Peripheral polyneuropathies and myopathies are not uncommonly inherited, and it can be very revealing to find a family history of similar neurologic symptoms. There is an autosomally dominant condition known as familial predisposition to pressure palsies (12).

PHYSICAL EXAMINATION

Whereas the history often contributes most significantly to establishing a differential diagnosis, physical examination is useful in providing more objective evidence of focal peripheral nervous system dysfunction.

In most cases, the four most important components of the examination are muscle strength, sensation, muscle stretch reflexes, and provocative signs. The strength examination should be directed to all four limbs to look for widespread abnormalities and to assess any underlying poor effort. Although weakness is severe in some cases, in most referrals the weakness is mild or subtle. Optimally, muscles should be tested at or near their "break" points as opposed to the large range at which resistance cannot be overcome. Thus, one must be sure to obtain a maximum mechanical advantage in performing the muscle strength testing. Useful techniques include applying force as far as possible from the joint to obtain a maximal lever arm, putting particularly strong muscles at added stretch to put them at a mechanical disadvantage, and using gravity and body weight as an aid to maximally stress antigravity muscles. Simply testing dorsiflexion or plantar flexion at the ankle against manual resistance, for example, is insufficient; one must have the patient walk on his or her heels and toes or perform 10 toe rises.

Sensory testing should be directed at eliciting subtle deficits in sensation. As opposed to the patient with spinal cord injury with whom one is looking for a very gross sensory level, patients with entrapment neuropathies often have mild or difficult-to-elicit sensory losses. Simply finding out whether the patient can distinguish pinprick from dull touch is usually insufficient for all but the most severe deficits. One should compare pinprick and light touch sensation in a questionable area with an asymptomatic area (such as the cheek or forehead) or with the other side if it is not symptomatic. A useful technique is to touch first the asymptomatic area and then the symptomatic area, while asking the patient, "If this (asymptomatic) area is 100%, how much is this (the symptomatic area)?" Two-point discrimination often detects more mild deficits in sensation that are missed with simple pinprick tests.

Muscle stretch reflexes are probably the most objective findings in examination of the peripheral nervous system, in that they are not easily influenced by patient cooperation or reporting (though they are influenced by the level of relaxation). Reflexes are usually normal in many focal entrapment neuropathies because they assess proximal (unaffected) areas, but they will help to rule out more proximal lesions.

There are several useful provocative tests that can be employed in the physical examination prior to electrophysiologic studies. Phalen's test is a moderately sensitive and specific test for detecting median nerve compression at the wrist; this is performed by keeping the wrist sustained in flexion for 60 seconds and monitoring for paresthesia. Tinel's sign (which was originally developed for detecting the distal-most site of peripheral nerve regeneration) is sensitive but not very specific. Tinel's sign can be elicited over the median nerve at the wrist or the ulnar nerve at the elbow in the case of entrapment, but many asymptomatic control subjects also have a positive test over unaffected peripheral nerves.

TIMING

Before embarking upon the electrodiagnostic examination, it is critical to appreciate the amount of time since the onset of symptoms. Falsely negative or misleading conclusions can result from not understanding or considering the influence of timing since the onset of the lesion.

The time course of electrodiagnostic changes after onset of a neuropathic lesion should always be considered when interpreting the electrophysiologic examination in the presence of focal neuropathies. Neurapraxia, demyelination, and severe axon loss produce electrophysiologic changes immediately if one can stimulate proximal to the lesion. More proximal lesions, which one cannot easily stimulate proximally, do not immediately produce changes on distal nerve conduction studies or electromyography (EMG). Moreover, distinction between neurapraxia and axonotmesis cannot be made until the time for wallerian degeneration has passed.

Day One After an Axon Loss Lesion

Immediately after onset of an axon loss lesion, electrophysiologic changes may be subtle. On needle EMG, the only potential abnormality is change in the recruitment, with reduced or discrete recruitment if there is enough axon loss. Mild lesions will not produce noticeable changes in recruitment. Nerve conduction studies distal to the site of the lesion will not be changed, but stimulation proximal to a lesion with recording distally may produce small-amplitude or absent responses. Otherwise, nerve conduction studies and EMG will be usually unremarkable at day one.

Days Seven to 10

Seven days after a complete nerve lesion, wallerian degeneration will have progressed such that distal stimulation of the affected motor axons elicits no motor response. Ten days after onset of a complete lesion, sensory nerve action potentials (SNAPs) will be absent as well (48). Incomplete lesions will produce less marked changes, but with similar timing. Therefore, seven to 10 days after onset, one can distinguish by nerve conduction studies (NCS) a neurapraxic injury (i.e., the distal amplitudes will be normal) from an axonotmetic lesion (the distal amplitudes will be reduced), primarily by looking at distal amplitudes.

Days 14 to 21

Two to three weeks after onset of injury, the needle EMG starts to show fibrillation potentials and positive sharp waves. Proximal muscles demonstrate these abnormalities earlier and distal muscles later.

Fibrillations and positive sharp waves may be persistent for several months or even many years after a single injury, depending upon the extent of reinnervation. Therefore, the presence of positive sharp waves or fibrillations does indicate that there has been some denervation but does not indicate that there is "active" or "ongoing" loss of axons over time. Fibrillation amplitudes are sometimes helpful in determining the chronology of the lesions; fibrillation potentials larger than 100 μV indicate a lesion probably less than one year old (38).

Reinnervation

The timing and type of electrophysiologic changes consequent to reinnervation will depend in part upon the mechanism of reinnervation. When reinnervation is a result of axonal regrowth from the site of the lesion, usually in complete injuries, the appearance of new motor unit action potentials (MUAPs) will not occur until motor axons have had sufficient time to regenerate the distance between the lesion site and the muscle (usually proceeding at roughly 1 mm/day or 1 inch/month). When these new axons first reach the muscle, they will innervate only a few muscle fibers, producing short-duration, small-amplitude potentials, formerly referred to as nascent potentials. With time, as more muscle fibers join the motor unit, the MUAPs will become larger, more polyphasic, and longer in duration.

Motor unit potential changes will also develop when reinnervation occurs by axonal sprouting from intact axons. Polyphasicity and increased duration develop first as newly formed, poorly myelinated sprouts supply the recently denervated muscle fibers. As the sprouts mature, large-amplitude, long-duration MUAPs develop and usually persist indefinitely.

PATHOPHYSIOLOGY

Whenever possible, it is helpful to provide to the referring physician some indication of the pathophysiology of the peripheral nerve lesion, e.g., neurapraxia, demyelination, or axon loss.

Neurapraxia is best demonstrated, assuming at least 7 days have passed, when there is focal conduction block on nerve conduction studies with a large-amplitude compound muscle action potential (CMAP) or SNAP elicited distal to the site of the lesion and a smaller or absent response with more proximal stimulation. Purely neurapraxic injuries have no electrophysiologic evidence for axon loss (fibrillation potentials or positive sharp waves) or reinnervation on needle EMG.

Axon loss lesions are usually demonstrated by evidence of denervation upon needle EMG examination as well as by small-amplitude CMAP and SNAP responses with stimulation and recording distal to the site of the lesion. Although needle EMG is a more sensitive indicator for the presence of *any* motor axon loss, measurement of the distal CMAP or SNAP amplitude is a better quantitative measure of the *degree* of axon loss and of prognosis. It is critical to remember that often there is a mixture of axon loss and neurapraxia in many focal neuropathies.

Demyelination is best demonstrated by slowing of conduction, often with conduction block. Slowing of conduction may take the form of slowed conduction velocities, prolonged distal latencies, or increased temporal dispersion. Slowing of conduction does not always mean that demyelination has occurred; axon loss, particularly of the faster-conducting fibers, will produce mild slowing of conduction as well.

ESTIMATING PROGNOSIS

Prognosis of a peripheral nerve lesion is related to the pathophysiologic process that has occurred, the degree of axon loss, if any, the time since onset, and the distance between the lesion and the target muscles. Those lesions that have had extensive axon loss are less likely to have full recovery of function.

Unfortunately, electrophysiologic measures cannot assess the integrity of supporting structures around the nerve and hence cannot distinguish axonotmesis from neurotmesis. Neurotmesis, which has marked disruption of supporting structures, carries a much worse prognosis for regeneration than axonotmesis, in which the supporting structures are largely intact. Therefore, careful, periodic re-examination of proximal muscles (those expected to reinnervate first) will give the best information to estimate prognosis for full reinnervation.

Those lesions that are predominantly neurapraxic have a much better prognosis; conduction block in these lesions rarely lasts more than 2 to 3 months. Demyelinating lesions also have a better prognosis than axon loss, but specific prognosis will depend often upon what intervention is taken, e.g., the release of entrapment sites.

When axon loss is present, there is a critical window of 18–24 months for peripheral nerve regeneration to occur before the target muscles cannot be reinnervated any longer. Because peripheral nerves regenerate roughly one inch per month, proximal lesions with a great deal of axon loss have a poor chance of reinnervating distal hand or foot muscles.

PRINCIPLES OF LOCALIZATION

A number of principles are useful for localizing peripheral nerve lesions based upon the electrophysiologic examination.

Conventionally in primarily axonal lesions or in proximal lesions where one cannot stimulate both proximal and distal to an entrapment site, needle EMG is often used to diagnose and localize abnormalities. Knowing the branch points along the nerve, one can examine muscles supplied by each branch and infer lesion localization based upon the point at which muscles change from normal to abnormal. Thus, localization is based upon finding abnormalities distal to a branch point with normal findings proximally.

This approach, however, sometimes provides an erroneous site. Sir Sidney Sunderland (72) has shown that fascicles within peripheral nerves intertwine considerably as they move proximally through the limbs. Fascicles supplying the flexor carpi ulnaris muscle, for example, are not uniquely placed proximally within the ulnar nerve as it joins the medial cord of the brachial plexus. However, fascicles do become organized within peripheral nerves several centimeters prior to branch points and, in this example, fascicles destined to supply the flexor carpi ulnaris become organized within the ulnar nerve several centimeters prior to supplying the muscle. Consequently, even though ulnar nerve entrapment at the elbow usually occurs proximal to the branch to the flexor carpi ulnaris, this muscle is usually spared in ulnar neuropathy at the elbow; it is thought that the fascicles for this muscle are isolated in a relatively protected area of the nerve at the entrapment site. If one were basing localization on needle EMG only using the known branch points, one would erroneously place these lesions distal to the branch point and in the forearm.

The ulnar nerve is not unique with regard to the intraneural topography causing potential problems in localization. There have been cases reported of peroneal neuropathy occurring proximally to the popliteal fossa but resulting in only deep peroneal lesions clinically (18). Sciatic neuropathies, even occurring near the hip joint, can result in predominantly peroneal nerve lesions clinically. The fascicular structure within the peroneal division of the sciatic nerve may make it more predisposed to injury than the tibial division (72). Thus, whereas EMG does make use of known anatomical branch points to arrive at localization, the electromyographer should be aware of the intraneural topography within the nerve, and that a partial lesion higher than expected could produce similar findings.

Nerve conduction studies are best at localizing the site of pathology when there is demyelination. As mentioned earlier, demyelination causes focal slowing and conduction block; when present, these findings can precisely localize a focal entrapment. A problem arises with localizing lesions based on NCS when there is predominantly axon loss and little demyelination. In these cases, conduction velocity throughout the nerve is mildly slowed owing to loss of the faster-conducting fibers, but it is not focally or markedly slowed. Although there is a diffuse reduction in CMAP or SNAP amplitude at all sites of stimulation (owing to axon loss and subsequent wallerian degeneration), there will be no focal drop in amplitude as one goes across the lesion site. Conduction block, in which there is a drop in amplitude of the CMAP as stimulation occurs distal and proximal to the lesion, is related only to demyelination and neurapraxia and will not be present in axon loss lesions once wallerian degeneration has occurred (about 7 days after onset).

ULNAR NEUROPATHY AT THE ELBOW (FIG. 10–1)

Case 1

Case History and Examination

A 46-year-old anesthesiologist has gradually noted mild but progressive weakness in his right hand and numbness in the ring and little finger. He comes at the prompting of a neurosurgical colleague who commented upon his wasting in the right first web space. The numbness is constant and involves both dorsal and palmar aspects of the little finger and palm, but does not extend proximal to the wrist. He denies any symptoms in the other upper limb or either lower limb. He denies neck pain except when working with selected surgeons in the operating room.

Physical examination reveals wasting in the hypothenar and first web space muscles. Strength is reduced (4/5) in finger abduction and adduction and thumb adduction. Strength is otherwise normal, including wrist flexion and flexion of the distal interphalangeal joints. Sensation to pinprick is decreased over the little finger and ulnar aspect of the palm on both the dorsal and palmar surfaces. Muscle stretch reflexes at the biceps, brachioradialis, and triceps are active and symmetrical.

Differential Diagnosis

The differential diagnosis includes ulnar neuropathy at the elbow, ulnar neuropathy at the wrist, and a lower brachial plexus lesion (lower trunk or medial cord), or C8 radiculopathy. The presentation is largely compatible with ulnar neuropathy at the elbow. The only findings that may at first glance appear inconsistent with this diagnosis are the normal wrist flexion (in part supplied by the flexor carpi ulnaris) and normal flexor digitorum profundus strength; however, these muscles are often spared in ulnar neuropathy at the elbow (Fig. 10–1). Ulnar neuropathy at the wrist is unlikely given sensory involvement of the dorsal aspect of hand, supplied by the dorsal ulnar cutaneous nerve, which branches before the wrist. Normal strength in the thenar muscles suggests focal ulnar neuropathy rather than lower brachial plexopathy or C8 radiculopathy (Table 10–1).

Clinical Presentation

Patients with ulnar neuropathy at the elbow typically report difficulty with sensation over

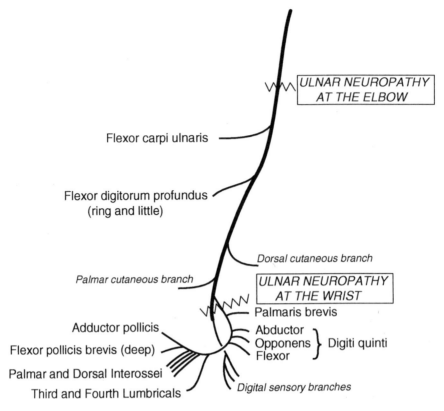

Figure 10–1. Ulnar nerve anatomy showing branches and common sites of focal neuropathy.

the ulnar two digits of the hand. This involves both palmar and dorsal aspects of the little finger and usually the ulnar half of the ring finger. There is, however, substantial variability in the sensory supply to the hand. In up to 20% of patients, the ulnar nerve may supply the entire ring finger and the ulnar half of the middle finger. Paresthesiae are typically in the same distribution and usually do not extend above the wrist, although patients may report some elbow pain. Weakness is often less common than sensory complaints on initial report, but patients may have difficulty holding onto objects, especially with a power grasp (such as using a hammer) because this requires using the hand in ulnar deviation.

On physical examination, sensory deficits are usually limited to the little finger and variably the ring finger and middle finger. Testing two-point discrimination is more sensitive than simply testing pinprick or light touch for detecting sensory deficits. In considering the differential diagnosis, it is important to accurately define the distribution of the sensory abnormalities. Patients with abnormal sensation limited to the palmar side of the hand are more likely to have an ulnar nerve lesion at the wrist because the dorsal ulnar cutaneous nerve, supplying the back of the hand, branches from the ulnar nerve in the distal forearm (proximal to the wrist). If patients have sensory abnormalities extending into the medial forearm, the area supplied by the medial antebrachial cutaneous nerve, ulnar neuropathy is less likely. Because this sensory branch derives from the medial cord of the brachial plexus, patients with clear-cut sensory abnormalities over the medial forearm are more likely to have a lower brachial plexus lesion, cervical radiculopathy, or a spinal cord lesion.

On physical examination, atrophy may be noted in the first dorsal interosseus and hypothenar muscles, with sparing of the thenar musculature. The forearm usually appears normal. In more advanced cases, a "claw hand" deformity may be present, with the medial two digits hyperextended at the metacarpal/phalangeal joints and flexed at the inter-phalangeal joints. The fingers involved in claw hand deformity vary because there is often anatomical variation in which lumbricals are supplied by the ulnar and median nerves.

Weakness can be demonstrated in the dorsal or palmar interossei and the adductor pollicis muscles. Froment's sign, which demonstrates difficulty or inability to perform lateral pinch, is due to weakness of the adductor pollicis and flexor pollicis brevis, as well as the first dorsal interosseus. When patients are asked to perform a lateral pinch between the thumb and index fingers, they are unable to do so; as the strength of the pinch increases, they compensate by using their long flexors (flexor pollicis longus and flexor digitorum

profundus). Thus, instead of using the sides of the thumb and index finger to grasp an object such as a piece of paper, they use the tips of the fingers.

Special note should be made of examining the ulnar-innervated muscles in the presence of a radial neuropathy. Two errors are often made in this examination. First, many patients with isolated radial neuropathy are mistakenly thought to also have ulnar neuropathy because of weakness in finger abduction. This weakness is simply an artifact of the metacarpal/phalangeal (MCP) joint flexion produced by the radial neuropathy. In this disadvantaged position, finger abduction is far weaker than it would be when the MCP joints are fully extended. In the presence of a radial neuropa-

Table 10–1
Electrodiagnostic Data for Case 1

		NERVE CONDUCTION STUDIES			
Nerve	Record	Stim	Distal Latency (msec)	Amplitude (µV)	Conduction Velocity (m/s)
R. Ulnar (motor)	ADM	Wrist	3.4	5,000	
		Below elbow		3,600	53
					46
		Above elbow		3,000	
					55
		Axilla		2,800	
R. Ulnar (sensory)	Little finger	Wrist	3.6	7	
R. Ulnar (motor)	ADM	4 cm below	7.6		
		2 cm below	7.9		
		medial epi.	8.3		
		2 cm above	9.1		
		4 cm above	9.5		

Needle EMG (all on right side)

	Spont. Activity			Motor Unit Action Potentials		
Muscle	PSWs	Fibs	Ampl.	Dur.	Phasicity	Recruitment
FDI	2+	1+	↑	↑	↑	reduced
ADM	2+	1+	↑	↑	↑	reduced
FCU	0	0	N	N	N	full
APB	0	0	N	N	N	full

PSWs: Positive sharp waves
Fibs: Fibrillation potentials
FDI: First dorsal interosseous
ADM: Abductor digiti minimi
FCU: Flexor carpi ulnaris
APB: Abductor pollicus brevis

thy, these ulnar-innervated muscles must be tested when the MCP joints are held into full extension by placing the hand flat on a table or desk. Second, patients with a complete isolated radial neuropathy are often thought to have radial nerve sparing because they can extend the interphalangeal joints of the fingers. This, however, is a movement supplied by the intrinsic hand muscles and does not indicate preservation of radial nerve function.

Many patients with ulnar neuropathy at the elbow will have a positive Tinel's sign over the elbow. However, so do many patients without ulnar neuropathy at the elbow. Although Tinel's sign is a sensitive finding on physical examination, it is very nonspecific, and many patients without the disease also have a positive finding.

Nerve Conduction Studies (Table 10-1)

Motor nerve conduction studies are often the most useful technique for localizing the site of ulnar neuropathy at the elbow and determining the pathophysiology of the lesion. Recording from the abductor digiti minimi is the most common method employed. Some authors, however, have found that recording from the first dorsal interosseus muscle, the most distal muscle supplied by the ulnar nerve, is more sensitive (28,56,70). A two-channel technique may be used to record from both muscles simultaneously so that extra stimulations are not required. The recording site for the first dorsal interosseus is usually described as the active electrode over the bulk of the muscle, with the reference distally over the MCP joint of the index finger. Such a recording arrangement often produces an initial positive deflection, which is difficult to interpret. An initial negative deflection is more commonly seen when the reference is placed over the carpometacarpal joint of the thumb. Alternatively, recording may be from the adductor pollicis, which usually gives an initial negative deflection as well.

Stimulation is usually performed at the wrist, below the elbow, above the elbow, and at the axilla. Although some electromyographers do not stimulate at the axilla routinely, the advantage of this technique is that it offers a conduction velocity across one more segment (the arm), which can be compared with the across-elbow conduction velocity. Study of the across-elbow segment requires much care in technique and interpretation. First, it is well known that the position of the elbow greatly influences the measured conduction velocity. When the elbow is extended, it is thought that the ulnar nerve may become redundant in the ulnar groove and surface measurements do not reflect the true distance of the underlying nerve. Typically, the more flexed the elbow, the slower the measured conduction velocity (4, 8). It is thought that flexing the elbow stretches the nerve to its full length, and measurement of the distance over the ulnar groove more closely reflects the distance along the nerve. There are advocates of both techniques (elbow flexed or extended). Clearly, the same technique that was used in deriving one's normative data should be used in clinical measurements.

The distance between the sites of stimulation above and below the elbow may also influence the accuracy of the conduction velocity measurement. Because surface measurements can be in error by many millimeters, use of short distances between stimulation sites means that there will be a relatively large percentage error in the distance and, hence, conduction velocity measurements. A 10-centimeter across-elbow distance is recommended to reduce this measurement error.

Although Martin-Gruber anastomosis is usually discussed in the context of median nerve conduction studies, it is probably far more important to recognize this anomaly when performing ulnar nerve conduction studies. This author is aware of patients who have been operated on for "ulnar neuropathy" when they have simply had Martin-Gruber anastomosis masquerading as a conduction block in the proximal forearm. When present, this anomaly will result in a much lower amplitude response with below-elbow stimulation when compared to that obtained with wrist stimulation. The inexperienced electromyographer may suspect a focal ulnar neuropathy in the proximal forearm that could even be "confirmed" by inching studies (as one inches along the ulnar nerve and across the anastomosis). However, in all such cases, the presence of a Martin-Gruber anastomosis can and should be ruled out simply by stimulating over the median nerve above the elbow and recording over the abductor digiti minimi (ADM) and first dorsal interosseus (FDI) muscles. Presence of any significant response with an initial negative takeoff indicates the presence of the anomaly.

How much slowing in the across-elbow segment is sufficient to diagnose ulnar neuropathy? This is best addressed by comparing the across-elbow segment to the forearm segment. Because there is room for considerable error in measurement of the across-elbow conduction velocity owing to distance measurements and elbow position, most electromyographers would allow up to an 11- to 15-m/s difference between the across-elbow and forearm segments before calling the finding "abnormal" (36). Thus, if the forearm conduction velocity were 56 m/s, the across-elbow segment velocity should be below 41–45 m/s before deciding that the result is "abnormal." In our laboratory, a 10- to 15-m/s difference is considered suspicious, and a difference of more than 15 m/s is considered abnormal. There are, however, some authors who prefer to use the absolute conduction velocity rather than a comparison between segments (56,73).

Slowed conduction velocity is not the only finding that should be considered diagnostic of ulnar neuropathy at the elbow. Patients with slowed conduction velocity may also have a drop in amplitude in the across-elbow segment or an increased temporal dispersion. Some authors state that an amplitude reduction of more than 10% in the across-elbow segment may be abnormal (36).

Although it was just stated that at least a 10-centimeter distance across the elbow is recommended for conduction velocity measurements, it is often found that study of very short segments yields a higher sensitivity for small, focal lesions. With short-segment studies, the area of demyelination occupies a higher percentage of the distance studied than the longer segments in which normal nerve dilutes the conduction measurement. Inching studies (or perhaps more appropriately called "centimetering" studies) can be performed by stimulating the nerve at two-centimeter increments across the elbow (31, 47). Landmarks are best

established by drawing a line between the medial epicondyle and the olecranon (7) and measuring two-centimeter increments distal and proximal to this line. Stimulation should be *just* supramaximal because overstimulation may cause nerve activation distal to the cathode and potentially distal to a lesion. Using this technique, a conduction delay of more than 0.7 msec across 2 cm segments is abnormal (31). More impressive are focal changes in amplitude or waveform morphology across a segment. Although inching studies may add sensitivity to the examination and may help in localization, it is not wise to stake one's professional reputation on a site determined by inching studies. It is easy to be off by one or more segments. In any event, a surgeon operating on the nerve likely will expose a long length of nerve.

Most of the abnormalities mentioned above require the presence of demyelination for localization. However, in many traumatic ulnar neuropathies in which there is only axon loss without demyelination, localization of ulnar neuropathy is far more difficult. In such cases, there will be diffuse mild slowing of conduction velocity without focal slowing, conduction block, or temporal dispersion; thus, there are no focal nerve conduction changes across the lesion. Needle EMG is only marginally helpful, because the two ulnar-innervated muscles in the forearm are often spared (see below) and there are no ulnar-innervated muscles in the arm. Therefore, despite one's best technique, there are significant numbers of patients with traumatic or vasculitic lesions of the ulnar nerve (in which there is only axon loss present) and in whom localization cannot be precisely determined.

Sensory nerve conduction studies are often of less localizing value than motor conduction studies. There are several technical problems that make this response more difficult to interpret. First, with stimulation of the ulnar nerve and antidromic recording over the little finger, there is sometimes a large-amplitude motor response (motor artifact), volume conducted to the recording electrodes, which makes accurate identification and measurement of the sensory nerve action potential difficult. Second, owing to phase cancellation (35), the amplitude of the sensory response falls dramatically over distance, and reductions of 50% are not unusual or abnormal in the wrist-to-elbow segment. Third, it is much harder to record sensory responses, particularly with proximal stimulation, when there is any significant ulnar neuropathy, and temporal dispersion is difficult to measure.

Nevertheless, sensory responses are often helpful for measuring the degree of sensory axon loss. A drop in the amplitude of the ulnar sensory nerve action potential (SNAP) is probably one of the more sensitive indicators of the ulnar neuropathy at the elbow (16). Of course, a drop in the amplitude of the sensory response in the wrist-to-little-finger segment is not localizing and means that there has been sensory axon loss at or distal to the dorsal root ganglion at C8.

Measurement of SNAPs may be helpful to exclude lesions other than ulnar neuropathy at the elbow. When attempting to distinguish ulnar neuropathy at the elbow from ulnar neuropathy at the wrist, measurement of the dorsal ulnar cutaneous sensory response can be of help. This nerve is involved with lesions at the elbow but not at the wrist (where it bypasses Guyon's canal). When this response is normal and symmetrical, it is more suggestive of ulnar neuropathy at the wrist. When the lesion is at the elbow, the dorsal ulnar cutaneous response is typically reduced in amplitude or absent (Fig. 10–2). Similarly, the medial antebrachial cutaneous nerve (MABCN) can be studied to rule out more proximal lesions like a lower brachial plexus lesion. Lower plexus lesions would be expected to have a small amplitude or an absent response, whereas this nerve is usually spared in ulnar neuropathies.

Needle EMG

Needle electromyography of the ulnar-innervated muscle is critical, both in determining whether any axon injury has occurred and in localizing lesions that may be purely axonal in

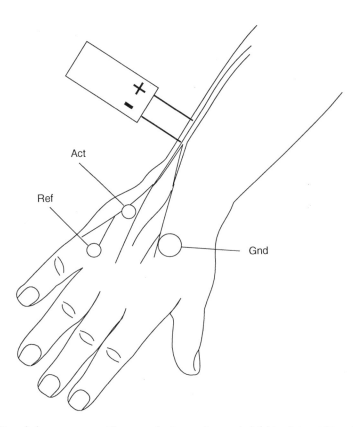

Figure 10–2. Dorsal ulnar cutaneous. Nerve conduction studies are helpful in distinguishing ulnar neuropathy at the wrist from ulnar neuropathy at the elbow.

nature. Thus, even if nerve conduction studies are entirely normal, needle EMG should be performed when ulnar neuropathy is clinically suspected. Two hand muscles very useful to assess are the abductor digiti minimi (ADM) and first dorsal interosseus (FDI), which are commonly involved in ulnar neuropathy at the elbow (Table 10–1) (28). Study of the flexor carpi ulnaris (FCU) and ulnar half of the flexor digitorum profundus (FDP) is marginally helpful. Although the branch to these forearm muscles usually comes off distal to most entrapment sites at the elbow, the fascicles supplying these muscles are in a relatively protected position within the nerve; consequently, these muscles are often spared.

Needle EMG of nonulnar-innervated muscles is often useful to rule out other lesions that may mimic ulnar neuropathy. Examination of the thenar muscles or the extensor indicis proprius offers the opportunity to compare C8/T1 muscles not innervated by the ulnar nerve. This can be useful to rule out lower cervical radiculopathies and lower brachial plexopathies. When interpreting abnormalities in the first dorsal interosseus muscle, it should be remembered that this is the muscle most commonly innervated by the Martin-Gruber anastomosis. Moreover, in many cases of Martin-Gruber anastomosis, the anomalous branch is derived from the anterior interosseus nerve (77). Thus, median neuropathy or anterior interosseus nerve syndrome should be considered when evidence of axon loss is found in the first dorsal interosseus and clinical presentation is not typical of ulnar neuropathy.

As with any other problem evaluated electrodiagnostically, one should always find normal nerves and normal muscles on the examination to exclude more widespread lesions. In particular, other things that often need to be thought of and ruled out include motor neuron disease, multifocal motor neuropathy, chronic inflammatory demyelinating polyradiculoneuropathy (CIDP), C8 radiculopathy, lower brachial plexus lesions, and spinal cord lesions such as syrinx or tumor.

Etiology

There are several different etiologies of ulnar neuropathy at the elbow. In cubital tunnel syndrome, a relatively common cause of ulnar neuropathy, the ulnar nerve (which normally travels deep to the two heads of the flexor carpi ulnaris) is entrapped by an aponeurotic band arising from the medial epicondyle of the humerus and attaching to the medial border of the olecranon. Tardy ulnar palsy occurs late after fracture or secondary to arthritis. Many believe that it is secondary to persistent cubitus valgus deformity, putting a chronic stretch on the ulnar nerve following a fracture. Also, osteophytes from old fractures or synovitis from rheumatoid arthritis may impinge upon the nerve, as may tumors in or around the elbow joint.

In some cases, trauma or external pressure is the cause of ulnar neuropathy at the elbow. A relatively minor trauma occurring directly over the ulnar groove may induce ulnar neuropathy without significant bony injury. Some believe that ulnar nerve subluxation predisposes to ulnar neuropathy. Childress determined that about 16% of 1000 normal people have recurrent subluxation when the elbow is flexed (9). Such patients may be more susceptible than others to ulnar neuropathy.

Several authors have reported ulnar neuropathy post-surgically. This is typically after intrathoracic or intra-abdominal operations (40,63). Although many patients do have ulnar-innervated hand muscle weakness after surgery, it is much more common for a lower trunk or medial cord lesion than for ulnar neuropathy to be responsible for these lesions (40). In such cases, extensive examination of median-innervated muscles, as well as the medial antebrachial cutaneous nerve, may help detect a more proximal lesion.

ULNAR NEUROPATHY AT THE WRIST (FIG. 10–1)

Case 2

Clinical History and Physical Examination

A 72-year-old man presents with the chief complaint of being unable to cup his left hand sufficiently to apply shaving cream. He denies pain, sensory loss anywhere, or weakness in any of the other limbs. He is referred to the electrodiagnostician to rule out motor neuron disease or ulnar neuropathy. Past medical history is remarkable only for essential hypertension. He is retired. Physical examination reveals marked weakness of palmar and dorsal interossei in the left hand and the hypothenar muscles. Thenar muscle strength (abduction and opposition) is normal. Wrist flexion and extension as well as all proximal muscle groups is 5/5 on strength testing. Sensation is normal to pinprick, light touch, vibration, and two-point discrimination. Reflexes are active and symmetrical in the upper limb.

Differential Diagnoses

The patient presents with painless weakness without complaints or sensory loss in the hand. Motor neuron disease may also present with painless weakness, starting in the distal upper or lower limb muscles, but the absence of hyperreflexia and the restriction to unilateral ulnar-innervated muscles controverts this, though not definitively. Spinal cord lesions or cervical root lesions would also be expected to produce pain or sensory loss in addition to the weakness.

Impression

Findings are consistent with ulnar neuropathy at the wrist affecting only the motor branches. Surgical evaluation and exploration later reveal a ganglion at the wrist that is compressing the ulnar nerve. This is surgically removed and the patient becomes symptomatically improved.

Review of Pertinent Anatomy

As the ulnar nerve extends through the distal forearm into the wrist, it gives off several branches (Fig. 10–1). These include the dorsal ulnar cutaneous nerve, which innervates the dorsal aspect of the ulnar side of the hand and the little and ring fingers; the palmar cutaneous branch, which innervates the ulnar side of the palm; the branches to the hypothenar muscles; the digital sensory branches; and the deep ulnar branch, which innervates the interossei (non-median innervated), lumbricals, and adductor pollicis. There are a variety of lesions that can occur in this area, injuring the braches either individually or in combination. Most commonly, the ulnar nerve is injured as it passes through Guyon's canal, which has boundaries of the transverse carpal ligament and the volar carpal ligament and on either side, the bony margins of the pisiform bone and the hook of the hamate. Guyon's canal contains the ulnar nerve along with the corresponding artery and vein, but does not contain any tendons (as does the carpal tunnel). Be-

cause the nerve often divides into motor and sensory branches within the canal, it is possible to have either isolated motor weakness or combined motor and sensory deficits. In addition to the site at Guyon's canal, it is possible to have ulnar nerve injury deep within the palm, affecting only the deep ulnar branch, or only isolated involvement of the dorsal ulnar cutaneous branch of the ulnar nerve.

Clinical Presentation

Clinical presentation of ulnar neuropathy at or near the wrist will depend upon which branches are affected. Commonly, there is isolated motor weakness without any sensory loss. When this is seen in the ulnar distribution, ulnar neuropathy at the wrist should be immediately suspected. Hypothenar muscles are often involved, but if the lesion is distal enough, these muscles may be spared. Only the interossei, lumbricals, and other distally innervated muscles may be weakened. Sensory loss will occur when the sensory branches are affected either in isolation or together with the motor branches, and the sensory distribution will depend upon which branches are most severely impaired.

Etiology

The most common etiologies of ulnar nerve entrapment at the wrist are ganglia and "occupational neuritis" (64). Occupational neuritis may be seen with metal polishers (in which one puts pressure over Guyon's canal chronically), pipecutters, mechanics, and professional cyclists (14,51,64). Other less common causes include laceration of the nerve, ulnar artery disease with thrombosis, and fracture of carpal or forearm bones.

Dorsal ulnar cutaneous nerve (DUCN) lesions are rare. They may be a result of repetitive wrist motion, handcuff neuropathy (27), or chronic pressure over the ulnar aspect of the wrist (69).

Nerve Conduction Studies (Table 10–2)

A combination of motor and sensory nerve conduction studies will be helpful in localizing the lesion and determining which branches

Table 10-2
Electrodiagnostic Data for Case 2

		NERVE CONDUCTION STUDIES			
Nerve	Record	Stim	Distal Latency (msec)	Amplitude (μV)	Conduction Velocity (m/s)
L. Ulnar (motor)	ADM	Wrist	5.4	4900	
		Below elbow		4600	53
		Above elbow		4300	51
L. Ulnar (motor)	FDI	Wrist	6.5	3700	
		Below elbow		3300	54
		Above elbow		3100	53
L. Ulnar	Little finger	Wrist	3.6	17	
L. Median (motor)	APB	Wrist	3.7	7200	
		Elbow		6900	55

Needle EMG (all on left side)

	Spont. Activity			Motor Unit Action Potentials		
Muscle	PSWs	Fibs	Ampl.	Dur.	Phasicity	Recruitment
FDI	2+	2+	↑	↑	↑	reduced
ADM	2+	1+	↑	↑	↑	reduced
FCU	0	0	N	N	N	full
APB	0	0	N	N	N	full

PSWs: Positive sharp waves
Fibs: Fibrillation potentials
FDI: First dorsal interosseous
ADM: Abductor digiti minimi
FCU: Flexor carpi ulnaris
APB: Abductor pollicus brevis

are the most severely involved (Table 10–2). When performing motor nerve conduction studies, it is critical when suspecting ulnar neuropathy at the wrist to record from both the ADM and FDI muscles. Because hypothenar muscles can often be selectively spared, recording from the ADM and not the FDI would miss a significant percentage of these lesions (13,66). One may see the slowing of forearm conduction velocity in some patients, sometimes confounding one's ability to precisely localize the site of demyelination; this slowing is probably similar to the forearm slowing of median nerve conduction seen in carpal tunnel syndrome.

Sensory nerve conduction studies recorded from the little finger help to determine whether the digital branches are involved. If an isolated DUCN lesion is suspected, or if differentiation between wrist and elbow lesions is difficult, recording from the DUCN will provide additional useful information.

Needle electromyography should be performed in ulnar-innervated muscles supplied by both the hypothenar branch and the deep ulnar branch (ADM and FDI, for example). Needle EMG should also include ulnar-innervated forearm muscles and median-innervated muscles to exclude more proximal lesions.

RADIAL NERVE LESIONS AT THE SPIRAL GROOVE (FIG. 10–3)

Case 3

Clinical History and Physical Examination

A 32-year-old, otherwise healthy man awoke two months ago with the sudden onset of right wrist drop and weakness in finger extension. He was intoxicated the night before the onset of symptoms and remembers waking up with his arm hanging over the wooden frame of his waterbed. He also reports mild pain in the mid-arm and numbness over the dorsal aspect of the right hand on the radial side.

Physical examination of the right upper limb reveals the following strength measurements:

Shoulder abduction	5/5
Shoulder flexion	5/5
Shoulder extension	5/5
Elbow flexion	5/5 (brachioradialis not palpable)
Elbow extension	5/5
Supination	4/5
Wrist extension	0/5
Wrist flexion	5/5
MCP extension	0/5
MCP flexion	5/5
Interphalangeal joint extension	4/5
Finger abduction	4+/5

Sensation is reduced over the radial aspect of the dorsum of the hand but is otherwise normal. Reflexes are active (2+) and symmetric at the biceps and triceps. Brachioradialis reflex is absent on the right and active (2+) on the left.

Differential Diagnosis

The differential diagnosis in this patient includes radial neuropathy as well as higher lesions at the posterior cord or the C7 root. However, the presence of normal triceps strength and shoulder abduction strength makes the second two possibilities unlikely.

Impression

These findings are consistent with a lesion of the radial nerve at the spiral groove distal to the innervation to the triceps (which starts off at the axilla) and proximal to the branch to the brachioradialis (Fig. 10–3). The presence of a large-amplitude CMAP from the extensor indicis proprius, even with needle recording (which is less reliable than surface electrode recording), suggests that there is a significant element of neurapraxia and axonal preservation (Table 10–3). Thus, prognosis is good for at least some element of recovery in the next several months.

Clinical Presentation

High radial nerve lesions typically present with weakness of wrist extension and finger extension. Because the radial nerve branch to the triceps comes off high near the axilla, elbow extension is spared in most lesions around

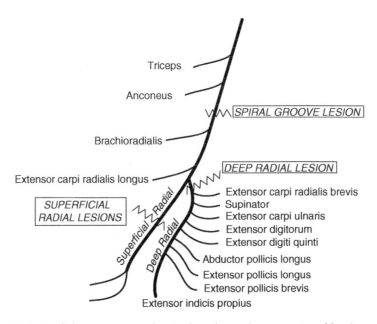

Figure 10–3. Radial nerve anatomy showing branches and common sites of focal neuropathy.

Table 10-3
Electrodiagnostic Data for Case 3

		NERVE CONDUCTION STUDIES			
Nerve	Record	Stim	Distal Latency (ms)	Amplitude (μV)	Conduction Velocity (m/s)
R. Radial (motor)	EIP (needle)	Forearm	4.2	5700	51
		Elbow		5400	
		Spiral groove		Absent response	
R. Radial (sensory)	Dorsum hand	Forearm	3.3	20	
R. Median (motor)	APB	Wrist	3.6	7600	55
		Elbow		7100	

Needle EMG (all on right side)

	Spont. Activity			Motor Unit Action Potentials		
Muscle	PSWs	Fibs	Ampl.	Dur.	Phasicity	Recruitment
EIP	2+	2+				None
EDC	2+	1+				None
ECR	1+	1+				None
BR	1+	1+				None
TRIC	0	0	N	N	N	full
DELT	0	0	N	N	N	full
FDI	0	0	N	N	N	full
APB	0	0	N	N	N	full

PSWs: Positive sharp waves
Fibs: Fibrillation potentials
FDI: First dorsal interosseous
APB: Abductor pollicus brevis
EIP: Extensor indicis proprius
EDC: Extensor digitorum communis
ECR: Extensor carpi radialis
BR: Brachioradialis
TRIC: Triceps brachii
DELT: Deltoid

the spiral groove. Occasional cases of crutch palsy, in which the radial nerve is injured at the axilla, will present with triceps weakness as well as more distal involvement. Sensory complaints usually involve the dorsum of the hand, although this distribution is variable; at times the lateral antebrachial cutaneous nerve (from the musculocutaneous nerve) supplies the area of skin often thought of as superficial radial.

On physical examination, the lesion can often be localized by testing the appropriate radial innervated forearm muscles. Unfortu-
nately, it is often difficult to detect weakness in the radial innervated elbow flexor, the brachioradialis. The strongest elbow flexors include the biceps and brachialis, which are innervated by the musculocutaneous nerve; thus, elbow flexion is typically normal. Brachioradialis function can best be assessed by having the patient flex the elbow in a neutral forearm position (neither pronated nor supinated) and palpating over the muscle. Although many patients with complete denervation to brachioradialis will still have normal or nearly normal elbow flexion strength in this

position, it is still possible to detect the lack of any muscle bulk upon the maneuver.

There are similar problems with testing supination of the forearm. Although the radial-innervated supinator muscle may be denervated in these cases, it is often missed because the strongest supinator in the forearm is the biceps, supplied by the musculocutaneous nerve. Wrist extension and MCP joint extension are reliably weak in radial neuropathies because there are no other muscles to substitute for these movements. It is easy, however, for the beginning clinician or electromyographer to mistake interphalangeal (IP) joint extension as indicating an incomplete radial neuropathy; this movement is, of course, supplied by ulnar-innervated muscles. It is also sometimes noted that finger abduction appears weak in the presence of radial neuropathy. This is because abduction is often tested when the MCP joints are flexed, in which position the muscles are at a mechanical disadvantage and joint motion is limited by the collateral ligaments. Finger abduction should be tested when the hand is flat against the table or desk so that the MCP joints can be maximally extended during the procedure.

Etiology

The vast majority of radial nerve lesions high in the arm are a result of trauma. The most common trauma is an external compression to the radial nerve as it passes through the spiral groove adjacent to the humerus. Saturday night palsy got its name from the condition resulting from an inebriated individual sleeping with his arm over a park bench on a Saturday night.

When humeral fractures are repaired with closed intramedullary nailing, there is also about a 10% to 15% incidence of radial nerve injuries (54), which are thought to result from incarceration of the radial nerve between fracture fragments as reduction is accomplished.

Improper use of axillary crutches may also result in radial nerve lesions, but these lesions are often high, sometimes additionally involving the triceps muscle. Better instruction of patients using axillary crutches (i.e., to not put the patient's weight through the axillary pad) will reduce the incidence of this neuropathy.

Nerve Conduction Studies (Table 10–3)

Motor nerve conduction studies are often technically suboptimal and difficult to perform for the radial nerve. The greatest problem with the technique is finding a suitable recording method. When surface electrodes have been used, it has been difficult to consistently find a surface recording site that produces a local response and is not volume-conducted from distant muscles within the forearm. Needle recording from the extensor indicis proprius (EIP) has been more satisfactory but has limitations. Using this technique, one can stimulate the radial nerve in the distal forearm, elbow, spiral groove, and axilla. It is, however, difficult with needle recording to interpret the amplitudes one obtains, because the amplitudes depend greatly upon needle position within the muscle. Moreover, any needle movement during the study may make it impossible to compare results obtained from one site of stimulation to another. Nevertheless, this technique can provide useful information about whether the lesion is neurapraxic or axonal and can localize the site of the conduction block.

Sensory nerve conduction studies may be performed with stimulation in the forearm and by recording over the dorsal aspect of the hand in the first web space (or on the thumb). Although these studies are usually not of localizing value, the presence of a reduced or absent response indicates the degree of sensory axon loss present. In rare cases, the lateral antebrachial cutaneous nerve innervates part of the dorsum of the hand and can contribute to or produce a SNAP in the presence of complete radial sensory axon loss.

Needle EMG provides the most useful localizing information in most radial neuropathies. Key muscles to examine include the triceps and occasionally the anconeus, brachioradialis, extensor carpi radialis (it is difficult to distinguish longus from brevis), and supinator. Although the degree of axon loss cannot be quantitatively estimated based on needle EMG studies, the distribution of denervation can help with localization.

DEEP RADIAL (FORMERLY POSTERIOR INTEROSSEOUS) NERVE LESIONS (FIG. 10–3)

A 42-year-old man presents with the gradual onset over two weeks of an inability to extend his fingers, weak wrist extension, and pain over the dorsal aspect of the forearm. He denies any sensory loss or paresthesias. He also denies any antecedent trauma. On physical examination, strength is

Shoulder abduction	5/5
Shoulder flexion	5/5
Shoulder extension	5/5
Elbow flexion	5/5
Elbow extension	5/5
Supination	5/5
Pronation	5/5
Wrist extension	3/5 (wrist deviated radially)
Wrist flexion	5/5
MCP extension	2/5
Thumb extension	2/5
Finger flexion	5/5

Sensation is normal to light touch, pinprick, and two-point discrimination. Reflexes are active (2+) and symmetrical at the biceps, brachioradialis, and triceps.

Differential Diagnosis

The differential diagnosis in this case includes radial neuropathy at the elbow (e.g., the deep radial nerve), high radial nerve lesions, and middle trunk or C7 root lesions. Presence of normal sensation suggests that the lesion spares the superficial radial sensory nerve and is affecting only the deep radial (formerly called posterior interosseous) branch.

Impression

The presence of denervation only in the distribution of the deep radial nerve (distal to the supinator and extensor carpi radialis muscles) suggests this is a deep radial nerve lesion (Fig. 10–3). The presence of normal and symmetrical findings in the radial sensory nerve action potentials controverts any higher radial neuropathy, although they could not exclude a preganglionic lesion. Normal findings in C7-innervated muscles outside the deep radial distribution eliminate cervical radiculopathy.

Clinical Presentation

Most patients with a deep radial nerve compression have a gradual onset of weakness and pain in the elbow or proximal forearm over several days to weeks. Typically, the nerve is compressed as it enters the supinator muscle under the arcade of Frohse. Alternatively, it can be compressed by tumors, ganglia, or elbow joint synovitis in this region. Because the radial nerve branches to the brachioradialis, supinator, and extensor carpi radialis leave the nerve before the site of compression, they are usually well preserved. However, muscles distant to the site are typically weak or completely paralyzed. These muscles include the extensor carpi ulnaris (selective weakness of this muscle produces radial deviation with wrist extension because the radialis is spared), the extensor digitorum, the extensor indicis proprius, the extensor pollicis longus and brevis, and the abductor pollicis longus. Sensation is usually spared.

The etiology of deep radial nerve syndrome is most commonly tumors or other mass lesions. Lipomas are frequent in this region and may be the most frequent cause of deep radial nerve syndrome (2,11,49); lipomas are usually painless. Trauma can cause deep radial neuropathy secondary to elbow dislocations, radial head fractures, or fractures of the ulna with radial head displacement. Ganglia and rheumatoid elbow synovitis have also been reported as causes of neuropathy (5,43,46). Entrapment at the arcade of Frohse is probably a result of entrapment of the radial nerve as it passes under the fibrous tendinous band of the supinator muscle.

Some authors have proposed the existence of radial tunnel syndrome, also called resistant tennis elbow (25,41,60,76). This syndrome presents predominantly with lateral elbow pain, although these patients have less marked weakness and electrophysiologic findings than other patients with deep radial nerve lesions.

Electrophysiologic Examination

Needle EMG is the most useful part of the electrophysiological examination because it can clearly demonstrate abnormalities in the deep radial distribution while other muscles supplied by the radial nerve and C7 myotome are uninvolved (Table 10–4). Although some studies have demonstrated prolonged motor latencies from the elbow to the extensor digitorum (32), it is unclear whether this provides any useful additional information compared to the needle EMG. Sensory nerve action potentials of the radial nerve should all be within normal limits.

SUPERFICIAL RADIAL NERVE LESIONS

Case 4

Clinical History and Physical Examination

A 52-year-old, 300-pound woman underwent gallbladder resection at a major teaching hospital. Although the medical student, intern, and resident were not able to secure IV access in the upper limb, the attending anesthesiologist was successful in putting in a central venous access line. The patient did well during surgery, but postoperatively woke up with pain and numbness over the radial aspect of the right forearm. Although the numbness has been troubling, the dysesthetic pain has been most disabling.

Physical examination reveals normal strength in both upper limbs. There is reduced sensation to pinprick and two-point discrimination over the radial aspect of the hand on the dorsal surface only. Reflexes are all active (2+) and symmetrical. A Tinel's sign is present over the radial aspect of the forearm directly over the radius, which causes severe pain.

Differential Diagnosis

In the absence of strength and reflex changes, a superficial radial nerve lesion is the most likely diagnosis. Other items in the differential, though, include a C6 radiculopathy or possibly upper brachial plexus lesion secondary to positioning during surgery.

Table 10–4
Electrodiagnostic Data for Case 4

NERVE CONDUCTION STUDIES					
Nerve	Record	Stim	Distal Latency (msec)	Amplitude (μV)	Conduction Velocity (m/s)
R. Radial (sensory)	Dorsum hand	Forearm (14 cm)	3.8	2	
R. Radial (sensory)	Thumb	Wrist (10 cm)	3.3	3	
R. Median (sensory)	Thumb	Wrist	2.8	22	

Needle EMG (all on right side)

Muscle	Spont. Activity		Motor Unit Action Potentials			Recruitment
	PSWs	Fibs	Ampl.	Dur.	Phasicity	
EIP	0	0	N	N	N	full
ECR	0	0	N	N	N	full
BR	0	0	N	N	N	full
TRIC	0	0	N	N	N	full
DELT	0	0	N	N	N	full
PT	0	0	N	N	N	full

PSWs: Positive sharp waves
Fibs: Fibrillation potentials
EIP: Extensor indicis proprius
ECR: Extensor carpi radialis
BR: Brachioradialis
TRIC: Triceps brachii
DELT: Deltoid
PT: Pronator teres

Impression

These findings are all consistent with an isolated superficial radial sensory neuropathy (Table 10–4). The absence of needle EMG abnormalities rules out a more proximal radial nerve lesion or brachial plexopathy.

Clinical Presentation

Lesions of the superficial radial nerve can be painful and disabling. Sensory loss is usually less problematic than the dysesthetic pain. Neuromas often form that recur despite repeated resection. The superficial radial nerve typically supplies the dorsum of the hand on the radial aspect, but there is considerable variation in the nerve supplying the region. At times this area can be supplied largely or wholly by the lateral antebrachial cutaneous nerve, the dorsal ulnar cutaneous nerve, or the median nerve or its palmar cutaneous branch (1,42). Although sensation is abnormal, strength and reflexes are always preserved in patients with these lesions. Tinel's sign is often present over the injured nerve and may elicit painful dysesthesias.

Etiology

By and large, injuries to the superficial branch of the radial nerve are traumatic in etiology. Tight casts, wrist watches, or wrist bands can be responsible for injuries, as may too-tight handcuffs (6,45,71). Iatrogenic causes include complications from deQuervain's tenosynovectomy or the attempted placement of intravenous lines or shunts for dialysis, especially near the level of the wrist.

Electrodiagnostic Evaluation (Table 10–4)

The only electrodiagnostic study available to assist in documenting this lesion is the SNAP (Table 10–4). The SNAP is often best recorded from the first web space with stimulation of the radial nerve proximally along the forearm. The superficial radial nerve can be palpated as it crosses over the extensor pollicis longus tendon; the active electrode can be placed directly over the nerve. High radial nerve lesions, brachial plexopathies, and cervical radiculopathies can best be excluded by performing needle EMG. Independent of the

electrodiagnostic abnormalities, the prognosis for recovering from continued pain is poor once neuroma formation has occurred.

MEDIAN NEUROPATHY NEAR THE ELBOW (FIG. 10–4)

Case 5

Clinical History and Physical Examination

A 27-year-old waiter reports vague forearm pain and weakness, particularly exacerbated by holding a food tray up over his head (when his forearm is in the pronated position). He reports numbness over the palmar aspect of the radial three digits of the right hand and weakness in his hand, noting that he often drops things.

Physical examination is remarkable for tenderness in the proximal forearm, particularly over the pronator teres muscle; this produces local pain as well as pain extending into the forearm and accompanied by numbness in the thumb, index, and middle fingers. Strength is normal in all muscle groups in the upper limb. Sensation is normal to light touch, pinprick, and two-point discrimination. Reflexes are active (2+) and symmetrical. No Tinel's sign could be elicited at the median nerve at the wrist or the ulnar nerve at the elbow.

Differential Diagnosis

The differential diagnosis includes musculoskeletal syndromes such as overuse syndromes and medial epicondylitis. Given the intermittent numbness, carpal tunnel syndrome median nerve entrapment at the elbow or C6 radiculopathy are also possible.

Impression

Although the electrodiagnostic findings in Table 10–5 are mild, the changes seen, when combined with the clinical presentation, are most suggestive of pronator syndrome. Important to note are the mild conduction block seen in the median nerve between the wrist and elbow and the mild evidence of denervation seen in the median innervated muscles distal to the pronator teres.

Clinical Presentation

There are multiple potential sites of compression of the median nerve at or near the elbow (78). Starting proximally (Fig. 10–4), the median nerve may be compressed by the ligament of Struthers, a fibrous structure running from an aberrant spur of bone on the distal humerus to the medial epicondyle. The median nerve and brachial artery and vein run under this ligament, which is present in about 1% to 3%

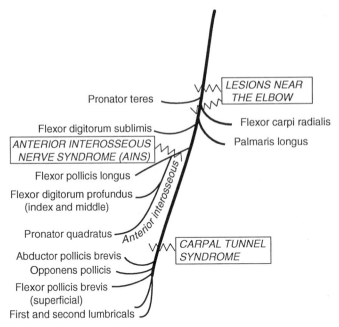

Figure 10–4. Median nerve anatomy showing branches and common sites of focal neuropathy.

of the general population (74). Compression at this site is rare and probably occurs in only a very small percentage of those individuals who have the ligament present (39). Distally, the nerve passes underneath the lacertus fibrosus, a fascial band normally present extending from the biceps tendon and broadening out to the forearm fascia. Although essentially this band is always present, in some people it is thickened and can cause compression of the underlying median nerve.

More distally, the median nerve can be compressed by a tendinous band within the pronator teres muscle as it dives between the two heads of the muscle (26,29). It may also be compressed distal to the pronator teres as it travels under the fibrous arch of the flexor digitorum superficialis.

Clinical presentation depends on the site of pathology, but usually the complaints are of aching pain in the forearm exacerbated by repetitive use. Sensory symptoms like paresthesia or dysesthesia are more rare than they would be in carpal tunnel syndrome and, when present, they are vague and ill defined.

Physical findings of weakness or sensory loss are rare, although Tinel's sign may be present when tapping over the site of compression (3).

Electrodiagnostic Evaluation (Table 10–5)

Although some patients may demonstrate focal slowing and conduction block of the median nerve at the site of the compression, most have minimal electrodiagnostic changes. When axon loss is present, motor or sensory amplitudes may be reduced with stimulation at the wrist and recording over the hand; this should not be confused with carpal tunnel syndrome (which usually produces prolonged distal latencies). Needle EMG typically shows minimal changes such as increased insertional activity or mild evidence of denervation, but most changes are not striking. Many times the diagnosis is made primarily on clinical grounds, with electrodiagnosis helping in large part to rule out other clinical syndromes.

ANTERIOR INTEROSSEOUS NERVE SYNDROME (AINS)

Case 6

Clinical History and Physical Examination

A 40-year-old construction worker presents with an inability to accurately direct traffic, which is part of his job. He stands in back of cement-pouring trucks, directing them as they back up, and is supposed to give the "OK" sign with his right hand when they have reached a good stopping point. About 3 weeks ago, he noticed the onset of right forearm pain and the sudden inability to make the "OK" sign with his right hand. He reported that he could not bend the distal joint of the index finger or the joint of his thumb sufficiently to make this sign. He denies any sensory loss or pain other than in the forearm. His other limbs are all asymptomatic.

Physical examination is remarkable for weakness of thumb flexion at the interphalangeal joint and weakness of flexion of the distal interphalangeal joint (DIP) of the index finger. All other finger and thumb flexion is normal. Pronation with the elbow extended is normal, although it is possibly weak with the elbow flexed. Sensation is within normal limits to pinprick, light touch, and two-point discrimination. Reflexes are active (2+) and symmetrical.

Differential Diagnosis

The differential diagnosis includes anterior interosseous nerve syndrome, idiopathic brachial plexitis (also known as neuralgic amyotrophy or Parsonage-Turner syndrome), and a high median nerve lesion. The absence of sensory symptoms or findings on clinical examination controverts a high median nerve lesion. Although the presentation is not classical for neuralgic amyotrophy, some patients with

Table 10–5
Electrodiagnostic Data for Case 5

NERVE CONDUCTION STUDIES					
Nerve	Record	Stim	Distal Latency (msec)	Amplitude (μV)	Conduction Velocity (m/s)
R. Median (motor)	APB	Wrist	3.6	7600	
		Elbow		5100	49
R. Median (sensory	Index finger	Wrist	3.4	23	
R. Ulnar (motor)	ADM	Wrist	3.4	7000	
		Below elbow		6600	53
		Above elbow		6000	51
					55
		Axilla		5800	
R. Ulnar (sensory)	Little finger	Wrist	3.3	19	

Needle EMG (all on right side)

Muscle	Spont. Activity		Motor Unit Action Potentials			
	PSWs	Fibs	Ampl.	Dur.	Phasicity	Recruitment
APB	1+	0	N	N	N	full
FCR	0	1+	N	N	N	full
FDS	1+	0	N	N	N	full
PT	0	0	N	N	N	full
FDI	0	0	N	N	N	full
EIP	0	0	N	N	N	full

PSWs: Positive sharp waves
Fibs: Fibrillation potentials
APB: Abductor pollicus brevis
FCR: Flexor carpi radialis
FDS: Flexor digitorum superficialis
PT: Pronator teres
FDI: First dorsal interosseous
EIP: Extensor indicis proprius

this disorder do have symptoms primarily in the anterior interosseous nerve distribution (34).

Impression
The findings of denervation localized to the anterior interosseous distribution, despite an extensive needle EMG, are most consistent with anterior interosseous nerve syndrome (AINS). Normal findings in the proximal median innervated muscles and the muscles supplied by other branches of the brachial plexus controvert a more widespread process (Fig. 10–4). Although there is some debate as to whether neuralgic amyotrophy may present with isolated anterior interosseous nerve deficits (17), there are a number of treatable causes of this lesion that should be considered (77).

Clinical Presentation

Typically, patients report the spontaneous onset of acute proximal forearm pain, which lasts several days. In some cases there is a history of trauma or overexertion prior to the onset of pain. Weakness is usually less bothersome to the patient than the pain, and patients only secondarily report a decrease in pinch strength.

Physical examination shows weakness in the flexor pollicis longus (which flexes the interphalangeal joint of the thumb) and the flexor digitorum profundus, supplying the index finger and sometimes the middle finger (which is sometimes innervated by the ulnar nerve). The pronator quadratus muscle is best tested by having the patient maximally flex the elbow (to reduce the contribution from the pronator teres) and assessing pronation strength. However, other muscles contribute to pronation (such as the flexor carpi radialis) and, even in patients with complete denervation of the pronator quadratus, strength testing of pronation may be normal (77). Because the Martin-Gruber median-to-ulnar nerve anastomosis is thought to frequently originate from the anterior interosseous nerve, patients with this anomaly or anterior interosseous nerve syndrome may be expected to exhibit weakness in the ulnar-innervated hand muscles as well as those muscles mentioned above.

Etiology

A number of anomalous or accessory muscles and tendons in the proximal forearm have been implicated in AINS and may be responsible for nearly half the lesions seen (77). Some-

times a repetitive movement or the strenuous use of the forearm muscles will provoke the onset of symptoms (50,58). More obvious trauma such as from fractures, gunshot wounds, or lacerations in the forearm have also been reported (52).

Some debate whether neuralgic amyotrophy may involve isolated peripheral nerves rather than just the brachial plexus. In their original report of neuralgic amyotrophy, Parsonage and Turner (55) reported a number of patients who had weakness limited to the flexor pollicis longus (FPL) and the median-innervated flexor digitorum profundus (FDP) but did not recognize that the weakness was in the anterior interosseous distribution. Kiloh and Nevin (34) later reported the neuralgic amyotrophy was within the distribution of a single peripheral nerve. England and Sumner (17) hypothesized that peripheral nerves (as opposed to only the brachial plexus) could be affected in neuralgic amyotrophy and that the anterior interosseous nerve was a particularly susceptible nerve. A substantial proportion of patients with AINS may actually have neuralgic amyotrophy rather than any extrinsic compression in the forearm.

Electrodiagnostic Examination (Table 10–6)

Needle EMG is usually the most helpful component of the electrodiagnostic evaluation (Table 10–6). The diagnosis depends upon finding evidence of denervation in the FPL, the FDP (median half), or the pronator quadratus. The latter muscle can be difficult to examine, but the access to this muscle is greatly facilitated if it is approached from its dorsal aspect when the forearm is in the neutral (not pronated) position (77). Muscles outside of this distribution are usually normal, although ulnar-innervated muscles may show evidence of denervation if a Martin-Gruber anomaly is present. Widespread examination of the limb is useful to exclude neuralgic amyotrophy or more diffuse nerve or plexus lesions.

Motor nerve conduction studies have been recorded from the pronator quadratus (50), although it is unclear whether this presents any useful information additional to that of the needle examination alone. Sensory nerve

Table 10–6
Electrodiagnostic Data for Case 6

NERVE CONDUCTION STUDIES

Nerve	Record	Stim	Distal Latency (msec)	Amplitude (μV)	Conduction Velocity (m/s)
R. Median (motor)	APB	Wrist	3.6	7800	55
		Elbow		7100	
R. Median (sensory	Index finger	Wrist	3.4	23	

Needle EMG (all on right side)

Muscle	Spont. Activity PSWs	Fibs	Motor Unit Action Potentials Ampl.	Dur.	Phasicity	Recruitment
APB	0	0	N	N	N	full
PQ	3+	2+	↑	↑	↑	reduced
FPL	3+	1+	↑	↑	↑	reduced
FCR	0	0	N	N	N	full
PT	0	0	N	N	N	full
FDI	0	0	N	N	N	full
EIP	0	0	N	N	N	full
DELT	0	0	N	N	N	full
IN-FRASPIN	0	0	N	N	N	full

PSWs: Positive sharp waves
Fibs: Fibrillation potentials
APB: Abductor pollicus brevis
PQ: Pronator quadratus
FPL: Flexor pollicis longus
FCR: Flexor carpi radialis
PT: Pronator teres
FDI: First dorsal interosseous
EIP: Extensor indicis proprius
DELT: Deltoid
INFRASPIN: Infraspinatus

conduction studies are typically normal but may be useful to rule out other potentially confusing diagnoses.

SCIATIC NEUROPATHY (FIG. 10–5)

Case 7

Clinical History and Physical Examination

A 48-year-old woman sustained injury to the left hip during a motor vehicle accident. X rays revealed an acetabular fracture, which was repaired with open reduction and internal fixation. Postoperatively, the patient awoke with a left foot drop. She

was referred for electrodiagnostic evaluation 3 weeks later. On physical examination, strength is

Hip flexion	5/5
Hip abduction	4/5
Hip extension	5/5
Hip adduction	5/5
Knee extension	5/5
Knee flexion	4+/5
Ankle dorsiflexion	1/5
Ankle plantar flexion	4+/5
Ankle eversion	3/5
Ankle inversion	4+/5

Sensation is reduced over the dorsum of the foot and lateral aspect of the leg. Reflexes are symmetrical and active (2+ at the knee), unelicitable at the medial hamstring on either side, and asymmetrically absent at the left ankle.

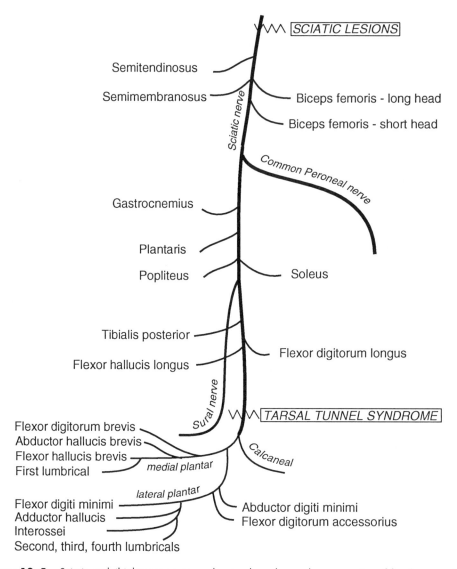

Figure 10–5. Sciatic and tibial nerve anatomy showing branches and common sites of focal neuropathy.

Differential Diagnosis

The differential diagnosis includes sciatic neuropathy (Fig. 10–5) as a result of the initial injury or the operative intervention; peroneal neuropathy, possibly as a result of prolonged external rotation in bed or pressure over the nerve; or L5 radiculopathy (hip abduction is weak, but this could result from the recent surgery).

Impression

The findings are consistent with a sciatic neuropathy that predominantly involves the peroneal distribution of the sciatic nerve (Table 10–7). The absence of denervation in proximal L5 muscles (the gluteus medius or tensor fasciae latae) controverts L5 radiculopathy; however, these muscles can be abnormal as a result of the direct trauma of surgery.

Although the abnormalities in the tibial distribution are relatively mild, predominance of peroneal abnormalities are not unexpected for a high sciatic neuropathy. Sciatic neuropathy in these cases likely results from the stretch on the sciatic nerve during the retraction required for surgical access to the hip joint.

Clinical Presentation

Sciatic neuropathies typically present with weakness and sensory loss in the sciatic distribution. However, it is not unusual and is probably even customary for the peroneal distribution to be much more affected than the tibial division. This may be related to differences in the fascicular structure of the nerve; the peroneal division has a few large fascicles with relatively little intervening fibrous tissue, and the tibial division carries many small fascicles cushioned by large amounts of fibrous tissue (72). In fact, in many cases it may be difficult to distinguish sciatic neuropathy from peroneal neuropathy on clinical grounds. Helpful findings are weakness of the knee flexors, absence of the ankle jerk, and subtle weakness in the tibial-innervated muscles. Sensory loss is also greater in the peroneal than the tibial distribu-

Table 10–7
Electrodiagnostic Data for Case 7

NERVE CONDUCTION STUDIES					
Nerve	Record	Stim	Distal Latency (msec)	Amplitude (μV)	Conduction Velocity (m/s)
L. Peroneal (motor)	EDB	Ankle	5.6	800	
		Below fib. head		700	37
					38
		Polp. fossa		650	
L. Peroneal (F wave)	EDB	Ankle	Absent response		
L. Tibial (motor)	AH	Ankle	4.7	2300	
		Polp. fossa		1900	40
L. Tibial (F wave)	EDB	Ankle	57.0		
L. Sural (sensory)	Ankle	Leg	4.3	1	

Needle EMG (all on left side)

Muscle	Spont. Activity		Motor Unit Action Potentials			
	PSWs	Fibs	Ampl.	Dur.	Phasicity	Recruitment
TA	3+	3+	N	N	↑	reduced
PL	3+	2+	N	N	↑	reduced
MG	1+	1+	N	N	N	
SOL	1+	0	N	N	N	
BICFEMsh	1+	1+	N	N	N	reduced
SEMITEM	1+	0	N	N	N	full
TFL	0	0	N	N	N	full
GLUTMED	0	0	N	N	N	full
VASTMED	0	0	N	N	N	full
LUMB Psps	0	0				

PSWs: Positive sharp waves
Fibs: Fibrillation potentials
BICFEMsh: Biceps femoris (short head)
SEMIMEM: Semitendinosis
TA: Tibialis anterior
PL: Peroneus longus
MG: Medial gastroc
SOL: Soleus
TFL: Tensor fascia lata
GLUTMED: Gluteus medius
VASTMED: Vastus medialis
LUMB Psps: Lumbar paraspinals

tion. Characteristically, the saphenous distribution (an extension of the femoral nerve) is spared along the medial leg and foot.

Etiology

Sciatic neuropathy can result from hip surgery, either hip replacement or other types of surgery in which retraction of the sciatic nerve is required to get access to the hip (75). Intraoperative monitoring is often helpful to avoid reversible sciatic nerve injury (22). Sciatic nerve injury may also result from injections in the gluteal muscles (10) and is particularly severe when irritating compounds are injected.

Piriformis syndrome is another possible etiology of sciatic neuropathy, although debate exists about its true frequency. In about 6% of cadaver specimens, the sciatic nerve passes within the piriformis muscle (57), although only a small fraction of this frequency can be expected to have clinical findings. In the cadaver specimens, hip internal rotation can cause compression of the sciatic nerve.

Electrodiagnostic Evaluation (Table 10–7)

With sciatic neuropathies, electrodiagnostic studies (Table 10–7) have several roles. They help with localizing the lesion, assessing the degree of axon loss and prognosis, and, in severe lesions, assessing the degree of reinnervation, if any, and allowing an informed decision about operative intervention.

Needle EMG is usually the best tool for localizing the lesion. Key muscles to study include the peroneal- and tibial-innervated muscles in the leg, the short head of the biceps femoris (supplied by the peroneal division of the sciatic nerve), other hamstring muscles (supplied by the tibial division of the sciatic nerve), and the gluteal-innervated muscles. If the gluteal muscles are involved, the diagnosis is more likely a lumbosacral plexopathy or radiculopathy rather than sciatic neuropathy. Examination of paraspinal muscles allows separation of sciatic neuropathy from radiculopathy.

Needle EMG is also useful for evaluating reinnervation after complete or very severe lesions. By examining muscles just distal to

the lesion, one can note if reinnervation is occurring in muscles previously completely denervated. When there are no signs of reinnervation, surgical nerve grafting may be indicated.

Nerve conduction studies are best at determining the degree of axon loss but are not as good in localizing the lesion. Abnormalities in both peroneal and tibial motor nerve conduction studies indicate that the lesion is above the bifurcation of the sciatic nerve. Similarly, late responses such as the F wave or the Hreflex can help to determine if both the tibial and peroneal branches are affected.

There are reports of sciatic nerve stimulation at the gluteal fold; however, this technique has been difficult in this author's experience. Surface stimulation rarely elicits a maximal response. The absence of a response to needle stimulation is often difficult to interpret, and it is unclear how to rule out technical problems with the procedure. SNAPs of the sural or superficial peroneal nerves are useful to distinguish a postganglionic lesion (e.g., sciatic nerve or lumbosacral plexus) from a preganglionic lesion (e.g., root or cauda equina).

PERONEAL NEUROPATHY AT THE KNEE (FIG. 10–6)

Case 8

Clinical History and Physical Examination

A 55-year-old woman reports the sudden onset of right-sided foot drop 3 weeks ago after waking up from sleeping on a chaise lounge outdoors at a party. She admits to drinking alcohol at the party. She reports difficulty walking and easily falling because of the right foot drop. She denies any back pain but does report a sensory loss over the dorsum of the right foot and the lateral aspect of the right leg. Significant past medical history includes a recent weight loss over the last three years, from 220 pounds to 140 pounds, secondary to intentional dieting (because of medical complications from being overweight).

Physical examination reveals 0/5 ankle dorsiflexion, 2/5 ankle eversion, 5/5 ankle inversion, and 5/5 ankle plantar flexion. Proximally, limb strength is all normal. Sensation is reduced to pinprick and light touch over the dorsum of the right foot, including the first web space, and over the lateral aspect of the right leg. Reflexes at the knees and ankles are active (2+) and symmetrical and the medial hamstring reflexes are 1+ and symmetrical.

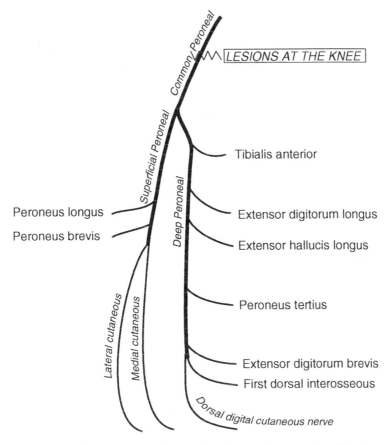

Figure 10-6. Peroneal nerve anatomy showing branches and common sites of focal neuropathy.

Differential Diagnosis

The differential diagnosis includes not only peroneal neuropathy at the fibular head, but also sciatic neuropathy or L5 radiculopathy (Figs. 10–5, 10–6). Of interest is the greater involvement of muscles innervated by the deep peroneal distribution than those innervated by the superficial peroneal nerve.

Impression

The electrodiagnostic findings in Table 10–8 are consistent with peroneal neuropathy at the fibular head (mostly neurapraxic), with a very good prognosis for recovery. The large-amplitude response with distal stimulation suggests that not much motor axon loss has occurred and the prognosis for recovery over the next 2 to 3 months is excellent, assuming no further compression or trauma occurs. The presence of abnormalities on needle EMG indicates that there may be some axon loss, but this is minimal given the good amplitude of the compound muscle action potential.

Clinical Presentation

Patients with peroneal neuropathy typically present with foot drop and weak ankle ever-

sion. Weakness is usually greater in the ankle dorsiflexors than in the everters, consistent with typically greater involvement of the deep peroneal distribution than of the superficial distribution. Ankle inversion and plantar flexion are strong in these patients, excluding a higher sciatic nerve or lumbosacral root lesion. In some cases, only the deep peroneal distribution is clinically affected, resulting in a small or unnoticed sensory loss (the web space between first and second toes) and marked weakness of ankle dorsiflexion and toe extension.

Etiology

The most common etiology of peroneal neuropathy at the fibular head is acute compression of the nerve. This can result from improperly fitting braces or casts, circumferential bandages at the level of the fibular neck, or the chronic external rotation of the lower limbs of patients who are unconscious and in bed. Improper positioning of the lower limb during surgical procedures may also be a predisposing factor. Previous weight loss is common in patients who develop an acute lesion (65). Occupations that involve chronic kneeling or squatting may also predispose to peroneal neuropathy at the fibular head (62). Tumors or cysts may occasionally involve the peroneal nerve.

Electrodiagnostic Examination (Table 10–8)

There are a variety of nerve conduction studies for localizing the site of peroneal neuropathy as well as assessing the prognosis. When significant demyelination is present in the peroneal nerve, motor nerve conduction studies are often of great value in localizing the lesion

Table 10–8
Electrodiagnostic Data for Case 8

NERVE CONDUCTION STUDIES

Nerve	Record	Stim	Distal Latency (msec)	Amplitude (μV)	Conduction Velocity (m/s)
L. Peroneal (motor)	EDB	Ankle	5.1	3800	
		Below fibular head		3700	43
		Popliteal fossa		250	38
L. Peroneal (F wave)	EDB	Ankle	Absent response		
L. Tibial (motor)	AH	Ankle	4.5	5300	
		Popliteal fossa		4900	42
L. Tibial (F wave)	EDB	Ankle	53.0		

Needle EMG (all on left side)

Muscle	Spont. Activity PSWs	Spont. Activity Fibs	Motor Unit Action Potentials Ampl.	Motor Unit Action Potentials Dur.	Motor Unit Action Potentials Phasicity	Recruitment
TA	2+	2+	N	N	N	discrete
PL	1+	1+	N	N	N	discrete
MG	0	0	N	N	N	
SOL	0	0	N	N	N	
BICFEMsh	0	0	N	N	N	full
SEMITEM	0	0	N	N	N	full
GLUTMED	0	0	N	N	N	full
VASTMED	0	0	N	N	N	full
LUMB Psps	0	0				

PSWs: Positive sharp waves
Fibs: Fibrillation potentials
BICFEMsh: Biceps femoris (short head)
SEMIMEM: Semitendinosis
TA: Tibialis anterior
PL: Peroneus longus
MG: Medial gastroc
SOL: Soleus
GLUTMED: Gluteus medius
VASTMED: Vastus medialis
LUMB Psps: Lumbar paraspinals

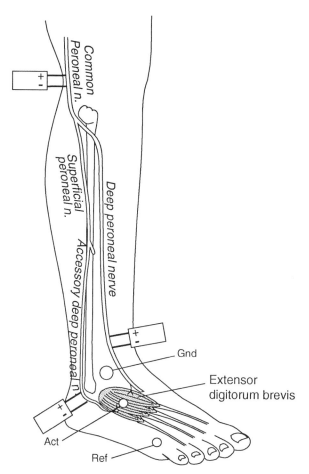

and assessing the degree of axon loss. Purely axonal lesions are more difficult to localize.

Recording for motor nerve conduction studies can be either at the extensor digitorum brevis (EDB) or the tibialis anterior (TA). The EDB is more commonly used. It has the advantage of permitting conduction velocity in the leg segment as well as proximally across the fibular head. It also is a well-isolated muscle with little chance of volume conduction from adjacent superficial peroneal-innervated muscles. On the other hand, there are disadvantages to using the EDB. The accessory peroneal nerve (which is present in about 20% of normal subjects) may cause difficulties in interpretation (23,24) (see Fig. 10–7). When this anomaly is present, a larger amplitude response from the EDB is recorded with stimulation at the fibular head than the response at the ankle. Although this anomaly is not likely to masquerade as conduction block (as opposed to the case of a Martin-Gruber anas-

tomosis and ulnar neuropathy), it can be technically confusing.

Recording from the TA also has advantages and disadvantages (Fig. 10–8). When the EDB response is absent or small-amplitude, the TA may be the only reliable muscle from which to record. There is some evidence that the response recorded from the TA may be more sensitive at detecting peroneal neuropathy at the fibular head than when recording from the EDB (33,59,67). In addition, the TA is a more important muscle functionally than the EDB; hence, any prognostic statements that can be made are more pertinent when applied to ankle dorsiflexion function. In this author's experience, the biggest problem with recording from the TA is volume conduction from the nearby peroneus longus (PL) muscle. Because the deep division of the peroneal nerve is typically more affected than the superficial branch, it is not uncommon to have complete denervation of the TA and preservation

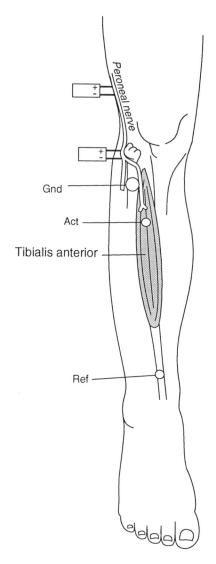

Figure 10-8. Peroneal NCV to tibialis anterior. Peroneal nerve may be studied by stimulating at the popliteal fossa and fibular head while recording over the tibialis anterior.

of the PL. Despite complete denervation of the TA, stimulation of the peroneal nerve at the fibular head can give a volume-conducted response at the TA. In these cases, recording from both the TA and the PL, with both surface and needle electrodes, can help to sort out which muscles are contributing to the surface-recorded CMAP over the tibialis anterior.

Independent of the recording site, the nerve should be stimulated both at the fibular head and proximally in the popliteal fossa. It is critical with popliteal fossa stimulation to avoid overstimulation of the tibial nerve. This becomes apparent when a) the amplitude with stimulation at the knee is larger than that at the fibular head; b) an initial positive deflection appears; or c) a nonsensical conduction

velocity is obtained for the across-fibular head segment (e.g., 100 meters per second). Stimulation in the popliteal fossa should occur laterally, just medial to the lateral hamstring tendons.

Evidence of demyelination is the most helpful finding for localization. Focal slowing, conduction block, or temporal dispersion may indicate the site of demyelination. However, in the majority of axon-loss lesions, amplitudes are small and conduction velocities mildly slowed throughout all segments of the nerve. In this event, the diagnosis is made largely on the distribution of findings with needle EMG.

Inching studies have been reported for the diagnosis of peroneal neuropathy and are probably more sensitive than long-segment studies, similar to the diagnosis for ulnar neuropathy (30). Latency changes over 2-cm segments exceeding 0.7 msec are thought to be abnormal. For amplitude drop, some authors have recommended using a 50% drop from the fibular head to knee stimulation sites to define abnormal (33), although smaller decrements are probably abnormal.

SNAPs are useful in demonstrating a postganglionic lesion and differentiating it from a preganglionic injury. However, sensory nerve responses can usually be obtained only from the superficial peroneal nerve. Thus, a normal superficial peroneal sensory nerve response can be seen with a neurapraxic lesion, a selective involvement of the deep peroneal branch, or a preganglionic lesion. Recordings of the SNAP from the superficial peroneal nerve are typically nonlocalizing but do provide some measure of the degree of sensory axon loss.

Needle EMG is the only way to localize a lesion that is purely axonal (Table 10–8). The PL and TA are excellent muscles to study in this regard. The EDB is not usually a reliable muscle for EMG because many asymptomatic subjects have fibrillation potentials or positive sharp waves. To exclude a more proximal lesion, the short head of biceps femoris (which is innervated by the peroneal division of the sciatic nerve) and hip abductors (the gluteus medius and tensor fasciae latae) are helpful. The tibialis posterior or flexor digitorum longus may also provide an opportunity to study L5-innervated nonperoneal muscles, although it is usually difficult to tell which of these two muscles the needle is in. Given the preponderance for more severe involvement of peroneal-innervated muscles in both sciatic neuropathy and L5 radiculopathy, the differential diagnosis of these disorders is not always straightforward and may require extensive examination.

TARSAL TUNNEL SYNDROMES (FIG. 10–5)

Case 9

Clinical History and Physical Examination

A 32-year-old, otherwise healthy woman fell from a ladder at work and sustained a severe eversion injury to the left foot. This was diagnosed as an ankle sprain to the medial ligaments. She was treated conservatively with casting but soon (several weeks) thereafter developed pain and paresthesias in the sole of the left foot.

Physical examination revealed normal strength in the lower limbs, including toe flexion. Sensory testing revealed decreased sensation to pinprick over the sole of the left foot compared to the right, but normal sensation elsewhere in the limb. Reflexes at the knee, medial hamstring, and ankles were active (2 +) and symmetrical. Tinel's sign was present with tapping over the ankle just posterior to the medial malleolus.

Differential Diagnosis

The symptoms are most suggestive of a focal lesion of the tibial nerve at the ankle. Although there are many other causes of foot and ankle pain, other neurogenic causes include entrapment of the medial plantar nerve distal to the tarsal tunnel, where the abductor hallucis originates from the calcaneus (37); higher tibial nerve lesions at the knee (such as from a Baker's cyst); or sciatic nerve or S1 root lesions (Fig. 10–5).

Impression

Prolongation of the compound nerve action potential latency and the compound muscle action potential latencies unilaterally are consistent with the diagnosis of tarsal tunnel syndrome or tibial neuropathy at the ankle (Table 10–9). Needle EMG of the intrinsic muscles in the foot suggests there may have been some axon loss, but it is common to see minor abnormalities in otherwise asymptomatic patients, and thus is not clearly indicative of axon loss from a focal neuropathy. Normal studies proximally in the tibial, sciatic, and S1 distributions controvert any significant higher lesion.

Clinical Presentation

The frequency of tarsal tunnel syndrome is often disputed (68). Some authors believe it appears frequently and is often missed electrodiagnostically. Other authors, including this one, believe that tibial neuropathy at the ankle occurs rarely in the absence of significant trauma.

Patients with tarsal tunnel syndrome typically report burning pain over the sole of the foot. They often report a recent history of significant injury such as fracture, ankle dislocation, or sprain (21). Physical examination may show atrophy of intrinsic foot muscles. Most intrinsic foot muscles are difficult to test for strength, although toe flexion may be the best maneuver to examine these muscles. The EDB should be relatively spared, because it is innervated by the deep peroneal nerve; it is one of the few nontibial-innervated intrinsic foot muscles.

Sensory loss is usually restricted to the sole of the foot. Because the tibial nerve divides into three branches as it is passing through the tarsal tunnel, any one or a combination of these three branches may be affected. The medial plantar branch supplies the medial sole of the foot and the first three-and-a-half toes; this is analogous to the median nerve in the hand. The lateral plantar branch supplies the lateral sole and the lateral one-and-a-half-toes; this is analogous to the ulnar nerve in the hand. These analogies also hold up in general terms when comparing muscle innervation. The calcaneal branch supplies the skin over the plantar surface of the heel and provides no muscular innervation.

Tinel's sign is often present over the tibial nerve behind the medial malleolus in patients with tarsal tunnel syndrome, but this sign generally is not specific. Some authors feel the presence of a Tinel's sign only indicates that there is a nerve under the area being tapped [Jun Kimura; personal communication].

Etiology

In tarsal tunnel syndrome, the tibial nerve is thought to be injured as it passes under the retinaculum and the lancinate ligament. Fractures and dislocations are the usual inciting events that lead to compression of the nerve (21), although joint hypermobility (20) may also play a role. Some investigators report that persistent ankle hyperpronation contributes as well, although this latter point is debatable.

Electrodiagnostic Examination (Table 10–9)

Because intrinsic foot muscles often show at least minor abnormalities in asymptomatic individuals, the majority of the diagnosis relies on nerve conduction studies. However, nerve conduction studies are not without technical difficulties, and side-to-side comparison is crucial. As with any other nerve conduction studies, the absence of a response is less convincing and diagnostic than a prolonged latency or other evidence of demyelination. An absent response, especially if present bilater-

ally, could simply be due to technical problems. In these cases every effort, including near-nerve recording, should be made to obtain a response.

Motor nerve conduction studies are the easiest to obtain, yet are less sensitive than compound nerve action potential studies. Stimulation is applied behind and superior to the medial malleolus, over the tibial nerve, with recording over the abductor hallucis for the medial plantar nerve and over the abductor digiti quinti for the lateral plantar nerve. The lateral plantar response is usually best recorded when the active recording electrode is placed over the bulk of the muscle belly rather than immediately below the lateral malleolus. It has been suggested that a difference in motor latency of more than 1.0 msec between the two feet may be abnormal (15).

Measuring compound nerve action potentials across the tarsal tunnel is more sensitive than simply measuring motor latencies but is more problematic. Stimulation of either nerve can occur at the sole of the foot 14 cm distal to the recording electrode, placed posterior and superior to the medial malleolus (61) (Fig. 10–9). This is a compound nerve action potential rather than a sensory nerve action potential because motor fibers supplying intrinsic foot muscles are also stimulated antidromically. Latencies longer than 3.8 msec, given a 14-cm distance, are probably abnormal, although skin temperature should be considered and side-to-side comparisons made. The most common technical problems with this technique are difficulty in stimulation through the sole of the foot and excessive stimulus artifact. Stimulation can best be accomplished by scrubbing the sole of the foot using pumice compound or even the edge of a 1.0-centimeter disk electrode. Needle stimulation may also be helpful if the needle is placed just under the corneum of the skin, very superficially. This author has attempted stimulation with a needle placed deeper through the sole of the foot, but the technique is too painful for the patient. Stimulus artifact can be improved by scrubbing the skin underneath the ground electrode and placing it directly between the stimulation and recording electrodes. Rotation of the stimulating electrode also helps to reduce the stimulus artifact.

Table 10–9
Electrodiagnostic Data for Case 9

		NERVE CONDUCTION STUDIES			
Nerve	Record	Stim	Distal Latency (msec)	Amplitude (μV)	Conduction Velocity (m/s)
L. Med Plant (motor)	AH	Ankle	6.0	2300	
		Popl. fossa		1900	42
L. Lat Plant (motor)	ADMP	Ankle	6.3	2400	
R. Med Plant (motor)	AH	Ankle	4.5	5300	
		Popl. fossa		4900	42
R. Lat Plant (motor)	ADMP	Ankle	4.5	3600	
L. Med Plant (CNAP)	Ankle	Sole	4.7	5	
L. Lat Plant (CNAP)	Ankle	Sole	4.9	3	
R. Med Plant (CNAP)	Ankle	Sole	3.6	12	
R. Lat Plant (CNAP)	Ankle	Sole	3.7	9	

Needle EMG

	Spont. Activity			Motor Unit Action Potentials		
Muscle	PSWs	Fibs	Ampl.	Dur.	Phasicity	Recruitment
L. FDIP	2+	2+	↑	↑	↑	
L. AH	1+	1+	↑	↑	↑	
L. MG	0	0	N	N	N	
L. SOL	0	0	N	N	N	
R. FDIP	1+	0	N	N	N	
R. AH	0	0	↑	↑	↑	

PSWs: Positive sharp waves
Fibs: Fibrillation potentials
MG: Medial gastroc
SOL: Soleus
FDIP: First dorsal inter (pedis)
AH: Abductor hallucis
ADMP: Abd. dig. minimi pedis

Pure study of the sensory nerves can also be accomplished by stimulating the great toe (for the medial plantar nerve) or the little toe (for the lateral plantar nerve) (53). Because the nerve action potential from toe stimulation is very small when recorded over the medial malleolus, it is usually necessary to perform near-nerve recording and averaging. Abnormalities may include either a prolonged latency or an increase in temporal dispersion of the potential. The relative sensitivity of these last two techniques, i.e., stimulation at the sole vs. stimulation at the toes, is not known; thus, it is unclear whether it is better to stimulate the toes or the sole of the foot, although the sole is probably technically easier.

Needle EMG should be performed to look for evidence of gross abnormalities. The two muscles that are best studied are the abductor hallucis (medial plantar innervation) and the

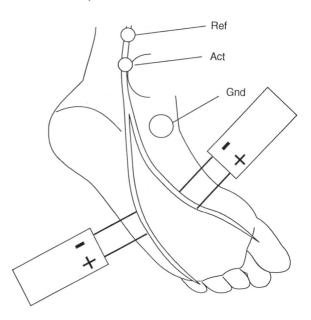

Figure 10-9. Compound nerve action potentials from medial and lateral plantar nerves are a sensitive measure for detecting tarsal tunnel syndrome.

first dorsal interosseus (lateral plantar innervation). These muscles are relatively protected from trauma and have a low incidence of positive sharp waves and fibrillations compared to other intrinsic foot muscles in asymptomatic individuals. Nevertheless, abnormalities in these muscles should be interpreted cautiously in the absence of changes on nerve conduction studies. There is still some debate as to whether this lesion is due to demyelination or primarily to axon loss (68).

Attempting to diagnose tarsal tunnel syndrome in the presence of an underlying polyneuropathy is exceedingly difficult, if not impossible. The diagnosis of tarsal tunnel syndrome in such a setting requires the demonstration of markedly more severe changes in one nerve than others or considerable asymmetry.

Conclusions

Entrapment neuropathies are a common reason for electrodiagnostic medical consultation. Clinical assessment is critical to forming a reasonable list of differential diagnoses. The electrodiagnostic evaluation is very helpful for localizing lesions, determining the extent of axon loss and the prognosis, and following reinnervation over time in more complete injuries.

ACKNOWLEDGMENT

Special thanks to Paula Mickelsen for the original artwork in this chapter.

References

1. Appleton AB: A case of abnormal distribution of the N. musculocutaneous with complete absence of the ramus cutaneous N. radialis. J Anat Physiol 46(89):1911–1912.
2. Barber KW Jr, Biano AJ Jr, Soule EH, et al.: Benign extramural soft tissue tumors of the extremities causing compression of nerves. J Bone Joint Surg 1962;48(A):98.
3. Bayerl W, Fischer K: The pronator teres syndrome. J Chir 1979;11(2):91.
4. Bielawski M, Hallet M: Position of the elbow in determination of abnormal motor conduction of the ulnar nerve across the elbow. Muscle Nerve 1989;12:803.
5. Bowen TL, Stone KH: Posterior interosseous nerve paralysis caused by a ganglion at the elbow. J Bone Joint Surg 1966;48(B):774.
6. Braidwood AS: Superficial radial neuropathy. J Bone Joint Surg 1975;57(B):380.
7. Campbell WW, Pridgeon RM, Sahni KS: Short segment incremental studies in the evaluation of ulnar neuropathy at the elbow. Muscle Nerve 1992; 15:1050–1054.
8. Checkles NS, Russakov AD, Piero DL: Ulnar nerve conduction velocity: Effect of elbow position on measurement. Arch Phys Med Rehabil 1971;52:362.
9. Childress HM: Recurrent ulnar nerve dislocation at the elbow. J Bone Joint Surg 1956;38(A):978.
10. Clark K, Williams P, Willis W, et al.: Injection injury of the sciatic nerve. Clin Neurosurg 1960; 17:111–125.

11. Dharapak C, Numberg GA: Posterior interosseus nerve of the forearm. J Bone Joint Surg 1966; 48(B):770.

12. Dubi J, Regli F, Bischoff A: Recurrent familial neuropathy with liability to pressure palsies. J Neurol 220:43,199.

13. Ebeling P, Gilliatt RW, Thomas PK: The clinical and electrical study of ulnar nerve lesion in the hand. J Neurol Neurosurg Psychiatry 1960;23:1.

14. Eckman PB, Perlstein G, Altrocchi PH: Ulnar neuropathy in bicycle riders. Arch Neurol 32:1304, 1975.

15. Edwards WG, Lincoln CR, Bassett FH: The tarsal tunnel syndrome: Diagnosis and treatment. JAMA 1969;207:716.

16. Eisen A: Early diagnosis of ulnar nerve palsy: An electrophysiologic study. Neurology 1974;24:256.

17. England JD, Sumner AJ: Neuralgic amyotrophy: An increasingly diverse entity. Muscle Nerve 1987; 10:60.

18. Esselman PC, Tomski MA, Robinson LR, et al.: Selective deep peroneal nerve injury associated with arthroscopic knee surgery. Muscle Nerve 1993;16:1188–1192.

19. Feindel W, Stratford V: Role of the cubital tunnel in tardy ulnar palsy. Can J Surg 1957;1:287.

20. Francis H, Nearch L, Terentz T, et al.: Benign joint hypermobility with neuropathy: Documentation and mechanism of tarsal tunnel syndrome. J Rheumatol 1987;14:577.

21. Goodgold J, Kopell HP, Speilholz NI: The tarsal tunnel syndrome. N Engl J Med 1965;273:742.

22. Gudmendsson GH, Pilgoard S: Prevention of sciatic nerve entrapment in trochanteric wiring following total hip arthroplasty. Clin Orthop 1985;196:215.

23. Gutmann L: AAEM Minimonograph #2: Important anomalous innervations of the extremities. Muscle Nerve 1993;16:339–347.

24. Gutmann L: Atypical deep peroneal neuropathy in presence of accessory deep peroneal nerve. J Neurol Neurosurg Psychiatry 1970;33:453.

25. Hagert CG: Entrapment of the posterior interosseous nerve, causing forearm pain. In: Proceedings of the Scandinavian Society for Surgery of the Hand. J Hand Surg 1977;2:486.

26. Hartz CR, Linscheid RL, Gramse RR, et al.: The pronator teres syndrome: Compressive neuropathy of the median nerve. J Bone Joint Surg 1981; 63(A):885.

27. Henderson M, Robinson LR: Dorsal ulnar cutaneous handcuff neuropathy. Muscle Nerve 1991; 14:905–906.

28. Jabre JF, Wilbourn AJ: The EMG findings in 100 consecutive ulnar neuropathies. Acta Neurol Scand 1979;60 (Suppl):73:91.

29. Johnson RK, Spinner M, Shrewsbury MM: Median nerve entrapment syndrome in the proximal forearm. J Hand Surg 1979;4:48.

30. Kanakamedala RV, Hong C-Z: Peroneal nerve entrapment at the knee localized by short segment stimulation. Am J Phys Med Rehabil 1989; 68:116–122.

31. Kanakamamedala RV, Simons DG, Porter RW, et al.: Ulnar nerve entrapment at the elbow localized by short segment stimulation. Arch Phys Med Rehabil 1988;69:959.

32. Kaplan PO: Posterior interosseous neuropathies: Natural history. Arch Phys Med Rehabil 1984; 65:399.

33. Katirji MB, Wilbourn AJ: Common peroneal mononeuropathy: A clinical and electrophysiological study of 116 lesions. Neurology 1988;38:1723.

34. Kiloh LG, Nevin S: Isolated neuritis of the anterior interosseous nerve. BMJ 1952;1:850.

35. Kimura J, Machida M, Ishida T, et al.: Relation between size of compound sensory or muscle action potentials and length of nerve segment. Neurology 1986;36:647–652.

36. Kincaid JC: AAEE Minimonograph #31: The electrodiagnosis of ulnar neuropathy at the elbow. Muscle Nerve 1988;11:1005–1015.

37. Kopell HP, Thompson WAL: Peripheral entrapment neuropathies. Baltimore: Williams & Wilkins, 1963.

38. Kraft GH: Fibrillation potential amplitude and muscle atrophy following peripheral nerve injury. Muscle Nerve 1990;13:814–821.

39. Laha RK, Dujovny M, DeCastro C: Entrapment of median nerve by supracondylar process of the humerus. J Neurosurg 1977;46:252.

40. Lederman RJ, Breuer AC, Hanson MR, et al.: Peripheral nervous system complications of coronary artery bypass surgery. Ann Neurol 1982;12:297–301.

41. Lister GD, Belsole RB, Kleivert HE: The radial tunnel syndrome. J Hand Surg 1979;4:52.

42. MacKinnon SE, Dellon AL: The overlap pattern of the lateral antebrachial cutaneous nerve and the superficial branch of the radial nerve. J Hand Surg 1985;10(A):522.

43. Marmar L, Lawrence JF, Dubois E: Posterior interosseous nerve paralysis due to rheumatoid arthritis. J Bone Joint Surg 1967;49(A):381.

44. Masear VR, Hill JJ, Cohen SM: Ulnar compression neuropathy secondary to the anconeus epitrochlearis muscle. J Hand Surg 1988;12(A):720.

45. Massey EW, Pleet AB: Handcuffs and cheiralgia paresthetica. Neurology 1978;28:1312.

46. Millender LH, Nalebuff EA, Holdsworth DE: Posterior interosseous nerve syndrome secondary to rheumatoid synovitis. J Bone Joint Surg 1973;55(A):753.

47. Miller RG: The cubital tunnel syndrome: Diagnosis and precise localization. Ann Neurol 1979;6:56.

48. Miller RG: AAEE Minimonograph #28: Injury to peripheral motor nerves. Muscle Nerve 1987; 10:698–710.

49. Moon N, Marmor L: Parosteal lipoma of the proximal part of the radius. J Bone Joint Surg 1964; 46(A):608.

50. Nakano KK, Lundergan C, Okihiro MM: Anterior interosseous nerve syndromes. Arch Neurol 1977;34:477.

51. Noth J, Dietz V, Mauritz HK: Cyclist's palsy. J Neurol Sci 1980;47:111.

52. O'Brien MD, Upton ARM: Anterior interosseous nerve syndrome: A case report with neurophysiolog-

ical investigation. J Neurol Neurosurg Psychiatry 1972;35:531.

53. Oh SJ, Kim HS, Ahmad BK: The near-nerve sensory nerve conduction in tarsal tunnel syndrome. J Neurol Neurosurg Psychiatry 1985;48:999–1003.

54. Packer JW, Foster RR, Garcia A, et al.: The humeral fracture with radial nerve palsy: Is exploration warranted? Clin Orthop 1972;88:34.

55. Parsonage MJ, Turner JW: Neuralgic amyotrophy: The shoulder girdle syndrome. Lancet 1948;1:973.

56. Payan J: Electrophysiological localization of ulnar nerve lesions. J Neurol Neurosurg Psychiatry 1969;32:208.

57. Pezina M: Contribution to the etiological explanation of the piriformis syndrome. Acta Anat 1979;105:181.

58. Rask MR: Anterior interosseous nerve entrapment (Kiloh-Nevin syndrome). Clin Orthop 1979; 142:176.

59. Redford JB: Nerve conduction in motor fibers to the anterior tibial muscle in peroneal palsy. Arch Phys Med Rehabil 1964;45:500.

60. Roles NC, Maudsley RH: Radial tunnel syndrome: Resistant tennis elbow as a nerve entrapment. J Bone Joint Surg 1972;54(B):499.

61. Saeed MA, Gatens PF: Compound nerve action potentials of the medial and lateral plantar nerves through the tarsal tunnel. Arch Phys Med Rehabil 1982;63:304–307.

62. Sandhu HD, Sandberg BS: Occupational compression of the common peroneal nerve at the neck of the fibula. Aust NZ J Surg 1976;46:160.

63. Seyfer AE, Nadja YG, Bogumill GP, et al.: Upper extremity neuropathies after cardiac surgery. J Hand Surg 1985;10(A):16–19.

64. Shea JD, McClain EJ: Ulnar nerve compression syndrome at and below the wrist. J Bone Joint Surg 1969;51(A):1095.

65. Sherman DG, Eason JD: Dieting and peroneal nerve palsy. JAMA 1977;238:230.

66. Simpson JA: Electrical signs in the diagnosis of carpal tunnel and related syndromes. J Neurol Neurosurg Psychiatry 1956;19:275.

67. Singh N, Behse F, Buchthal F: Electrophysiological study of peroneal palsy. J Neurol Neurosurg Psychiatry 1974;37:1202.

68. Spindler HA, Reischer RA, Felsenthal G: Electrodiagnostic assessment in suspected tarsal tunnel syndrome. In: Physical medicine and rehabilitation clinics of North America: New developments in electrodiagnostic medicine 1994;5(3):595.

69. Spinner M: Injuries to the major branches of peripheral nerves of the forearm. 2nd ed. Philadelphia: WB Saunders, 1978.

70. Stewart JD: The variable clinical manifestations of ulnar neuropathies at the elbow. J Neurol Neurosurg Psychiatry 1987;50:252.

71. Stopford JSB: Neuritis produced by a wristlet watch. Lancet 1922;1:993.

72. Sunderland S: Nerves and nerve injuries. 2nd ed. Edinburgh: Churchill-Livingstone, 1968.

73. Tackmann W, Vogel P, Kaeser HE, et al.: Sensitivity and localizing significance of motor and sensory electroneurographic parameters in the diagnosis of ulnar nerve lesions at the elbow. J Neurol 1984;231:204.

74. Terry RJ: A study of the spuracondyloid process in the living. Am J Phys Anthropol 1921;4:129.

75. Weber ER, Daube JR, Coventry MB: Peripheral neuropathies associated with total hip arthroplasty. J Bone Joint Surg 1976;58(A):66.

76. Werner CO: Lateral elbow pain and posterior interosseous nerve entrapment. Acta Orthop Scand, Supplementum 1979;174:1.

77. Wertsch JJ: AAEM Case Report #25: Anterior interosseous nerve syndrome. Muscle Nerve 1992; 15:977–983.

78. Wertsch JJ, Melvin J: Median nerve anatomy and entrapment syndromes: A review. Arch Phys Med Rehabil 1982;63:623–627.

Chapter 11

Assessment of the Brachial Plexus and the Phrenic Nerve

Asa J. Wilbourn

BRACHIAL PLEXUS ASSESSMENT

A 6-week-old girl has demonstrated marked right shoulder girdle weakness since her birth. Diagnosis: obstetric paralysis. A 15-year-old boy has experienced transient burning dysesthesia and weakness of his entire left upper extremity for several weeks, whenever he has been struck forcibly on the head or left shoulder during football games. Diagnosis: burner syndrome. A 22-year-old man has had a very painful, anesthetic, flail right upper extremity and a right Horner's syndrome since he was involved in a motorcycle accident 2 years ago. Diagnosis: extensive avulsion injury. A 30-year-old woman who has had intermittent mild aching along her left medial forearm and hand for many years was recently noted to have weakness and wasting of that hand, particularly of the lateral thenar imminence; cervical spine x-rays have revealed a rudimentary cervical rib on the left side. Diagnosis: true neurogenic thoracic outlet syndrome. A 41-year-old woman awoke after undergoing a cholecystectomy 8 weeks ago with bilateral shoulder girdle weakness and paresthesias along the lateral forearms; her symptoms have decreased considerably over the past 2 weeks. Diagnosis: "classic" postoperative paralysis. A 53-year-old man has experienced right-hand weakness and progressive pain in his right shoulder, radiating down the medial forearm to the hand, for the last 4 months; he has an ipsilateral Horner's syndrome, and a recent chest x-ray showed a small density at the apex of the right lung, along with a bony obstruc-

tion of the nearby first rib and vertebrae. Diagnosis: Pancoast's syndrome. A 64-year-old woman has experienced slowly progressive paresthesias, sensory loss, and weakness of her left upper extremity for the last several years; she underwent radiation for left breast cancer 10 years ago. Diagnosis: radiation-induced brachial plexopathy. A 75-year-old man has been unable to elevate his right upper extremity from his side since he fell and dislocated his right shoulder 2 months ago; the dislocation was successfully reduced the day of injury, and the rotator cuff was not torn. Diagnosis: infraclavicular plexopathy involving the axillary terminal nerve.

Even though each of the above clinical vignettes has a different diagnostic label, they all are due to abnormalities of the same peripheral nervous system (PNS) structure: the brachial plexus. This series of cases illustrates several points about brachial plexopathies. First, they occur in persons of all ages, unlike many other PNS disorders, which tend to be limited to certain age ranges. Second, they affect persons of either gender; and although some subgroups have an approximately equal gender incidence (e.g., obstetric paralysis), others have a marked tendency to affect just men (e.g., avulsion injuries), or just women (e.g., radiation-induced plexopathy). Third, they have a remarkable variety of causes. Although closed trauma is the most common etiology, virtually every process known to affect any other localized portion of the PNS has been reported to affect the brachial plexus as well, ranging from neoplasms and radiation to gunshot wounds and lacerations to compartment syndromes and malpositioning on the operating table. Fourth, their presentations can be strikingly diverse. They can affect one or both forequarters and, if bilateral, they can be symmetric or asymmetric. Their major symptoms include weakness, sensory loss, paresthesias, pain, or any combination thereof. Their onset timing ranges from very abrupt to very slow. Their severity may extend from being a minor annoyance (e.g., paresthesias restricted to the index finger with early radiation-induced brachial plexopathy) to a major disability (e.g., a flail, anesthetic, and painful limb with multiple root avulsions). Their clinical course can be maximal at onset followed by no, slow, or rapid improvement; rapidly or slowly progressive; or stepwise. Finally, their recovery potential, regardless of the severity of initial weakness and sensory loss, ranges from no recovery to complete recovery (37).

Brachial plexopathies are relatively common PNS lesions that can present in a myriad of ways and often are mistaken for other, more frequently occurring upper extremity disorders. Consequently, almost every electromyographer will encounter them. Therefore, the optimal electrodiagnostic (EDX) assessment of brachial plexopathies is important. Before we discuss this, however, we will review the anatomy and characteristic pathophysiologic responses to injury of the brachial plexus.

Anatomy

The brachial plexus is a large PNS structure extending from the base of the neck to the axilla, through which passes the nerve supply to essentially the entire upper limb and much of the shoulder girdle. A rather stereotyped description of the brachial plexus appears in anatomy textbooks. They report that it consists of five components: 1) Five roots: the C5 through T1 ventral primary rami (VPR); 2) Three trunks: upper, middle, and lower; 3) Six divisions: three anterior and three posterior; 4) Three cords: lateral, posterior, and medial; 5) Various—three to five—terminal nerves, which are the very proximal portions of the major nerves that arise from the cords of the brachial plexus (7,8,46) (Fig. 11–1). In contrast to the anatomists' concept of the brachial plexus, surgeons who deal extensively with brachial plexopathies have a somewhat different perspective. First, they disagree with the anatomists concerning what constitutes the "roots" of the bracial plexus. Rather than restricting its most proximal component to the C5 through T1 VPR, which are completely extraforaminal structures, they also include the C5–T1 ventral and dorsal primary roots, arising from the spinal cord, as well as the C5–T1 mixed spinal nerves, formed by fusion of the primary roots. Thus, the surgeons con-

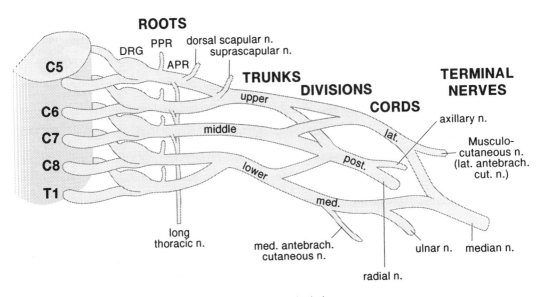

Figure 11–1. Brachial plexus.

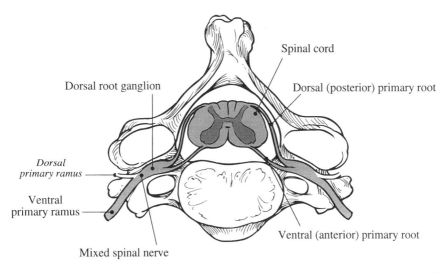

Figure 11-2. Components of the first portion of the brachial plexus, the roots, as envisioned by brachial plexus surgeons. Anatomists include only the ventral primary rami under this designation (see text).

sider the "roots" to be more extensive structures, and they envision the most proximal portion of the plexus to be within the intraspinal canal (Fig. 11–2). This is why they classify avulsion injuries, i.e., the "tearing away" by severe traction of one or more of the primary roots from the spinal cord, as "brachial plexopathies."

Second, these surgeons clinically subdivide the brachial plexus in a manner that is often unmentioned in anatomy texts. Because, when the arm is at the side, the clavicle overlies the third component of the brachial plexus (the divisions), they subdivide the brachial plexus into "supraclavicular" and "infraclavicular." The supraclavicular plexus consists of the primary roots, the VPR, and trunks, whereas the infraclavicular plexus consists of the cords and terminal nerves; lesions involving these particular areas are labeled "supraclavicular plexopathies" and "infraclavicular plexopathies," respectively (Fig. 11–3). (Although it would have been more logical to refer to these two plexus regions as "supradivisional" and "infradivisional," such designations are never used.) Lesions of the divisions themselves, i.e., "subclavicular" or "retroclavicular" plexopathies, are mentioned infrequently, because they seldom occur in isolation; e.g., even with traumatic clavicular fractures, the supraclavicular plexus elements usually sustain far more

traction damage than do the divisional elements.

Third, plexus surgeons further apportion supraclavicular plexopathies based on both their longitudinal and their vertical locations. Longitudinally, they subdivide these lesions into "preganglionic" (also referred to as "supraganglionic" or "intradural") and "postganglionic" (also referred to as "infraganglionic," "extradural," or "extraforaminal"). These designations literally apply only to the location of the lesions along the sensory fibers in relation to their dorsal root ganglia (DRG), but conventionally they are used to describe lesions of both the sensory and motor axons occurring either within the intraspinal canal or external to it. The surgeons also subdivide supraclavicular plexopathies in a vertical fashion. This is because it frequently is difficult with some plexopathies, particularly those caused by violent trauma, to determine on the initial evaluation which supraclavicular components—the primary roots, mixed spinal nerves, VPR, or trunks—sustained injury. Thus, depending upon whether the abnormalities are in the distribution of fibers derived from the C5 and C6 roots, the C7 root, or the C8 and T1 roots, the surgeons subclassify supraclavicular plexopathies as "upper plexus lesions," "middle plexus lesions," and "lower plexus lesions" (Fig. 11–4). Although these

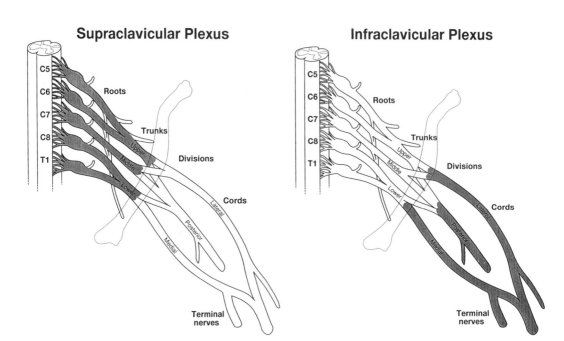

Figure 11–3. Supraclavicular and infraclavicular plexus. The former consists of the *C5–T1* roots (primary roots, mixed spinal nerves, ventral primary rami) and the trunks. The latter consists of the cords and terminal nerves.

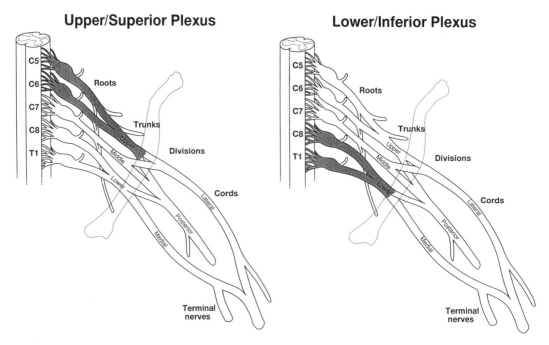

Figure 11–4. Upper and lower plexus portions of the supraclavicular plexus. (The middle plexus portion is not darkened.)

terms are deliberately indefinite in regard to specific lesion sites, they facilitate communication (1,19,20,24,32).

FIVE ROOTS OF THE BRACHIAL PLEXUS

In this and the following sections, the "roots" of the brachial plexus will be considered in their expanded sense (i.e., as envisioned by brachial plexus surgeons). Therefore, they consist of a) the C5, C6, C7, C8, and T1 dorsal and ventral primary roots, which arise from the spinal cord and are situated within the intraspinal canal; the cell bodies for the peripheral sensory fibers are in the DRG, which are located along the very distal end of the dorsal roots, immediately before they fuse with the ventral roots to form mixed spinal nerves; b) the C5 through T1 mixed spinal nerves, which are located within the intervertebral foramina; c) the C5 through T1 VPR, which originate when the mixed spinal nerves, soon after exiting the intervertebral foramina, terminate by dividing into ventral and dorsal primary rami; the VPR are situated between the scalenus anticus and the scalenus medius muscles, deep in the inferior lateral aspect of the neck, beneath the sternocleidomastoid muscle(8,39,46) (Fig. 11–2).

Two points regarding the roots that contribute to the brachial plexus require discussion. First, among the various anomalies of the brachial plexus, one of the most frequently mentioned is its root contributions. Often, the C4 or the T2 root supplies small branches to the brachial plexus. Occasionally, the C4 root contribution is considerable whereas that from the T1 root is reduced, resulting in a "pre-fixed" plexus; in other instances the situation is reversed, with a contribution from the T2 root being substantial and that from the C5 root being correspondingly reduced, resulting in the "post-fixed" plexus. Moreover, at times both the C4 and the T2 root contributions are relatively large, resulting in the root origin of the brachial plexus expanding rather than shifting superiorly or inferiorly. A debate exists about how much clinical impact these anomalies actually have, in part because of their relatively low incidence (1,17,20,37).

The second point is that because of structural differences, the primary roots within the intraspinal canal are much more vulnerable to traction forces than are the more distal portions of the brachial plexus: the fibers composing the primary roots are short (particularly those of C5 through C7); the roots lack epineural and perineural sheaths; and they are arranged in parallel bundles, rather than in a lattice network. Compared to the C8 and T1 roots, the 5th, 6th, and 7th roots are under tension at rest and are therefore more readily injured by traction forces. Nonetheless, their most proximal portions are more protected from severe traction injuries than are those of the C8 and T1 primary roots because they are secured immediately upon leaving the foramen (in the gutter of their transverse processes) by their epineural sheaths, the prevertebral fascia, and various fibrous slips and musculotendinous attachments of the transverse processes. In contrast, both the C8 and T1 roots lack these anchors. Consequently, traction placed upon them is transmitted centripetally to the primary roots, and thus they are relatively much more susceptible to avulsion injuries (34). This explains the somewhat paradoxical fact that although, overall, the C5 through C7 roots are more commonly injured by traction, they are avulsed less often than are the C8 and T1 roots whenever severe traction injuries occur.

Several motor nerve branches arise from the VPR. From proximal to distal, these include 1) From the C5 through C8 VPR, very close to where they exit from the intervertebral foramina, the nerves to the scalene muscles and the longus colli; 2) From the C5, C6, and C7 VPR, the fibers that compose the long thoracic nerve, which innervates the serratus anterior muscle; 3) From the C5 VPR, the most caudal contribution to the phrenic nerve, that supplies the diaphragm; 4) From the C5 VPR, the dorsal scapular nerve that innervates the rhomboid major, rhomboid minor and, partially, the levator scapulae. No somatic nerve fibers arise from the T1 VPR. However, the preganglionic sympathetic fibers that supply the ipsilateral head and neck are situated in the C8 and T1 mixed spinal nerves. Almost as soon as the latter exit the intervertebral foramina and terminate as ventral and dorsal primary rami, these autonomic fibers pass to the inferior cervical ganglion through a white ramus communicans. They can be interrupted by very proximal C8 and T1 root lesions (i.e., of the primary roots or mixed spinal nerves), causing ipsilateral miosis, ptosis head vasodilatation, and anhydrosis (Horner's syndrome). Conversely, if the distal C8 and T1 roots, i.e., the C8 and T1 VPR, are injured, the sympathetic fibers for the ipsilateral head are not affected, whereas the bulk of the postganglionic sympathetic fibers destined for the arm, and particularly the hand, are compromised (8,34,37,46).

THREE TRUNKS OF THE BRACHIAL PLEXUS

The three trunks—upper, middle, and lower—are named for their relationship to one another. The C5 and C6 VPR fuse to form the upper trunk; the C7 VPR continues as the middle trunk; and the C8 and T1 VPR join together to form the lower trunk. The trunks begin near the lateral border of the scalene muscles and are situated in the anteroinferior portion of the posterior triangle of the neck. Their more distal portions, located in the supraclavicular fossa, are relatively superficial and so are vulnerable to external injury. The lower trunk is near the subclavian artery and the apex of the lung. Two peripheral nerves arise from the plexus at the trunk level. Both nerves arise at or near the origin of the very proximal upper trunk: 1) the subclavian nerve, which innervates the subclavian muscle; and 2) the suprascapular nerve, which innervates the supraspinatus and infraspinatus muscles. No branches arise from either the middle trunk or the lower trunk (8,39,46).

The trunk region is important to electromyographers because the brachial plexus can be stimulated percutaneously no further proximal than the midtrunk level. Consequently, focal conduction blocks situated proximal to that level cannot be definitely localized by standard motor nerve conduction studies (NCS), whereas those located distal to it can be. All percutaneous plexus stimulation at the mid-trunk level frequently and incorrectly is referred to as "Erb's point stimulation." In fact, "Erb's point" refers to a specific small area at the base of the neck that overlies the site where the C5 and C6 VPR join to form the

upper trunk (2,5). Consequently, it is "Erb's point stimulation" only if motor NCS responses are being recorded from C5, C6-innervated muscles, e.g., the biceps or deltoid muscles. If the trunk is being stimulated to activate ulnar or median motor hand fibers, as it typically is, terms such as "trunk stimulation" or "supraclavicular stimulation" more accurately describe the stimulation site.

SIX DIVISIONS OF THE BRACHIAL PLEXUS

The six divisions are formed when each of the three trunks divides into an anterior and a posterior division. Anatomically, the divisions are between the mid portion of the clavicle in front and the first rib behind. No nerve branches arise from the divisions and they are injured less often than the other brachial plexus components. The divisions are very important for two reasons. First, at this level the axons that will supply the ventral and the dorsal aspects of the upper extremity separate from one another. Consequently, proximal to the divisions, each plexus element contains motor fibers that will ultimately innervate both extensor and flexor muscles, whereas distal to the divisions each plexus element essentially contains motor fibers that will innervate either one or the other type of muscle group. Second, as noted, when the arm is at the side the clavicle overlies the divisions, so that anatomically the brachial plexus can be considered under two broad subgroups: the supraclavicular plexus and the infraclavicular plexus (8,20,39).

Supraclavicularly, the brachial plexus fibers are arranged in a segmental fashion, excluding the few named peripheral nerves that arise from the VPR and the upper trunk. Consequently, supraclavicular plexopathies typically produce motor and sensory deficits in the distribution of one or more spinal cord segments (i.e., in myotome and dermatome distributions), and clinically they often are mistaken for radiculopathies. The segmental character of the brachial plexus is lost distal to the divisions so that infraclavicular plexopathies typically involve various components of one or more peripheral nerves. Consequently, infraclavicular plexopathies readily are mistaken clinically for more distal peripheral nerve lesions, particularly when only one terminal nerve is affected (17,39).

Subdividing lesions of the brachial plexus into "supraclavicular plexopathies" and "infraclavicular plexopathies" has clinical relevance because lesions at these different levels differ significantly in incidence, severity, and prognosis for both etiologic and anatomic reasons. Supraclavicular plexopathies are the more common of the two; in several large series, more than 60% of all brachial plexopathies involved the supraclavicular plexus. Moreover, severe supraclavicular lesions are less likely to recover completely than are infraclavicular ones, partly because of the differing nature of the injuries that produced them. Brachial plexopathies frequently can be classified as either supraclavicular or infraclavicular based on their etiology alone (Table 11–1) (1,20,24).

THREE CORDS OF THE BRACHIAL PLEXUS

The anterior divisions of the upper and middle trunks join to form the lateral cord, while the anterior division of the lower trunk continues as the medial cord. All three posterior divisions fuse to form the posterior cord. The cords are located in the apex of the axilla, where they are closely associated with the second portion of the axillary artery; each cord is named for its position relative to that arterial segment. The cords are the longest of all the plexus components, and from them originate all the major peripheral nerves that supply the upper extremity (as opposed to the shoulder girdle) (8,39,46).

Because of the intimate relationship between the axillary artery and the cords, coexisting involvement of both, i.e., neurovascular lesions, is common. Moreover, the cords are near some of the axillary lymph nodes and thus often are the first plexus component that manifests abnormalities with radiation-induced plexopathy.

The lateral cord fibers derive from the C5, C6, and C7 roots, through the upper and middle trunks and the upper two anterior divisions. Distally, they form the musculocutaneous nerve and the lateral head of the median

Table 11–1
The Portion of the Brachial Plexus Most Affected by Brachial Plexopathies

Supraclavicular Plexopathies

   Closed traction lesions (violent trauma)

   Obstetrical paralysis

   "Classic" postanesthesia paralysis

   Burner syndrome

   Metastatic plexus lesions

   Postmedian sternotomy plexopathies

   True neurogenic TOS

   Post disputed neurogenic TOS surgery

   Penetrating injuries

Infraclavicular Plexopathies

   Lesions 2° to:

      Humeral head fractures/dislocations

      Attempted humeral head reductions

      Other orthopedic procedures

   Radiation-induced plexopathies

   Compartment syndromes 2° to:

      Axillary anteriograms

      Axillary plexus blocks

      Penetrating injuries

      Blunt trauma

   Penetrating injuries

   Blunt trauma

Note that the plexus, particularly the infraclavicular portion, can be injured by penetrating injuries and blunt trauma both directly and indirectly; with the latter, the blood vessels sustain initial damage and then produce compartment syndromes.

nerve. The lateral cord contains all the axons that traverse the more distal upper and middle trunks, excluding those that exit at the division level to join the posterior cord via the upper two posterior divisions. The posterior cord is composed of axons that traverse the C5 through C8 roots, all three trunks, and all three posterior divisions. Four peripheral nerves arise from the posterior cord: the subscapular, thoracodorsal, axillary, and radial nerves. The axons forming the medial cord derive from the C8 and T1 roots, through the lower trunk and the lower anterior division. Distally, these axons form the medial brachial and medial antebrachial cutaneous nerves, the ulnar nerve, and the medial head of the median nerve. The medial cord primarily is a continuation of the lower trunk, minus the C8 component of the radial nerve that departed in the lower posterior division to join the posterior cord (8,17,46).

The lateral pectoral and medial pectoral nerves originate from the proximal lateral and medial cords, respectively, near the points where the latter arise from the divisions. Branches of the lateral and medial pectoral nerves fuse, permitting both nerves to provide innervation to the pectoralis muscles (8,46).

TERMINAL BRANCHES OF THE BRACHIAL PLEXUS

Three to five of the peripheral nerves (the exact number varying with the anatomy textbook source) that arise from the cords are designated the "terminal nerves" of the brachial plexus: the median, ulnar, radial, and sometimes musculocutaneous and axillary nerves (7,8,46). Although all anatomy books list the terminal nerves as being the most distal component of the brachial plexus, none provides an answer to the following question. "How long a segment of each of these peripheral nerves, after it originates from a cord, can be considered a portion of the brachial plexus; i.e., exactly where is the dividing line, proximal to which it is designated a part of the brachial plexus, and distal to which it is simply a peripheral nerve trunk?" Presumably only Narakas, a well-known peripheral nerve surgeon, has made a definite statement on this point: Those portions of these peripheral nerves "at their origin and a few centimeters below" constitute the most distal portion of the brachial plexus. Thus, very proximal lesions of these peripheral nerve trunks are classified as "infraclavicular plexopathies," even when only one of them, such as the axillary or the median nerve, is affected (24).

PATHOLOGY/ PATHOPHYSIOLOGY

The axons that compose the brachial plexus can be damaged by an almost infinite variety of injurious agents. Nonetheless, their pathologic responses and even more so their patho-

physiologic responses to such trauma are limited. Essentially, the myelinated fibers—the only nerve fibers assessed in the EDX laboratory—have two primary responses to focal trauma, whereas the unmyelinated fibers have only one. Regardless of etiology, if a lesion is severe enough it causes axon degeneration that affects the nerve fiber not only at the localized point of injury but also along its entire segment distal to that site; both large myelinated fibers and small unmyelinated nerve fibers undergo axon degeneration whenever they are sufficiently traumatized. Discrete lesions of lesser severity can affect the myelinated fibers in a different manner, by producing focal demyelination that is restricted to the lesion site; thus, in contrast to what occurs with axon loss, the segment of nerve fiber distal to the point of injury remains intact. Focal myelin damage can result in a focal disturbance of conduction limited to the affected portion of the nerve fiber, manifested as either conduction slowing or conduction block depending upon the degree of myelin compromise (25,39,43).

Axon Loss/Axon Degeneration and Focal Demyelination

AXON LOSS/AXON DEGENERATION

With the majority of brachial plexopathies, particularly those of more than a few weeks duration, axon loss is the underlying pathology. It typically involves both myelinated and unmyelinated fibers and can affect any percentage (from 1% to 100%) of the axons composing any brachial plexus element. In most instances, it is the sole type of pathology present, e.g., with avulsion injuries and neoplastic plexopathies. In a minority of patients, it coexists with focal demyelination, characteristically manifested as conduction block. Examples of this type of plexopathy include many traumatic plexopathies (including those of iatrogenic origin) early in their course, most radiation-induced plexopathies, and the rarely encountered multifocal conduction block syndrome.

Even though a process causing axon loss may directly injure only a very small longitudinal portion of the brachial plexus (e.g., a transection of the lower trunk by a scalpel), its effects never remain so localized because the entire nerve segment peripheral to the lesion site undergoes wallerian degeneration. When sufficient axons degenerate, both clinical and electrodiagnostic signs occur. Clinical deficits include muscle paresis or paralysis, sensory loss involving all modalities (including pain and temperature sensation mediated over unmyelinated and lightly myelinated fibers), and autonomic disturbances. Axon segments that have undergone wallerian degeneration manifest conduction failure and can neither be activated by nerve stimuli nor transmit impulses from more proximal, viable segments of nerve with which they are continuous. Consequently, on NCS, axon loss lesions affect almost solely the amplitudes of the responses. Generally, they do not substantially alter either the latencies or the nerve conduction velocities (NCVs), because the latter are being determined along the surviving fibers, which are conducting at their normal rate. Nonetheless, the distal latencies may be mildly prolonged and the NCVs slightly slowed with severe but incomplete lesions of recent onset, owing to loss of the fastest conducting fibers, and with very remote, complete lesions, owing to the regenerating axons having a smaller diameter and a thinner myelin sheath (39).

The Effect of Axon Loss on NCS Amplitudes

Three points regarding axon loss and its effect on NCS amplitudes are pertinent in regard to brachial plexopathies. First, the amplitudes of the motor NCS responses, the compound muscle action potentials (CMAPs), can be decreased by lesions located at any point along the motor axon, up to and including its cell body of origin located within the anterior horn of the spinal cord. In contrast, the amplitudes of the sensory NCS responses, the sensory nerve action potentials (SNAPs), are affected only by those axon loss lesions located at or distal to the DRG, where their cell bodies of origin reside. Thus, a focal injury of any portion of the brachial plexus, if it produces enough axon loss, will affect the CMAP amplitudes. However, only those injuries located interforaminally or extraforaminally will alter the SNAP amplitudes, i.e., the SNAP amplitudes will not decrease with lesions involving the dorsal sensory roots proximal to the DRG, such as avulsion injuries.

Second, with incomplete axon-loss brachial plexopathies located inter- or extraforaminally, the SNAP amplitudes often are more severely affected than are the corresponding CMAP amplitudes. With moderate axon loss lesions, for example, the amplitudes of the sensory NCS that assess the involved fibers frequently will be low, whereas the corresponding motor NCS amplitudes will still be within the normal range. With more severe axon loss, the sensory NCS responses often become unelicitable at a time when the motor NCS responses are still present but low in amplitude. Why this amplitude dissociation occurs is unknown, but its practical effect is that the SNAP amplitudes generally are the most sensitive component of the motor and sensory NCS for detecting axon loss. For this reason, extensive sensory NCS often are indicated whenever a brachial plexopathy is suspected. Moreover, with mild, unilateral brachial plexopathies, it often is of benefit to perform at least some sensory NCS bilaterally so that the results from the two limbs can be compared; this is particularly helpful when a critical sensory NCS performed on the symptomatic limb yields a SNAP of borderline low amplitude. When sensory NCS are performed bilaterally, a SNAP amplitude of 50% or less than that of the corresponding one obtained from the contralateral, normal limb is considered abnormal, even when it is within the normal range of values for the EMG laboratory.

Third, with abrupt-onset brachial plexopathies, as with abrupt-onset peripheral nerve lesions in general, the NCS results are unreliable until, if axon loss has occurred, the distal stump fibers have had time to degenerate and cease to conduct impulses. When sufficient motor axon loss occurs, the CMAP amplitudes begin to drop on the second or third day but do not reach their nadir until 7 days after injury. Conversely, the SNAP amplitudes do not begin to drop until day five post-injury, and do not reach their nadir until 10 or 11 days after lesion onset. Hence, the results of the NCS can be misleading with proximal axon loss lesions, such as plexopathies, if studies are performed along the distal segments of the affected nerve fibers before conduction failure supervenes. For example, 6 days after a moderately severe, axon-loss lower trunk plexus lesion is sustained, the ulnar and median CMAPs will be low in amplitude but the ulnar SNAP amplitude will still be nearly unchanged, even though ultimately the SNAP will be much smaller. Based on these misleading interim NCS results, the patient may mistakenly be considered to have an avulsion injury when, in fact, the lesion is extraforaminal (38,39).

The changes in the NCS amplitudes that occur with conduction failure correlate highly with the clinical symptoms of muscle weakness and loss of sensory modalities mediated over large myelinated fibers. This correlation is particularly impressive for motor nerves, at least with lesions of recent onset (i.e., those lesions studied before substantial collateral sprouting has had time to occur). If the CMAP amplitude is approximately half of normal, for example, then the strength of the recorded muscle, on clinical testing, usually is about half of normal (grade 4). If, instead, no motor NCS response can be elicited, the recorded muscle usually is paralyzed or nearly so. Whenever a muscle appears clinically to be much weaker than the CMAP amplitude recorded from it suggests that it should be, the possibility that some of the weakness is due to proximal demyelinating conduction block, rather than to axon loss, must always be considered (see Demyelination Conduction Block, below).

The needle electrode examination (NEE) with axon-loss brachial plexopathies can reveal fibrillation potentials, motor unit potential (MUP) dropout, suggestive reinnervational MUPs, and chronic neurogenic MUPs, depending upon the severity and duration of the lesion and, if it is progressive, upon how active it is at the time of the EDX study.

The Needle Electrode Examination and Axon Loss

Several points regarding the NEE and axon loss need to be emphasized. First, because fibrillation potentials may require up to 3 weeks to appear in denervated muscles, performing NEEs on plexus lesions of 1 or 2 weeks' dura-

tion can yield very misleading results. Second, the density of fibrillation potentials seen in a denervated muscle often is a poor indicator of the severity of axon loss present. For example, a severely denervated muscle—as determined by its clinical weakness and by it generating a very low CMAP amplitude during motor NCS—may show only a moderate number of fibrillation potentials, even when the NEE is performed 3 to 6 weeks after injury onset (25). Conversely, in a muscle that has lost only an insignificant amount of its innervation, fibrillation potentials sometimes may be found in rather abundant numbers. Third, fibrillation potentials should never be present in the cervical and high thoracic paraspinal muscles with extraforaminal lesions, but logically they should be prominent in those muscles with cervical intraspinal canal lesions. Nonetheless, for uncertain reasons, fibrillation potentials frequently are not detectable in the paraspinal muscles with known root avulsions even when they are abundant in the limb muscles. Consequently, with proximal brachial plexus lesions, if the NCS results and the paraspinal muscle NEE findings are at a variance—i.e., the CMAP responses are not elicitable whereas the SNAPs are normal or low in amplitude, suggesting a preganglionic or mostly preganglionic lesion, but fibrillation potentials cannot be found in the paraspinal muscles, suggesting a postganglionic lesion—it is *always* more prudent to consider the NCS results to be the more reliable of the two. Fourth, the MUP firing pattern with many plexus lesions is not helpful; because of pain on attempted activation, lack of sensory input, etc., the MUPs fire in decreased numbers but at a slow-to-moderate rate. This is a nonspecific finding in contrast to the MUPs firing in decreased numbers at a rapid rate, which is indicative of a substantial lower motor neuron deficit (because of either axon loss or demyelinating conduction block). Fifth, a lesion may consist of two separate pathophysiologic processes—axon loss and demyelinating conduction block—and the latter may be responsible for most of the patient's symptoms. In these instances, the NEE findings—fibrillation potentials and substantial MUP dropout—are misleading because they are readily misinterpreted as indicative of severe axon loss. In fact, the mild axon loss component of the lesion causes the fibrillation potentials, whereas the severe demyelinating block component produces the MUP dropout. Such a mistake is readily avoided in most situations if a motor NCS response is recorded from the clinically weak muscle using surface recording electrodes while stimulating the nerve supplying the muscle distal to the lesion. The CMAP amplitude obtained in this manner, when compared to either the EMG laboratory normal values or the CMAP amplitude obtained by studying the corresponding, unaffected nerve in the opposite extremity, is a much more reliable indicator of the degree of motor axon loss present than is the dropout of MUPs noted on NEE. For some plexus elements (e.g., the axillary terminal nerve with infraclavicular injury), such studies cannot be performed because it is not possible to stimulate distal to the lesion site, moreover for all plexus motor fibers, this procedure only becomes reliable after enough time has elapsed (7 days) for all the distal stump segments to have become unexcitable if the lesion is one of axon loss (38,39).

Overall, axon-loss brachial plexopathies are not progressive in nature, the major exceptions being neoplastic plexopathies, radiation-induced plexopathies, and compartment syndromes. Most are due instead to an injurious force being applied to various plexus elements over a brief period of time. Such abrupt-onset lesions characteristically are maximal at injury onset, and the majority of lesions tend to improve as time passes. The amount of spontaneous recovery that ultimately occurs following an axon-loss brachial plexus lesion depends on several interrelated factors, including the grade of injury, the particular elements of the plexus affected, and the completeness of the lesion for each element.

Designations of Axon-Loss Lesions

Regarding the grade of injury, an extremely broad range (0% to 100%) of recovery can ultimately result from axon-loss lesions of the same initial clinical severity. The reason for this is that although all such lesions share in common axon death with subsequent wallerian degeneration of the distal segment, they can vary markedly in the amount of damage sustained at the lesion site by the supporting structures of the nerve: the endoneurium, perineurium, and epineurium. The more severely these structures are injured, the more difficult it is for the regenerating axons to traverse the lesion site to reach the distal segment of the nerve and, consequently, the poorer the degree of ultimate recovery. Depending upon the amount of this supporting structure damage, axon-loss lesions often are designated as "low grade" and "high grade." At one end of the spectrum is the most benign type, in which the axon is killed at the point of injury but all of its supporting elements at that site remain intact. In the classifications of focal peripheral nerve injuries proposed decades ago by Seddon and Sunderland, this low-grade lesion is designated an "axonotmesis" lesion or a "second-degree injury," respectively (31,34). The regenerating axons readily traverse the damaged segment of the nerve because their endoneurial tubes have not been disturbed, and the only limiting factor to complete recovery is the distance that the motor fibers must grow to reach denervated muscles (see below). At the opposite end of the spectrum is the most severe lesion type, Seddons' worst "neurotmesis" lesion or Sunderland's "fifth-degree injury," in which not only the axon but also all of its supporting structures are irreparably damaged at the injury site owing to physical separation, e.g., the transection of fibers caused by cutting, or the rupture (tearing apart), or avulsion of fibers caused by traction. No recovery occurs spontaneously with these high-grade lesions and, unfortunately, surgical repair sometimes cannot be done or is of little benefit. There is a level of injury immediately below the worst neurotmesis/fifth-degree lesion in severity in which the gross continuity of the brachial plexus elements is preserved but no spontaneous recovery occurs. With this severe "neurotmesis lesion" or "fourth-degree injury," which is a high-grade axon-loss lesion "in continuity," the endoneurium and perineurium of the damaged segment are so disrupted that even though that segment is still bridged by its epineurium, or external covering—and thus appears grossly intact to visual inspection—very few, if any, of the regenerating axons can grow through it (19,31,34,37).

Two Mechanisms of Reinnervation

Following an axon-loss lesion, denervated muscle fibers can be reinnervated and sensation restored by two separate mechanisms: 1) the progressive, proximal to distal advancement of regenerating motor and sensory axons from the site of injury; and 2) the collateral sprouting from nearby intact motor and sensory axons. Both methods of regeneration have limitations. A major limitation of proximodistal regeneration has already been discussed: high-grade lesions that prevent the regenerating axons from traversing the lesion site. Another serious limitation, at least for motor fibers, is the "time-distance factor": regenerating motor nerve fibers progress distally from the site of injury at approximately one inch per month, whereas denervated muscle fibers survive approximately 20–24 months without a nerve supply before they degenerate. Consequently, whenever a distance of more than approximately 2 feet separates the lesion site from the motor point of the denervated muscle, proximodistal regeneration is unlikely to result in more than minimal regeneration. It is because of the time-distance factor that, following diffuse brachial plexus injuries, reinnervation occurs much sooner and often is more complete for proximal limb muscles, e.g., shoulder girdle and arm muscles, than for more distal muscles, i.e., proximal forearm muscles. In adults, the intrinsic hand muscles are so distant from the lesion site with either lower trunk or medial cord plexus lesions that they rarely can be reinnervated by progressive proximodistal regeneration. The major limitation of the second mechanism of reinnervation, collateral sprouting, is that it is critically dependent upon the completeness of the lesion. By definition, collateral sprouting from axons that escaped injury can only occur with partial rather than complete lesions; if all or nearly all of the axons supplying a particular muscle have degenerated, then few, if any, intact axons are available to send out sprouts to adopt the denervated muscle fibers. Moreover, the grade and completeness of a focal nerve lesion frequently are interrelated: incomplete lesions often are low grade, whereas complete lesions tend to be high grade (19,37,39).

Based on the above, it is obvious that the determining factor concerning restoration of innervation to the intrinsic hand muscles following axon-loss lesions of the lower trunk and medial cord is the completeness of the lesion; the grade of injury is of little significance in these instances because adequate proximodistal regeneration from the lesion site cannot occur owing to the adverse time-distance factor.

FOCAL DEMYELINATION

One of the defining differences between lesions producing axon loss and those producing focal demyelination is that the latter actually are focal in their effect. They generally involve a relatively small segment of axon and they do not alter the endoneurium, perineurium, or epineurium at that site nor cause degeneration of either the axon or the myelin distal to it. Depending upon the degree of demyelination, nerve transmission through the lesion site is either slowed or blocked. It is important to distinguish between these two types of pathophysiology, because their clinical and EDX presentations are quite different.

Focal Demyelinating Conduction Slowing

With demyelinating conduction slowing, all the nerve impulses traverse the site of injury to reach their destinations, although they move at less than their normal rates across the damaged segment. Focal demyelinating slowing alone typically produces no symptoms; it causes neither clinical weakness when it affects motor fibers nor sensory deficits when it involves sensory fibers. However, when the rate of conduction through the lesion site is slowed to different degrees along the various fibers, yielding "differential slowing," then the results of those physical examination procedures that assess the ability of the PNS to transmit synchronized volleys of nerve impulses (e.g., deep tendon reflex and vibratory testing) will be abnormal. Thus, demyelinating conduction slowing causes primarily EDX and neurologic examination changes rather than clinical disturbances. For this reason, despite the fact that evidence of conduction slowing is frequently sought in the EMG laboratory, such slowing is rarely found with undisputed brachial plexopathies because almost all patients with actual lesions have clinical deficits. Of note is that some focal demyelinating lesions along sensory fibers cause ectopic impulse generation and thereby produce sensory disturbances such as paresthesias. This is an independent manifestation of focal demyelination. It can, however, coexist with demyelinating slowing or demyelinating conduction block, but the sensory disturbance also can occur when neither conduction abnormality is present (6,23,39).

Focal Demyelinating Conduction Block

Focal demyelinating conduction block, in contrast to focal demyelinating slowing, produces symptoms that are mainly identical to those that result from axon loss. Whenever it affects a sufficient number of motor fibers, it causes clinical weakness that is indistinguishable from that found with the same degree of axon loss. Whenever it involves sufficient sensory fibers, it disrupts large sensory nerve functions (e.g., vibration and position sense). In contrast to axon loss, however, it does not materially alter pain or temperature sensation, because the axons subserving those sensory modalities are unmyelinated or only lightly myelinated. Thus, paresthesias (caused by ectopic generators) are often prominent, but pain, particularly persistent causalgic pain, generally is not a feature of demyelinating conduction block.

Demyelinating conduction block is found with only a distinct minority of brachial plexopathies. Moreover, it seldom occurs in insolation. Instead, it usually is accompanied by varying amounts of axon loss. Nonetheless, it may be the predominant pathophysiology and, therefore, responsible for the majority of the clinical manifestations. Typically, it is seen early in the course of the injury (e.g., usually only during the first 6 to 12 weeks or so) with many acute-onset traumatic plexopathies, such as those that result from childbirth, operation, and high-velocity trauma (e.g., falls; roadway accidents; gunshot wounds). In these situations, the demyelinating conduction block is referred to clinically as "neurapraxia," a term popularized by Seddon; Sunderland subsequently labeled it a "first-degree injury" (31,34). This is the mildest type of lesion that is clinically apparent in Seddon's and Sunderland's classifications of focal nerve injuries. (As already noted, demyelinating focal slowing is a less-severe lesion, but because it produces EDX changes almost solely and does not cause clinical signs, it is not included in any clinical classification of focal nerve injuries [37,39].)

There are two types of chronic, gradual-onset brachial plexopathies in which demyelinating conduction block is the prominent pathophysiology: 1) radiation-induced (except in advanced cases, when axon degeneration frequently has supervened); and 2) multifocal conduction block syndrome. With these disorders, it is not appropriate to use the term "neurapraxia" to describe the underlying demyelinating conduction blocks because the latter are of a far different, and usually a much more ominous, nature than those that may initially follow traumatic plexopathies. With radiation-induced plexopathies, for example, demyelinating conduction blocks typically persist for long periods of time and then often convert to axon loss; in any case, they never resolve (39).

The possibility that demyelinating conduction block is present should always be considered with recent onset, traumatic brachial plexopathies (although it is very unlikely to be the pathophysiology with low-velocity injuries, such as those resulting from stab wounds), with radiation-induced plexopathies, and with slowly progressive plexopathies of unknown cause, which may represent multifocal conduction block syndrome. Moreover, the possibility that conduction block may be responsible for at least some of the clinical deficits caused by any type of brachial plexus lesion must always be entertained whenever, 7 days or more after onset, a weak muscle generates a CMAP on motor NCS that is disproportionately preserved, compared to both the degree of its clinical weakness and the amount of MUP dropout found on the NEE of it. In these instances, the axons supplying the weak muscle(s) should be stimulated both in the axilla and supraclavicularly. A marked CMAP amplitude drop on supraclavicular stimulation will demonstrate that the demyelinating conduction block lesion involves the distal trunk, cord, or proximal terminal nerve fibers. Conversely, if the CMAP amplitude on supraclavicular stimulation is similar to that found on more distal stimulations, then the lesion must be situated proximal to the mid-trunk stimulation site. Two examples of conduction block are encountered with some frequency. First, with many radiation-induced plexopathies, conduction block along the various cord elements is readily demonstrated by supraclavicular stimulation of the median, ulnar, musculocutaneous, radial, and axillary nerves. Second, with many postmedian sternotomy "lower trunk" brachial plexopathies, supraclavicular stimulation of the ulnar fibers reveals no focal abnormality from the mid-trunk level distally, indicating that the responsible lesion is proximal to the supraclavicular stimulation site. (It probably affects the C8 VPR; see below [39]). Finally, it is important to note that these lesions are rarely "pure." Almost invariably, they are accompanied by some axon loss which, although clinically insignificant, is often sufficient to produce a number of fibrillation potentials. This is because any motor nerve lesion that is severe enough to cause demyelinating conduction block along most of the fibers generally is severe enough to have killed at least a few of them (12). In these instances, as already mentioned, the NEE findings can be very misleading because of the combination of fibrillation potentials and severely decreased numbers of MUPs, firing rapidly, mistakenly being attributed to substantial axon loss (38,39).

ELECTRODIAGNOSTIC ASSESSMENT OF BRACHIAL PLEXOPATHIES—GENERAL

The brachial plexus is a very vulnerable structure that can be damaged at many points along its course by a great variety of both internal and external insults. Overall, the most common of these are traction injuries, resulting from the great mobility of the nearby shoulder joint, shoulder girdle, and neck. Brachial plexopathies are diagnosed by clinical evaluation, neuroimaging studies, and EDX examination. Regarding the laboratory investigative procedures, neuroimaging studies have not proven to be nearly as beneficial for assessing the extraforaminal components of the brachial plexus as for evaluating the intraspinal canal structures. For various reasons, computerized axial tomography (CAT) scans are of relatively little value, and magnetic resonance imaging (MRI) studies commonly are normal in the presence of profound clinical deficits. In some

instances (e.g., true neurogenic thoracic outlet syndrome) plain x rays may be more informative than any of the "cutting edge" neuroimaging techniques available. The best laboratory procedure for brachial plexus assessment, overall, is the EDX examination. It often can provide objective, accurate evidence regarding the location, pathophysiology, and severity of a brachial plexus lesion, thereby playing a significant role in both diagnosis and management. Assessing the brachial plexus in the EMG laboratory, however, generally is a more formidable task than assessing most peripheral nerve lesions, because it is situated quite proximally and its anatomy is complex. Regarding the latter, the brachial plexus is not a homogenous structure, similar to a single giant peripheral nerve, that can be examined satisfactorily by performing one or two upper extremity NCS and sampling a few random limb muscles on NEE. In fact, it is one of the largest PNS structures, through which thousands of axons travel many different routes with much intermixing and ultimately exit at different points. Consequently, its optimal evaluation depends on the fact that the axons that more distally compose the various peripheral nerves travel known pathways through it; by performing NCS on many of those nerves and by sampling, on NEE, the muscles the motor fibers of those nerves innervate, the electromyographer may uncover a pattern of abnormalities that points to a particular component of the plexus as the site of the lesion (25,38,39).

ELECTRODIAGNOSTIC ASSESSMENT OF BRACHIAL PLEXOPATHIES—SPECIFIC ELEMENTS

Supraclavicular Plexopathies

UPPER PLEXUS (C5, C6 PRIMARY ROOTS, MIXED SPINAL NERVES, OR VPR; UPPER TRUNK)

The upper portion of the supraclavicular brachial plexus is damaged more often than any other portion. It is solely or principally affected by a number of disorders, including obstetric paralysis, classic post-anesthesia paralysis, pack palsy, the burner syndrome, and, particularly, high-velocity closed trauma (e.g., as sustained in vehicular accidents). Upper plexus lesions may occur in isolation, but frequently are accompanied by middle plexus lesions. A disorder involving upper plexus fibers should be considered whenever the shoulder girdle and forearm flexor muscles are weak or there is sensory loss along the lateral forearm and thumb (19,20,24,37).

ELECTRODIAGNOSTIC FEATURES (TABLE 11–2)

Nerve Conduction Studies

The upper plexus usually is not assessed by the "routine" upper extremity NCS. The axons studied during the median motor NCS, the ulnar motor NCS, and the ulnar sensory NCS never traverse the upper plexus, whereas those evaluated by the median sensory NCS, recording the index finger (median S-D2), do so in only 20% of the limb. (They are much more likely to traverse the middle plexus because their cell bodies of origin usually are in the C7 DRG). Consequently, to adequately evaluate the upper plexus, other "nonstandard" upper extremity motor and sensory NCS must be performed. These include median sensory, recording/stimulating the thumb (median S-D1) (Fig. 11–5); lateral

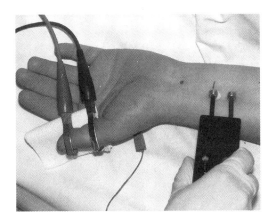

Figure 11–5. Median sensory nerve conduction study (NCS), recording thumb (D1). This NCS assesses sensory fibers derived from the C6 dorsal root ganglion (DRG). Along with the lateral antebrachial cutaneous NCS, it is the preferred sensory NCS for detecting axon loss upper trunk plexus lesions. This NCS also assesses the lateral cord for axon loss.

antebrachial cutaneous (LAC) (Fig. 11–6); musculocutaneous motor, recording the biceps (musculocutaneous m.-biceps) (Fig. 11–7); and axillary motor, recording the deltoid (axillary m.-deltoid) (Fig. 11–8). In addition, the radial motor, recording the proximal extensor forearm muscles, i.e., the brachioradialis and extensor carpi radialis, often is abnormal with lesions at this level, and the radial SNAP, recording from the thumb base (radial S-BT) is abnormal in approximately 60% of the ganglionic and postganglionic lesions affecting the upper plexus sensory fibers. (In the other 40% of these lesions, the radial sensory fibers apparently are derived from the C7 DRG and, therefore, traverse the middle trunk.) The median S-D1 NCS, the LAC NCS, or both, should be performed whenever there is a question of an upper plexus lesion. They will be normal with preganglionic lesions regardless of the severity of motor axon loss; however, with interforaminal or extraforaminal axon loss lesions of at least moderate severity, almost invariably they will be abnormal, i.e., either low in amplitude or unelicitable. Typically, the SNAPs obtained with these two studies are affected to the same degree for any particular lesion. Hence, for screening purposes, performing only one of them usually is sufficient. One of the major drawbacks of the median S-D1 NCS is that

Table 11–2
Muscles Affected by Upper Plexus Lesions*

Nerve Conduction Studies	Needle Electrode Examination
Sensory	Pronator teres
Lat. antebrachial cutaneous	Brachioradialis
Median—D1 (thumb)	Biceps brachii
Radial—thumb base (60%) of limbs)	Brachialis
	Deltoid
Motor	Infraspinatus
Axillary—deltoid muscle	Supraspinatus
Musculocutaneous— biceps muscle	Serratus anterior
	Rhomboids
(Radial—proximal extensor forearm)	Paraspinals

*Nerve conduction studies and muscles (on needle electrode examination) that may show abnormalities, on electrodiagnostic assessment, with (supraclavicular) upper plexus lesions.

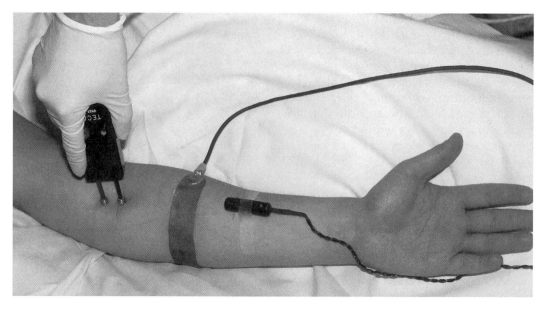

Figure 11–6. Lateral antebrachial cutaneous NCS. This NCS assesses sensory fibers derived from the C6 DRG. Along with the median sensory NCS, recording thumb, it is the optimal sensory NCS for detecting axon loss, upper trunk plexus lesions. This NCS also assesses the lateral cord for axon loss.

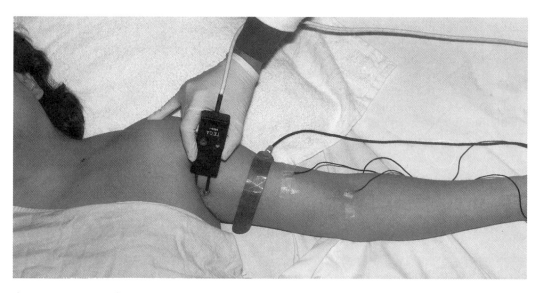

Figure 11–7. Musculocutaneous motor NCS, recording biceps. This NCS assesses motor axons derived from the C5 and C6 roots. Along with the axillary motor NCS, recording deltoid, it is the optimal motor NCS for evaluating the upper plexus for axon loss; this NCS also assesses the lateral cord for axon loss.

its usefulness in brachial plexus assessment is lost in the presence of an ipsilateral carpal tunnel syndrome (CTS), unless the CTS is quite mild and not detectably affecting the median SNAP amplitudes as determined by performing median S-D2 and median sensory, recording/stimulating the middle finger (me-

dian S-D3). The musculocutaneous m.-biceps NCS and the axillary m. deltoid NCS, should be performed whenever the recorded muscles are clinically weak or prominent MUP dropout is seen on the NEE of them. One or the other may be substantially more affected with severe but partial axon-loss upper plexus le-

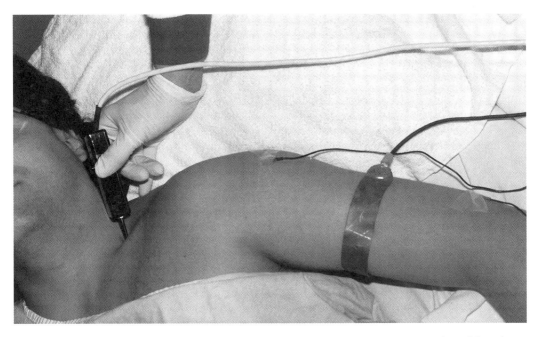

Figure 11-8. The axillary motor NCS, recording deltoid. This NCS assesses motor axons derived from the C5 and C6 roots. Along with the musculocutaneous motor NCS, recording biceps, it is the optimal motor NCS for evaluating the upper plexus for axon loss; this NCS also assesses the posterior cord for axon loss.

sions, so sometimes it is helpful to perform both (11,39).

Needle Electrode Examination

The muscles likely to show abnormalities with upper plexus lesions if only the mid- or distal upper trunk is affected include the pronator teres, brachioradialis, biceps, brachialis, and deltoid muscles. If the lesion involves the very proximal upper trunk, the supraspinatus and infraspinatus muscles may also be denervated, whereas if the lesion is even more proximal along the upper plexus fibers (usually within the intraspinal canal), the rhomboid major, rhomboid minor, and serratus anterior muscles may show abnormalities. Assessing and interpreting the findings of these proximal muscles often is more difficult with the rhomboids. This is because the rhomboids are deep to the trapezius, which is not innervated by the brachial plexus and, therefore, not affected with brachial plexopathies. At times it is difficult to determine exactly which of these muscles is being studied on the NEE. If the needle electrode is in the trapezius, but mistakenly thought to be in the rhomboids, then the normal findings that result can cause the plexus

lesion to be localized more distally than it actually is. Consequently, an NEE of the serratus anterior muscle often produces more reliable information. Whenever NEE abnormalities are found in the limb muscles innervated by the upper plexus, 1) the muscles innervated by the median and radial nerves via other portions of the plexus—e.g., the flexor pollicis longus (FPL), the abductor pollicis brevis (APB), the triceps, and the extensor indicis proprius (EIP)—should always be surveyed, to demonstrate that the median and radial nerves themselves are not affected; and 2) the proximal extent of the lesion should always be ascertained by consecutive NEE of the spinati, the serratus anterior and rhomboids, and the paraspinal muscles (39).

The next section reviews some specific entities in which upper plexus fibers characteristically are affected.

Closed Traction Lesions, Including Obstetric Paralysis

Early in the course of these disorders, demyelinating conduction block may be responsible for a substantial amount of the clinical weakness present. However, typically this process cannot be demonstrated on NCS because the lesion is proximal to the mid-trunk, supraclavicular stimulation point. Nonetheless, its presence may be inferred if normal or near-normal CMAP amplitudes can be recorded from the clinically weak muscle(s) (e.g., biceps/brachialis; deltoid) 5 or more days after onset. The amount of axon loss is highly variable. If it is substantial, as it frequently is, the amplitudes of the NCS that assess the upper plexus are affected. With postganglionic lesions, both the CMAPs and SNAPs will be abnormal, whereas with "pure" preganglionic lesions, only the CMAPs will be affected. However, "two-level" lesions can occur, so even though the SNAPs are unelicitable, if the serratus anterior muscle show abnormalities on NEE, the ipsilateral mid- and low cervical paraspinal muscles should be assessed as well.

When closed traction is the etiology, combined upper and middle plexus lesions probably are as common as upper plexus lesions alone. Often the middle plexus component is not recognized clinically, because its fibers are less involved. Consequently, in these situations, EDX evidence of coexisting middle plexus involvement should always be sought by performing median S-D3 NCS and by sampling on the NEE the triceps, pronator teres, and flexor carpi radialis (FCR) muscles, most of which are also innervated by the upper plexus to varying degrees (see the section on Middle Plexus, below) (2,18,19,20,37,39).

The Burner Syndrome

This disorder is essentially restricted to young males engaged in contact sports (e.g., football; wrestling). Generally, the patients are not referred for EDX studies until they experience multiple episodes of transient upper limb dysesthesia, often with more persistent weakness with each athletic contest. The EDX examination characteristically reveals a mild axon-loss lesion. The amplitudes of all the NCS, motor and sensory, that assess the upper plexus are normal (37). One group has reported finding prolonged motor NCS distal latencies when recording with needle electrodes from various shoulder girdle muscles (21). Why this would occur is unclear, because it is quite unusual to encounter conduction slowing with an acute-

onset lesion, especially one causing weakness. An NEE usually reveals only a modest number of fibrillation potentials in the deltoid, biceps, spinati, and brachioradialis. Some authorities contend that the burner syndrome is not due to an upper trunk brachial plexopathy, but rather to a C6 radiculopathy (27); unfortunately, this disagreement regarding lesion location cannot be resolved by EDX studies, primarily because only a modest amount of axon loss typically occurs with this disorder.

"Classic" Post-Anesthesia Paralysis

This rather rarely studied disorder, an operative complication, was first described about 1900. Initially it was attributed to some toxic effect of the anesthetic agents but, subsequently, its real etiology was understood: malpositioning on the operating table. The typical patient awakens from anesthesia following a surgical procedure often performed at a distance from the brachial plexus (e.g., an abdominal or pelvic operation) with weakness and anesthesia in an upper plexus distribution or a pan-plexus distribution initially, with the mid and lower plexus findings rapidly resolving. Demyelinating conduction block is the predominant pathophysiology. One clinical clue to this is that pain—indicative of small axon involvement—generally is conspicuously absent. The majority of patients recover rapidly and are never assessed in the EDX laboratory (37). Among the distinct minority of patients in whom weakness is still present, the musculocutaneous m. biceps NCS and the axillary m.-deltoid NCS are abnormal: supraclavicular stimulation of the musculocutaneous and axillary fibers yield low-amplitude CMAPs, whereas axilla stimulation of the musculocutaneous fibers may produce a CMAP of much higher, normal amplitude. (The axillary nerve cannot be stimulated below the level of the lesion.) Usually only modestly decreased amplitudes are found on median S-D1 and LAC NCS, indicating that substantial axon loss has not occurred. This is confirmed by the NEE, which reveals a modest number of fibrillation potentials in several upper trunk-innervated limb muscles, but not the spinati, rhomboids, or serratus anterior. MUP dropout typically is prominent in the affected muscles if the conduction block component of the lesion is still present at the time of the examination; otherwise, only fibrillation potentials are seen. Both the NCS and NEE changes suggest that the lesion involves the distal upper trunk (37,44).

Upper Trunk Simulators

Several disorders, including some involving the PNS, are often mistaken for upper plexus lesions. These will now be reviewed.

1. *C5 or C6 Compressive Radiculopathies.* These root lesions can produce pain, paresthesias and sensory loss, and deep tendon reflex changes similar to those found with upper plexus lesions. However, interscapular pain and neck stiffness, characteristic of compressive radiculopathies, do not occur with plexus lesions; conversely, frank muscle weakness and wasting are more common with plexus than compressive root lesions. The median S-D1 and LAC NCS are normal with compressive radiculopathies, but this often is of relatively little help in lesion localization. This not only is because neither assesses the C5 component of the upper plexus, but also because the typical differential diagnosis is between a C5/C6 radiculopathy and a mild axon-loss upper trunk lesion, i.e., one in which the appropriate SNAPs would be unaffected, even with an extraforaminal lesion. However, in unusual cases, a compressive radiculopathy produces an unusually severe amount of axon loss, and the fact that these sensory NCS responses are normal in the presence of low-amplitude musculocutaneous m.-biceps and axillary m.-deltoid NCS responses, localizes the lesion to the primary roots within the intraspinal canal. The NEE can be very helpful in these situations if it reveals fibrillation potentials in the mid or low cervical paraspinal muscles.

2. *Rotator Cuff Tears.* These disorders, most often seen in middle-aged and elderly men, commonly are mistaken for upper plexus lesions because they cause weakness and wasting (owing to disuse) of various shoulder girdle muscles, particularly the spinati. The EDX studies readily distinguish the two, however, because no abnormalities are found with rotator cuff tears. Specifically, the CMAP amplitude of the axillary m. deltoid NCS is normal, regardless of the amount of deltoid wasting present. The median S-D1 and LAC NCS are normal, and the NEE of the deltoid and spinati as well as other upper plexus-innervated muscles shows no evidence of a lower motor neuron lesion. Only an MUP firing abnormality is seen: a decreased number of MUPs, firing at a moderate rate on maximal effort, consistent with pain on activation.

3. *Spinal Accessory Neuropathies.* These extraplexal nerve lesions are relatively uncommon; most are iatrogenic in nature, owing to injuries sustained during minor surgical procedures (e.g., lymph node biopsies; "lumpectomies") performed in the posterior triangle of the neck. Spinal accessory nerve damage at this location affects only the branch to the trapezius because the motor branch supplying the sternocleidomastoid muscle arises cephalad to the injury site. Unlike almost all other acute severe PNS lesions, many spinal accessory mononeuropathies initially are asymptomatic. In these instances, several weeks to a few months often pass before the patient seeks medical attention for either obvious shoulder deformity or weakness of arm elevation; by that time a link between the current symptoms and the remote minor neck operation frequently is overlooked by both the patient and his physician. Consequently, many patients with this disorder are referred to the EMG laboratory with the diagnosis of axillary neuropathy, suprascapular neuropathy, dorsal scapular neuropathy or, particularly, upper trunk brachial plexopathy. All of the above are readily excluded by EDX studies. The actual diagnosis, however, can prove elusive unless the upper trapezius is

sampled during the NEE. Once fibrillation potentials and MUP loss are found in this muscle, the mid and lower trapezius can be assessed, as well as the sternocleidomastoid and contralateral upper trapezius; moreover, spinal accessory NCS can be performed bilaterally to determine the severity of axon loss present.

4. *Neuralgic Amyotrophy.* This curious PNS disorder, also called acute brachial neuropathy and Parsonage-Turner syndrome, almost always is classified under brachial plexopathies, although it probably is not one; instead, it most likely is due to involvement of one or more peripheral nerves of the shoulder girdle or extremity. Neuralgic amyotrophy generally affects adults; it can be both familial and acquired, although the latter is far more common. In most patients it appears to be triggered by some nonspecific antecedent event, such as a nondescript upper respiratory infection, an inoculation, hospitalization for any reason (including childbirth, infectious diseases, and surgical procedures), and various types of trivial trauma. Unilateral involvement is more common than bilateral involvement; when the latter does occur, the two sides can be affected either simultaneously or sequentially and typically the abnormalities are asymmetrical. A relatively small percentage of patients experience recurrent bouts, weeks to months apart. The characteristic presenting symptom is pain, which is abrupt in onset, very severe, and most often localized to the shoulder. It frequently begins at night, awakening the patient from sleep, and usually reaches its maximum within a few hours. Typically, within a few days of onset, weakness and subsequent wasting of various shoulder girdle and upper extremity muscles are apparent. In some patients, the abnormalities are solely in the distribution of one or a few peripheral nerves, particularly the suprascapular, long thoracic, axillary, anterior in-

terosseous, and musculocutaneous nerves. In other patients, however, multiple nerves are involved and they all commonly derive from the upper trunk of the brachial plexus. It is for this reason that neuralgic amyotrophy is so often considered an upper trunk brachial plexopathy. Sensory loss usually is either undetectable or restricted to a small patch on the lateral shoulder in the axillary nerve territory (26,37).

The diagnosis of neuralgic amyotrophy depends mainly on the clinical and EDX examinations, because neuroimaging studies are of no value. On EDX examination, the routine motor and sensory NCS usually are normal, because they do not assess the particular nerve fibers most often involved. However, the axillary and musculocutaneous CMAP amplitudes are low if those nerves are substantially affected, and sometimes the LAC SNAP is abnormal as an isolated sensory NCS finding. The NEE typically shows severe axon loss in the distribution of one, two, or several peripheral nerves, particularly motor nerves supplying the shoulder girdle and upper limb muscles. Frequently, the EDX examination demonstrates that the disorder is more extensive than clinically appreciated, with NEE abnormalities being seen in clinically uninvolved muscles of the affected limb or the contralateral limb. Several findings, often more apparent on EDX than clinical examination, are very suggestive of neuralgic amyotrophy, including a) severe involvement of only some muscles innervated by a particular peripheral nerve, e.g., near-total denervation of the supraspinatus muscle, with minimal to no involvement of the infraspinatus muscle, or vice versa; b) severe involvement of the pronator teres and FCR muscles, with no accompanying involvement of other C7 or median nerve-innervated muscles; c) involvement of muscles not innervated by the brachial plexus, e.g., the serratus anterior, innervated by the long thoracic nerve; the trapezius (and rarely the sternocleidomastoid) muscle, innervated by the spinal accessory nerve; and occasionally the diaphragm, innervated by the phrenic nerve. In some patients in whom neuralgic amyotrophy appears to involve the upper trunk, the LAC SNAP is abnormal but the median S-D1 SNAP is not. This dissociation of sensory NCS responses that assess the upper trunk suggests that multiple peripheral nerves derived from the upper trunk (e.g., suprascapular, axillary, musculocutaneous) actually are affected, rather than the upper trunk itself. That NEE changes often are found in these patients in the spinati, deltoid, and biceps but not the brachioradialis or pronator teres supports this view (9,38).

MIDDLE PLEXUS (C7 PRIMARY ROOT, MIXED SPINAL NERVE, OR VPR; MIDDLE TRUNK)

Lesions of this portion of the supraclavicular plexus are rare in isolation. This is fortunate because they produce limb symptoms and signs identical to those caused by C7 radiculopathies, which are the most common of the cervical radiculopathies. When middle plexus fiber lesions are present, they usually coexist with lesions of the upper plexus, the lower plexus, or both, and involvement of the latter elements usually dominates the clinical picture. Sometimes the coexisting middle plexus fiber injury is unappreciated until EDX studies are performed. Middle plexus lesions should be suspected whenever forearm extension and pronation is substantially impaired or sensory loss extends to the middle finger (19,20,24,37).

ELECTRODIAGNOSTIC FEATURES (TABLE 11–3)

Nerve Conduction Studies
The interforaminal and extraforaminal portions of the middle plexus are readily assessed for axon loss by the median S-D2 and, particularly, the median S-D3 (Fig. 11–9). Also, in approximately half of the limbs, the radial S-BT NCS will be abnormal with more distal plexus lesions. There apparently is no satisfactory motor NCS for assessing middle plexus fibers. Intuitively, it would seem that the radial motor NCS should evaluate primarily these fibers, but when that study is performed while recording from the proximal extensor forearm, the CMAP is being generated primarily by C5, C6-innervated muscles, and when the distal extensor forearm is used as a recording

Table 11–3
Muscles Affected by Middle Plexus Lesions*

Nerve Conduction Studies	Needle Electrode Examination
Sensory	Triceps
Median—D3 (middle)	Anconeus
Median—D2 (index) (80% of limbs)	Pronator teres
	Flexor carpi radialis
(Radial—thumb base) (40% of limbs)	Paraspinals
Motor	
*	

*Nerve conduction studies and muscles (on needle electrode examination) that may show abnormalities, on electrodiagnostic assessment, with (supraclavicular) middle plexus lesions. No satisfactory motor NCS is available for assessing the middle trunk (see text).

site, the principle generators of the motor response are C8-innervated muscles (11,39).

Needle Electrode Examination
The triceps, anconeus, pronator teres, and FCR typically show NEE abnormalities with axon-loss lesions involving the middle plexus. Unfortunately, all of these muscles are also in the C6 myotome to a greater or lesser extent, so sometimes it is difficult to distinguish severe upper plexus lesions from combined upper and middle plexus lesions by NEE. Involvement or noninvolvement of the appropriate median sensory NCS responses may be more helpful in this differentiation than the NEE findings (39).

LOWER PLEXUS (C8, T1 PRIMARY ROOTS, MIXED SPINAL NERVES, VPR; LOWER TRUNK)

Lesions of this portion of the supraclavicular plexus are sustained less frequently than those of the upper plexus. They occur both in isolation and as a portion of a more extensive process (combined middle and lower plexus lesions; pan-plexus lesions). The lower plexus is solely or preferentially involved with a variety of plexopathies, including closed traction injuries, neoplastic plexopathies, post-median sternotomy plexopathies, true neurogenic thoracic outlet syndrome (TOS), and post-disputed neurogenic TOS surgery. A lower

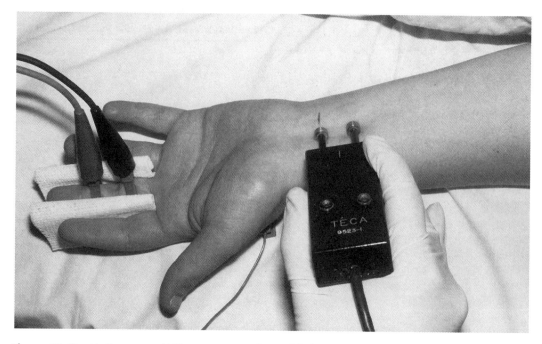

Figure 11–9. Median sensory NCS response, recording middle finger (D3). This NCS most often assesses sensory fibers derived from the C7 DRG. This is the optimal NCS for detecting axon loss, middle plexus lesions; this NCS also assesses the lateral cord for axon loss. The median sensory NCS, recording index finger (D2), and the radial sensory NCS, recording thumb base, also detect axon loss, middle plexus lesions in some patients (see text).

plexus disorder should be considered whenever the intrinsic hand muscles and some forearm muscles are weak or sensory loss is present along the medial forearm or hand, and fingers, or both (19,20,24,37).

ELECTRODIAGNOSTIC FEATURES (TABLE 11–4)

Nerve Conduction Studies

This is the only portion of the supraclavicular plexus that is adequately evaluated by the standard upper extremity NCS. The "routine" median motor NCS, ulnar motor NCS, and ulnar sensory recording/stimulating the fifth finger (ulnar S-D5) NCS all assess axons that traverse the lower plexus. Consequently, although additional NCS can be performed— e.g., ulnar motor, recording the first dorsal interosseus (FDI); ulnar sensory, recording the dorsum of the hand (ulnar S-DH); ulnar sensory, recording the fourth finger—they seldom provide additional useful information. An exception is the medial antebrachial cutaneous (MAC) NCS (Fig. 11–10). The fibers assessed by this study usually originate from

Table 11–4
Muscles Affected by Lower Plexus Lesions*

Nerve Conduction Studies	Needle Electrode Examination
Sensory	Abductor pollicis brevis
Ulnar—D5 (little)	Opponens pollicis
Ulnar—D4 (ring)	Flexor pollicis longus
Ulnar dorsal cutaneous	First dorsal interosseus
Medial antebrachial cutaneous	Adductor pollicis
	Abductor digiti minimi
Medial	Flexor carpi ulnaris
Motor	Flexor digitorum profundus 4,5
Ulnar—hypothenar	
Ulnar—first dorsal interosseus	Extensor indicis proprius
Median—thenar	Extensor pollicis brevis
(Radial—distal extensor forearm)	Paraspinals

*Nerve conduction studies and muscles (on needle electrode examination) that may show abnormalities, on electrodiagnostic assessment, with (supraclavicular) lower plexus lesions.

the T1 DRG, as opposed to the ulnar sensory fibers (those studied by both ulnar S-D5 and ulnar S-DH), which appear to derive almost solely from the C8 DRG. All of these motor and sensory NCS tend to be involved to approximately the same degree with high velocity, traumatic lower trunk brachial plexopathies. Nonetheless, presumably because individually these studies tend to assess fibers derived from either one or the other, rather than both, nerve roots that form the lower trunk (i.e., the median motor and MAC NCS, C8; the ulnar motor and sensory NCS, T1), very different clinical and EDX presentations are seen with two so-called "lower trunk" brachial plexopathies: 1) those caused by a cervical band (true neurogenic TOS); and 2) those that occur during open heart surgery (post-median sternotomy brachial plexopathy). Both are discussed below (11,39).

Needle Electrode Examination

Many muscles are innervated by the lower plexus, and most are readily assessed during the NEE. These include a) all of the C8(T1)/ulnar nerve-innervated forearm and hand muscles, e.g., the FDI, abductor digiti minimi (ADM), flexor carpi ulnaris (FCU), and flexor digitorum profundus-4,5 (FDP-4,5); b) several (C8) T1/median nerve-innervated muscles, including the APB, opponens pollicis, and FPL; and c) several C8/radial nerve-innervated muscles, including the EIP, extensor pollicis brevis (EPB), and sometimes the extensor digitorum communis (EDC). Because the NCS changes with lesions of the medial cord are usually identical to those of the lower trunk, the only means the electromyographer has for distinguishing one from another is to demonstrate NEE abnormalities in the radial nerve-innervated muscles with lower trunk lesions. For this reason, the EIP and EPB muscles or other C8/radial nerve-innervated muscles, should *always* be assessed whenever a lower plexus lesion is suspected. This is particularly important with post-median sternotomy brachial plexopathies. The characteristic EDX presentation of several lower plexus lesions are reviewed below (36,38,39).

Closed Traction Lesions

The lower plexus fibers are injured rather infrequently by closed traction. Nonetheless, when such lesions occur they often are severe and, regrettably, frequently preganglionic in location (i.e., avulsion injuries) (37). Typically,

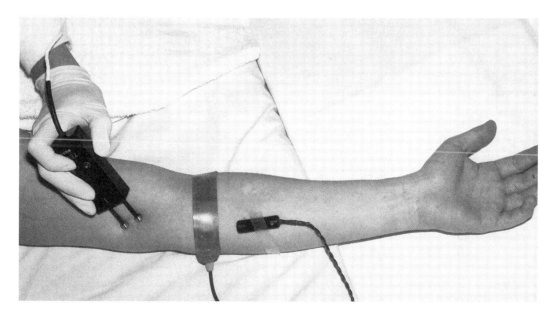

Figure 11–10. The medial antebrachial cutaneous NCS. This NCS assesses sensory fibers derived from the T1 DRG. Along with the ulnar sensory NCS, it is the optimal sensory NCS for detecting axon loss in lower trunk and medial cord lesions. However, because its cells of origin are in the T1 DRG rather than the C8 DRG as are the ulnar sensory fibers, it is particularly likely to be severely affected with true neurogenic thoracic outlet syndrome (see text).

with lower plexus lesions of this type, the median and ulnar CMAPs are equally affected and occasionally, with very severe lesions, the radial motor NCS response, recording from the distal extensor forearm, is also low in amplitude. The ulnar sensory and MAC NCS responses characteristically are spared with "pure" preganglionic lesions, but typically are abnormal with postganglionic lesions. The uniformity of abnormalities carries over to the NEE, with changes generally present in all the lower plexus-innervated muscles; of particular note is that the ulnar nerve-innervated forearm muscles usually are as abnormal or more abnormal than the ulnar nerve-innervated hand muscles, a pattern of NEE findings seldom seen with ulnar neuropathies at the elbow. Although closed traction can produce isolated lower plexus lesions, more often combined lower plexus and middle plexus lesions occur. In these situations, NEE changes also are seen in the middle plexus-innervated muscles and, if the lesion is inter- or extraforaminal, the median S-D3 SNAP and often the median S-D2 SNAP are affected, as well as the radial S-BT SNAP.

Neoplastic Brachial Plexopathies

Most plexopathies of this type are due to the spread of primary malignant lung or breast neoplasms. Any portion of the supraclavicular plexus can be affected and diffuse lesions are common when the process is advanced. Nonetheless, in their early stages these neoplasms most often involve lower plexus fibers, usually those of the lower trunk, and present with C8/T1 dermatomal pain and a weak hand. With Pancoast's syndrome, however, pre- and postganglionic lesions can coexist along the lower plexus fibers, adding a Horner's syndrome. Customarily, as with closed traction lesions, both the NCS and the NEE changes tend to be rather uniform in a lower plexus distribution. Frequently, axon loss is severe at the time of the initial EDX examination (37,38).

Post-Median Sternotomy Brachial Plexopathies

The direct cause for the lower plexus lesions that occur during open heart surgery is unknown. Most investigators believe the process is triggered by the sternal retraction that

allows access to the heart; very proximal first rib fractures have been reported. Clinically, patients typically complain of hand weakness and pain and paresthesias along the medial aspect of the hand, occasionally extending to the medial forearm. Unlike the "lower trunk" lesions already described, this particular type of brachial plexopathy characteristically injures the ulnar motor and sensory fibers more severely than the other lower plexus fibers. Consequently, on NCS, sometimes only the ulnar responses are abnormal. The ulnar CMAPs typically are somewhat low in amplitude, whereas the ulnar S-D5 and S-DH SNAPs are low or very low in amplitude. In contrast, the amplitudes of the median CMAP and the MAC SNAP may be low or within the normal range. On NEE, abnormalities characteristically are found in all the ulnar nerve-innervated muscles in both the hand and forearm and usually in the lower trunk/radial nerve-innervated muscles also. However, they are found in the lower trunk/median nerve-innervated muscles, particularly the lateral thenar muscles, in only a slight majority of affected limbs. Because of the disproportionate involvement of the ulnar fibers, post-median sternotomy brachial plexopathies frequently are mistaken clinically for postoperative ulnar neuropathies. A similar misdiagnosis readily occurs on the EDX examination unless the EIP and EPB muscles are assessed on the NEE.

The striking dichotomy between the findings in the ulnar nerve distribution and those in the median motor nerve and MAC nerve distributions suggests that the lower trunk per se is not involved but, rather, it is one of the VPR that contributes to the lower trunk. That this is the C8, rather than the T1, VPR is likely because, in many respects, the combination of changes seen with this disorder are the reverse of those that occur with true neurogenic TOS (see below), for which it has been established that the T1 VPR is more, if not solely, affected as compared to the C8 VPR. Many patients with post median-sternotomy plexopathies, when studied soon after onset, have weakness of the ulnar nerve-innervated hand muscles that is disproportionately severe compared to the CMAP amplitudes that can be recorded from those muscles on ulnar motor NCS. The

CMAP amplitudes recorded are also at variance with the prominent MUP dropout noted in those muscles on the NEE. This constellation of clinical and EDX changes suggests that demyelinating conduction block is responsible for a substantial amount of the motor disability present, a suspicion confirmed by the rapid, although often only partial, improvement that soon ensues. However, such a block almost never can be demonstrated on supraclavicular stimulation of the lower trunk fibers, indicating that the lesion is proximal to the mid-trunk level. (This finding is also consistent with the premise that the lesion site is the C8 VPR [11].)

True Neurogenic Thoracic Outlet Syndrome
This disorder, also known as classic neurogenic TOS (N-TOS) and the cervical rib and band syndrome, was first recognized in 1903, but was soon confused with then-unknown CTS, because both cause lateral thenar wasting. Its classical clinical and radiographic presentations finally were well defined in 1970 by Gilliatt and coworkers, who also described its typical EDX presentation (13). True N-TOS occurs rarely, and almost always unilaterally. It is found far more commonly in women than men. In affected patients, the distal T1 VPR or very proximal lower trunk fibers are stretched and angulated around a congenital anomaly: a fibrous band extending from the first rib to the tip of a rudimentary cervical rib. Sometimes the C8 VPR is distorted as well, but it is never as affected as the T1 VPR. Patients with this disorder typically seek medical attention as young to middle-aged adults, whenever they or someone else notices that one of their hands is wasted. In approximately one-fourth of patients, the atrophy is restricted to the lateral thenar eminence (i.e., the median nerve-innervated APB and opponens pollicis muscles), although the whole hand is weak. In the majority of patients, however, the entire hand is weak and wasted, but the lateral thenar muscles consistently are the most severely affected. Many patients report, when questioned, having experienced intermittent aching along the medial forearm, sometimes extending into the hand, for periods ranging from a few weeks to many years; most of them never sought medical attention for these sensory symptoms, however (13,37).

The typical findings on EDX examination are as follows. On NCS, the median motor CMAP is very low in amplitude, often below 2 millivolts; the MAC SNAP is unelicitable; the ulnar sensory SNAPs are low or relatively low in amplitude; the ulnar motor CMAPs are within the normal range, although sometimes they are somewhat lower than the corresponding responses obtained on studying the contralateral hand, particularly those recording from the FDI. On the NEE, evidence of a chronic, axon-loss lower plexus lesion is found. The APB and opponens pollicis invariably are the most severely affected muscles; usually only a modest number of fibrillation potentials and a few MUPs, showing very prominent chronic neurogenic changes (with amplitudes sometimes greater than 10 millivolts) and firing at a rapid rate, are seen in them. Similar but less severe MUP changes, sometimes accompanied by a minimal number of fibrillation potentials, are found in the FDI, ADM, and FPL muscles. In most patients, similar but often less severe MUP changes are in the FCU and FDP (4,5) as well as the EIP and EPB muscles. In some patients, however, the latter muscles appear normal (43). The fact that the lower plexus/radial nerve-innervated muscles do not show abnormalities does not mean, as has been suggested in one recent syllabus concerned with brachial plexus assessment, that the lesion involves the medial cord rather than the lower plexus (36); it is anatomically impossible for the medial cord, an infraclavicular structure, to be injured by a cervical band at the high supraclavicular level. A more logical interpretation for the lack of involvement of these muscles is that their motor innervation, derived primarily from the C8 VPR, has been spared; essentially, only the T1 VPR fibers have been injured in these particular patients.

Disputed N-TOS
Almost as soon as true N-TOS was first recognized, the concept arose that similar brachial plexus compromise could occur in patients who lacked a cervical rib and band. Based on this theory, several distinct TOS "syndromes" have been described over the years. Typically,

each has enjoyed a period of popularity and then been abandoned, although some have been resurrected at a later date. The scalenus anticus syndrome was one such entity. Described in 1935, it was thoroughly discredited in the decade from 1945 to 1955 when other, undisputed causes for the symptoms attributed to it were discovered—e.g., cervical radiculopathies; CTS—and when the operation proposed to treat it, anterior scalenotomy, was shown to have a low success rate. Nonetheless, essentially the same concept reappeared in 1962 when still another syndrome was described: "disputed N-TOS" or "symptomatic N-TOS." As initially proposed, its symptoms were produced by the lower plexus being compressed between the normal first thoracic rib and some other structure. In 1966, a surgical procedure, transaxillary first rib resection, was devised to treat this lower plexus type of disputed N-TOS, and soon that operation became even more popular than anterior scalenotomies had been a few decades earlier to treat its predecessor. In the early 1980s, a second type of disputed N-TOS was reported, in which the upper plexus was reputedly compressed by the scalene muscles. To treat this version, a different operation was devised: anterior scalenectomy. The title somewhat understates this aggressive surgery, however, because not only is the anterior scalene removed (rather than cut), but so is the middle scalene and often the omohyoid muscle (28,37,43).

Disputed N-TOS is the most amorphous, and the only controversial, subgroup of TOS. It is also by far the one most frequently diagnosed. It reportedly most often is caused by trauma, particularly vehicular and work place accidents, and affects women (especially young women) more than men. Clinically, almost every forequarter symptom imaginable has been attributed to it by its various proponents, although its most common stated symptomatology has been vague shoulder and upper extremity pain and paresthesias, sometimes in a indistinct C8/T1 distribution (28). In contrast to true N-TOS, objective findings characteristically are absent; convincing organic weaknesses is rarely encountered and frank muscle wasting, essentially never.

Some proponents of this N-TOS subgroup have been attempting to prove its existence, by means of objective, verifiable EDX changes, for over three decades. The particular EDX studies employed for this purpose have varied. Initially, NEE findings in the affected limb were said to be characteristic. Later, retroclavicular or infraclavicular ulnar motor NCS slowing, demonstrated on supraclavicular and axilla stimulations, reportedly provided "objective evidence" of its presence. More recently, C8 root stimulation, F waves, F loops, and somatosensory evoked potentials have all been championed, by one proponent or another, as the optimal ancillary EDX test for diagnosis (40). Unfortunately, none of these procedures has had its reputed value confirmed in major EMG laboratories. Consequently, disputed N-TOS remains a clinical diagnosis. Moreover, although some proponents acknowledge that EDX studies assist in the evaluation of these patients by helping to exclude other causes for their symptoms (e.g., CTS; ulnar neuropathy; cervical radiculopathy), other proponents deny their value. They contend that EDX studies are painful, expensive, and yield "confusing" results (28). Presumably, the results are confusing whenever a patient diagnosed as having TOS is shown to have CTS on EDX studies, thereby calling into question the need for any TOS surgery. Regardless, it is during operations to treat disputed N-TOS that almost all intraoperative plexus lesions associated with TOS surgery occur.

Post-Disputed TOS Surgery
Brachial Plexopathy

As noted, a great number of people are diagnosed as having disputed N-TOS. Many of them undergo first rib resection, anterior scalenectomy, or both, and some sustain intraoperative brachial plexopathies during these procedures. Most often the operation has been a transaxillary first rib resection, and the injured plexus elements have been the C8 or T1 VPR or the proximal lower trunk. Hand weakness and wasting is a common finding, but the most disabling feature is the causalgic pain that characteristically occurs.

The EDX findings typically are indicative of an axon-loss lower trunk plexus lesion. On NCS, the median and ulnar CMAPs are low in amplitude, and the ulnar S-D5 and MAC

SNAPs are low in amplitude or unelicitable. On NEE, fibrillation potentials and rather prominent MUP dropout are found in a lower trunk distribution. In some cases, the T1 component appears to be more severely affected, and the NCS abnormalities are similar to those seen with true N-TOS. However, the NEE findings are suggestive of an abrupt onset, rather than a slowly progressive lesion; i.e., fibrillation potentials usually are abundant, and although MUP dropout is often severe, prominent suggestive chronic neurogenic MUP changes usually are not seen. (An exception is when these patients are studied years after their injurious TOS operations; in these instances, because of the chronicity of the lesions, the EDX changes occasionally can be almost indistinguishable from those seen with true N-TOS [41].)

PAN TRUNK LESIONS

There are relatively few causes for involvement of all three trunks. These include diffuse trauma, often severe; end-stage neoplastic lesions; end-stage radiation-induced lesions, and early post-anesthesia paralysis. Combined upper, middle, and lower plexus lesions should be suspected whenever a patient presents with a flail, anesthetic, and sometimes painful, upper extremity. With traumatic lesions, a Horner's syndrome should always be sought because frequently this presentation is a manifestation of C5-T1 root avulsions (19,20,37).

ELECTRODIAGNOSTIC FEATURES

If CMAPs of normal or near-normal amplitude can be recorded from any of the weak limb muscles 6 days or more after onset, demyelinating conduction block is responsible for at least some of the patient's symptoms. Usually, however, axon loss is the main or sole pathophysiology, and the findings are as described below.

Nerve Conduction Studies
Characteristically, all the upper extremity motor NCS responses, both routine and "nonstandard," are unelicitable or very low in amplitude. With "pure" preganglionic lesions, all the corresponding sensory NCS responses are normal, whereas with interforaminal and

extraforaminal lesions, or two-level lesions, they are usually unelicitable, including the median S-D1 and the LAC SNAPs, both of which assess C6 sensory fibers; the median S-D3 SNAP, which assesses C7 fibers; the radial S-BP SNAP, which assesses C6 and C7 fibers; the ulnar SNAPs, which assess C8 fibers; and the MAC SNAP, which assesses T1 fibers.

Needle Electrode Examination
Typically, all the arm and shoulder girdle muscles show severe changes, including fibrillation potentials and unelicitable MUPs or only a few MUPs firing at a rapid rate. Depending upon the level of the lesion, the spinati, rhomboids, serratus anterior, and cervical/high thoracic paraspinal muscles may show abnormalities as well (39).

Infraclavicular Plexopathies

THE CORDS

Lesions of this portion of the infraclavicular plexus probably are sustained somewhat less frequently than terminal nerve lesions; an appreciable number are iatrogenic in nature. Radiation-induced brachial plexopathies, in our experience, often are initially symptomatic owing to cord involvement, particularly of the lateral cord. Iatrogenic cord lesions also result from infraclavicular placement of intravenous lines and during breast operations. Noniatrogenic etiologies include blunt or penetrating axilla trauma and sustained axilla compression.

Disorders of the various cords present clinically as motor and sensory deficits in the distribution of two or more peripheral nerves or portions of peripheral nerves (17).

Lateral Cord
This infraclavicular plexus element is composed of the axons which will form the musculocutaneous nerve and the lateral head of the median nerve. The musculocutaneous nerve innervates the biceps and brachialis muscles and supplies sensation, via the LAC nerve, to the lateral aspect of the forearm; the lateral head of the median nerve innervates the pronator teres and FCR muscles and supplies sensation to the median nerve-innervated fingers (at least the lateral three) (8,37,46).

Table 11-5
Muscles Affected by Middle Plexus Lesions*

Nerve Conduction Studies	Needle Electrode Examination
Sensory	Biceps brachii
Median—D1 (thumb)	Brachialis
Median—D2 (index)	Pronator teres
Median—D3 (middle)	Flexor carpi radialis
Lat. antebrachial cutaneous	
Motor	
Musculocutaneous— biceps muscle	

*Nerve conduction studies and muscles (on needle electrode examination) that may show abnormalities, on electrodiagnostic assessment, with (infraclavicular) lateral cord lesions.

Lateral cord lesions should be suspected whenever there is weakness of forearm pronation, elbow flexion, and radial hand flexion, accompanied by sensory changes along the lateral forearm and sometimes the thumb, but rarely the other median-innervated fingers (37).

EDX Studies (Table 11-5)

Only one of the four "routine" upper extremity NCS, the median S-D2, assesses the lateral cord. Consequently, to optimally study this plexus element, nonstandard NCS are required. They help to confirm that the abnormalities are in a lateral cord distribution rather than an upper trunk or posterior cord distribution. Also, they aid in excluding a main trunk median nerve lesion.

On NCS, with axon loss lesions that are at least moderately severe, the musculocutaneous m. biceps CMAP, the LAC SNAP, and the various median SNAPs are affected. On NEE, abnormalities are found in the biceps, brachialis, pronator teres, and FCR muscles (38,39).

Lateral cord lesions must always be distinguished from the more common upper trunk lesions and from median nerve lesions by demonstrating that certain NCS and muscles are not involved, including the routine median CMAP, the axillary m. deltoid CMAP, and the radial S-BT SNAP (which is affected in approximately 50% of patients with upper trunk lesions.) On NEE, pertinent muscles that should appear normal include the bra-

chioradialis, the deltoid, the spinati, and the muscles innervated by the medial head of the median nerve via the lower trunk/medial cord of the plexus, e.g., the FPL and APB (39).

Posterior Cord

This portion of the infraclavicular plexus is composed principally of axons that subsequently will be components of the thoracodorsal, axillary, and radial nerves. Posterior cord lesions result in impairment of arm abduction, extension, full elevation, internal rotation, and external rotation, as well as extension of the forearm, hand, and fingers. Somewhat surprisingly, sensory disturbances often are incomplete, with loss apparent only over a small area overlying the deltoid and, occasionally, the base of the thumb (17,19,20,37).

EDX Studies (Table 11-6)

Similar to the assessment of several other portions of the brachial plexus, nonstandard NCS must be performed to assess the posterior cord. These include the axillary m. deltoid; the radial motor, recording from the proximal or distal extensor forearm; the radial S-BT, and the posterior antebrachial cutaneous. (We rarely find it necessary to perform the last study in our EMG laboratory). The NEE should demonstrate abnormalities in all radial-innervated muscles, regardless of their

Table 11-6
Muscles Affected by Posterior Cord Lesions*

Nerve Conduction Studies	Needle Electrode Examination
Sensory	Deltoid
Radial—thumb base	Teres minor
Post. antebrachial cutaneous	Triceps
	Anconeus
Motor	Brachioradialis
Axillary—deltoid m.	
Radial—prox. extensor forearm	Extensor carpi radialis
	Extensor digitorum communis
Radial—distal extensor forearm	Extensor indicis proprius
	Extensor pollicis brevis

*Nerve conduction studies and muscles (on needle electrode examination) that may show abnormalities, on electrodiagnostic assessment, with (infraclavicular) posterior cord lesions.

trunk innervation (e.g., the brachioradialis, upper trunk; triceps, middle trunk; and the EIP, lower trunk), as well as in the deltoid and teres minor muscles. To confirm the presence of a posterior cord lesion, other nerves in the limb, derived from the trunks via the anterior divisions, must be shown to be unaffected, including the musculocutaneous, median, and ulnar nerves. On NCS, the standard upper extremity studies are helpful in this regard, particularly when supplemented by the median S-D1 and median S-D3 responses. The NEE should include median and ulnar nerve-innervated intrinsic hand muscles as well as the pronator teres and biceps. Because two muscles innervated by the upper trunk, the brachioradialis and deltoid, are abnormal with posterior cord lesions, it is helpful to confirm on NEE that the spinati, in addition to the biceps and the brachialis, are unaffected (39).

Medial Cord

This portion of the infraclavicular plexus is composed of the medial cutaneous nerve, the MAC nerve, the ulnar nerve, and the medial head of the median nerve. Lesions of the medial cord result in weakness of some of the median and ulnar nerve-innervated forearm muscles, e.g., the FPL, FCU, and FDP (4,5), and of all of the intrinsic hand muscles. Sensory loss often is present along the medial arm, forearm, and hand (17,19,20,37).

EDX Studies (Table 11–7)

Because the median cord derives from the lower trunk, it is adequately assessed by the standard upper extremity NCS: median motor, ulnar motor, and ulnar S-D5. The only additional NCS that may be beneficial is the MAC NCS. On NEE, abnormalities are found in all the ulnar nerve-innervated muscles, as well as the median nerve-innervated APB and FPL. Median nerve fibers that traverse the lateral head of the median nerve via the lateral cord and radial nerve fibers derived from the lower trunk must be examined and shown to be unaffected. Thus, pertinent studies include any of the median sensory NCS and the NEE of at least the pronator teres or FCR and also the EIP and EPB (11,39).

Occasionally, the radial nerve component of the lower trunk is spared with lower trunk

Table 11–7
Muscles Affected by Medial Cord Lesions*

Nerve Conduction Studies	Needle Electrode Examination
Sensory	Abductor pollicis brevis
Ulnar—D5 (little)	Opponens pollicis
Ulnar—D4 (ring)	Flexor pollicis longus
Ulnar dorsal cutaneous	First dorsal interosseus
Med. antebrachial cutaneous	Adductor pollicis
	Abductor digiti minimi
Motor	Flexor carpi ulnaris
Ulnar—hypothenar	Flexor digitorum profundus 4,5
Ulnar—first dorsal interosseus	
Median—thenar	

*Nerve conduction studies and muscles (on needle electrode examination) that may show abnormalities, on electrodiagnostic assessment, with (infraclavicular) medial cord lesions.

lesions, especially with some true N-TOS, resulting in both the clinical and EDX presentations mimicking a medial cord lesion.

Pan-Cord

Co-existing lesions of all three cords are occasionally encountered. One of the more common causes for these, in our experience, is radiation. This type of pan-cord plexopathy is discussed below.

Radiation-induced Brachial Plexopathy

These disorders first appeared in the 1960s, soon after megavoltage radiation therapy replaced orthovoltage therapy; much higher voltages were utilized, and peak dosages were delivered far below the skin level, so skin changes were no longer a limiting factor. Most of the patients with radiation-induced brachial plexopathy are women who were treated for breast carcinoma. The onset of the symptoms of the brachial plexus injury in relation to the radiation therapy can vary remarkably, from before the radiation treatment is completed to decades later (16,37).

Probably the most common presenting symptom has been paresthesias, initially involving one or more of the median nerve-innervated fingers. There is a marked divergence of opinion regarding when, or even if, pain occurs. The typical clinical picture is one of slow progression, initially of sensory and then of motor disturbances. In some patients, the symptoms plateau for varying periods, occasionally indefinitely. Far more often, they ultimately progress until the patient is left with a useless limb. At this advanced stage, the diagnosis usually is obvious. However, early in its course, radiation-induced brachial plexopathy almost always must be differentiated from neoplastic brachial plexopathy because the radiation therapy was initially used to treat a neoplasm. This differentiation often proves difficult. Abnormalities on neuroimaging studies may be found with both, but frequently they are nondiagnostic. In addition, the EDX examination may not be helpful if it shows only an axon-loss brachial plexopathy. However, with radiation-induced plexopathies, conduction blocks often are demonstrable on motor NCS, myokymic discharges are noted on NEE, or both; these are due to focal demyelination, which is rarely seen with plexus neoplasms but is common with radiation-induced lesions (16,37,42).

Nerve Conduction Studies

The NCS findings are extremely variable, depending upon the severity and extent of the disorder which, in turn, often is dependent upon its duration. NCS performed soon after onset may be normal, or show only minimal changes, such as a low amplitude or a relatively low-amplitude median SNAP, recorded from just one of the median nerve-supplied fingers. As time passes, it is characteristic that progressively more of the sensory NCS responses become abnormal. The median sensory and LAC SNAPs are affected initially much more often than are the ulnar sensory and MAC SNAPs. Ultimately, however, all the upper extremity sensory NCS can be unelicitable. As soon as clinical weakness develops, the motor NCS usually become abnormal. In most instances, conduction blocks can be demonstrated on several, and sometimes all, of the upper extremity motor NCS, including ulnar, median, radial, musculocutaneous, and axillary. Excluding the axillary m. deltoid NCS, for which there is no infraclavicular stimulation site, these conduction blocks can be shown to involve the plexus fibers at some point between the supraclavicular and axilla stimulation sites; i.e., the distal trunk, divi-

sions, or cords (16,42). Such conduction blocks can persist for years. We have followed one patient, for example, who has been weak primarily because of them for over a decade (42). Eventually, however, axon loss often supervenes; as this occurs, the CMAPs that assess the affected fibers begin to decrease in amplitude on distal stimulation. Even when the limb is essentially useless, motor NCS responses usually are still present; the major cause for disability in many of these patients is sensory ataxia of the limb, not total motor axon loss, as when flail upper extremities result from neoplastic brachial plexopathies.

Needle Electrode Examination

The NEE findings with radiation-induced brachial plexopathies, similar to the NCS findings, are extremely variable. Some of the earliest findings, in our experience, are fibrillation potentials in the pronator teres muscle. This, along with the earliest NCS change usually being a low-amplitude median SNAP, suggests that the lateral cord is the initial site of injury. Fibrillation potentials usually are widespread when the disorder is advanced, although they rarely are present in abundant numbers. Nonetheless, they are the single most common type of spontaneous activity seen. Fasciculation potentials also are a common finding, particularly an unusual type of *regularly* firing repetitive fasciculation, which could be designated a "simple repetitive discharge." Myokymic discharges are less commonly seen, overall, than are fibrillation potentials and fasciculation potentials; moreover, they seldom are an early finding. Nonetheless, because they are not found with neoplastic plexopathies, they help confirm the underlying etiology of the lesion. (In our experience, repetitive fasciculation potentials do the same, and they are more common.) The MUP firing pattern is altered with the more advanced radiation-induced brachial plexopathies. The MUPs fire in decreased numbers at a rapid rate with both conduction block and axon loss. In addition, with long-standing lesions in which sensory dysfunction is severe, the patients experience difficulty with both activating and sustaining MUP firing because of sensory ataxia; this difficulty can be mistaken for deliberate poor voluntary effort. Often having the patient look at the body structure he or she is to move and the muscle he or she is to activate (e.g., to watch the index finger when asked to move it while the needle recording electrode is resting in the FDI muscle), yields a better MUP firing pattern. Chronic neurogenic MUP changes are usually prominent after several years. In advanced cases, these may be found in almost every muscle of the limb (42).

THE TERMINAL NERVES

Elements of the terminal nerves, the most distal portion of the brachial plexus, are injured in a variety of ways. These include fractures and dislocations of the humeral head and attempted reduction of humeral head dislocations; both of these usually injure at least the axillary terminal nerve. The terminal nerves also are injured by both blunt and penetrating trauma to the axilla region and by prolonged axilla compression; e.g., a person becomes unconscious with his arm draped over the back of a chair. With open injuries, the infraclavicular brachial plexus can sustain both direct and indirect (but often very severe) trauma, the latter owing to initial vascular injury with subsequent hematoma or pseudo-aneurysm formation. Iatrogenic causes include axillary arteriograms and axillary plexus blocks (20,37). This type of "neurovascular lesion" has recently been designated the "medial brachial fascial compartment syndrome" (33). One to several nerves can sustain extensive permanent damage. The median nerve is always involved. This is not surprising, considering that it is formed by the fusion of its medial and lateral heads virtually on top of the third portion of the axillary artery. With many infraclavicular plexopathies, two or more terminal nerves are injured simultaneously, and frequently such lesions are difficult to distinguish from cord lesions. Moreover, extensive infraclavicular lesions, involving two or more cords, multiple terminal nerves, or a combination of both, are not uncommon. Such "diffuse infraclavicular plexopathies" or "pan cord/terminal nerve lesions," often are mistaken for "pan-trunk lesions," based on the clinical examination or EDX studies alone, i.e., without taking into account the etiology of the lesion. That such

confusion occurs is understandable, because the only difference between a diffuse lesion of the mid or distal trunks and a diffuse lesion of the cords or terminal nerves is that the pectoralis muscles should show abnormalities with the former but generally not the latter, unless the extreme proximal medial and lateral cords are involved (39).

Electrodiagnostic Features
With all infraclavicular terminal nerve lesions, it must be demonstrated that the EDX abnormalities are restricted to the distribution of the affected nerve or nerves. How readily this can be accomplished on NCS depends upon the particular nerve involved. If only the median motor and sensory NCS are abnormal, the lesion must be affecting the median nerve fibers distal to the cord level, because the axons that are assessed by these NCS do not become contiguous in the plexus until the termination of the lateral and medial cords. In contrast, if only the ulnar motor and ulnar sensory NCS are abnormal, the lesion could be affecting the ulnar terminal nerve, but it could also be involving the lower trunk or medial cord because the ulnar motor and sensory axons are contiguous throughout the plexus. To assess lesions involving terminal nerves other than the median and ulnar, nonstandard NCS must be performed: the radial motor (recording either the proximal or distal extensor forearm) and radial S-BT NCS for radial nerve assessment; the musculocutaneous motor and LAC NCS for musculocutaneous nerve assessment; and the axillary motor NCS for axillary nerve assessment. On NEE, two criteria must be met. First, abnormalities must be demonstrated in several muscles innervated by the affected nerve, always including muscles supplied by its most proximal branches, i.e., the FCU and FDP (4,5) for ulnar; the pronator teres and FCR for median; and the triceps and anconeus for radial. Because no motor branches arise proximal to the elbow from either the median or ulnar nerves, it is impossible, using EDX studies, to distinguish an infraclavicular plexus lesion from a proximal (i.e., arm) peripheral nerve lesion of those nerves. Second, several muscles, innervated by the same root(s) as the affected muscles but by other than the involved terminal

nerve(s), must be shown to be normal. Thus, with a terminal median nerve infraclavicular plexopathy, the APB ((C8)T1-innervated), FPL (C8,T1-innervated), and pronator teres (C6,C7-innervated) should be abnormal on the NEE, whereas the FDI (C8,T1/ulnar-innervated), EIP (C8/radial-innervated), and triceps (C6,C7/radial-innervated) should be normal (39).

Finally, multiple terminal nerve lesions can be difficult to distinguish from cord lesions on EDX examination, just as on clinical examination.

Brachial Plexus Assessment—Some Guidelines

Electromyographers lacking experience in assessing patients with possible brachial plexopathies should appreciate the following points.

1. NCS, both motor and sensory, and NEE should be performed on every patient, because neither one alone provides all the relevant information available.
2. Whenever possible, sensory NCS should be recorded from areas where there are sensory complaints, and motor NCS should be recorded from muscles that are clinically weak. Often, this means nonroutine NCS must be performed.
3. The amplitude of the CMAP recorded from a weak muscle usually is a much more reliable indicator of the amount of axon loss that muscle has undergone than are the changes seen on the NEE of the muscle. The two major exceptions to this are a) With very recent-onset lesions, i.e., those of less than 7 days' duration, the distal stump can still conduct impulses; and b) With very remote or slowly progressive lesions, marked collateral sprouting may have occurred in the interim, causing the motor NCS amplitudes to be deceptively high compared to the amount of MUP dropout and chronic MUP changes found on the NEE.
4. Whenever an NCS amplitude is borderline low or in the lower range of

normal, the same NCS on the contralateral normal limb should be performed to obtain control data; any amplitude 50% or less than that found in the corresponding opposite limb is abnormal, even though it may be within the normal range for the EMG laboratory.
5. The duration of the lesion should be considered when performing the EDX examination and interpreting its results. In general, with acute onset lesions, EDX studies should not be done too soon after onset, before all changes caused by axon loss have had sufficient time to manifest themselves. Unless a conduction block is demonstrable on supraclavicular stimulation, the results of any NCS performed during the first 2 days after lesion onset will simply reflect the pre-injury state. Moreover, NCS performed 5–6 days post-injury can be quite misleading, because the CMAP, but not the SNAP, amplitudes will have had time to reach their nadir. Finally, fibrillation potentials typically require 3 weeks or more to develop in limb muscles, so the full extent of a lesion, or even its very presence, can be missed if the NEE is performed too early.
6. It helps to think anatomically. Using the history and clinical examination, it can be decided before the EDX examination is initiated whether the lesion is most likely supraclavicular or infraclavicular in location. This can influence what NCS are performed and what muscles are sampled on the NEE, because it permits predicting the distribution of the EDX abnormalities. If the results turns out to be other than anticipated, the tentative pre-EDX examination localization must be revised.
7. Supraclavicular stimulation should be done whenever there is a possibility that a conduction block is present. It can be demonstrated if it involves the distal supraclavicular, the subclavicular, or the infraclavicular plexus, but not if it is more proximal. Moreover, supraclavicular stimulation also should

be performed whenever the degree of weakness on clinical examination and the dropout of MUPs on NEE of a paretic muscle are not consistent with the CMAP amplitude recorded from it during motor NCS.

8. In regard to axon loss, although the basic upper extremity NCS—median motor and sensory; ulnar motor and sensory—assess the lower trunk and medial cord well, and the middle trunk and lateral cord often adequately, they usually do not assess the upper trunk, and never the posterior cord. Consequently, in many instances additional NCS must be performed.

9. Unelicitable CMAPs in the presence of normal or even low-amplitude SNAPs that assess the same plexus elements are very indicative of an intraspinal canal lesion, usually an avulsion injury, even if paraspinal fibrillation potentials cannot be found.

10. The longitudinal location of a lesion should be determined whenever possible. Thus, if fibrillation potentials are present in the median- and ulnar-innervated hand muscles, among the possible lesion locations are the lower trunk and medial cord; the latter can be excluded by demonstrating similar abnormalities in the C8/radial nerve-innervated muscles. Similarly, if abnormalities are found in the biceps, deltoid, and brachioradialis, the spinati should be assessed. If they are also abnormal, the serratus anterior and possibly the rhomboids should be sampled. If they, in turn, show fibrillation potentials, the paraspinal muscles must be studied.

11. EDX localization of brachial plexopathies can be faulty, especially when only a modest amount of axon loss has occurred or the process is of very remote onset and static. Characteristically, in this instance, the lesion is mislocalized more distal along the plexus than it actually is.

12. The value of EDX studies in brachial plexus assessment can be compromised by many confounding factors. These include such diverse processes as prior or coexisting peripheral nerve lesions; open wounds, intravenous lines, bandages and casts overlying stimulation and recording sites; and patients being unable to tolerate the limb placement necessary for a particular study, NCS or NEE.

13. Finally, whenever "shoulder" weakness is present but the upper plexus EDX assessment is normal, performing NEE on the upper trapezius muscle may reveal an unsuspected spinal accessory mononeuropathy.

PHRENIC NERVE ASSESSMENT

The phrenic nerve, composed of two-thirds motor fibers and one-third sensory fibers, is the major nerve originating from the cervical plexus. Its motor component innervates the diaphragm and thus is the principal nerve of respiration (3,7).

Anatomy

The phrenic nerve derives principally from the C4 VPR, with contributions from the C3 and C5 VPR. It is formed from the more caudal cervical plexus, on the lateral superficial surface of the anterior scalene muscle. It then descends on that muscle, covered partly by the sternomastoid muscle. After passing between the subclavian artery and vein, it leaves the neck and enters the thorax behind the sternoclavicular joint. It then continues inferiorly through first the superior mediastinum, near the root of the lung, and then the middle mediastinum, along the lateral aspect of the pericardium, to reach the diaphragm. Its motor branches innervate the diaphragm, whereas its sensory branches supply the diaphragm, a portion of both the mediastinal and costal pleura, and the pericardium (7,8).

PHRENIC NERVE LESIONS

The phrenic nerve can be injured by both blunt and penetrating neck trauma (7). It may also be damaged during surgical procedures, particularly during open heart surgery, in which several etiologies—traction, instrumentation, hypothermia (owing to cold cardioplegia)—may be operative. It can also be affected by neoplasms and other space-occupying lesions (3,7,34,37,45). Occasionally, neuralgic amyotrophy involves one or both phrenic nerves (3,7,34,40,45). Unilateral phrenic nerve involvement generally causes few, if any, symptoms (7). To treat brachial plexus avulsion injuries, for example, one surgical group has used the phrenic nerve as a donor nerve for neurotization; i.e., they have sectioned the phrenic nerve and connected its proximal end to the avulsed motor axons supplying the biceps and other muscles to partially reinnervate them (15). Bilateral phrenic nerve involvement, in contrast, is always marked by major symptoms, including dyspnea on exertion, constant use of the accessory respiratory muscles, and an inability to cough. The last disability frequently leads to pneumonia (7).

ELECTRODIAGNOSTIC ASSESSMENT

Difficulty with breathing is a relatively common disorder, particularly in postsurgical and critical care units, where the inability to wean patients from mechanical ventilators occurs with some frequency. There are many causes for such respiratory difficulties, including primary lung disease, airway or chest wall problems, lack of central nervous system respiratory drive, phrenic nerve dysfunction, and weakness of the respiratory musculature, including the diaphragm. The last two etiologies—phrenic nerve and diaphragmatic muscle abnormalities—often can be diagnosed in the EMG laboratory by performing both phrenic NCS and NEE of the diaphragm (3,4). At present, neither of these EDX procedures is standardized; instead, several techniques for performing each have been described and are being used by various investigators. Assessing the phrenic nerve is difficult by any means, including EDX studies. Its sensory component cannot be evaluated, and the muscle it innervates, the diaphragm, not only is relatively inaccessible but also is situated near structures that generally will not tolerate even minor injuries by a needle recording electrode without serious complications ensuing. Moreover, phrenic nerve assessments all-too-often are requested on patients who have, from the EDX viewpoint, the worst possible physiognomy: thick necks and barrel chests.

Phrenic NCS

Various techniques have been used during this procedure for phrenic nerve assessment, both for stimulating the phrenic nerve and for recording the resulting CMAP from the diaphragm, including the use of needle stimulating and recording electrodes as well as esophageal recording electrodes (3,22,29,35). Surface electrodes are used in most EMG laboratories for both stimulating and recording. The nerve is stimulated along the posterior border of the sternocleidomastoid muscle, with the exact site varying among different investigators. Some prefer to stimulate along the mid portion of that muscle, on a line with the upper border of the thyroid cartilage, whereas others stimulate more inferiorly, immediately above the clavicle. The most significant variation in phrenic NCS, from one EMG laboratory to another, is in the recording sites employed. Bolton, for example,

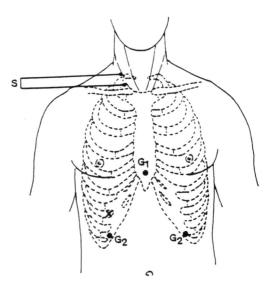

Figure 11–11. Phrenic nerve motor NCS (technique of Bolton). The active (*G1*) electrode is over the mid-inferior sternum, 5 cm superior to the xiphoid, whereas the reference electrodes (*G2*) are located 16 cm laterally and inferiorly, on the lower costal margin. The nerve is stimulated (*S*) immediately above the clavicle. (Reprinted with permission from Bolton CF: Electromyography in the critical care unit. In: Brown WF, Bolton CF, eds. Clinical electromyography, 2nd ed. Boston: Butterworth-Heineman, 1993.)

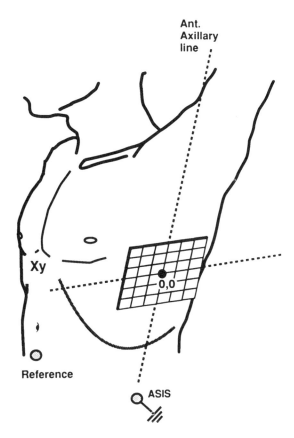

Ant.
Axillary
line

Xy

0,0

Reference

ASIS

Figure 11-12. Phrenic nerve motor NCS (technique of Swenson and Rubenstein). The active (*G1*) electrode is located either over the xiphoid (*Xy*) or on the lateral chest wall, at a point (*O,O*) where the anterior axillary line intersects with a transverse plane through the xiphoid. With both techniques, the G2 electrode (*reference*) is located on the abdominal midline, halfway between the umbilicus and the pubis. (Reprinted with permission from Swenson MR, Rubenstein RS: Phrenic nerve conduction studies. Muscle Nerve 1992; 15:597–603.)

places the G1 (active) electrode in the midline over the inferior sternum, 5 cm above the xiphoid, and the G2 (reference) electrode 16 cm inferiorly laterally, on the lower costal margin (Fig. 11–11) (3,4). Swenson and Rubenstein, in contrast, have used as their G1 site both the xiphoid and a point on the lateral chest wall where the anterior axillary line intersects with the transverse plane through the xiphoid; with both techniques, their G2 electrode has been located on the abdomen in the midline, halfway between the umbilicus and the pubis (Fig. 11–12) (35). Probably the majority of investigators have used the xiphoid as their active electrode site, with various intercostal spaces near the costochondral junction serving as the reference point. Regardless of the method employed, the CMAP obtained in normal persons is usually less than 1.0 millivolt in amplitude, with the average often being between 0.3 to 0.5 millivolts. The distal latencies have ranged from approximately 4 to 9 milliseconds, with an average of 6 to 8 milliseconds; latencies of greater than 10 millisec-

onds generally are considered abnormal. Confounding factors have included variation in the CMAP with the respiratory cycle, EMG artifact from chest wall muscles (caused by accidental stimulation of some brachial plexus fibers during phrenic nerve stimulation), and EKG artifact (3,4,35).

Needle Electrode Examination

At least two different techniques are used for the NEE of the diaphragm muscle. With the method of Goodgold and of Saadeh et al., the recording needle electrode is inserted through the abdominal wall and then angulated upward under the costal margin (14,30). With the technique first described by Koepke and then reintroduced by Bolton, the recording needle electrode is inserted through an intercostal space, between the anterior axillary and medial clavicular lines (3,4). When it is inserted immediately above the costal margin, it does not enter the plural space. On the NEE, the diaphragmatic MUPs fire in regular bursts with each inspiration. They are lower in amplitude and of shorter duration than limb muscle MUPs and are quite numerous during each burst. Whenever diaphragmatic NEE is performed on patients who are on mechanical ventilation, the latter must be discontinued for a brief period. Although several structures—the lung, spleen, liver, and colon—can be injured accidentally during attempted NEE of the diaphragm, probably the most common complication, albeit still rare (1 per 500 studies), is pleural cavity penetration with the production of a pneumothorax. For this reason, patients undergoing diaphragmatic NEE should be observed for at least one hour following the procedure; if any evidence of a pneumothorax appears, further evaluation is necessary (3,4).

Electrodiagnostic Findings

With generalized disorders, the findings with phrenic nerve assessment usually mirror those seen during the general EDX examination. In patients who suffer respiratory insufficiency caused by either amyotrophic lateral sclerosis or axon-loss polyneuropathies (e.g., porphyric polyneuropathy), the phrenic CMAP usually is of low amplitude or unelicitable and the distal latency, if a response is obtainable, generally is normal. Diaphragmatic NEE reveals fibrillation potentials and MUP dropout. If MUPs can be activated then, depending upon the chronicity of the lesion, they either are normal in appearance or they show chronic neurogenic changes. With demyelinating polyradiculoneuropathies (e.g., Guillain-Barré syndrome), the phrenic CMAP usually is low in amplitude or unelicitable soon after onset and low in amplitude, dispersed, and prolonged in distal latency during later stages. Diaphragmatic NEE may show only MUP dropout but often, as with the limb muscles, some associated axon loss has occurred and fibrillation potentials are seen. With neuromuscular transmission disorders (e.g., myasthenia gravis), slow repetitive stimulation studies can be performed on the phrenic nerve and may reveal a defect. However, this type of study is seldom done because of technical difficulties in its interpretation; the phrenic motor NCS amplitudes normally vary during the respiratory cycle, and they can also change because of superimposed EKG artifact. With

primary myopathies, the phrenic CMAP amplitude can be affected, although the distal latency remains normal. Diaphragmatic NEE is helpful with those myopathies in which spontaneous activity, such as fibrillation potentials or myotonic discharges, occur. However, assessing the MUPs of the diaphragm for "myopathic" changes is extremely difficult because of their normal "myopathic" morphology, attributed to their low innervation ratio (3,4).

It is when phrenic nerve assessment is used to detect unilateral or bilateral phrenic nerve lesions that the reported results become both variable and sometimes perplexing. Theoretically with acute phrenic nerve injury, only the amplitude of the phrenic CMAP is affected. With complete focal lesions, no response is obtained (i.e., the amplitude is "0"); therefore, a distal latency cannot be determined. Incomplete lesions yield a low-amplitude response with a distal latency that most often is normal but may be somewhat prolonged, owing to the loss or inactivation of the fastest conducting fibers. In addition with unilateral lesions, the CMAP amplitude obtained by performing motor NCS on the contralateral phrenic nerve should serve as a normal control. Although some reports have described the CMAP amplitudes as being essentially equal from one side to the other in normal persons (as intuitively they should be), Swenson and Rubenstein, following very detailed studies, have made the disturbing observation that side-to-side correlations for both CMAP amplitude and waveform are poor. As a result, they consider the uninvolved side to be an unreliable standard for comparison when assessing for unilateral partial phrenic nerve lesions (35). Moreover, some physicians do not consider the amplitudes at all during phrenic motor NCS, preferring instead to focus only on the distal latencies (10, 29, 45). This approach seems inherently flawed, because patients with suspected acute phrenic nerve lesions invariably are studied because of presumed diaphragmatic weakness; yet, of the various components of the phrenic motor NCS, only the amplitude has any consistent correlation with weakness of the recorded muscle. The distal latencies, by contrast, are affected by axon loss only whenever the fastest conducting fibers happen to be among those that degenerate. Consequently, prolonged distal latencies are an inconsistent, and therefore unreliable, finding whenever the recorded muscle is weak. This undoubtedly is the explanation for reports of normal phrenic distal latencies "inexplicably" being found in patients with ipsilateral diaphragmatic paresis. On NEE of the diaphragm, MUP dropout is present with phrenic nerve weakness, regardless of whether the primary pathophysiology is axon loss or demyelinating conduction block. (The primary pathophysiology is never just demyelinating focal slowing.) In addition, if axon loss has occurred, fibrillation potentials are present.

References

1. Alnot JY: Traumatic paralysis of the brachial plexus: Pre- operative problems and therapeutic indications. In: Terzis JK, ed. Microreconstruction of nerve injuries. Philadelphia: WB Saunders 1987;325–345.
2. Aston JW: Brachial plexus birth injury. Orthopedics 1979; 2:594–601.
3. Bolton CF: AAEM minimonograph #40: Clinical neurophysiology of the respiratory system. Muscle Nerve 1993; 18: 809–818.
4. Bolton CF: Electromyography in the critical care unit. In: Brown WF, Bolton CF, eds. Clinical electromyography. 2nd ed. Boston: Butterworth-Heineman, 1993; 759–773.
5. Brody IA, Wilkins RH: Erb's palsy. Arch Neurol 1969; 21:442–444.
6. Burke D: Value and limitations of nerve conduction studies. In: Delwaide PJ, Gorio A, eds. Clinical neurophysiology in peripheral neuropathies. Amsterdam: Elsevier, 1985;91–102.
7. Chusid J: Correlative neuroanatomy and functional neurology. 16th ed. Los Altos: Lange Medical Pub., 1976.
8. Clements CD, ed: Gray's anatomy of the human body. 30th American ed. Philadelphia: Lea and Febiger, 1985.
9. Cwik VA, Wilbourn AJ, Rorick M: Acute brachial neuropathy: Detailed EMG findings in a large series. Muscle Nerve 1990; 13: 859.
10. DeVita MA, Robinson LR, Rehder J, et al.: Incidence and natural history of phrenic neuropathy occurring during open heart surgery. Chest 1993; 103: 850–856.
11. Ferrante MA, Wilbourn AJ: The utility of various upper extremity sensory nerve conduction responses in assessing brachial plexopathies. Muscle Nerve 1995 (in press).
12. Fowler TJ, Danta G, Gilliatt RW: Recovery of nerve conduction after a pneumatic tourniquet; observations on the hind limb of the baboon. J Neurol Neurosurg Psychiatry 1958; 21: 109–118.
13. Gilliatt RW, LeQuesne PM, Logue V, et al.: Wasting of the hand associated with a cervical rib and band. J Neurol Neurosurg Psychiat 1970; 175–178.
14. Goodgold J: Anatomical correlates of clinical electromyography. 2nd ed. Baltimore: Williams & Wilkins, 1984:41.
15. Gu YD, Wu MM, Zhen YL, et al.: Phrenic nerve transfer for treatment of root avulsion of the brachial plexus. Chinese Med J (Peking) 1990;103:267–270.
16. Harper CM, Thomas JE, Casino TL, et al.: Distinction between neoplastic and radiation-induced brachial plexopathy with emphasis on the role of EMG. Neurology 1989; 39:502–506.
17. Haymaker W, Woodhall B: Peripheral nerve injuries. 2nd ed. Philadelphia: WB Saunders, 1953.
18. Johnson EW, Alexander MA, Koenig WC: Infantile Erb's palsy (Smellie's palsy). Arch Phy Med Rehabil 1977; 58: 175–178.
19. Kline DG, Hudson AR: Nerve injuries. Philadelphia: WB Saunders, 1995.
20. Leffert RD: Brachial plexus injuries. New York: Churchill- Livingstone, 1985.
21. Markey KL, DiBenedetto M, Curl WW: Upper trunk brachial plexopathy: The stinger syndrome. Am J Sports Med 1993; 21: 650–655.
22. Markland ON, Kincaid JC, Pourmand RA, et al.: Electrophysiological evaluation of diaphragm by transcutaneous phrenic nerve stimulation. Neurology 1984; 34: 604–614.
23. McDonald WI: Physiological consequences of demyelination. In: Sumner A, ed. The physiology of peripheral nerve disease. Philadelphia: WB Saunders, 1980;265–286.
24. Narakas AO: Traumatic brachial plexus lesions. In: Dyck PJ, Thomas PK, Lambert EH, et al., eds. Peripheral Neuropathy. 2nd ed. Philadelphia: WB Saunders 1984;2:1394–1409.
25. Parry GJ: Electrodiagnostic studies in the evaluation of peripheral nerve and brachial plexus lesions. Neurol Clin 1992; 10: 921–934.
26. Parsonage MJ, Turner AJW: Neuralgic amyotrophy: The shoulder girdle syndrome. Lancet 1948; 1:973–978.
27. Poindexter DP, Johnson EW: Football shoulder and neck injury: A study of the "stinger." Arch Phys Med Rehabil 1984;65:601–603.
28. Roos DB: The place for scalenectomy and first rib resection in thoracic outlet syndrome. Surgery 1982;92:1077–1085.
29. Russell RIR, Mulvey D, Laroche C, et al.: Bedside assessment of phrenic nerve function in infants and children. J Thorac Cardiovasc Surg 1991;101: 143–147.
30. Saadeh PB, Sosner J, Wolf E: Needle EMG of the diaphragm: A new technique. Arch Phys Med Rehabil 1987;68:599–601.
31. Seddon H: Surgical disorders of the peripheral nerves. 2nd ed. Edinburgh: Churchill-Livingstone, 1972.
32. Sedel L: Repair of severe traction lesions of the brachial plexus. Clin. Orthop Related Research, 1988; 237:62–66.

33. Smith DC, Mitchell DA, Peterson GW, et al.: Medial brachial fascial compartment syndrome: Anatomic basis of neuropathy after transaxillary arteriography. Radiology 1989;173:149–154.

34. Sunderland S: Nerve and Nerve Injuries. 2nd ed. Edinburgh: Churchill-Livingstone, 1978.

35. Swenson MR, Rubenstein RS: Phrenic nerve conduction studies. Muscle Nerve 1992;15:597–603.

36. Swift TR: Diagnosing and evaluating plexopathies. In syllabus: Course #441: Clinical EMG. Minneapolis, MN: American Academy of Neurology, 1994; 29–55.

37. Wilbourn AJ: Brachial plexus disorders. In: Dyck PJ, Thomas PK, eds. Peripheral neuropathy. 3rd ed. Philadelphia, WB Saunders, 1993;2:911–950.

38. Wilbourn AJ: Electrodiagnosis of plexopathies. Neurol Clin 1985;3:511–520.

39. Wilbourn AJ: The brachial plexus: Anatomy, pathophysiology, and electrodiagnostic assessment. 1994 AAEM Course C: Brachial plexus assessment. Rochester MN: American Association of Electrodiagnostic Medicine, 1994;7–30.

40. Wilbourn AJ: Thoracic outlet syndrome. In syllabus: Course D: Controversies in entrapment neuropathies. Rochester, MN: American Association of Electromyography and Electrodiagnosis, 1984; 28–38.

41. Wilbourn AJ: Thoracic outlet syndrome surgery causing severe brachial plexopathy. Muscle Nerve 1988;11:66–74.

42. Wilbourn AJ, Levin KH, Lederman RJ: Radiation-induced brachial plexopathy; Electrodiagnostic changes over 13 years. Muscle Nerve 1994;17:1108.

43. Wilbourn AJ, Porter JM: Thoracic outlet syndrome. Spine: state of the art reviews. 1988;2:597–626.

44. Wilbourn AJ, Shields RW: Classic post-operative brachial plexopathy-the electrodiagnostic features. Neurology 1993;43:PA322.

45. Wilcox PG, Paré PD, Pardy RL: Recovery after unilateral phrenic nerve injury associated with coronary artery revascularization. Chest 1990;98:661–666.

46. Williams PL, Warwick R: Functional neuroanatomy in man. In: Gray's anatomy (neurology). Br. 35th ed. Philadelphia: WB Saunders, 1975.

Chapter 12

Evaluation of the Patient with Suspected Peripheral Neuropathy

James W. Albers

The clinical electromyographer is referred a patient with slowly progressive extremity weakness, mild sensory loss, and areflexia. The referring physician asks only, "Does the patient have neuropathy?" After evaluation, the possible responses could include "Yes," "No," or "I'm not sure," or you, the electromyographer, could use your combined clinical and electrodiagnostic skills to help explain the patient's symptoms and signs. The evaluation of patients with suspected polyneuropathy (subsequently referred to as "neuropathy"), is relatively straightforward. The evaluation consists of a combination of clinical, electrophysiologic, and laboratory studies, with the expectation that the electromyographer will integrate this combined information. It is no longer sufficient to simply confirm the presence of abnormality or to conclude that findings are consistent with neuropathy.

Evaluation of suspected neuropathy is among the most frequent investigations performed in the electromyography (EMG) laboratory, and the electromyographer plays an important role in establishing not only the presence but also the etiology of neuropathy (3). The patient's history and clinical findings provide important clues in establishing the diagnosis or suggesting studies important in identifying etiology, and the electromyographer's role in performing a neuromuscular

consultation includes paying careful attention to relevant clinical information. Knowledge of potential exposures (occupational, social, or pharmacologic) or recognition of a systemic illness may suggest the cause of a patient's neuropathy, although symptomatic neuropathy may appear before recognition of a systemic disorder. The electromyographer frequently is the physician most experienced in making these important associations.

The electrodiagnostic examination is in many ways an extension of the clinical neurologic evaluation. It is derived from sound neurophysiologic principles, and provides objective information useful in confirming clinical findings; in addition, it localizes abnormalities to a degree not clinically possible. In the evaluation of neuropathy, electrodiagnostic results often suggest the underlying pathophysiology, providing additional clues in establishing etiology. A complete electrodiagnostic study includes evaluation of sensory and motor nerve conduction studies, late responses, and needle electromyography. Almost all patients with neuropathy demonstrate large fiber dysfunction, making the EMG examination a powerful clinical tool for evaluating suspected neuropathy. Classification of neuropathy using electrophysiological information focuses the differential diagnosis and the subsequent evaluation, and often offers a specific diagnosis or class of disorders (27). Unfortunately, many neuropathies are characterized by non-specific axonal loss, increasing the importance of clinical information in establishing a diagnosis. Nevertheless, several of the most common treatable polyneuropathies do have characteristic electrodiagnostic features, yet were rarely

Portions of the unreferenced material in this chapter are modified from Albers JW: Evaluation of polyneuropathy. American Association of Electrocardiagnostic Medicine; Course D: Fundamentals of Electrocardiagnostic Medicine, October 9, 1993; and Donofrio PD, Albers JW: AAEM Minimonograph #34: Polyneuropathy. Classification by nerve conduction studies and electromyography. Muscle Nerve 1990;13:889–903.

diagnosed 25 years ago. Awareness of these disorders relates to the increased utilization of clinical electrophysiology and the identification of characteristic electrodiagnostic features that result in the disorders' recognition.

The following section reviews the underlying pathophysiology associated with neuropathy, defines expectations of the electromyographer, outlines a recommended evaluation, and identifies distinguishing electrical and clinical features useful in defining specific classes of neuropathy. For each classification, specific clinical examples are included.

PATHOPHYSIOLOGIC FEATURES OF NEUROPATHY

Few major pathophysiologic changes are important in the clinical electrodiagnostic evaluation of neuropathy. The most important include axonal degeneration, axonal atrophy, demyelination (uniform and multifocal), and metabolic changes that alter nerve conduction (2,27).

Axonal Lesions

Axonal degeneration results from disorders of the nerve cell (neuronopathy) or the axon (axonopathy). Pathophysiologic findings resemble those associated with nerve transection, varying only in degree (2). Separation of the distal axon from the nutritive cell body produces distal axonal degeneration and breakdown of the myelin sheath (wallerian degeneration). Landau reported that muscle contraction to nerve stimulation distal to the lesion persisted for several days after transection, but then disappeared (59). Sensory and motor responses similarly remain normal for several days with stimulation distal to the transection. Within days, sensory nerve action potential (SNAP) and compound muscle action potential (CMAP) motor amplitudes diminish and ultimately disappear, although conduction along individual axons remains relatively normal before disappearance.

Needle EMG initially shows absent voluntary activity but no other findings. Gilliatt and Taylor (41) demonstrated spontaneous discharge (i.e., fibrillation potentials) of individual muscle fibers beginning 1 to 4 weeks after

axonal degeneration, depending upon their proximity to the transection. Fibrillation potentials reflect muscle fiber hypersensitivity to acetylcholine (ACh) and are associated with the proliferation and migration of extrajunctional acetylcholine receptors (AChRs) on the muscle membrane (31). Initial findings include increased muscle fiber sensitivity to mechanical stimulation (typically in the form of positive waves), followed by sustained spontaneous activity at rest. The amplitude of fibrillation potentials and positive waves diminishes over time, proportional to muscle fiber atrophy, providing a useful marker for assessing the duration of partial denervation.

Findings with partial or incomplete axonal lesions are similar, with decreased (instead of absent) sensory and motor responses, normal conduction along surviving axons, and reduced voluntary motor unit action potential (MUAP) recruitment (2). Abnormal spontaneous activity appears in denervated muscle fibers. After partial denervation, some denervated muscle fibers eventually are reinnervated by collateral sprouts from surviving axons, resulting in large motor units at the same time the total number of motor units is reduced (93). Acetylcholine hypersensitivity resolves once muscle fibers are reinnervated, and abnormal spontaneous activity disappears. Ballantyne and Hansen demonstrated that regenerating axons produced new motor units by reinnervating muscle fibers shed by the abnormally large motor units (15).

The most common morphologic response to a variety of disorders producing neuropathy is a distal axonopathy (2). A variety of mechanisms exist to explain distal axonal degeneration in neuropathy, including the failure of axonal transport of some nutrient required for maintenance of the distal axon, as proposed by Schaumburg and associates (79). Axonal atrophy is controversial, but may represent a form of incomplete axonal lesion appearing before axonal degeneration. It is described at the terminal axon as a reduced caliper of the distal axon (i.e., axonal stenosis). Because conduction velocity is proportional to axonal diameter, action potential propagation is reduced proportional to the size of the atrophic distal axon. Unlike axonal degeneration, sensory and motor amplitudes are not substantially reduced, and muscle membrane excitability is unaffected.

Myelin Sheath Lesions

Disorders of the myelin sheath produce conduction abnormalities similar to those associated with focal nerve compression. Conduction may be slowed or blocked across the site of compression without producing axonal degeneration (67, 69). In experimental models using a compressing tourniquet, Ochoa and associates identified localized defects beneath the edges of the tourniquet, with telescoping of one myelin segment beneath the next at the node of Ranvier (38, 68). This structural abnormality is thought to reduce or block ionic current flow by occluding the node, thereby slowing or preventing action potential propagation (67). Paranodal demyelination is associated with a variety of conditions including focal compression and neuropathy, and conduction block is attributed to localized demyelination and intramyelin edema. Ochoa and Marotte demonstrated that chronic nerve compression produces similar findings, with distorted myelin segments (segmental demyelination), exposed axons, and paranodal remyelination with short internodal distances (69). Membrane excitability does not increase substantially with demyelinating lesions. Conduction slowing or block across a compressive lesion is relevant to the evaluation of generalized neuropathy; findings attributed to acquired demyelinating neuropathies have similar myelin abnormalities distributed throughout the peripheral nervous system, combining demyelination and remyelination, short internodes, and reduced conduction velocity.

Metabolic Lesions

Reduced conduction velocity does not always indicate histologic abnormality such as axonal stenosis or demyelination, because metabolic disorders may produce conduction slowing without identifiable structural abnormalities (2). In patients with hyperglycemia, increased conduction velocity 6 hours after normalizing glucose levels suggests that nonstructural changes account partially for conduction slowing (89). In the neuropathy associated with chronic diabetes mellitus, hyperglycemia is associated with a decrease in nerve myo-inositol and increased polyol-pathway activity related to the increased conversion of glucose to sorbitol by aldose reductase. The reduced nerve myo-inositol leads to reduced Na^+/K^+-ATPase activity and a resultant increase in intracellular Na^+ (44). In isolation, the resultant mild depolarization of the resting membrane potential decreases conduction velocity independent of structural alteration. Additional changes, including inactivation of sodium channels and axoglial disjunction also contribute to conduction velocity abnormalities (82).

WHAT IS EXPECTED OF THE ELECTROMYOGRAPHER?

The electromyographer or electrodiagnostic medicine consultant plays an important role in the evaluation of suspected peripheral disorders. It is expected that the electromyographer does more than confirm the presence of abnormality or conclude that findings are consistent with a neuropathy; possible etiologies should be suggested to complete the consultation. The electromyographer is a neuromuscular specialist with experience in the evaluation and treatment of patients with neuropathy. It is this clinical experience, combined with electrophysiologic information, that is useful in deriving a diagnosis. The emphasis of this chapter is on the application and interpretation of electrodiagnostic information. However, the study begins with a focused history and neurologic examination. Features of the clinical examination particularly important to the evaluation of neuropathy are summarized in Table 12–1.

The electrodiagnostic information is useful only when collected appropriately. Several components of the examination can be standardized. In the examination, the electromyographer must attend to these components, which are covered in the following questions.

1. Are the clinical findings consistent with the electrodiagnostic evaluation?
2. Were the limb temperatures monitored and cool limbs warmed to at least 31° to 32°C?

Table 12-1
Important Features of the Clinical Examination in Suspected Neuropathy

General information:
      Onset and temporal profile of motor, sensory, and autonomic complaints.
      Type and distribution of paresthesia, hyperesthesia, and hyperpathia.
      Distribution of weakness.
      Industrial and medical history for toxin or drug exposures.
      Family history, including bony deformities such as pes cavus or hammer toes.
      Social habits, including recreational drug use.
      Antecedent illness or symptoms of underlying disease.

Clinical examination
    General:
        Findings most prominent in distal lower extremities.
        Relative symmetry.
        Associated findings, such as tremor, skin lesions, bony deformities (pes cavus or hammer toes).
        Peripheral nerves palpated for tenderness, paresthesia, hypertrophy.
    Motor (emphasis upon distal muscles):
        Intrinsic hand muscles; finger and wrist extensors.
        Toe extensors and foot dorsiflexors.
    Sensory:
        Demonstrate distal-to-proximal sensory loss gradient.
        Identify involved modalities.
            Large fiber: vibration, light-touch, touch-pressure (common); joint position sensation (JPS) when severe.
            Small fiber: temperature, pin-pain, deep pain.
        Discriminative sensations less helpful in peripheral disorders.
        Absence of sensory level on the trunk.
        Vibratory loss to iliac crest and JPS loss may suggest spinal cord lesion.
    Reflexes:
        Achilles reflexes usually absent.
        Diffusely hypoactive reflexes not necessarily abnormal.
        Absence of pathologic reflexes (e.g., Babinski's reflex or sign).
    Autonomic nervous system:
        Postural hypotension.
        Abnormality of sweating.

Modified with permission from Albers JW: Numbness, tingling, and weakness. Making sense of the neuropathies. AAEM Course for Primary Care Physicians, Rochester, Minnesota: American Association of Electrodiagnostic Medicine, September 28, 1994.

3. Were the measurement techniques described?

4. Were normal values provided?

5. Was the evaluation sufficient to both document the problem and exclude alternative explanations (avoiding errors of omission)?

6. Were appropriate negative findings described?

7. Is the EMG interpretation consistent with the clinical findings?

Although clinical skills are important in documenting the distribution and magnitude of a suspected neuropathy, the electromyographer's role is to help identify the underlying pathophysiology and focus the differential diagnosis so that appropriate laboratory investigations are ordered. Basis questions that should be addressed by the electrodiagnostic study in the evaluation of neuropathy are listed in Table 12–2. These listed questions also extend those addressed by the clinician prior to performing the study.

One of the most important tasks of the electromyographer is to distinguish axonal loss lesions from lesions characterized by uniform or multifocal demyelination. This allows identification of acquired demyelinating neuropathies, which are important because they are treatable and frequently associated with a systemic illness. The electromyographer must also exclude disorders that mimic neuropathy but are difficult to identify clinically. For example, identifying fibrillation potentials in paraspinal muscles differentiates a distal neuropathy from a polyradiculopathy or a polyradiculoneuropathy. Another example is distinguishing neuropathy from a confluent mononeuritis multiplex. Although clinically difficult, the diagnosis of an underlying vasculitis may be suggested by characteristic EMG findings, distinguishing it from an otherwise typical distal neuropathy. The answers to questions addressed in Table 12–2 form the basis of the electrodiagnostic classification of neuropathy, which is described below.

CLINICAL ELECTROMYOGRAPHY

Nerve conduction studies and needle electromyography evaluate slightly different components of the peripheral nervous system. Nerve conduction studies are noninvasive and provide the most useful information in documenting and establishing the etiology of neuropathy, whereas the needle examination is more

Table 12–2
Expectations For the EMG Evaluation of Neuropathy

Document evidence of a peripheral abnormality:
    Detect presence.
    Document location (diffuse, focal, multifocal).

Identify peripheral modalities involved:
    Sensory fibers.
    Motor fibers.
    Autonomic fibers.

Identify the predominant pathophysiology:
    Axonal loss lesions.
    Uniform demyelination.
    Multifocal demyelination with partial or complete conduction block.
    Conduction slowing suggestive of membranopathy.
    Combination of the above.

Establish temporal profile when possible (acute, chronic, old, ongoing).

Exclude accompanying or alternative disorders.

Determine prognosis.

Modified with permission from Albers JW: Numbness, tingling, and weakness. Making sense of the neuropathies. AAEM Course for Primary Care Physicians. Rochester, Minnesota: American Association of Electrodiagnostic Medicine, September 28, 1994.

useful in documenting the magnitude and distribution of axonal loss lesions and identifying disorders clinically indistinguishable from neuropathy.

Nerve Conduction Studies

SNAPs and CMAPs are recorded using surface electrodes and percutaneous electrical stimulation (Figs. 12–1 and 12–2) (2). Amplitudes and latencies are measured, and conduction velocities are calculated in nerve conduction studies. Conduction over an entire motor nerve is evaluated by F-wave latency (Fig. 12–3). F-wave measures accentuate mild generalized slowing because of the long conduction distances. Most normal values are age-dependent and some vary according to patient size (18, 73, 86, 88). Improper electrode placement, inaccurate measurements, and failure to monitor and control limb temperature influence the results (2). Limb temperature is particularly important in the evaluation of neuropathy. Cooling decreases conduction velocity and increases amplitude, a combination of findings atypical for most pathologic processes. Limb temperature should be monitored, and cool limbs should be warmed to between 32° and 36°C (surface temperature).

Needle Electromyography

The needle examination plays a limited but important role in suspected neuropathy (2). The needle examination evaluates insertional activity (i.e., positive waves and fibrillation potentials) and volitional MUAP recruitment, size, and configuration. As a sensitive indicator of denervation, the needle examination documents the distribution of axonal lesions, providing information from muscles inaccessible to nerve conduction study (e.g., the paraspinal muscles). Recruitment refers to the sequential introduction of additional MUAPs into the interference pattern as force is increased. In the evaluation of neuropathy, the needle examination provides an indication of ongoing or previous denervation. It also is used to define the distribution of axonal lesions, identifying disorders sometimes confused with or superimposed upon a generalized polyneuropathy. The amplitude of positive waves or

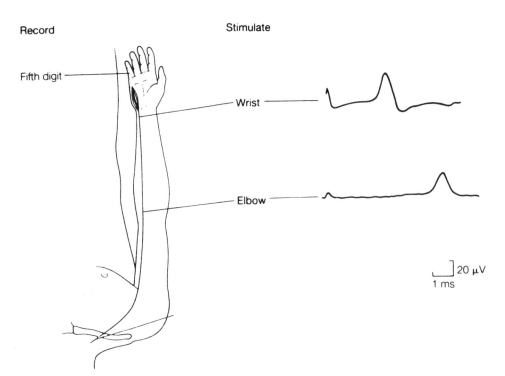

Figure 12–1. Representative sensory nerve conduction study. Sensory nerve action potentials recorded from the fifth digit following ulnar nerve stimulation at the wrist and elbow. (Caliber: 1 msec, 20 μV.) (Reprinted with permission from Albers JW, Leonard JA Jr: Nerve conduction studies and electromyography. In: Crockard A, Hayward R, Hoff JT, eds. Neurosurgery: The scientific basis of clinical practice. 2nd ed. Oxford, England: Blackwell Scientific Publications Ltd., 1992;2:735–757.)

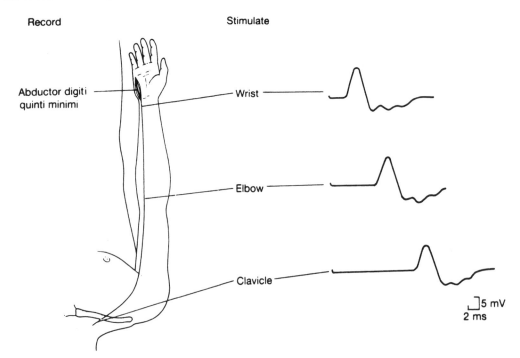

Figure 12–2. Representative motor nerve conduction study. Compound muscle action potentials recorded from hypothenar muscles following ulnar nerve stimulation at the wrist, elbow, and clavicle. (Caliber: 2 msec, 5 mV.) (Modified from Albers JW, Leonard JA Jr: Nerve conduction studies and electromyography. In: Crockard A, Hayward R, Hoff JT, eds. Neurosurgery: The scientific basis of clinical practice. 2nd ed. Oxford, England: Blackwell Scientific Publications Ltd., 1992;2:735–757.)

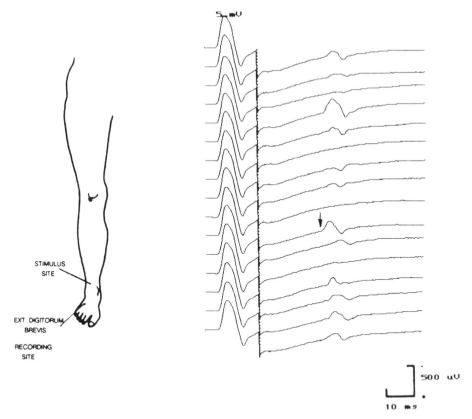

Figure 12-3. Representative F waves following antidromic peroneal nerve stimulation. (Reprinted with permission from Albers JW: Clinical neurophysiology of generalized polyneuropathy. J Clin Neurophysiol 1993;10: 149–166.)

fibrillation potentials and the configuration of MUAPs are used to distinguish acute from chronic disorders and estimate the progression of axonal loss.

Electrodiagnostic Evaluation in Suspected Neuropathy

Patients commonly are referred for evaluation because of symptoms or signs suggestive of neuropathy. Occasionally, asymptomatic patients are referred because of an underlying illness associated with neuropathy. Some patients referred for other reasons are found to have an unsuspected neuropathy. Regardless of the reason for referral, the initial evaluation for possible neuropathy is based upon the patient's history and clinical findings. Initial impressions are confirmed or altered, and the study is modified to accept or reject additional considerations until a final diagnosis is achieved.

Protocols for the evaluation of suspected polyneuropathy are straightforward (Table 12–3). When signs are mild, one directs the evaluation toward the most sensitive or susceptible sites (e.g., the distal lower extremity sensory nerves). When severe, evaluation of less-involved sites is important because absent responses provide no information about the presence or absence of demyelination. Bilateral studies are performed on some nerves to evaluate symmetry, although a superimposed focal abnormality (e.g., entrapment) should not exclude the diagnosis of neuropathy. The needle examination provides information supplementary to that obtained from the conduction studies. The examination evaluates muscles inaccessible to conduction study, such as paraspinal muscles in suspected radiculopathy, and the results are used to demonstrate a proximal-to-distal abnormality gradient in neuropathy.

Table 12–3
Representative Electrodiagnostic Protocol for Evaluating Polyneuropathy

Nerve Conduction Studies*
1. Test the most involved site if mild or moderate, the least involved site if severe.
2. Evaluate peroneal motor nerve (extensor digitorum brevis); stimulate ankle, below fibular head, and knee. Measure F-wave latency.†
3. If abnormal, evaluate tibial motor nerve (abductor hallucis); stimulate ankle and knee. Measure F-wave latency.
4. If no responses, evaluate:
   a. Peroneal motor nerve (anterior tibialis); stimulate below fibular head and knee.
   b. Ulnar motor nerve (hypothenar); stimulate wrist and below elbow. Measure F-wave latency.
   c. Median motor nerve (thenar); stimulate wrist and elbow. Measure F-wave latency.
5. Evaluate sural nerve (ankle); stimulate calf.
6. Evaluate median sensory nerve (index finger); stimulate wrist and elbow. If response is absent or focal entrapment is suspected, record from wrist and stimulate midpalm; evaluate ulnar sensory nerve (fifth digit); stimulate wrist.
7. If distal CMAP amplitude is substantially larger (greater than 15%) than proximal CMAP amplitude, evaluate for abnormal temporal dispersion of partial conduction block.
   a. Measure CMAP duration (distal and proximal) to identify abnormal dispersion.
   b. Evaluate CMAP amplitude and duration over short segments (few mm) to identify partial conduction block.
   c. If capability exists, measure CMAP negative phase area (distal and proximal).
8. Evaluate additional nerves if findings are equivocal. Definite abnormalities should result in:
   a. Evaluation of contralateral extremity.
   b. Evaluation of specific suspected abnormality.

Needle Examination
1. Examine anterior tibialis, medial gastrocnemius, abductor hallucis, vastus lateralis, biceps brachii, first interosseous (hand), and lumbar paraspinal muscles.
2. Confirm any abnormality by examination of at least one contralateral muscle looking for symmetry.

*Muscles in parentheses indicate recording site for conduction studies.
†All F-wave latency measurements are for distal stimulation sites. Record as absent if no response after 10 to 15 stimulations.
Modified with permission from John Wiley & Sons, Inc., ©1985. Albers JW, Donofrio, PD, McGonagle TK. Sequential electrodiagnostic abnormalities in acute inflammatory demyelinating polyradiculopathy. Muscle Nerve 1985;8:528–539.

Interpretation of Findings

The initial goal is to determine the presence and location of sensory or motor involvement (Table 12–2). Clinically apparent sensory loss may reflect a lesion proximal to the dorsal root ganglia, whereas abnormal SNAPs document peripheral involvement at or distal to the dorsal ganglia (2). Weakness and atrophy in combination with low CMAP amplitudes reflect abnormality of the lower motor neuron, but in isolation cannot localize the lesion more precisely (64,91). The distribution of needle examination abnormalities is helpful in further localizing the abnormality.

The next goal is to identify the primary pathophysiology (axonal degeneration or demyelination) (2). Axonal neuropathies are easily identified. They are characterized by reduced amplitudes, little evidence of conduction slowing, and neurogenic changes on needle electromyography with evidence of active denervation and reinnervation (i.e., the decreased MUAP recruitment and increased MUAP amplitude, duration, and polyphasia). Using a computerized model of the peripheral nerve, expected CMAP responses for a normal nerve are shown in Figure 12–4. Motor conduction abnormalities associated with axonal degeneration are shown in Figure 12–5. With a loss of 75% of the axons, the CMAP amplitude is markedly diminished, but conduction velocity is reduced only to the extent that is related to the loss of the largest myelinated axons. There is no evidence of abnormal temporal dispersion.

Although primary demyelination is characterized by conduction slowing, overemphasis of mild or focal slowing is a common error in establishing the presence of demyelination (2). Important differences exist between hereditary and acquired demyelination. Hereditary disorders of peripheral myelin (e.g., hereditary motor sensory neuropathy, or HMSN type I) have uniform involvement of all myelinated fibers. Conduction along individual fibers may be greatly reduced, but slowing is uniform; abnormal temporal dispersion is present only if conduction velocities are markedly slowed and there is substantial phase cancellation. Conduction slowing is disproportionate to the relatively preserved evoked response amplitudes with distal and proximal stimulation (60). Conduction block is not a typical feature of hereditary demyelination unless conduction velocities are very slow and produce substantial phase cancellation.

Acquired demyelination is characterized by multifocal, nonuniform abnormalities. The

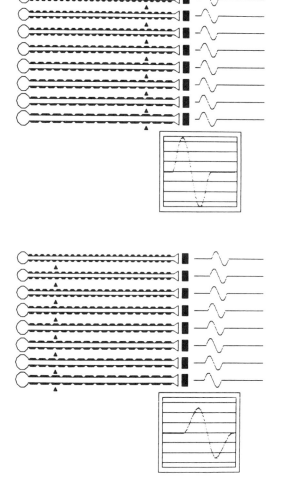

Figure 12–4. Peripheral motor nerve model, demonstrating the resultant compound muscle action potential (CMAP) produced by summation of eight individual muscle fiber action potentials. Individual axons differ in size and therefore conduct at different rates. Arrows represent stimulation sites. *Top*: CMAP (shown in screen) following distal stimulation. *Bottom*: CMAP following proximal stimulation. (Reprinted with permission from Albers JW: Inflammatory demyelinating polyradiculoneuropathy. In: Brown WF, Bolton CF, eds. Clinical electromyography. Boston: Butterworth, 1987.)

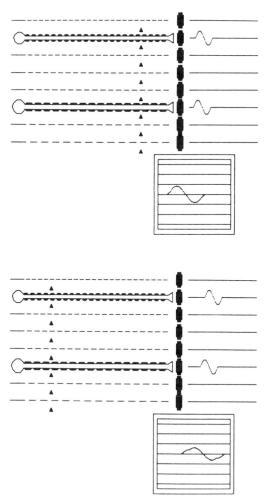

Figure 12–5. Model of axonal degeneration in motor nerve model described in Figure 12–4, demonstrating CMAPs after random loss of 75% of axons. Arrows represent stimulation sites. CMAPs following distal (upper screen) and proximal (lower screen) stimulation. (Reprinted with permission from Albers JW: Inflammatory demyelinating polyradiculoneuropathy. In: Brown WF, Bolton CF, eds. Clinical electromyography. Boston: Butterworth, 1987.)

disproportionate involvement of some myelinated fibers compared to others produces increased CMAP duration and a characteristic dispersion of the CMAP (Fig. 12–6) (7). Partial conduction block results from transmission failure along the axon. Because the likelihood of conduction block in any given fiber is length-dependent, there is abnormal dispersion of the response and evidence of partial conduction block when the results of proximal stimulation are compared to those from distal stimulation. This is demonstrated in the

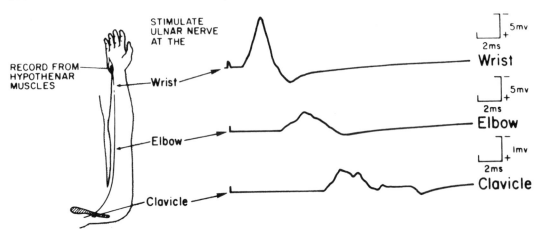

Figure 12–6. Compound muscle action potentials recorded from hypothenar muscles following ulnar nerve stimulation at distal and proximal sites. Responses from patient with an acquired demyelinating neuropathy, demonstrating abnormal temporal dispersion with partial conduction block, increased duration, and decreased conduction velocity. (Reprinted with permission from John Wiley and Sons, Inc. ©1989. Albers JW, Kelly JJ Jr.: Acquired inflammatory demyelinating polyneuropathies: Clinical and electrodiagnostic features. Muscle Nerve 1989;12:435–451.)

model in Figure 12–7 after random, multifocal demyelination, in which propagation is slowed across a single demyelinated internode and blocked if two adjacent internodes are demyelinated (shown by the absence of the myelin sheath). Distal stimulation produces a CMAP of slightly reduced amplitude and increased duration because of increased dispersion. The area beneath the negative phase of the CMAP is only slightly reduced. Proximal stimulation produces a low-amplitude, highly dispersed CMAP because of the variable amounts of demyelination in some fibers compared to others, producing an increased range of conduction velocities. The initial component of the CMAP is greatly separated from the trailing portion of the CMAP (representing the slowest conducting axon). Phase cancellation of the dispersed responses produces an additional reduction in the proximal CMAP amplitude. Conduction block in two of the axons further reduces the CMAP amplitude to a greater extent than could be explained by abnormal temporal dispersion alone.

Criteria exist to identify acquired demyelination (Table 12–4), but all of the criteria have limitations (7,21,24). In some criteria,

Table 12–4
Electrodiagnostic Criteria Suggestive of Chronic Acquired Demyelination

Evaluation should satisfy at least three of the following in motor nerves (with exceptions noted below):

1. Conduction velocity less than 75% of the lower limit of normal (two or more nerves).*

2. Distal latency exceeding 130% of upper limit of normal (two or more nerves).†

3. Evidence of unequivocal temporal dispersion (an increase in negative component duration exceeding 15% for proximal vs. distal stimulation) or a proximal-to-distal amplitude ratio less than 0.7 (one or more nerves).†,††

4. F-wave latency exceeding 125% of upper limit of normal (one or more nerves).*,†

*Excluding isolated ulnar or peroneal nerve abnormalities at the elbow or knee, respectively.
†Excluding isolated median nerve abnormality at the wrist.
††Excluding the presence of anomalous innervation (e.g., median-to-ulnar nerve crossover).
Modified with permission from John Wiley & Sons, Inc., © 1989. Albers JW, Kelly, JJ Jr.: Acquired inflammatory demyelinating polyneuropathies; Clinical and electrodiagnostic features. Muscle Nerve 1989;12:435–451.

conduction velocity and distal latency thresholds are amplitude-dependent. In general, conduction velocities that are less than 70% of the lower limit of the normal range cannot be attributed to axonal loss alone (7). The presence of fibrillation potentials and neurogenic MUAP findings does not exclude the diagnosis of demyelinating polyneuropathy, because most hereditary and acquired demyelinating neuropathies have some superimposed axonal degeneration.

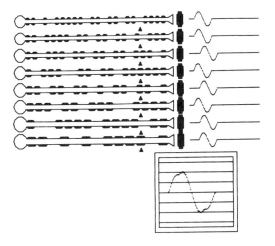

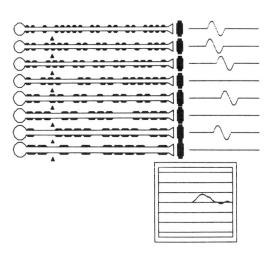

Figure 12–7. Model of focal demyelination in motor nerve model described in Figure 12–4. Arrows represent stimulation sites. CMAPs following distal (upper screen) and proximal (lower screen) stimulation. The reduced amplitude with proximal stimulation reflects increased temporal dispersion and conduction block in some axons. (Reprinted with permission from Albers JW: Inflammatory demyelinating polyradiculoneuropathy. In: Brown WF, Bolton CF, eds. Clinical electromyography. Boston: Butterworth, 1987.)

The remaining goals of the electromyographic examination are to characterize the neuropathy's distribution, severity, rate of progression, and prognosis. Neuropathic distribution is usually defined clinically, not electrodiagnostically, except for the needle examination of paraspinal muscles in polyradiculopathy or the intrinsic foot muscles in mild axonal polyneuropathy. Neuropathic severity is best related to CMAP and SNAP amplitudes, because they are proportional to the extent of abnormality, particularly in axonal disorders. The needle examination is useful in documenting very mild axonal neuropathies, as noted above. Defining severity in demyelinating neuropathy is difficult because conduction slowing is not usually associated with functional impairment. Conduction block results in weakness, but may be difficult to distinguish from abnormal temporal dispersion. Serial studies are used to estimate the rate of progression, although a mixture of large and small amplitude fibrillation potentials suggests active and chronic denervation.

ELECTRODIAGNOSTIC CLASSIFICATION OF NEUROPATHY

Neuropathy is classified by a variety of means, including clinical, biochemical, pathologic, electrodiagnostic, or a combination thereof. The electrodiagnostic results provide information additional to that obtained from the clinical evaluation and are used to assign patients with suspected neuropathy to general categories, thereby directing the subsequent clinical examination. The classification that follows separates disorders into broad categories based upon electrodiagnostic evidence of sensory or motor involvement, combined with uniform or multifocal demyelination versus pure axonal loss (27). This classification scheme is not inclusive and there is substantial overlap between categories. Nevertheless, when combined with the clinical history and examination, it may suggest a specific diagnosis or direct the subsequent evaluation. Selected examples are provided in each category; a more extensive discussion exists elsewhere (27).

Motor Greater Than Sensory Neuropathy; Uniform Conduction Slowing (Table 12–5)

Case 1

A 23-year-old male presents with a several-year history of progressive ankle weakness and clumsiness. Examination reveals that he has distal weakness of his upper and lower extremities with footdrop, hammer toes and high arches, mild sensory loss to vibration and touch, areflexia, and large firm nerves. Nerve conduction and needle EMG studies are shown in Table 12–6, characterized by reduced CMAP and SNAP amplitudes, prolonged distal and F-wave latencies, and substantially reduced conduction velocities (well below 50% of the lower limit of normal). Initial findings of prolonged distal latency that could have been explained by distal entrapment were excluded by demonstrating similar abnormalities in all the nerves examined. There was little change in the configuration (amplitude, duration, or shape) of the CMAP with distal and proximal stimulation; there was no evidence of abnormal temporal dispersion or partial conduction block. Chronic neurogenic changes were recorded on needle examination of distal extremity muscles. The findings provided electrodiagnostic evidence of a moderately severe sensorimotor neuropathy of the demyelinating type, with mild superimposed axonal degeneration. The markedly reduced conduction velocity without evidence of abnormal temporal dispersion or partial conduction block is most consistent with a hereditary neuropathy.

The classic example of a neuropathy characterized by a uniform peripheral myelinopathy is hereditary motor sensory neuropathy type I (HMSN I), or the demyelinating form of Charcot-Marie-Tooth disease. HMSN I is a dominantly inherited hypertrophic neuropathy that presents with the insidious onset of distal weakness and sensory loss in young adult life. The diagnosis is clinically suggested by findings of enlarged nerves, distal weakness with hammer toes and pes cavus, abnormal vibratory sensation, and hyporeflexia (34).

The characteristic electrodiagnostic finding is markedly reduced conduction velocity in all tested nerves, often as low as 25 m/s or less (34,35). Conduction velocities typically are below 70% of the lower limit of normal, and therefore cannot be explained by axonal loss alone. Abnormal temporal dispersion and partial conduction block usually are not present because of the uniform involvement of all fibers. Nevertheless, when conduction velocities are extremely slow, phase cancellation may result in findings suggestive of abnormal temporal dispersion (60). F waves are present unless the CMAP

amplitude is very reduced, and latencies are prolonged proportional to conduction velocity slowing. Sensory nerves demonstrate similar conduction abnormalities, but low-amplitude responses often preclude conduction velocity measurement. Most patients show at least some degree of axonal loss, and it sometimes is severe. Needle electromyography demonstrates decreased MUAP recruitment proportional to weakness, fibrillation potentials and positive waves, and increased MUAP amplitude and duration, reflecting chronic reinnervation. Abnormalities are most prominent distally. The patient presented was found to have an asymptomatic sibling with mild ankle weakness, absent ankle reflexes, equivocal sensory loss, and definite slowing of motor conduction velocities.

Disorders other than HMSN I, many of which also are familial, present with similar electrodiagnostic findings (32). Several disorders are not associated with primary myelin abnormalities but reflect selective loss of large myelinated fiber with preservation of smaller myelinated axons. One example is the neuropathy attributed to amiodarone (39). Amiodarone is associated with a slowly progressive motor neuropathy with prominent conduction slowing, often in the range of 20 m/s to 30 m/s. Abnormal temporal dispersion and partial conduction block are not features of this neuropathy; slowing reflects preferential loss of the largest myelinated fibers.

Table 12–5
Motor Greater Than Sensory; Uniform Conduction Slowing

Adrenomyeloneuropathy

Amiodarone

Charcot-Marie-Tooth disease (hereditary motor sensory neuropathy Type I)

Congenital hypomyelinating neuropathy

Cytosine arabinoside (ara-C)

Dejerine-Sottas disease (hereditary motor sensory neuropathy Type III)

Doxorubicin

Hexacarbons

Metachromatic leukodystrophy

Methyl n-butyl ketone

N-hexane

Perhexiline maleate

Sodium channel blockers (e.g., tetrodotoxin)

Modified with permission from John Wiley & Sons, Inc., ©1990. Donofrio PD, Albers JW: Polyneuropathy: Classification by nerve conduction studies and electromyography. Muscle Nerve 1990; 13:889–903.

Table 12–6
(Case 1)

Nerve Stimulate (record)	Nerve Conduction Studies		Latencies (msec)	
	Amplitude (μV)	Conduction Velocity (m/sec)	Distal	F wave
Motor				
R median (thenar)				
Wrist	4000		7.0	44.5
Elbow	3800	18		
R ulnar (hypothenar)				
Wrist	6000		6.1	NR
Elbow	5700	21		
R peroneal				
Ankle	400		7.8	
Knee	400	17		NR
R tibial				
Ankle	NR			
Sensory				
R median (index)	12	23	5.8	
R ulnar (fifth)	5		5.2	
R sural (ankle)	NR			

Muscle	Electromyography			Motor Unit Action Potential	
	Insertional Activity	Fib	Fasc	Recruitment	Amplitude/Duration
R first dorsal interosseous (hand)	Normal	0	0	Reduced	Mild increase
R anterior tibialis	Increased	+	0	Reduced	Mild increase
R abductor hallucis	Increased	++	0	Reduced	Moderate increase
L abductor hallucis	Increased	++	0	Reduced	Moderate increase
R vastus medialis	Normal	0	0	Normal	Normal

Neurotoxins that block sodium channels include tetrodotoxin derived from the puffer fish and saxitoxin derived from contaminated shell fish (red tide) (61). Sodium channel blockade decreases the local electrical currents associated with action potential propagation (an effect similar to that seen with reduced temperature), thereby slowing conduction velocity. Motor amplitudes are reduced, but there is no abnormal temporal dispersion or partial conduction block.

Several hexacarbons are implicated in neuropathy after occupational or recreational exposures (12,22,54). N-hexane and methyl n-butyl ketone are metabolized to 2,5-hexanedione, the likely neurotoxic agent. The neuropathy is characterized by progressive distal sensory loss, reduced or absent reflexes, and eventual weakness and atrophy. Individuals who voluntary inhale n-hexane sometimes develop a motor greater than sensory neuropathy. Motor and sensory amplitudes are reduced and conduction slowed, suggestive of primary demyelination. However, conduction slowing is attributed to secondary myelin damage associated with axonal lesions, similar to the neuropathy associated with

several solvents; these neuropathies are characterized by giant axonal swellings filled with neurofilaments (46,85). Positive waves and fibrillation potentials are recorded on needle EMG, and motor units are reduced in number but of increased amplitude. Additional examples of neuropathies that demonstrate evidence of uniform conduction slowing are listed in Table 12–5.

Motor Greater Than Sensory Neuropathy, Multifocal Conduction Slowing (Table 12–7)

Case 2

A 42-year-old female has a 3-year history of progressive weakness, gait unsteadiness, and uncomfortable extremity dysesthesias. On examination, she has increased skin pigmentation, generalized distal atrophy and weakness, diminished sensation

Table 12-7
Motor Greater Than Sensory, Multifocal Conduction Slowing

Arsenic (acute intoxication)

Guillain-Barré syndrome

Chronic inflammatory demyelinating polyneuropathy (CIDP)

Chronic disimmune polyneuropathy myelin
    Monoclonal gammopathy of undetermined significance (MGUS)
    Osteosclerotic myeloma
    Multiple myeloma (substantial proportion are axonal)
    Systemic lupus erythematosus
    Waldenstrom's macroglobulinemia
    Cryoglobulinemia
    Castleman's disease
    Lymphoma
    HIV infection

Hereditary neuropathy with liability to pressure palsies

Multifocal motor neuropathy (MMN) with conduction block

Modified with permission from John Wiley & Sons, Inc., ©1990. Donofrio PD, Albers JW: Polyneuropathy: Classification by nerve conduction studies and electromyography. Muscle Nerve 1990; 13:889–903.

The inflammatory demyelinating neuropathies are the prototype disorders associated with multifocal conduction slowing. They are acquired immune diseases of peripheral nerves and nerve roots. Included in this group are acute (acute inflammatory demyelinating polyneuropathy [AIDP] and Guillain-Barré syndrome [GBS]) and chronic (CIDP) forms. CIDP is thought to be the most common treatable neuropathy seen in most neuromuscular clinics. Identification of CIDP in patients with suspected neuropathy is important, not only because it is treatable, but because a subgroup of these patients has an underlying systemic illness (plasma cell dyscrasias, Waldenstrom's macroglobulinemia, gamma heavy chain disease, cryoglobulinemia, lymphoma, systemic lupus erythematosus, Castleman's disease, occult malignancy, and HIV-1 infection) (7). Acquired demyelinating neuropathies are characterized by progressive weakness, areflexia, diminished distal sensation, dysautonomia, and elevated cerebral spinal fluid (CSF) protein (13,14,52).

The most prominent electrodiagnostic feature suggestive of an acquired demyelinating neuropa-

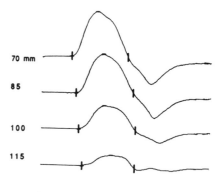

to all modalities except deep pain, and areflexia. Nerve conduction and needle EMG studies are shown in Table 12–8. An initial median motor conduction study demonstrated marked slowing of conduction velocity (approximately 50% of the lower limit of normal), as well as a prominent change in the CMAP configuration with proximal compared to distal configuration. These abnormalities were confirmed in the ulnar nerve, but lower extremity motor responses were unobtainable. A representative motor conduction study is shown in Figure 12–6, demonstrating the abnormal temporal dispersion and partial conduction block that followed stimulation at a distal and more proximal site. A sural response was unobtainable, but upper extremity responses demonstrated low amplitudes, reduced conduction velocities, and prolonged distal latencies. Needle electromyography demonstrated evidence of chronic partial denervation and reinnervation, most prominent in the distal lower extremities. Paraspinal muscles were spared. The combined studies were interpreted as providing evidence of an acquired sensorimotor neuropathy of the demyelinating type with superimposed axonal degeneration. The presence of abnormal temporal dispersion and partial conduction block is typical of multifocal involvement and characteristic of an acquired demyelinating neuropathy such as seen in chronic inflammatory demyelinating polyneuropathy (CIDP).

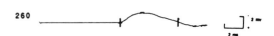

Figure 12–8. Compound muscle action potentials (CMAPs) recorded from thenar muscles following percutaneous stimulation of median nerve at multiple sites from patient with an acquired inflammatory demyelinating polyneuropathy. The distance from stimulation to recording site (millimeter) is indicated at the left of individual tracings. Although there is evidence of abnormal temporal dispersion over long stimulation distances, small incremental increases in the stimulation distance confirm partial conduction block with an abrupt decrease in CMAP amplitude (and area) with little increase in CMAP duration (less than 10%). (Reprinted with permission from Albers JW: Clinical neurophysiology of generalized polyneuropathy. J Clin Neurophysiol 1993;10: 149–166.)

**Table 12–8
(Case 2)**

Nerve Stimulate (record)	Nerve Conduction Studies			
	Amplitude (μV)	Conduction Velocity (m/sec)	Latencies (msec)	
			Distal	F wave
Motor				
R median (thenar)				
Wrist	4000		6.5	42.3
Elbow	1200	25		
R ulnar (hypothenar)				
Wrist	3000		5.6	44.5
Below elbow	1500	26		
R peroneal				
Ankle	NR			
R tibial				
Ankle	NR			
Sensory				
R median (index)	8		5.5	
R ulnar (fifth)	10	34	5.4	
R sural (ankle)	NR			

Muscle	Electromyography				
	Insertional Activity	Fib	Fasc	Motor Unit Action Potential	
				Recruitment	Amplitude/Duration
R first dorsal interosseous (hand)	Increased	+	0	Reduced	Mild increase
R biceps brachii	Normal	0	0	Normal	Normal
R anterior tibialis	Increased	++	0	Reduced	Moderate increase
R abductor hallucis	Increased	+++	0	Reduced	Severe increase
L abductor hallucis	Increased	+++	0	Reduced	Severe increase
R vastus medialis	Increased	+	0	Reduced	Mild increase
R gluteus medius	Normal	0	0	Normal	Normal
R paraspinal (lumbar)	Normal	0	0	Normal	Normal

thy is abnormal temporal dispersion or partial conduction block. Decreases in the ratio of the CMAP amplitude or the area beneath the negative potential following proximal and distal stimulation of up to 50% may result from dispersion and resultant phase cancellation (7). Reductions exceeding 50% require at least some degree of conduction block. Changes in the CMAP duration reflect abnormal temporal dispersion, and increases exceeding 15% over short segments and 20% over longer segments indicate abnormality (21,50). The site of partial conduction block can sometimes be demonstrated by making small incremental changes in the stimulation site and observing the resultant CMAP (Fig. 12–8). Although it is sometimes difficult to distinguish abnormal temporal dispersion from partial conduction block, the distinction is clinically unnecessary because both indicate acquired demyelination. Reduced conduction velocity and prolonged distal latency also reflect demyelination; however, abnormalities must be interpreted in relation to

other information, including response amplitude and disease duration, so one should not give undue significance to mild conduction slowing. Whenever possible, evaluation should include nerves with reasonably preserved CMAP amplitudes. Absent F responses are a nonspecific finding in isolation; reliance on such findings is inappropriate (5).

The combination of an abnormal median response with a normal sural response is a relatively common finding in acquired demyelinating polyneuropathy (20). The discrepancy between sural and median sensory responses may be due to the more proximal sural recording site, because the location of greatest initial abnormality may involve the distal, thinly myelinated fibers. An abnormal median sensory with normal sural response occurs more commonly with AIDP (39%) than with CIDP (28%) (7, 20).

The needle examination is secondary in the evaluation of demyelinating neuropathy. Most patients develop at least some evidence of axonal degenera-

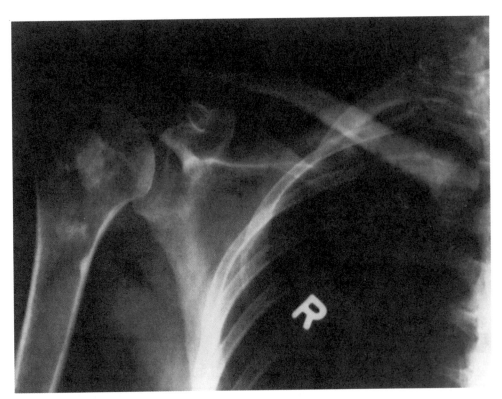

Figure 12–9. Multiple scattered sclerotic bone lesions within the right humerus and clavicle of patient (case 2). (Reproduced by permission from John Wiley and Sons, Inc. ©1984. Donofrio PD, Albers JAW, Greenberg SH, et al.: Peripheral neuropathy in osteosclerotic myeloma: Clinical and electrodiagnostic improvement with chemotherapy. Muscle Nerve 1984;7:137–141.)

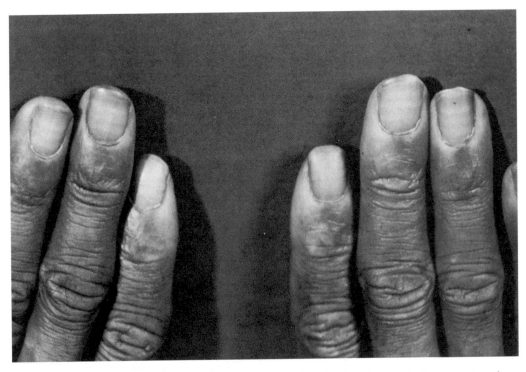

Figure 12–10. Mees' line in a patient with documented arsenical neuropathy. Photograph taken approximately one month after the most recent acute exposure. Note the multiple set of Mees' lines, documenting multiple prior exposures.

tion, and the presence of fibrillation potentials and positive waves does not exclude the diagnosis of a demyelinating polyneuropathy. The needle examination is useful in estimating the extent, distribution, and duration of axonal degeneration, but is a relatively insensitive measure of severity (4).

The patient described above was believed to have an acquired demyelinating neuropathy. The resultant clinical evaluation disclosed an abnormal skeletal survey (Fig. 12–9) and biopsy evidence of osteosclerotic myeloma. Her systemic disease responded dramatically to melphalan and prednisone treatments. Serial electrodiagnostic studies documented resolution of her neuropathy over approximately 2 years (28).

Table 12–7 lists several other disorders associated with a neuropathy characterized by multifocal or nonuniform conduction slowing. Acute arsenical neuropathy presents as part of a systemic illness characterized by nausea, vomiting, diarrhea, dermatitis, cardiomyopathy, pancytopenia with basophilic stippling, and abnormal liver function tests. The interesting neurologic deficit progresses over weeks and may suggest a diagnosis of AIDP (30). Because Mees' lines (Fig. 12–10) do not appear on the nails until approximately one month after exposure to arsenic, they are not helpful during the initial phase of the evaluation if the patient has had a single arsenic exposure. As with AIDP, CSF protein becomes elevated several weeks after onset of arsenical neuropathy, whereas basophilic stippling identified in a laboratory suggests a toxic etiology. Initial EMG studies show reduced conduction velocity, abnormal temporal dispersion, partial conduction block, and low amplitude or absent sensory responses. Serial studies demonstrate a dying-back neuropathy with progressive axonal degeneration, and initial findings are probably related to generalized axonal failure.

Motor or Motor Greater Than Sensory Neuropathy; Axonal Loss (Table 12–9)

Case 3

A 50-year-old man with dermatitis herpetiformis has a 6-month history of painless, progressive hand weakness and atrophy. Previous electrodiagnostic examinations have diagnosed multiple entrapment neuropathies. In addition to profound distal upper extremity weakness and atrophy (Fig. 12–11), he has bilateral weakness of foot dorsiflexion and intrinsic foot muscles. Sensation is normal. Reflexes are hypoactive. Nerve conduction and needle EMG studies are shown in Table 12–10. They demonstrate relatively symmetric but scattered reduction of CMAP amplitudes, with some prolonged motor distal latencies, minimally reduced motor conduction velocities, and no sensory

abnormalities. The needle examination demonstrated chronic neurogenic changes consisting of small-amplitude fibrillation potentials, decreased recruitment, and MUAPs of increased amplitude and duration. The findings were interpreted as representing a moderately chronic motor neuropathy, although the findings are indistinguishable from those associated with multifocal motor neuron disease.

Motor greater than sensory neuropathies are relatively uncommon, and identification suggests a relatively small differential diagnosis. Most neuropathies in the differential have metabolic or toxic etiologies, often involving medications. The prototype disorder of an axonal motor greater than sensory neuropathy is hereditary motor sensory neuropathy type II (HMSN II), the axonal form of Charcot-Marie-Tooth disease (34). HMSN II is an autosomal dominant polyneuropathy characterized by slowly progressive weakness and sensory loss, usually beginning in the third or fourth decade of life. Distal atrophy may be severe, producing an inverted champagne bottle appearance to the legs. Other symptoms include pes cavus, hammer toes, hyporeflexia, and mild sensory loss. CMAP amplitudes are reduced with normal or minimally slowed conduction velocities. SNAPs are absent in about 50% of patients; when present, differentiation from a familial progressive muscular atrophy is difficult. The needle examination as described by Dyck and Lambert demonstrates nonspecific neurogenic changes with a distal predilection (34).

The patient described above had a negative family history. His medications, however, included dapsone, a medication he had taken for over 16 years with a cumulative dose exceeding 650 grams.

Table 12–9
Motor or Motor Greater Than Sensory, Axonal Loss

Charcot-Marie-Tooth disease (hereditary motor sensory neuropathy Type II)

Dapsone

Disulfiram

Guillain-Barré syndrome (axonal form)

Hyperinsulinism

Nitrofurantoin

Organophosphates

Porphyria

Paraneoplastic (lymphoma or carcinoma)

Vincristine

Modified with permission from John Wiley & Sons, Inc., ©1990. Donofrio PD, Albers JW. Polyneuropathy: Classification by nerve conduction studies and electromyography. Muscle Nerve 1990;13:889–903.

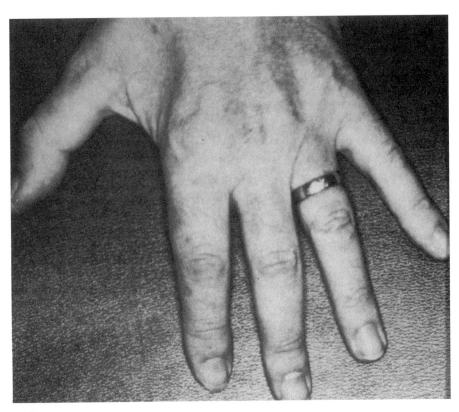

Figure 12–11. Photograph of hand of patient (case 3) prior to discontinuing dapsone, demonstrating severe atrophy of the intrinsic hand muscles.

Dapsone is associated with a slowly reversible neuropathy that is primarily motor and usually occurs after prolonged periods (years) of daily use. The neuropathy may be related to abnormal metabolism. Dapsone is metabolized by N-acetyl transferase, the same enzyme that acetylates isoniazid, and susceptible patients may be slow acetylators (1). Weakness and wasting sometimes involve the arms more than the legs, and mild sensory abnormalities may be present. Electrodiagnostic evaluation is characterized by low-amplitude CMAPs with normal sensory studies (45). Any conduction slowing presumably relates to the loss of the largest motor fibers. Needle examination demonstrates evidence of chronic denervation and reinnervation. The predilection of upper extremity involvement mimics multiple entrapment neuropathies, although the sensory normality would be atypical for a true mononeuropathy multiplex. Dapsone was discontinued and initial evidence of improvement was apparent within 4 months, with almost complete resolution over the next 3 years.

The hepatic porphyrias include acute intermittent porphyria, hereditary coproporphyria, and variegate porphyria and are characterized by the symptomatic triad of abdominal pain, psychosis, and polyneuropathy (17,76). Porphyric neuropathy resembles AIDP with quadriparesis, areflexia, dysautonomia, and elevated CSF protein, but its distinguishing features include an initial proximal predilection, asymmetry, and electrophysiologic features of an axonal polyneuropathy or polyradiculoneuropathy. Typical findings include reduced CMAP amplitude, minimally reduced conduction velocity, profuse fibrillation potentials after the fourth week, and decreased MUAP recruitment (9). Some rare studies fulfill criteria for primary demyelination, but these results may represent secondary demyelination associated with axonal death. Sensory responses occasionally are spared. The early appearance of fibrillation potentials in paraspinal muscles localizes the lesion to the root or neuron.

Other axonal motor greater than sensory polyneuropathies include the axonal form of AIDP (36,37), the remote-effect motor neuropathy associated with lymphoma (80) or carcinoma (94), hypoglycemic neuropathy (49,58), and several toxic neuropathies, including those associated with disulfiram (70), organophosphates (26,62,81), nitrofurantoin (25,47,72), and vincristine (19).

Hypoglycemic neuropathy is associated with insulin excess and almost always occurs after hypoglycemic coma (49,58). Like dapsone, the resultant neuropathy sometimes involves the upper more than the lower extremities and usually involves motor fibers. The etiology and underlying pathophysiology are poorly understood, but aspects of this neuropathy are consistent with isolated anterior horn cell involvement. Disulfiram (Antabuse) is metabolized to acetaldehyde when combined with alcohol, which should be a deterrent to alcohol use. Disulfiram is associated with a neuropathy characterized by predominant weakness, mild sensory involvement, and areflexia (25). Weakness usually appears slowly but occasionally onset is abrupt, mimicking AIDP (70). Neuropathy develops in approximately 0.2% of nitrofurantoin-treated patients (25). Initial sensory involvement with paresthesias and sometimes pain is common, although the most characteristic feature is rapid onset of severe weakness in elderly women with impaired renal function and presumably high blood nitrofurantoin levels (47, 72).

Organophosphates (OP) are used as pesticides and nerve gases, producing slowly reversible inactivation of acetylcholinesterase and acetylcholine accumulation in cholinergic neurons (26,62). Muscarinic overactivity results in miosis, increased secretions, sweating, gastric hyperactivity, and bradycardia, whereas nicotinic overactivity results in fasciculations and weakness. Following resolution of its acute effects, some OPs may produce a rapidly progressive neuropathy that begins 2 to 4 weeks after exposure (62,81). OP-induced delayed

Table 12–10
(Case 3)

Nerve Stimulate (record)	Nerve Conduction Studies				
	Amplitude (μV)	Conduction Velocity (m/sec)	Latencies (msec)		
			Distal	F wave	
Motor					
R median (thenar)					
Wrist	400		4.7	NR	
Elbow	400	50			
L median (thenar)					
Wrist	1200		4.2	NR	
R ulnar (hypothenar)					
Wrist	5000		3.1	30.5	
Below elbow	4500	55			
R peroneal					
Ankle	300		6.2	NR	
Below knee	300	42			
R tibial					
Ankle	2300		5.4		
Sensory					
R median (index)	25	64	3.2		
R ulnar (fifth)	20	58	3.4		
R sural (ankle)	12	44	3.8		

Muscle	Electromyography				
	Insertional Activity	Fib	Fasc	Motor Unit Action Potential	
				Recruitment	Amplitude/Duration
R FDI (hand)	Increased	++	0	Reduced (3+)	Moderate increase
L FDI (hand)	Increased	+++	0	Reduced (3+)	Moderate increase
R abd. pollicis brevis	Increased	++++	0	Reduced (4+)	Severe increase
L abd. pollicis brevis	Increased	++	0	Reduced (2+)	Moderate increase
R biceps brachii	Normal	0	0	Normal	Normal
R anterior tibialis	Increased	+	0	Reduced (1+)	Slight increase
R FDI (pedis)s	Increased	++++	0	Reduced (4+)	Severe increase
L FDI (pedis)s	Increased	++++	0	Reduced (4+)	Severe increase
R vastus medialis	Increased	0	0	Normal	Normal
R paraspinal (lumbar)	Normal	0	0	Normal	Normal

neuropathy (OPIDN) has been associated with ingestion of triorthocresyl-phosphate (TOCP) in adulterated Jamaican ginger extract (jake paralysis) and contaminated cooking oil in Morocco (66,83). OPIDN presents with dysesthesias and progressive distal greater than proximal weakness. Reflexes are reduced at the ankles, but may be normal or brisk elsewhere, and spasticity may become a late feature. During acute OP intoxication, repetitive CMAPs occur after a single stimulus, presumably from recurrent postsynaptic depolarization by persistent acetylcholine. Other electrodiagnostic findings are those of axonal degeneration of motor and sensory fibers. Conduction velocities remain essentially normal, but evoked amplitudes are reduced and there is needle EMG evidence of denervation characterized by fibrillation potentials in the distal mus-

Table 12–11
Sensory, Axonal Loss

Cisplatin	Pyridoxine
Congenital	Sjogren's syndrome
Metronidazole	Styrene
Paraneoplastic	Thalidomide
Friedreich's ataxia	Tabes dorsalis

Modified with permission from John Wiley & Sons, Inc., ©1990. Donofrio PD, Albers JW: Polyneuropathy: Classification by nerve conduction studies and electromyography. Muscle Nerve 1990;13:889–903.

cles (62,81). Vincristine typically produces an axonal sensorimotor neuropathy with sensory greater than motor involvement, although there are reports of weakness rapidly progressing to functional quadriplegia associated with vincristine (18). In some patients, the arms initially may be involved more than the legs, and the disorder resembles a pure motor neuropathy or neuronopathy.

Sensory, Axonal Loss (Neuropathy or Neuronopathy; Table 12–11)

Case 4

A 43-year-old woman with ovarian cancer was treated monthly with cisplatin. After the sixth and final chemotherapy treatment, she noted the subacute onset of progressive clumsiness and profound sensory loss. Examination confirmed the presence of large fiber sensory loss (reduced vibration and joint position sensations) and areflexia without weakness. Nerve conduction and needle EMG studies are shown in Table 12–12. All sensory amplitudes were unobtainable, but the motor conduction studies and needle examination were normal other than the irregular activation of MUAPs attributed to poor sensation. Examination of a single sensory nerve in this setting would be insufficient to document an abnormality in this setting, because local entrapment or a variety of technical factors

Table 12–12
(Case 4)

Nerve Stimulate (record)	Nerve Conduction Studies			
	Amplitude (μV)	Conduction Velocity (m/sec)	Latencies (msec) Distal	F wave
Motor				
R median (thenar)	8000	63	3.4	26.8
R ulnar (hypothenar)	9000	61	3.1	28.5
R peroneal	12000	57	4.8	48.5
Sensory				
R median (index)	6	44	4.1	
R ulnar (fifth)	NR			
R radial	NR			
R sural (ankle)	NR			

Muscle	Electromyography			Motor Unit Action Potential	
	Insertional Activity	Fib	Fasc	Recruitment	Amplitude/Duration
R FDI (hand)	Normal	0	0	Normal	Normal
R biceps brachii	Normal	0	0	Normal	Normal
R anterior tibialis	Normal	0	0	Normal	Normal
R abductor hallucis	Normal	0	0	Normal	Normal

could result in a false-positive result. Evaluation of several sensory nerves provided confirmation that a diffuse abnormality of peripheral sensory function existed in this patient. The combined abnormalities were interpreted as characteristic of a pure sensory neuropathy or neuronopathy.

Sensory involvement is common in most forms of neuropathy, but exclusive, severe sensory involvement is unusual. Acquired axonal sensory neuropathies or neuronopathies include those associated with pyridoxine (11,78) and cisplatin (74), as well as those associated with Sjogren's syndrome (57), paraneoplastic syndromes (e.g., oat cell carcinoma) (29), vitamin E deficiency (48), tabes dorsalis, idiopathic sensory ganglionitis, Friedreich's ataxia (65), and perhaps the Miller-Fisher variant (40) of AIDP. All present subacutely with unpleasant paresthesias and evidence of reduced vibration and joint position sensations, areflexia, and minimally decreased pain sensation. Pyridoxine (vitamin B_6) is occasionally taken in large amounts to treat a variety of nonspecific syndromes. Schaumburg and associates demonstrated that neurotoxicity is dose related, owing either to long-term cumulative exposure or the short-term administration of large doses (78). With large doses, sensory loss may be complete and irreversible, including the facial and mucous membrane areas (10). Cisplatin is an antineoplastic agent associated with a dose-related sensory neuronopathy (74). Cisplatin sensory neuronopathy is indistinguishable from the paraneoplastic sensory neuronopathy associated with small cell lung carcinoma and antineuronal nuclear antibodies (53). Carcinomatous sensory polyneuropathy is the most distinctive remote-effect polyneuropathy (29). It presents with paresthesias and dysesthesias and large fiber sensory loss in association with areflexia, gait ataxia, and choreoathetoid movements. Electrodiagnostic findings include markedly reduced or absent SNAPs with normal motor studies. Sequential studies demonstrate a progressive reduction of SNAP amplitude without motor conduction abnormality or any needle EMG evidence of denervation. In Friedreich's ataxia, there typically are additional motor abnormalities consisting of slowing of conduction velocity related to the loss of large myelinated fibers. There also may be mild chronic neurogenic changes on needle electromyography, differentiating this from the sensory neuropathies described above.

Styrene and thalidomide also have been associated with a sensory neuronopathy (56,75). Styrene is an organic solvent associated with acute behavioral effects and possible peripheral effects (distal paresthesias) after chronic styrene exposure. Electrodiagnostic evaluations demonstrate mild SNAP abnormalities compatible with axonal loss but no motor abnormalities (75). Thalidomide was initially introduced as a tranquilizer but was rarely used after 1961 because of teratogenic effects. Recently, thalidomide has been reintroduced for the treatment of systemic lupus erythematosus dermatitis. Thalidomide is associated with a small-fiber-greater-than-large-fiber neuropathy that is characterized by diminished pin and temperature appreciation, normal reflexes, and reduced SNAP amplitudes even in asymptomatic patients (56).

Sensory Greater Than Motor Neuropathy, Axonal Loss (Table 12–13)

Case 5

A 58-year-old man with a long history of ethanol abuse reports the insidious onset of painful distal paresthesias, numb feet, and clumsiness. On examination, he has evidence of midline cerebellar gait ataxia and abnormal heel-to-knee testing, with distal sensory loss to all modalities, areflexia, and weakness. Nerve conduction and needle EMG studies are shown in Table 12–14, demonstrating reduced SNAP and CMAP amplitudes with borderline-prolonged distal latencies but without other evidence suggestive of conduction slowing. An isolated sural abnormality could reflect technical factors, but the absent contralateral sural response and the borderline-low median and ulnar SNAP amplitudes confirmed a widespread abnormality. Chronic neurogenic changes are present on needle examination, predominantly involving the distal lower extremities. The findings are those of a nonspecific sensorimotor neuropathy of the axonal type. A diagnosis of ethanol-associated neuropathy was made, based in part on the absence of other contributing factors, the association of other ethanol-related findings including midline-cerebellar degeneration (confirmed on cranial magnetic resonance imaging [MRI]), and the systemic and laboratory evidence of ethanol-toxicity.

The majority of neuropathies present with predominant sensory abnormalities in association with mild but unequivocal motor abnormalities. Sometimes the motor abnormalities are only apparent on needle EMG examination. Examples described in the preceding section that fit into this classification equally well include neuropathies associated with the Miller-Fisher variant of GBS, Friedreich's ataxia, and rheumatoid arthritis. Most toxic-metabolic neuropathies are characterized by distal axonal degeneration (dying-back) of sensory and motor axons (84). Unfortunately, they are all physiologically similar, limiting the usefulness of electrodiagnostic studies in establishing etiology. Sensory symptoms and signs predominate with dysesthesias, paresthesias, distal sensory loss, and loss of distal reflexes. Weakness and atrophy of distal muscles develop subsequently. Sensory amplitudes are usually abnormal early in the course of the disease; motor amplitudes become abnormal later, oc-

Table 12–13
Sensory Greater Than Motor, Axonal Loss

Acromegaly

Amyloidosis

Chronic illness neuropathy

Connective tissue diseases
    Rheumatoid arthritis
    Periarteritis nodosa
    Churg-Strauss syndrome (vasculitis)

Degenerative disorders
    Friedreich's ataxia
    Olivopontocerebellar atrophy

Gout

Hypothyroidism

Metals
    Arsenic (chronic)
    Gold
    Lithium
    Mercury

Myeloma

Myotonic dystrophy

Nutritional
    B_{12} deficiency
    Folate deficiency
    Post-gastrectomy
    Thiamine deficiency

Pharmaceuticals
    Amitriptyline
    Colchicine
    Ethambutol
    INH
    Metronidazole
    Nitrous oxide
    Phenytoin
    Thallium
    Vincristine

Polycythemia vera

Sarcoidosis

Toxic
    Acrylamide
    Carbon disulfide
    Ethyl alcohol
    Hexacarbons (glue sniffing)
    Organophosphorus esters

Modified with permission from John Wiley & Sons, Inc., ©1990. Donofrio PD, Alberts JW. Polyneuropathy: Classification by nerve conduction studies and electromyography. Muscle Nerve 1990;13:889–903.

curring in the distal lower extremities first. Conduction velocities remain essentially normal. Fibrillation potentials and positive waves appear distally.

Ethyl alcohol is generally identified as the most common cause of neuropathy in the United States. Neuropathy appears in association with several neurologic findings related either to the direct neurotoxic effects of alcohol or its metabolites, nutritional disorders, genetic factors, or combinations thereof (16,23,90). The role of alcohol in neuropathy is controversial because individuals who consume large amounts of alcohol often are nutritionally compromised, and clinically similar neuropathies occur with vitamin deficiency states (e.g., thiamine and other B vitamin deficiencies) (90). Some evidence suggests that an alcohol neuropathy can occur with normal nutrition. Paresthesias and painful distal dysesthesias are common early symptoms. The neuropathy progresses slowly, and distal weakness, unsteady gait, and areflexia appear, often in association with dysautonomia.

The electromyographer's contribution to the evaluation of axonal sensorimotor neuropathies is in confirming the presence of neuropathy and identifying other findings, such as Mees' lines, that may suggest a cause. Axonal sensorimotor neuropathies with features suggesting a specific diagnosis include a painful neuropathy with superimposed carpal tunnel syndrome in amyloidosis (51), tremor and neuropathy with lithium (71) or mercury intoxication (6), preservation of reflexes with abnormal corticospinal tract signs with vitamin B_{12} deficiency (63), and the coexistence of neuropathy and myopathy associated with colchicine (55). Familiarity with the associated disorders listed in Table 12–13 may prove helpful in identifying potential causes for neuropathy in the individual patient with a nonspecific sensory greater than motor axonal neuropathy.

Sensory Greater Than Motor Neuropathy; Conduction Slowing (Table 12–15)

Case 6

A 32-year-old man with a 12-year history of insulin-dependent diabetes mellitus presents with the gradual onset of very painful distal paresthesias, numb feet, clumsiness, impotence, and orthostatic lightheadedness. On examination, he has evidence of sensory ataxia, distal sensory loss to all modalities, absent reflexes, and mild distal weakness. His feet do not appear to sweat, and he has a 15 mm Hg orthostatic drop in his blood pressure without an increase in his pulse rate. The nerve conduction and needle EMG studies shown in Table 12–16 demonstrate reduced SNAP amplitudes and mod-

Table 12–14
(Case 5)

Nerve Stimulate (record)	Nerve Conduction Studies		Latencies (msec)	
	Amplitude (μV)	Conduction Velocity (m/sec)	Distal	F wave
R median (thenar)				
Wrist	5000		4.1	30.9
Elbow	4500	55		
R ulnar (hypothenar)				
Wrist	7000		3.3	30.1
Below elbow	6500	57		
R peroneal				
Ankle	2000		5.2	NR
Below knee	1800	44		
R tibial				
Ankle	2300		5.4	
Sensory				
R median (index)	12	54	3.7	
R ulnar (fifth)	8	56	3.5	
R sural (ankle)	NR			
L sural (ankle)	NR			

Muscle	Electromyography			Motor Unit Action Potential	
	Insertional Activity	Fib	Fasc	Recruitment	Amplitude/Duration
R FDI (hand)	Increased	++	0	Reduced (2+)	Slight increase
R abd. pollicis brevis	Increased	++	0	Reduced (2+)	Slight increase
R Extensor digitorum	Normal	0	0	Normal	Normal
R biceps brachii	Normal	0	0	Normal	Normal
R anterior tibialis	Increased	++	0	Reduced (1+)	Slight increase
R median gastrocnemius	Increased	+++	0	Reduced (1+)	Slight increase
R FDI (pedis)s	Increased	+++	0	Reduced (4+)	Severe increase
R vastus medialis	Increased	0	0	Normal	Normal
R paraspinal (lumbar)	Normal	0	0	Normal	Normal

erate slowing of sensory and motor conduction velocities without clear evidence of abnormal temporal dispersion or partial conduction block. F-wave latencies are prolonged in upper and lower extremities. Skin potential responses are unobtainable. Isolated median abnormalities could have been explained by a focal median mononeuropathy at the wrist with the mild conduction velocity slowing related to conduction block of large myelinated fibers. However, similar findings of borderline-prolonged distal latencies and conduction velocities near the lower limit of normal were present in all of the motor nerves examined. The absent skin potential responses, sometimes called sympathetic skin responses, provide evidence of autonomic dysfunction but do not localize the level of abnormality more precisely. The needle examination demonstrates chronic neurogenic changes in the distal lower extremities and fibrillation potentials throughout the paraspinal muscles. The combined findings were interpreted as those of a moderately severe sensorimotor neuropathy with superimposed dysautonomia and polyradiculopathy. The conduction slowing was insufficient to fulfill crite-

Table 12–15
Sensory Greater Than Motor, Conduction Slowing

Diabetes mellitus	End-stage renal disease

Modified with permission from John Wiley & Sons, Inc. ©1990. Donofrio PD, Albers JW: Polyneuropathy: Classification by nerve conduction studies and electromyography. Muscle Nerve 1990;13:889–903.

Table 12–16
(Case 6)

Nerve Stimulate (record)	Nerve Conduction Studies Amplitude (μV)	Conduction Velocity (m/sec)	Latencies (msec) Distal	F wave
R median (thenar)				
Wrist	5000		4.2	33.9
Elbow	4600	47		
R peroneal				
Ankle	1500		6.1	NR
Below knee	1400	39		
R tibial				
Ankle	3300		5.8	
		40		
Sensory				
R median (index)	10	49	3.8	
R ulnar (fifth)	5	50	3.7	
R sural (ankle)	NR			

Muscle	Insertional Activity	Fib	Fasc	Motor Unit Action Potential Recruitment	Amplitude/Duration
R FDI (hand)	Increased	+	0	Reduced	Slight increase
R biceps brachii	Normal	0	0	Normal	Normal
R anterior tibialis	Increased	+	0	Reduced	Slight increase
R median gastrocnemius	Increased	+	0	Reduced	Slight increase
R vastus medialis	Increased	0	0	Normal	Normal
R FDI (pedis)s	Increased	++	0	Reduced	Moderate increase
L FDI (pedis)s	Increased	++	0	Reduced	Moderate increase
R paraspinal (lumbar)	Increased	++	0		
R paraspinal (thoracic)	Increased	++	0		

ria for primary demyelination, but was more characteristic of the loss of large myelinated nerve fibers or of a membranopathy. The combined abnormalities were characteristic of those frequently associated with diabetes mellitus.

In early symmetric diabetic neuropathy, sensory complaints and signs predominate with distal dysesthesias, paresthesias, and sensory loss. When present, weakness is most prominent in the distal lower extremities. Early signs of diabetic neuropathy include decreased vibration and pain sensations in the distal lower extremities. Joint position sensation may be impaired in severe neuropathy. Ankle reflexes are usually absent, and other reflexes hypoactive. Atrophy and weakness of distal muscles develop, followed by more proximal involvement.

Most asymptomatic, neurologically intact diabetic patients demonstrate conduction slowing with conduction velocities around the lower limit of normal (42,92). F-wave latencies are typically prolonged. As severity of the neuropathy increases, sensory amplitudes disappear in the lower extremities and motor amplitudes become reduced in asso-

ciation with the further reduction of conduction velocities (92). Abnormal temporal dispersion and partial conduction block are not prominent. Most patients with isolated sensory abnormalities and all patients with generalized sensorimotor diabetic neuropathy have fibrillation potentials distally.

The pathophysiology of reduced conduction velocity in symmetric distal diabetic polyneuropathy is complex and probably reflects chronic demyelination with remyelination, axonal stenosis, and a primary metabolic abnormality. Increased conduction velocity hours after normalizing glucose levels suggests that metabolic changes are related to the conduction abnormalities (43,89). Decreased nerve myo-inositol and increased polyol pathway activity related to increased conversion of glucose to sorbitol by aldose reductase are associated with reduced Na^+/K^+-ATPase activity, increased intracellular Na^+, and decreased conduction velocity, independent of structural alteration (44). Axoglial disjunction and the loss of channels also contribute to reduced conduction velocity (82). Intensive diabetes therapy delays the onset of clinical neuropathy and the electrophysiologic attributes of diabetic neuropathy in patients with insulin-dependent diabetes mellitus (87).

Patients with renal failure independent of diabetes mellitus develop a sensorimotor neuropathy characterized by low-amplitude motor and sensory responses, sometimes in association with pronounced conduction slowing (33). This is most apparent in patients with end-stage renal disease (ESRD). The magnitude of slowing is greater than expected from the loss of large myelinated fibers, and chronic demyelination and remyelination plus membrane changes contribute to the slowing (77). Although nerve conduction studies are important in the diagnosis of ESRD neuropathy, they are not required to evaluate the effectiveness of dialysis. Determination of adequate dialysis is complicated, and the primary indicators of adequate treatment are clinical, not electrodiagnostic. Dialysis and renal transplantation are generally effective in improving ESRD neuropathy, but electrodiagnostic improvement is a late finding.

References

1. Ahrens EM, Meckler RJ, Callen JP: Dapsone-induced peripheral neuropathy. Int J Dermatol 1986;25: 314–316.
2. Albers JW: Clinical neurophysiology of generalized polyneuropathy. J Clin Neurophysiol 1993;10: 149–166.
3. Albers JW: Evaluation of polyneuropathy. In: 1993 AAEM Course D: Fundamentals in electrodiagnostic medicine. New Orleans, Louisiana: AAEM, 1993;17–28.
4. Albers JW: Inflammatory demyelinating polyradiculopathy. In: Brown WF, Bolton CF, eds. Clinical electromyography. Boston: Butterworth, 1987; 209–244.
5. Albers JW, Donofrio PD, McGonagle TK: Sequential electrodiagnostic abnormalities in acute inflammatory demyelinating polyradiculopathy. Muscle Nerve 1985;8:528–539.
6. Albers JW, Kallenbach LR, Fine LJ, et al.: Neurological abnormalities associated with remote occupational elemental mercury exposure. Ann Neurol 1988;24:651–659.
7. Albers JW, Kelly JJ Jr: Acquired inflammatory demyelinating polyneuropathies; clinical and electrodiagnostic features. Muscle Nerve 1989;12:435–451.
8. Albers JW, Leonard JA Jr: Nerve conduction and electromyography. In: Crockard A, Hayward R, Hoff JT, eds. Neurosurgery: The scientific basis of clinical practice. 2nd ed. Oxford, England: Blackwell Scientific Publications Ltd., 1992.
9. Albers JW, Robertson WC, Daube JR: Electrodiagnostic findings in acute porphyric neuropathy. Muscle Nerve 1978;1:292–296.
10. Albin RL, Albers JW: Long-term follow-up of pyridoxine-induced acute sensory neuropathy-neuronopathy. Neurology 1990;40:1319.
11. Albin RL, Albers JW, Greenberg HS, et al.: Acute sensory neuropathy-neuronopathy from pyridoxine overdose. Neurology 1987;37:1729–1732.
12. Allen N, Mendell JR, Billmaier DJ, et al.: Toxic polyneuropathy due to methyl n-butyl ketone: An industrial outbreak. Arch Neurol 1975;32:209–218.
13. Arnason BGW, Soliven B: Acute inflammatory demyelinating polyradiculopathy. In: Dyck PJ, Thomas PK, Griffin JW, et al., eds. Peripheral Neuropathy. Philadelphia: WB Saunders, 1993;1437–1497.
14. Asbury AK, Arnason BGW, Karp HR, McFarlin DE: Criteria for diagnosis of Guillain-Barre syndrome. Ann Neurol 1978;3:565–566.
15. Ballantyne JP, Hansen S: A quantitative assessment of reinnervation in the polyneuropathies. Muscle Nerve 1982;5:S127–S134.
16. Behse F, Buchthal F: Alcoholic neuropathy: Clinical, electrophysiological, and biopsy findings. Ann Neurol 1977;2:95–110.
17. Bloomer JR, Bonkovsky HL: The porphyrias. Dis Mon 1989;35:1–54.
18. Bolton CF, Carter KM: Human sensory nerve compound action potential amplitudes: Variation with sex and finger circumference. J Neurol Neurosurg Psychiatry 1980;43:925–928.
19. Bradley WG, Lassman LP, Pearce GW, et al.: The neuromyopathy of vincristine in man. J Neurol Sci 1970;10:107–131.
20. Bromberg MB, Albers JW: Patterns of sensory nerve conduction abnormalities in demyelinating and axonal peripheral nerve disorders. Muscle Nerve 1993;16:262–266.
21. Brown WF, Feasby TE: Conduction block and denervation in Guillain-Barré polyneuropathy. Brain 1984;107:219–239.
22. Chang YC: Neurotoxic effects of n-hexane on the human central nervous system: Evoked potential abnormalities in n-hexane polyneuropathy. J Neurol Neurosurg Psychiatry 1987;50:269–274.
23. Charness ME, Simon RP, Greenberg DA: Medical Progress: Ethanol and the nervous system. N Engl J Med 1989;321:442–454.
24. Cornblath DR, Sumner AJ, Daube J, et al.: Conduction block in clinical practice. Muscle Nerve 1991;14:869–871.
25. Davey R: Macrodantin: A cautionary tale. Med J Aust 1986;145:476–477.
26. Davis CS, Johnson MK, Richardson DJ: Organophosphorus compounds. In: O'Donoghue JL, ed. Neurotoxicity of industrial and commercial chemicals. Vol. II. Boca Raton: CRC Press, Inc., 1985; 1–24.
27. Donofrio PD, Albers JW: Polyneuropathy: Classification by nerve conduction studies and electromyography. Muscle Nerve 1990;13:889–903.
28. Donofrio PD, Albers JW, Greenberg HS, et al:: Peripheral neuropathy in osteosclerotic myeloma: Clinical and electrodiagnostic improvement with chemotherapy. Muscle Nerve 1984;7:137–141.

29. Donofrio PD, Alessi AG, Albers JW, et al.: Electrodiagnostic evolution of carcinomatous sensory neuronopathy. Muscle Nerve 1989;12:508–513.

30. Donofrio PD, Wilbourn AJ, Albers JW, et al.: Acute arsenic intoxication presenting as Guillain-Barré-like syndrome. Muscle Nerve 1987;10:114–120.

31. Drachman DB: Pathophysiology of the neuromuscular junction. In: Asbury AK, McKhann GM, McDonald WI, eds. Diseases of the nervous system. Clinical neurobiology. Philadelphia: WB Saunders, 1986;258–259.

32. Dyck PJ: Inherited neuronal degeneration and atrophy affecting peripheral motor, sensory, and autonomic neurons. In Dyck PJ, Thomas PK, Lambert EH, et al., eds. Peripheral neuropathy. Philadelphia: WB Saunders, 1984;1600–1655.

33. Dyck PJ, Johnson WJ, Nelson RA, et al.: Uremic neuropathy. III. Controlled study of restricted protein and fluid diet and infrequent hemodialysis versus conventional hemodialysis treatment. Mayo Clin Proc 1975;50:641–649.

34. Dyck PJ, Lambert EH: Lower motor and primary sensory neuron diseases with peroneal muscular atrophy. I. Neurologic, genetic, and electrophysiologic findings in hereditary polyneuropathies. Arch Neurol 1968;18:603–619.

35. Dyck PJ, Lambert EH, Mulder DW: Charcot-Marie-Tooth disease: Nerve conduction and clinical studies of a large kinship. Neurology 1963;13:1–11.

36. Feasby TE, Gilbert JJ, Brown WF, et al.: An acute axonal form of Guillain-Barré polyneuropathy. Brain 1986;109:1115–1126.

37. Feasby TE, Hahn AF, Brown WF, et al.: Severe axonal degeneration in acute Guillain-Barré syndrome: Evidence of two different mechanisms? J Neurol Sci 1993;116:185–192.

38. Fowler TJ, Ochoa J: Unmyelinated fibers in normal and compressed peripheral nerves of the baboon. Neuropathol Appl Neurobiol 1975;1:247–255.

39. Fraser AG, McQueen INF, Watt AH, et al.: Peripheral neuropathy during long-term high-dose amiodarone therapy. J Neurol Neurosurg Psychiatry 1985;48:576–578.

40. Fross RD, Daube JR: Neuropathy in the Miller-Fisher syndrome: Clinical and electrophysiologic findings. Neurology 1987;37:1493–1498.

41. Gilliatt RW, Taylor JC: Electrical changes following section of the facial nerve. Proc R Soc Med 1959;52:1080–1083.

42. Gilliatt RW, Willison RG: Peripheral nerve conduction in diabetic neuropathy. J Neurol Neurosurg Psychiatry 1962;25:11–18.

43. Graf RJ, Halter JB, Pfeifer MA, et al.: Glycemic control and nerve conduction abnormalities in non-insulin dependent diabetic subjects. Ann Intern Med 1981;94:307–311.

44. Greene DA, Sima AAF, Albers JW, et al.: Diabetic neuropathy. In: Rifkin H, Porte D, eds. Diabetes Mellitus. New York: Elsevier, 1990;710–755.

45. Gutmann L, Martin JD, Welton W: Dapsone motor neuropathy—An axonal disease. Neurology 1976; 26:514.

46. Herskowitz A, Ishii N, Schaumburg HH: N-hexane neuropathy: A syndrome occurring as a result of industrial exposure. N Engl J Med 1971;285:82–85.

47. Holmberg L, Boman G, Bottiger LE, et al.: Adverse reactions to nitrofurantoin. Analysis of 921 reports. Am J Med 1980;69:733–738.

48. Iannaccone ST, Sokol RJ: Vitamin E deficiency in neuropathy of abetalipoproteinemia. Neurology 1986;36:1009.

49. Jaspan JB: Hypoglycemic peripheral neuropathy in association with insulinoma; Implications of glycopenia rather than hyperinsulinism. Medicine 1982; 61:33–44.

50. Kelly JJ Jr: Differential diagnosis of demyelinating polyneuropathies. In: American Academy of Neurology annual course no. 146, clinical EMG. Minneapolis: American Academy of Neurology, 1989; 107–124.

51. Kelly JJ Jr, Kyle RA, O'Brien PC, et al.: The natural history of peripheral neuropathy in primary systemic amyloidosis. Ann Neurol 1979;6:1–7.

52. Kennedy RH, Danielson MA, Mulder DW, et al.: Guillain-Barré syndrome. A 42-year epidemiologic and clinical study. Mayo Clin Proc 1978;53:93–99.

53. Kiers L, Altermatt HJ, Lennon VA: Paraneoplastic anti-neuronal nuclear IgG autoantibodies (type I) localize antigen in small cell lung carcinoma. Mayo Clin Proc 1991;66:1209–1216.

54. Korobkin R, Asbury AK, Sumner AJ, et al.: Glue-sniffing neuropathy. Arch Neurol 1975;32:158–162.

55. Kuncl RW, Duncan G, Watson D, et al.: Colchicine myopathy and neuropathy. N Engl J Med 1987; 316:1562–1568.

56. Lagueny A, Rommel A, Vignolly B, et al.: Thalidomide neuropathy: An electrophysiologic study. Muscle Nerve 1986;9:837–844.

57. Laloux P, Brucher JM, Guerit JM, et al.: Subacute sensory neuronopathy associated with Sjogren's sicca syndrome. J Neurol 1988;235:352–354.

58. Lambert EH, Mulder DW, Bastron JA: Regeneration of peripheral nerves with hyperinsulin neuronopathy: Report of case. Neurology 1960;10:851.

59. Landau WM: The duration of neuromuscular function after nerve section in man. J Neurosurg 1953; 10:64–68.

60. Lewis RA, Sumner AJ: Electrodiagnostic distinctions between chronic familial and acquired demyelinative neuropathies. Neurology 1982;32:592–596.

61. Long RR, Sargent JC, Hammer K: Paralytic shell fish poisoning: A case report and serial electrophysiologic observations. Neurology 1990;40: 1310–1312.

62. Lotti M, Becker CE, Aminoff MJ: Organophosphate polyneuropathy: Pathogenesis and prevention. Neurology 1984;34:658–662.

63. McCombe PA, McLeod JG: The peripheral neuropathy of vitamin B_{12} deficiency. J Neurol Sci 1984; 66:117–126.

64. McGonagle TK, Levine SR, Donofrio PD, et al.: Spectrum of patients with EMG features of polyradiculopathy without neuropathy. Muscle Nerve 1990;13:63–69.

65. McLeod JG: An electrophysiological and pathological study of peripheral nerve in Friedreich's ataxia. J Neurol Sci 1971;12:333–349.

66. Morgan JP, Penovich P: Jamaica ginger paralysis. Arch Neurol 1978;35:530–532.

67. Ochoa J: Nerve fiber pathology in acute and chronic compression. In: Omer GE, Spinner M, eds.: Management of peripheral nerve problems. Philadelphia: WB Saunders, 1980;487–501.

68. Ochoa J, Fowler TJ, Gilliatt RW: Anatomical changes in peripheral nerves compressed by a pneumatic tourniquet. J Anat 1972;113:433–455.

69. Ochoa J, Marotte L: Nature of the nerve lesion underlying chronic entrapment. J Neurol Sci 1973; 19:491–495.

70. Palliyath SK, Schwartz BD, Gant L: Peripheral nerve functions in chronic alcoholic patients on disulfiram: A six-month follow-up. J Neurol Neurosurg Psychiatry 1990;53:227–230.

71. Pamphlett RS, Mackenzie RA: Severe peripheral neuropathy due to lithium intoxication. J Neurol Neurosurg Psychiatry 1982;45:656–661.

72. Penn RG, Griffin JP: Adverse reactions to nitrofurantoin in the UK, Sweden and Holland. Brit Med J 1982;284:1440–1442.

73. Rivner MH, Swift TR, Crout BO, et al.: Toward more rational nerve conduction interpretations: The effect of height. Muscle Nerve 1990;13:232–239.

74. Roelofs RI, Hrushesky W, Rogin J, et al.: Peripheral sensory neuropathy and cisplatin chemotherapy. Neurology (Minneap) 1984;34:934–938.

75. Rosen I, Haeger-Aronson B, Rehnstrom S, et al.: Neurophysiological observations after chronic styrene exposure. Scand J Work Environ Health 1978;4(Suppl 2):184–194.

76. Sack GHJ: Acute intermittent porphyria. JAMA 1990;264:1290–1293.

77. Said GHJr, Boudier L, Selva J, et al.: Different patterns of uremic polyneuropathy. Neurology 1983; 33:567–574.

78. Schaumburg HH, Kaplan J, Windebank AJ, et al.: Sensory neuropathy from pyridoxine abuse: A new megavitamin syndrome. N Engl J Med 1983; 309:445–448.

79. Schaumburg HH, Spencer PS, Thomas PK: Anatomical classification of PNS disorders. Philadelphia: FA Davis Company, 1983;7–23.

80. Schold SC, Cho ES, Somasundaram M, et al.: Subacute motor neuropathy: A remote effect of lymphoma. Ann Neurol 1979;5:271–287.

81. Senanayake N, Karalliedde L: Neurotoxic effects of organophosphorus insecticides. N Engl J Med 1987; 316:761–763.

82. Sima AAF, Lattimer SA, Yagihashi S, et al.: "Axoglial dysjunction." Novel structural lesion that accounts for poorly reversible slowing of nerve conduction in the spontaneously diabetic BB rat. J Clin Invest 1986;77:474–484.

83. Smith HV, Spalding JMK: Outbreak of paralysis in Morocco due to ortho-cresyl phosphate poisoning. Lancet 1959;2:1019–1021.

84. Spencer PS, Schaumburg HH: Central peripheral distal axonopathy—The pathology of dying-back polyneuropathies. In Zimmerman H, ed. Progress in Neuropathology, Vol. III. New York: Grune & Stratton, 1976;253–250.

85. Spencer PS, Schaumburg HH: Experimental neuropathy produced by 2,5-hexanedione—A major metabolite of the neurotoxic industrial solvent methyl n-butyl ketone. J Neurol Neurosurg Psychiatry 1975;38:771–775.

86. Stetson DS, Albers JW, Silverstein BA, et al.: Effects of age, sex, and anthropometric factors on nerve conduction measures. Muscle Nerve 1992;15:1095–1104.

87. The Diabetes Control and Complications Trial Research Group: The effect of intensive treatment of diabetes on the development and progression of long-term complications in insulin-dependent diabetes mellitus. N Engl J Med 1993;329:977–986.

88. Trojaborg WT, Moon A, Andersen BB, et al.: Sural nerve conduction parameters in normal subjects related to age, gender, temperature, and height: A reappraisal. Muscle Nerve 1992;15:666–671.

89. Troni W, Carta Q, Cantello R, et al.: Peripheral nerve function and metabolic control in diabetes mellitus. Ann Neurol 1984;16:178–183.

90. Victor M: Neurologic disorders due to alcoholism and malnutrition. In: Joynt RJ, ed.: Clinical neurology. Philadelphia: JB Lippincott Company, 1989; 1–94.

91. Wilbourn AJ: Generalized low motor-normal sensory conduction responses: The etiology in 55 patients. Muscle Nerve 1984;7:564–565.

92. Wilbourn AJ: The diabetic neuropathies. In Brown WF, Bolton CF, eds.: Clinical electromyography. Boston: Butterworth, 1987;329–364.

93. Wolfart G: Collateral regeneration from residual motor fibers in amyotrophic lateral sclerosis. Neurology 1957;7:124–133.

94. Yamada M, Shintani S, Mitani K, et al.: Peripheral neuropathy with predominantly motor manifestations in a patient with carcinoma of the uterus. J Neurol 1988;235:368–370.

Chapter 13
Generalized Weakness
Daniel Clinchot and Charles Levy

The clinical electromyographer is often consulted to help determine the specific neuromuscular abnormalities in patients who present with weakness when weakness can be localized to a particular nerve distribution, which often makes the electrophysiologic evaluation succinct and the diagnosis and prognosis are usually clear. However, when the complaints are of a more generalized nature, the patient evaluation and diagnosis become more complex. A thorough history and physical examination are indispensable in choosing the proper electrophysiologic approach to the problem. The electrophysiologic evaluation of patients who present with generalized weakness requires a combination of motor and sensory nerve stimulation studies and a needle examination. An adequate sampling of sensory and motor nerves is essential, making sure to include distal and proximal nerve segments, frequently including long latency responses. The needle examination often requires sampling of both distal and proximal muscles in order to acquire adequate information about the distribution of pathology. In patients with mild-to-moderate symptoms, an evaluation of the involved extremity is often most productive. However, in patients with severe symptoms, an evaluation of the least involved limbs may have more diagnostic yield.

Case One

A 56-year-old-carpenter-presents with a 6-month history of slowly progressive weakness and "tiredness" in his lower limbs and hand cramps. On further questioning, he admits to difficulty swallowing for the past 2 months. He denies any sensory changes. His bowel and bladder function have not been affected.

Physical examination reveals normal mentation, a mixture of upper and lower motor neuron findings, and subtle tongue fasciculations. Although the patient's sensory examination is normal, he has diffuse weakness that is somewhat greater distally.

Diseases that involve the degeneration of the alpha motor neuron are best considered along a continuum. Primary lateral sclerosis results from the degeneration of upper motor neurons. It usually presents with a spastic gait and evolves slowly. Eventual progression leads to upper limb weakness, bulbar findings, and bowel and bladder dysfunction. Progressive bulbar palsy involves patients who present with oromotor dysfunction. Usually these patients have dysarthria and eventually they develop swallowing dysfunction. Patients with progressive muscular atrophy primarily present with a progressive lower motor neuron picture. Amyotrophic lateral sclerosis presents with a clinical picture of upper and lower motor neuron and bulbar findings. Patients usually develop all of these findings, although at the time of presentation they may primarily have upper motor neuron, lower motor neuron, or bulbar symptoms. Progression is usually over the course of 12 to 24 months. Voluntary motor weakness with minimal sensory findings predominate. Bowel and bladder function and cognition usually remain normal throughout the course of the disease. Amazingly, autonomic functions usually are well preserved.

The electrophysiologic evaluation of the patient with suspected motor neuron disease (MND) consists of nerve stimulation studies and needle examination, usually of three limbs, the paraspinal muscles, and a more cephalad muscle such as the tongue (Table 13–1). Cervical spinal disease, which mimics motor neuron disease, must be considered during the evaluation. In trying to delineate these two disease processes, abnormalities in craniofacial muscles would suggest a cranial process. Thus, the usefulness of EMG evaluation of these muscles can be appreciated. Sensory studies including distal latencies, sensory nerve action potential (SNAP) amplitudes, nerve excitability, and conduction are usually normal for MND. In advanced MND, the

Table 13-1
Electrophysiologic Approach in Suspected Motor Neuron Disease

Select a muscle with clinical weakness in mild involvement. Select muscles with least clinical weakness in severe involvement.

1. Perform nerve stimulation studies in varied distribution using multiple limbs. Include at least two motor and three sensory studies. Make note of compound muscle action potential (CMAP) amplitudes.

2. Perform needle examination of three limbs. Note insertional activity, spontaneous potentials, and the feel of the muscle. Look for changes in the motor unit action potentials.

3. If there are widespread fibrillation potentials, positive waves, and fasciculation potentials, examine a more proximal muscle. The tongue is a good choice in this scenario.

4. If all of the above are normal, consider repetitive nerve stimulation to evaluate neuromuscular junction disorders and F waves.

motor nerve conduction velocity is often reduced, as eventually there will be loss of some of the fastest conducting fibers. However, because these fibers are no more vulnerable than the rest of the motor neuron pool, it is rare to find motor conduction velocity below 75% of normal (31,36). The amplitude of the compound muscle action potential (CMAP) becomes reduced as more and more anterior horn cells are lost. Repetitive nerve stimulation in motor neuron disease often reveals a decremental response at slow stimulation rates of 2 Hz–3 Hz (6,26). As with myasthenia gravis, post-tetanic potentiation and exhaustion are also present. A reduced amplitude of the distal CMAP and a decremental response with repetitive stimulation portend a more rapid progression for patients with MND (25,36) (Fig. 13–1).

Needle examination in the early stages of the disease reveals minimal fibrillation potentials and positive waves. This is due to the fact that motor neurons are capable of innervating (by sprouting) up to five times their normal number of motor fibers. Thus, as some motor neurons degenerate and denervate their motor fibers, the fibers will be incorporated into the territory of the remaining viable motor neurons. As a result, the remaining motor units are characterized by increased motor unit amplitude, duration, and variability (Fig. 13–2). These changes in the motor unit characteristics are often present before the clinical onset of weakness. As the disease progresses, motor neuron degeneration exceeds the capacity of the remaining motor neurons to compensate. This is accompanied by the emergence of fibrillation potentials and

positive waves and continued increases in amplitude, duration, and motor unit action potential (MUAP) variability.

Variability of motor unit size and shape is commonly seen in motor neuron disease. Inconsistency of the MUAP amplitude, configuration, and duration is thought to represent an intermittent failure or slowing of nerve conduction over the newly sprouted axon to recently reinnervated muscle fibers (10). These MUAPs often display an increase in the number of phases and occasionally will have associated satellite potentials. Overall, the MUAPs will be reduced in number with a proportional reduction in recruitment, reflecting ongoing loss of motor neurons. The motor units will fire rapidly, reflecting a discrete pattern that is typical late in MND. However, increased recruitment frequency (see Chapter 1) is an early finding. The increased amplitude and duration reflects an increased territory of the remaining motor neuron pool and the loss of synchronous fiber depolarization (10).

Case Two

A 25-year-old man, referred for evaluation, presents with the insidious onset of bilateral hand and foot weakness. He has noticed significant stiffness in his hands, especially when trying to release an object grasped. He has been in special education classes for most of his life and has recently had surgical extraction of bilateral cataracts.

Physical examination shows a balding male with wasting of the bilateral temporalis muscles and

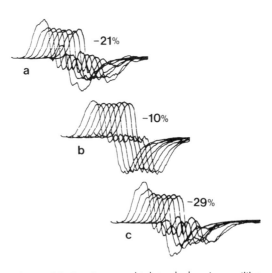

Figure 13-1. Amyotrophic lateral sclerosis: repetitive supramaximal stimulation of the peroneal nerve at 2 Hz, recording from a severely denervated anterior tibialis. *A.* Before exercise. *B.* Immediately after 30- second exercise. *C.* Two minutes after exercise.

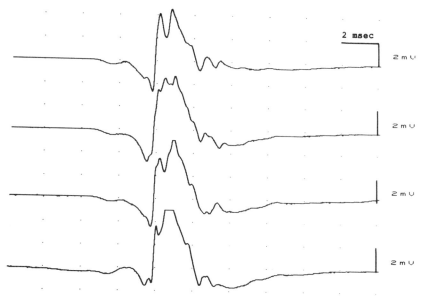

Figure 13–2. A first recruited MUAP in an ALS patient of increased amplitude and duration, polyphasic and unstable with repetitive discharge. (Monopolar recording 20 Hz to 10 Khz.)

weakness of the periocular and perioral musculature. He presents with mild dysarthria and has a swan-neck appearance to his cervical spine when viewed in the sagittal plane. He has evidence of testicular atrophy. Percussion of his muscles shows a quick contraction with a very slow relaxation. This is more evident upon first examination, but after warming the patient's hands, it appears to be less evident. Myotonia refers to the clinical observation of delayed muscle relaxation after voluntary activation or percussion.

The presenting signs and symptoms of the patient in this case suggest the diagnosis of myotonic dystrophy. Myotonic dystrophy, one of the most common of the myotonic syndromes, is inherited in an autosomal-dominant fashion with incomplete penetrance. Classically, a patient with myotonic dystrophy will present with complaints other than myotonia, and in fact as the disease progresses, the myotonia may be less evident to the clinical examiner. Bulbar pathology will often lead to difficulty with speech and swallowing. These symptoms are usually worse in patients who present earlier in life. Wasting of facial, masseter, and temporalis muscles results in the classic "hatched face" appearance. Myotonic dystrophy is one of the few myopathic processes that presents with distal rather than proximal weakness. The electrophysiologic evaluation is an integral component of the evaluation of patients suspected of having myotonic dystrophy (Table 13–2). It has been found to be efficacious in patients with subclinical or fully expressed disease (7). The electrophysiologic evaluation should include both nerve stimulation studies and

Table 13–2
Electrophysiologic Approach in Suspected Myotonic Dystrophy

Select a muscle with clinical weakness. Make sure that the patient has a skin temperature of at least 32° in the hands and 28° in the feet.

1. Perform nerve conduction studies (NCS) in a varied distribution of multiple limbs. Be sure to include two motor and three sensory nerves.

2. Perform examination of selected proximal and distal muscles of three limbs. Examining two or three muscles in each limb is usually sufficient. Look closely during insertions for evidence of myotonic discharges.

3. Make a quantitative assessment of the motor unit action potentials.

    If the motor units are normal and there is myotonia, consider myotonia congenita, paramyotonia, or hyperkalemic periodic paralysis.

    If the motor units are myopathic, consider myotonic dystrophy or inflammatory myopathy.

    If the motor units are neuropathic, review NCS data and consider proximal nerve pathology.

needle examination. Nerve stimulation studies usually reveal normal distal latencies as well as sensory and motor nerve conduction. However, when the myopathic process is severe, the distal CMAP amplitude will be reduced. Long latency responses (F waves, H reflexes) are usually normal. Repetitive nerve stimulation in myotonic dystrophy reveals a decremental response at low rates of stimulation, with eventual recovery. This decremental response is due to depolarization block. That is, the hyperirritable muscle cell membranes are still depolarized as the subsequent stimulation occurs, resulting in a decremental response. Usually this decrement is less than 30%.

The needle examination reveals small polyphasic MUAPs with reduced recruitment frequencies (Fig. 13–3). Electrically, myotonia appears as positive waves or spike discharges and occasionally can appear as triphasic potentials. The duration is usually variable, and the amplitudes of discharges will range from 10 μV–1000 μV. Myotonia usually fires at frequencies of 4 Hz–100 Hz with a waxing and waning rhythm (Fig. 13–4). Although myotonic dystrophy may have a greater incidence of myotonia than do the other myotonic syndromes, myotonia is often present only in affected muscles. Thus, myotonia will not be present in all muscles sampled during the electrophysiologic exam. The EMG doublet discharge of voluntary MUAPs are present in myotonic dystrophy, whereas they usually are not present in most other myopathies (28).

Other myotonic syndromes are thought to include myotonia congenita, generalized myotonia, paramyotonia congenita, and hyperkalemic periodic paralysis (32). Myotonia congenita (Thomsen's Disease, named after the Danish physician with the disease who described it in detail) is an autosomal dominantly inherited disease. It's hallmark feature is widespread disabling myotonia i.e., "stiffness" or difficulty with relaxing grip. This "stiffness" resolves with further activity, and is known as a "warm-up phenomenon". Myotonia is usually found in all muscles, although rarely patients will only be affected in a few muscles. Myotonia congenita is nonprogressive. Examination of recruitment may be complicated by the abundance of myotonic discharges triggered by voluntary activity; nevertheless, recruitment is normal (not myopathic).

Generalized myotonia, in contrast to myotonia congenita, is inherited in an autosomal recessive fashion. This disorder is of a more progressive nature than myotonia congenita and often will show a myopathic process upon needle examination. There are no clinical associations in these patients as is seen with myotonic dystrophy. Patients will usually complain of limb weakness or "stiffness" with a predilection for the lower limbs and proximal musculature. Paramyotonia is inherited in an autosomal dominant fashion. It is distinguished from the other myotonic syndromes by the worsening of myotonia and stiffness with cold. Repeated activation of a cooled muscle in such patients will result in paralysis of that muscle. Paramyotonia has no associated motor unit changes. Abortive trains of positive waves in most muscles were called "EMG disease" in the past. Wiechers and Johnson (35)

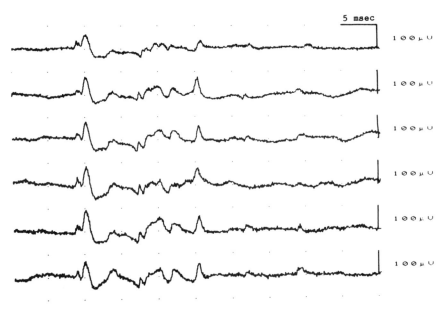

Figure 13-3. Long duration MUAP recorded from a teenage boy with Becker dystrophy. (Monopolar recording 20 Hz to 10 KHz.)

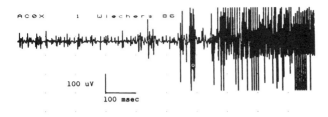

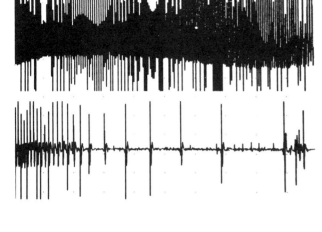

Figure 13-4. Myotonic discharge recorded from a patient with myotonic dystrophy.

suggested that these patients could have a "forme fruste" of paramyotonia congenita because they found families with dominant genetic patterns. Hyperkalemic periodic paralysis is an autosomal dominant disorder whereby elevated potassium levels result in muscle paralysis. These patients will have normal nerve stimulation studies and MUAPs between attacks, although needle examination may reveal the presence of myotonia. In the presence of elevated serum, potassium spontaneous electrical activity will occur and the CMAP amplitude and motor unit action potentials progressively reduce in size. Eventually all of these parameters will return to normal.

Case Three

A 35-year-old woman, referred for electrodiagnostic evaluation, presents with a 1-week history of bilateral hand tingling. The patient remembers having an upper respiratory illness 3 weeks prior. She reports that her legs and arms feel weak and she has difficulty walking. Her bowel and bladder functions are normal.

Physical examination reveals facial and upper and lower limb weakness with an essentially normal sensory exam. Deep tendon reflexes are reduced in the upper and lower limbs.

Acute inflammatory demyelinating polyneuropathy (AIDP), also known as Guillain-Barré syndrome, results from an aberrant immune response directed at components of the peripheral nerve.

It is preceded by a viral illness a few weeks prior to the onset of symptoms in about two-thirds of patients. Associated viruses include cytomegalovirus, Epstein-Barr virus, HIV, and vaccinia. Much recent interest has focused on the bacteria Campylobacter jejuni, which has been implicated in 12%–60% of AIDP cases. AIDP usually presents as rapidly progressive weakness in the presence of hyporeflexia. In fact, the early loss of muscle stretch reflexes strongly reinforces the clinical diagnosis of AIDP, whereas the presence of normal muscle stretch reflexes casts serious doubt on the diagnosis. Autonomic dysfunction and cerebral spinal fluid (CSF) protein elevations are commonly seen in the disease. The illness usually progresses to a point at which the patient is at his or her weakest at approximately 2–3 weeks after the symptoms first appear (2). The development of diagnostic criteria have been useful in the evaluation of the patient suspected of having AIDP (1–3).

AIDP characteristically involves short-segment demyelination along various sensory and motor nerves with a predilection for the nerve roots (Table 13–3). This demyelination results in conduction block and slowing of nerve conduction; thus, the electromyographer should assess the proximal and distal components of various nerves. F responses can be prolonged or difficult to elicit early in the course of the illness (2). This is thought to be secondary to the predilection for nerve root involvement in the disease. Distal and proximal evoked potentials will allow the clinician to determine the presence of conduction block, temporal dispersion, prolonged distal latencies, and reduced excitability of nerves, which are classic findings with AIDP. Criteria have been established to assist in the electrophysiologic diagnosis of AIDP (1–3). There is a high incidence of electrophysiologic abnormalities in AIDP, with peak incidence at approximately 4–12 weeks (17).

The needle examination in patients with AIDP reveals a reduced interference pattern. MUAPs are often of increased duration with polyphasia (17). Spontaneous activity is commonly found with an increased prevalence in the more proximal muscles. A type of AIDP primarily presents as an axonal degeneration. In this form of the disease, positive waves and fibrillation potentials predominate and nerve conductions may be prolonged (1). As the disease progresses and reinnervation proceeds, MUAPs will increase in size and duration. Along with these spontaneous potentials, myokymic discharges can be seen in AIDP. These discharges are believed to result from ephaptic transmission in localized areas of demyelination.

Nerve stimulation studies are helpful in determining the prognosis for the patient with AIDP. Poor recovery correlates with reduced amplitude of distal CMAP at the disease nadir. In fact, CMAP amplitudes that are less than 20% of the lower limit of normal correlate with a poorer prognosis (2). Reduced motor nerve conduction velocity and denervation on the needle examination also correlate with a poorer prognosis (1,17). Other portents of a lesser recovery include the clinical observation of extensive muscle atrophy, a failure to improve within one month of the disease's onset, and the need for mechanical ventilation.

Table 13–3
Electrophysiologic Evaluation in Suspected Acute Inflammatory Demyelinating Polyneuropathy

Select nerves with muscle weakness in their distribution.

1. Select nerve stimulation studies in both sensory and motor distribution. Stimulate on several points along the nerve to determine the presence of conduction block.

   Note distal latency.

   Note temporal dispersion.

2. Long latency responses in median or ulnar and peroneal distribution.

   Note if the F-wave latency exceeds 120% of the upper limit of the normal range.

3. Perform needle examination of involved muscles, looking for degree of membrane irritability and changes in the morphology of the motor unit action potential.

Case Four

A 32-year-old woman is referred for electrophysiologic evaluation with a 6-month history of difficulty chewing and swallowing. She reports being easily fatigued and is no longer able to chew gum. There is no family history of weakness. Her bowel and bladder functions are normal.

Physical examination reveals a slight degree of bilateral ptosis, a slight generalized weakness, and no atrophy. Muscle stretch reflexes and sensory examination are normal. When asked to chew a piece of gum, the patient initially has no problem but then develops an obvious weakening of the muscles of mastication.

Neuromuscular junction disorders are an important consideration in the patient who presents with generalized weakness. The neuromuscular junction consists of a presynaptic nerve terminal containing acetylcholine (Ach) stored in vesicles, a postsynaptic endplate zone located on the targeted muscle containing folds of Ach receptors, and the synaptic cleft in the space between (Fig. 13–5). It is normal for a few vesicles to spontaneously release their Ach into the cleft, causing small, nonpropagated depolarizations called miniature endplate potentials (MEPPs). However, when an action potential reaches the presynaptic nerve terminal, it causes a voltage-sensitive influx of calcium ions, which triggers approximately 50–60 vesicles to pour their contents into the synaptic cleft. The resulting MEPPs summate to form endplate potentials (EPP). When the EPP reaches electrical threshold in the postsynaptic membrane, a muscle action potential is created and muscle contraction ensues.

Neuromuscular junction disorders occur when there are defects in the presynaptic release or postsynaptic reception of Ach molecules. In myasthenia gravis, the body produces antibodies to the postsynaptic Ach receptors. With less postsynaptic receptors available, the postsynaptic membrane has greater difficulty reaching electrical threshold. Botulism, Lambert-Eaton myasthenic syndrome (LEMS; also known as myasthenic syndrome), and neuromuscular junction toxins cause dysfunction in the presynaptic release of Ach quanta. This then indirectly impairs the postsynaptic membrane's ability to reach electrical threshold.

Repetitive nerve stimulation is a useful tool for the electromyographer when evaluating a patient for a disorder of neuromuscular transmission (Table 13–4). Stimulating a normal nerve at 2 Hz–3 Hz often results in a slight decrease in the EPP amplitude by decreasing the available stores of Ach. This can result in very small reductions in the CMAP amplitude (usually less than 10% of the lower limit of normal for that muscle). Careful attention must be paid to technique when performing repetitive nerve stimulation to avoid spurious decremental responses (Fig. 13–6). Stimulating

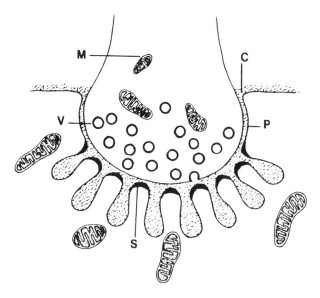

Figure 13–5. Simplified schematic representation of the junctional apparatus: mitochondrium (*M*), synaptic vesicle (*V*), synaptic cleft (*C*), postsynaptic membrane (*D*), and receptor site (*S*).

Table 13–4
Repetitive Stimulation in Suspected Neuromuscular Junction Disease

Select a muscle with clinical weakness or a facial muscle if ocular features predominate. Firmly affix electrodes to the skin for recording and stimulation. Control muscle movement.

1. Set supramaximal stimulation to 25% above that just producing the maximal compound muscle action potential (CMAP).

2. Stimulate at 2 Hz or 3 Hz for six to nine stimulations.

3. Observe the decrement of amplitude by comparing the first response to the fourth or fifth response.

4. Have the patient perform maximum isometric exercise of the muscle for 15 seconds. (If patient is unable to exercise, go to step #10 below.)

5. Immediately repeat the series of stimuli as in step #2.

> Note any increment or decrement. An increased amplitude of the first response suggests ELMS. Correction of the decrement suggests myasthenia gravis.

6. Wait one minute.

7. Repeat stimulation as in step #2, noting any increment or decrement.

8. Wait one minute.

9. Repeat stimulation as in step #2 (if able to complete, omit step #10).

> Note any increment or decrement. In myasthenia gravis, the decrement will be greater than in step #3. Decrement will tend to be stable in other diseases.

10. If patient is unable to cooperate with voluntary exercise, then stimulate the muscle at 20 Hz for 10 seconds.

> A progressive increment of 50% to 100% suggests botulism.

> A progression increment of 200% or more suggests Eaton-Lambert Myasthenic syndrome.

at rates higher than 5 Hz or pre-exercising the muscle to be tested usually increases the EPP amplitude and results in a slight increase in the CMAP amplitude owing to the increased incidence of Ach quanta being released. This occurs because the calcium that is released with each depolarization requires 100 msec to 200 msec to diffuse away from the nerve terminal. Therefore, stimulation that arrives at rates greater than 5 Hz–10 Hz will cause calcium to accumulate, facilitating vesicle release. After more extensive exercise or stimulation at very high frequencies, the expected increment in the

CMAP amplitude (which lasts for about 1 minute) is followed by a period of postactivation exhaustion in which the EPP amplitudes decrease and there is a reduction in the CMAP amplitude. This period usually lasts 10–15 minutes.

LEMS results from a defect in neuromuscular transmission. Although this disease can be found in patients without carcinoma, it is more frequently found in patients with small cell carcinoma of the bronchus and other cancers. The presentation is usually one of muscle weakness and fatigue. There may be associated ptosis or bulbar symptoms. Patients usually initially present with proximal weakness, but as the disease progresses the weakness usually involves the distal muscles as well.

Electrophysiologically there is a reduction in the CMAP on single stimulation. This reduction can be seen in any muscle sampled and thus usually is not localized to symptomatic muscles. There is often a decremental response to repetitive nerve stimulation at slow rates. With high rates of stimulation (Fig. 13–7) or after exercise, there is an exaggerated facilitation (Fig. 13–8). This facilitation usually reaches 200% and often brings the CMAP amplitude into the normal range.

Botulism presents an electrophysiologic picture

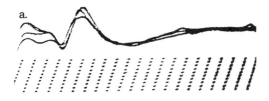

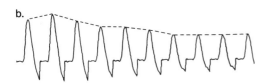

Figure 13–6. Repetitive stimulation at 2 Hz showing spurious decremental responses in normal subjects: *A.* Facial nerve to nasalis owing to movement of the recording electrode. *B.* Median nerve to thenar muscles owing to movement of the recording electrode. Note erratic display (highlighted by dotted line) resulting from faulty technique. When superimposed as in *A*, note that the baseline fluctuates, as well as the action potential (AP).

similar to that of myasthenic syndrome except that the CMAP obtained with single stimuli is often normal. In addition, no decremental response is seen in botulism (13,18). The postactivation facilitation seen in botulism is of a much smaller magnitude than that seen in myasthenic syndrome (18,27). In botulism, the abnormalities are scattered and are of a severity proportional to the degree of intoxication, in contrast to LEMS, in which abnormalities are found in all muscles sampled (18).

Myasthenia gravis usually presents with muscle fatigue and generalized weakness. In over 90% of cases, the levator palpebrae or extraocular muscles are involved, resulting in a drooping of the eyelids and intermittent diplopia. The muscles of facial expression, mastication, swallowing, and speech are involved in 80% of cases, leading to an altered facial appearance and difficulty eating. Muscles of the neck, shoulder girdle, trunk, and hips may also be involved. Sometimes patients will present with primarily ptosis or bulbar symptoms but then progress to generalized complaints. Sensory symptoms do not predominate, and there usually are no complaints of bowel or bladder dysfunction.

The role of electrodiagnosis is evident in the evaluation of the patient with suspected myasthenia gravis. Nerve stimulation studies produce normal sensory and motor latencies and conduction. The amplitude of the distal CMAP is usually normal except in severe cases in which the amplitude may be slightly reduced. The needle examination is often normal, although myopathic findings of reduced duration of MUAPs have been reported (11,30). Variability of voluntary MUAP amplitude is commonly seen in myasthenia gravis (Fig. 13–9).

Repetitive stimulation is the mainstay in the electrodiagnosis of patients suspected of having myasthenia gravis. In general, the proximal musculature tends to have a greater yield than the more distal muscles. Axillary, musculocutaneous, and facial nerve stimulation appear to have the best yield. Reduction of the amplitude, or more precisely the area of the maximal CMAP with repetitive stimulation rates at low frequencies (i.e., 2 Hz–3 Hz), can usually be seen by comparing the amplitudes of the first and fifth responses (11,15,30). A change in amplitude of greater than 10% is considered significant. This decrement is believed to be secondary to neuromuscular junction blocking of many neuromuscular junctions (18). Postactivation facilitation in myasthenia gravis refers to the exaggerated response of myasthenic muscles 10 to 15 seconds after tetanic or strong voluntary contraction. Last-

Figure 13–7. Lambert-Eaton myasthenia syndrome: repetitive supramaximal stimulation of the median nerve at *A* (5 Hz), *B* (10 Hz), *C* (20 Hz), and *D* (40 Hz); recordings from thenar muscles.

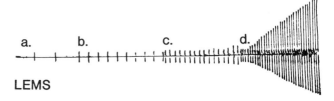

LEMS

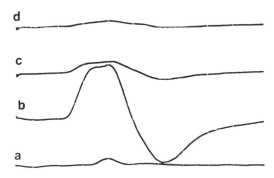

Figure 13-8. Lambert-Eaton myasthenic syndrome: single supramaximal stimulus (ulnar hypothenar). *A.* At rest. *B.* Immediately after 10-second exercise. *C.* 15 seconds after exercise. *D.* 30 seconds after exercise.

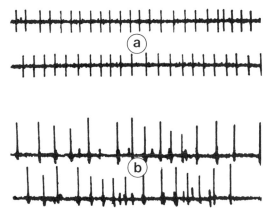

Figure 13-9. Single motor unit potential firing repetitively under voluntary control. *A.* Stable amplitude of a potential of a normal subject. *B.* Fluctuating amplitude of a potential of a patient with myasthenia gravis.

ing only 15–30 seconds, this facilitation is usually a short-lived phenomenon (11,30). Low-frequency repetitive stimulation during this period generally reveals a dampened decremental response.

High rates of repetitive stimulation or 10–15 seconds of maximal isometric muscle contraction will often result in post-tetanic exhaustion. This exhaustion occurs as a result of the progressive blocking of muscle fibers (11,30).

Disorders of neuromuscular transmission are an important consideration in the evaluation of the patient presenting with generalized weakness. Careful use of repetitive nerve stimulation will allow for an effective evaluation of the neuromuscular junction.

Case Five

A 20-year-old man is referred for an electrodiagnostic evaluation with a history of progressive difficulty rising from a chair. He denies any sensory

symptoms. His bowel and bladder functions are normal.

Physical examination reveals weakness of the hip and shoulder musculature. The biceps muscles appear to be atrophic and there is winging of the scapula bilaterally. Muscle stretch reflexes are reduced symmetrically. The sensory examination gives normal results.

Limb girdle dystrophy is a generic term representing a variable number of illnesses that have different clinical presentations and outcomes. Those with genetic links are often inherited in an autosomal recessive pattern, although sporadic cases also occur. The illness can progress slowly or rapidly over the course of a few years. Muscle enzyme elevations are usually found early in the disease process. Muscle biopsy will reveal fiber-splitting, variable fiber size, whorled fibers, multiple nuclei, and moth-eaten fibers. Eventual reduction in the ability to ambulate is universal. Other neuromuscular disorders can be mistaken for limb girdle dystrophy, especially Becker-type muscular dystrophy and spinal muscular atrophy (14). It is therefore of utmost importance for the clinician to incorporate the various diagnostic tools available to ensure that the correct diagnosis is made. Careful family histories, physical examination, electrophysiologic studies, and muscle biopsies should be the mainstay in the evaluation of the patient with suspected limb girdle dystrophy.

The electrophysiologic evaluation of the patient with suspected limb girdle dystrophy usually reveals a myopathic picture with a proximal distal gradient (Table 13–5). Sensory and motor stimulation studies are usually normal, and long latency potentials are not prolonged. In end-stage disease, there may be a reduction in CMAP amplitude. The needle examination reveals a typical myopathic pattern with short-duration, low-amplitude polyphasic

Table 13-5
Electrophysiologic Evaluation in Suspected Limb Girdle Dystrophy

Select muscle with clinical weakness. Make sure that the patient has a skin temperature of at least 32° in the hands and 28° in the feet.

1. Perform nerve stimulation studies in a varied distribution of multiple limbs. Be sure to include two motor and three sensory nerves.

2. Perform needle examination sampling muscles in three or four limbs. Look closely during insertions for evidence of abnormal discharges.

3. Make a quantitative assessment of the motor unit action potentials.

   Note any gradient in the severity of findings. Abnormalities concentrating around the shoulder and pelvic girdle is suggestive of limb-girdle dystrophy

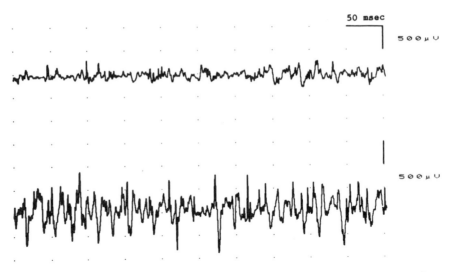

Figure 13–10. *Top.* Low threshold contraction reveals an increased number of MUAPs recruited per strength. *Bottom.* High threshold contraction reveals a reduced number of MUAPs or muscle fibers recruited.

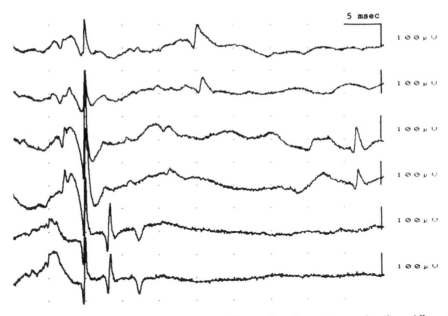

Figure 13–11. Long duration MUAPs from an 8-year-old boy with Duchenne's dystrophy. Three different MUAPs; two recordings of each to emphasize late components. Note second MUAPs in recordings are 3 msec and 4 msec total duration when including late components. (Monopolar recordings 20 Hz to 10 KHz.)

MUAPs. These potentials usually recruit early (Fig. 13–10). As the disease progresses, MUAPs will increase in duration as the motor unit territory increases. These potentials will often develop late components (Fig. 13–11). This occurs when motor units sprout to incorporate muscle fibers that have lost innervation owing to fiber degeneration. Positive waves, fibrillation potentials, and complex repetitive discharges, although rare, can be found in muscles that are severely affected.

Case Six

A 40-year-old man reports for an electromyographic examination with a 3-week history of difficulty getting out of a car. He has noted a deep aching pain in the large muscles of the arms and legs. He denies any sensory or bowel and bladder dysfunction.

Physical examination immediately reveals an erythematous telangiectatic rash over the patient's hands, neck, and thorax. He has proximal upper and lower limb weakness. The muscles of his shoulders and hips appear swollen. The sensory examination gives normal results and the muscle stretch reflexes are normal. His muscles are not tender to palpation.

Inflammatory myopathies commonly present with proximal limb weakness that has progressed over the course of weeks or, more insidiously, months. Cardiac, respiratory, and gastrointestinal involvement have been associated with these myopathies. Pain in the muscles is not always present. However, when present, the pain is described as a deep aching sensation within the muscle itself. Patients with dermatomyositis often develop an erythematous rash in the periocular, malar, cervical, or thoracic distributions. Thickened skin often develops over the dorsal surfaces of the ankles, elbows, and hands. Myositis can have associations with malignancy, HIV, or connective tissue disorders, or they may be idiopathic. Likewise, distinctions are made between the juvenile and adult forms of the disease. Associations with malignancy are often found in persons more than 50 years old with dermatomyositis. Specific classifications and diagnostic criteria have been developed for both polymyositis and dermatomyositis (20). Elevations in muscle enzymes, especially the creatinine kinase, are usually seen with inflammatory myopathies. These enzymes usually increase before the onset of clinical weakness and normalize before the onset of strength gains (29). In patients with dermatomyositis or polymyositis, muscle biopsy reveals fiber necrosis, fiber regeneration, variability in fiber size, and inflammatory infiltration. Special histocompatibility markers reveal differences between the types of myositis, especially in the Class 1 major histocompatibility complex (16,20).

The electrophysiologic findings in patients with myositis correlate with the pathophysiology of the disease itself (Table 13–6). Fiber necrosis leaves segments of the muscle fiber without innervation. These fibers fibrillate without their neural connection. Thus, early in the course of the disease there are fewer fibers per motor unit, creating MUAPs of shorter duration and smaller amplitude. Normal sensory and motor nerve stimulation studies are

the rule in myositis except in severe cases in which the amplitude of the CMAP may be reduced. Long-latency responses are usually normal. Needle examination reveals a proximal greater than a distal gradient and symmetrical involvement. Positive waves and fibrillation potentials in conjunction with short-duration low-amplitude polyphasic MUAPs are classic findings in inflammatory muscle disease. These motor unit action potentials will have a myopathic recruitment. Occasionally, complex repetitive discharges or perhaps myotonia can be seen in the muscles examined. There appears to be a predilection for the paraspinals in myositis, and thus these usually provide a high yield for abnormal findings (24).

SUMMARY

In the electrophysiologic evaluation of the patient who presents with generalized weakness, careful attention to historic and physical findings will lead the electromyographer to the appropriate examination. A combination of nerve stimulation studies and needle examination, as well as repetitive nerve stimulation, are often required for a thorough exam. These studies must be interpreted in conjunction with the patient's history and physical findings, providing the clinician not only with the diagnosis, but also information on disease extent and prognosis.

References

1. Albers JW: AAEM case report #4: Guillain-Barré syndrome. Muscle Nerve 1989;12:705–711.
2. Albers JW: Inflammatory polyneuropathies: clinical and electrodiagnostic features. AAEM course C. American Association of Electrodiagnostic Medicine. Rochester, MN.
3. Albers J, Donofrio P, McGonagle T: Sequential electrodiagnostic abnormalities in acute inflammatory demyelinating polyradiculoneuropathy. Muscle Nerve 1985;8:528–539.
4. Barchi RL: Myotonia. Neurol Clin 1988;6(3): 473–482.
5. Barkhaus P, Nandedkar D, Sanders D: Quantitative EMG in inflammatory myopathy. Muscle Nerve 1990;13:247–253.
6. Bernstein LP, Antel JP: Motor neuron disease: Decremental responses to repetitive nerve stimulation. Neurology 1981;31:202–204.
7. Brunner HG, Smeets HJ, Nillesen W, et al. : Myotonic dystrophy predictive value of normal results on clinical examination. Brain 1991;114:2303–2311.
8. Bruchthal F, Kamieniecka Z: The diagnostic yield of quantified electromyography and quantified muscle biopsy in neuromuscular disorders. Muscle Nerve 1982;5:265–280.
9. Coers C, Telerman-Toppet N: Differential diagnosis

Table 13–6
Electrophysiologic Evaluation in Suspected Polymyositis

Select muscles with clinical weakness for EMG and NCS. Be sure to include the paraspinal muscles.

1. Perform nerve stimulation studies of multiple nerves in a random distribution. Include at least two motor and three sensory nerves in the evaluation.

2. Perform a needle examination of at least two limbs and the paraspinals.

of limb-girdle muscular dystrophy and spinal muscular atrophy. Neurology 1979;29:957–972.

10. Daube JR: AAEM Minimonograph #11: Needle examination in clinical electromyography. Muscle Nerve 1991;14:685–700.

11. Desmedt JE: The neuromuscular disorder in myasthenia gravis. I. Electrical and mechanical response to nerve stimulation in the hand muscles. In: New Developments in EMG and Clinical Neurophysiology, Vol 1. Karger: Basel, 1973;241–342.

12. DeVere R, Bradley W: Polymyositis: Its presentation, morbidity, and mortality. Brain 1975;98:637–666.

13. Fakadej AV, Gutmann L: Prolongation of post-tetanic facilitation in infant botulism. Muscle Nerve 1982;5:727–729.

14. Fowler WM, Nayak NN: Slowly progressive proximal weakness: Limb-girdle syndromes. Arch Phys Med Rehabil 1983;64:527–538.

15. Hutter OF: Post-tetanic restoration of neuromuscular transmission blocked by D-tubocurarine. J Physiol 1952;118:216–227.

16. Karpati G, Pouliot Y, Carpenter S: Expression of immunoreactive major histocompatibility complex products in human skeletal muscles. Ann Neurol 1988;23:64–72.

17. Kaur U, Chopra JS, Prabkakar S, et al. : Guillain-Barré syndrome: A clinical and biochemical study. Acta Neurol Scand 1986;73:394–402.

18. Keesey JC: AAEM Minimonograph #33: Electrodiagnostic approach to defects of neuromuscular transmission. Muscle Nerve 1989;12:613–626.

19. Kimura J: Proximal versus distal slowing of motor nerve conduction velocity in the Guillian-Barré syndrome. Ann Neurol 1978;3:344–350.

20. Kingston W, Moxley R: Inflammatory myopathies. Neurol Clin 1988;6(3):545–561.

21. Koh ET, Seow A, Ong B, et al. : Adult onset polymyositis/dermatomyositis: Clinical and laboratory features and treatment response in 75 patients. Ann Rheum Dis 1993;52:857–861.

22. Lacomis D, Chad A, Smith T: Myopathy in the elderly: Evaluation of the histopathologic spectrum and the accuracy of clinical diagnosis. Neurology 1993;43:825–828.

23. Mechler F, Csenker E, Fekete I, et al. : Electrophysiological studies in myotonic dystrophy. Electromyogr Clin Neurophysiol 1982;22:349–356.

24. Mitz M, Chang G, Albers J, et al. : Electromyographic and histologic paraspinal abnormalities in polymyositis/dermatomyositis. Arch Phys Med Rehabil 1981;62:118–121.

25. Mulder DW: Electrodiagnostic techniques, their role in the diagnosis, prognosis, and study of aetiology of motor neuron disease. In: Rose FC: Research progress in motor neuron disease. London: Pitman Books, 1984;99–104.

26. Mulder DW, Lambert EH, Eaton LM: Myasthenic syndrome in patients with amyotrophic lateral sclerosis. Neurology 1959;9:627–631.

27. Oh SJ: Botulism: Electrophysiologic studies. Ann Neurol 1977;1:481–485.

28. Partanen VSJ: Double discharges in neuromuscular diseases. J Neurol Sci 1978;36:377–382.

29. Robinson L: AAEM Case Report #22: Polymyositis. Muscle Nerve 1991;14:310–315.

30. Somnier FE, Trojaborg W: Neurophysiological evaluation in myasthenia gravis. A comprehensive study of a complete patient population. Electroencephalogr Clin Neurophysiol 1993;89:73–87.

31. Stålberg E: Recent progress in ALS neurophysiology. Excerpta Medica International Congress Series No. 1988;769:155–160.

32. Streib EW: AAEE Minimonograph #27: Differential diagnosis of myotonic syndromes. Muscle Nerve 1987;10:603–615.

33. Streib EW, Sun SF: Distribution of electrical myotonia in myotonic muscular dystrophy. Ann Neurol 1983;14:80–82.

34. Tanimoto K, Nakano K, Kano S, et al. : Classification criteria for polymyositis and dermatomyositis. J Rheumatol 1995;22:668–674.

35. Wiechers D, Johnson E: Syndrome of diffuse abnormal insertional activity. Arch Phys Med Rehabil 1982;63:538.

36. Williams DB, Windebank AJ: Motor neuron disease (amyotrophic lateral sclerosis). Mayo Clin Proc 1991;66:54–82.

Appendix
Practical Examination

Paulette A. Smart
Ernest W. Johnson
William S. Pease

This test evaluates one's knowledge of electromyography and nerve conduction studies. Each question illustrates one principle. There is one correct answer per question.

1. Calibration for figure below: Each square = 10 msec (horizontal); 1 mV (vertical). Needle stimulation of spinal nerve at the posterior superior iliac spine with recording electrode over the soleus muscle.

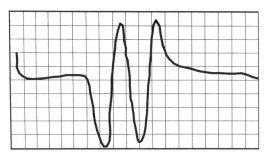

What is the second action potential (positive peak)?

  a. M wave of soleus
  b. H wave
  c. F wave
  d. M wave of gluteus maximus
  e. None of the above

2. If a low pass filter setting of 500 Hz and a high pass setting of 10 KHz are used for recording in motor nerve conduction studies, which of the following will be most apparent?

  a. Increased amplitude
  b. Reduced amplitude
  c. Decreased latency
  d. Increased latency
  e. None of the above

3. Trace is marked (interrupted) at 1-msec intervals; 1 cm on photo = 5 mV. Surface recording of abductor pollicis brevis. The trace to the left is median nerve stimulation at the wrist (motor). The trace to the right is median nerve stimulation at the elbow (motor). Distance = 20 cm. Stimulus initiates the trace.

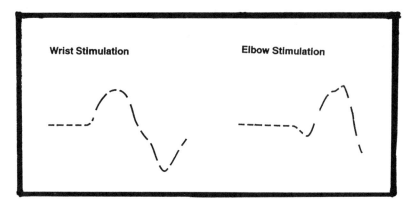

Which of the following is suggested?

a. Mild carpal tunnel syndrome (CTS)
b. Severe CTS
c. Martin-Gruber anastomosis
d. A and C are correct
e. Normal study

4. Calibration on figure below: Top trace is ulnar nerve stimulation at the wrist; middle trace is ulnar nerve stimulation below the elbow; bottom trace is ulnar nerve stimulation above the elbow. Surface recording of abductor digiti 5 stimulation occurs after 1-msec delay.

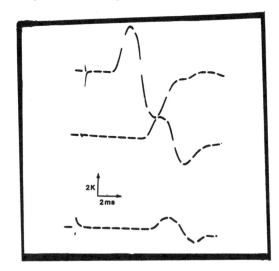

What is the most appropriate description of the ulnar nerve conduction?

a. Neurapraxic block
b. Axonotmesis
c. Partial axonal death
d. Combined conduction block, slowing, and axonal loss
e. Normal tracing

5. In a median nerve study, what would you expect to find in an individual who does not have carpal tunnel syndrome but has a Martin-Gruber anastomosis?

    a. Initial positive deflection on elbow stimulation
    b. False increase in conduction velocity
    c. Larger compound muscle action potential (CMAP) on wrist stimulation
    d. Smaller CMAP on elbow stimulation
    e. None of the above

6. Calibration of figure below: Each slanted line = 10 msec. Height = 50 μV. Monopolar needle in the first dorsal interosseous muscle.

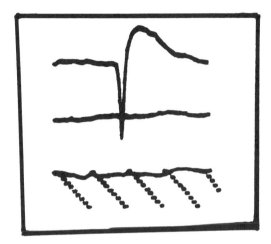

What is the origin of the waveform?

    a. Motor unit
    b. Single muscle fiber
    c. End-plate
    d. Intramuscular nerve
    e. Technique error

7. Refer to the figure above. In which area/condition was this likely recorded?

    a. Edematous subcutaneous tissue
    b. Near or on periosteum
    c. At end-plate zone
    d. Type II muscle atrophy
    e. Fibrotic muscle

8. Calibration on figure: Needle electrode in the brachioradialis. The bottom trace is first, the middle trace is second, and the top trace is third. What is the firing rate of the complex MUP?

    a. 1 Hz
    b. 8 Hz
    c. 13 Hz
    d. 18 Hz
    e. 22 Hz

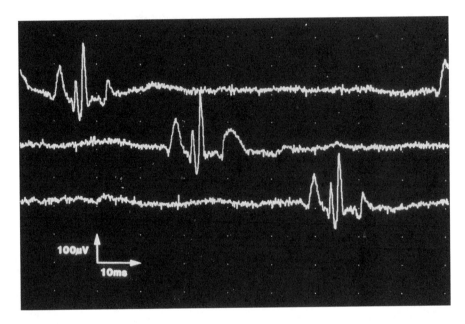

(Reprinted with permission of Pease WS: Recording of motor unit potentials and spontaneous activity. In: Kraft G, MacLean I, eds. Electromyography: A Guide for the Referring Physician. Phys Med Rehabil Clin NA 1990;1(1):27–42. Courtesy of W. B. Saunders Co.)

9. Refer to the figure above. What is the duration of the action potential in the second trace?

    a. 6 msec
    b. 10 msec
    c. 14 msec
    d. 18 msec
    e. 22 msec

10. Which of the stimulation parameters below are optimal for eliciting the "H" wave?

    a. 50 V; 0.1 msec
    b. 300 V; 1 msec
    c. 50 V; 1.0 msec
    d. 150 V; 5 Hz
    e. 300 V; 5 Hz

11. Calibration for figure below: 1 cm = 10 μV; 1 msec. There is no change in calibration between the top and bottom figures.

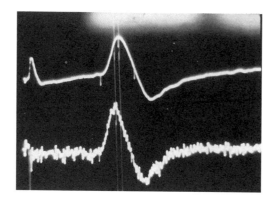

Which filter is interposed in the top trace, making it different from the bottom trace?

a. Band-pass setting of 100 Hz to 10 KHz
b. Band-pass setting of 500 Hz to 5 KHz
c. Band-pass setting of 100 Hz to 5 KHz
d. Band-pass setting of 2 Hz to 2 KHz
e. Band-pass setting of 2 Hz to 10 KHz

12. Refer to the question above. Which of the following electrical activities would be most affected by this change in the filter?

a. Positive wave
b. Fasciculation potential
c. Fibrillation potential
d. H-wave latency
e. CMAP

13. Which is the most frequent source of noise in electromyography?

a. Poor electrode contact
b. 60 Hz
c. Transcutaneous nerve stimulation (TENS) unit
d. Fluorescent lights
e. FM radio

14. Which statement best describes a fibrillation potential?

a. Positive-negative spike; firing at 10 Hz
b. Biphasic spike with 50-μV amplitude and 5-msec duration
c. Negative-positive spike; firing at 1 Hz
d. Triphasic spike with 1-mV amplitude and 6- to 7-msec duration
e. Biphasic spike firing at 50 Hz

15. What would be the earliest electrodiagnostic abnormality in minimal L5 radiculopathy?

a. Prolonged H-wave latency
b. Reduced number of motor units as compared to strength of contraction
c. Positive waves in the paraspinals; at appropriate level
d. Fibrillation potentials in proximal L5 innervated muscles
e. Prolonged F-wave latency in muscles innervated by the peroneal nerve

16. Calibration for figure below: Each slanted line = 50 μV (vertical); 1 msec (horizontal). Monopolar needle in the abductor pollicis brevis.

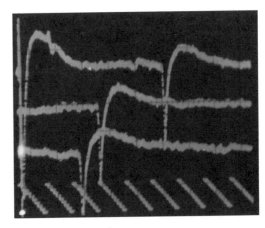

With which of the following conditions was this likely recorded?

a. Type II muscle atrophy
b. C8 radiculopathy 10 days after onset
c. Pronator teres syndrome 18 days after onset
d. Anterior interosseous syndrome
e. Normal (at end-plate)

17. Which of the following contributes most to the distal motor latency?

a. Delay at myoneural junction
b. Conduction along nerve segment between distal stimulation and recording site
c. Depolarization down the muscle fiber
d. Slowing along small-diameter and unmyelinated axon branches
e. None of the above

18. In the figure below, A and R represents G1 and G2 recording electrodes, respectively.

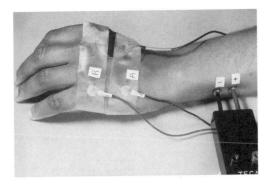

An abnormal finding from a nerve conduction study using the technique pictured would be most consistent with the diagnosis of which condition?

a. Median nerve entrapment
b. Radial nerve entrapment at the wrist
c. C8 radiculopathy
d. Ulnar nerve entrapment at Guyon's canal
e. Ulnar nerve entrapment proximal to the wrist

19. Calibration for the figures below: Each slanted line = 10 msec; height = 200 μV. Monopolar needle is in the deltoid muscle.

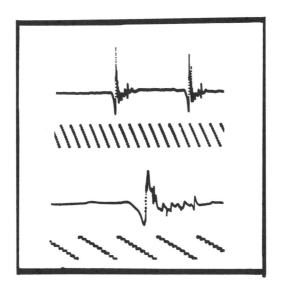

Which diagnosis is suggested?

a. C6 Radiculopathy 1 week after onset
b. Brachial plexitis 1 week after onset
c. Axillary nerve injury 3 months after onset
d. Myasthenia gravis
e. Early polymyositis

20. Calibration for figure below: Each slanted line = 1 msec; height = 20 μV. Antidromic sensory nerve action potential (SNAP) to digit IV. The top trace represents ulnar nerve stimulation at the wrist (14 cm). The bottom trace represents median nerve stimulation at the wrist (14 cm).

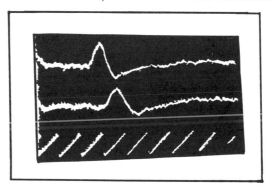

What is your conclusion?

a. Normal tracing
b. Mild CTS
c. Cold hand
d. Diabetic peripheral neuropathy
e. Severe CTS

21. Choose the best answer. How can one identify an action potential as a SNAP and not a volume-conducted motor potential?

    a. Amplitude
    b. Latency
    c. Duration of the negative spike
    d. Number of phases
    e. Initial deflection of the action potential

22. Calibration for figure below: Each slanted line = 10 msec; height = 5 mV. Tracing represents ulnar nerve stimulation at the wrist (8 cm, trace A), below the elbow (28 cm, trace B), and above the elbow (38 cm, trace C).

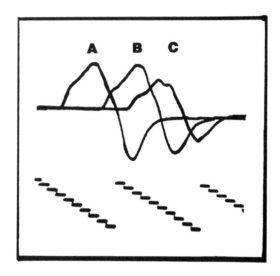

What can you infer from the tracing?

    a. Entrapment at the elbow
    b. Diabetic neuropathy
    c. Anatomic anomaly
    d. Early Guillain-Barré syndrome
    e. Normal study

23. What technique in CTS diagnosis is shown below?

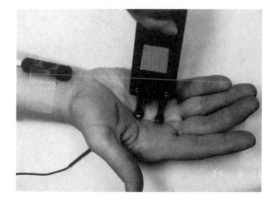

    a. Orthodromic sensory latency
    b. Antidromic motor latency
    c. Mixed nerve latency
    d. Orthodromic motor latency
    e. Recurrent median nerve stimulation

24. Calibration on the figure below: 1-cm vertical height = 1 mV; variable stimulation frequency along x-axis. Surface recording is over abductor pollicus brevis.

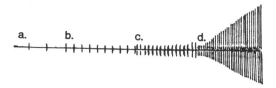

What is the diagnosis?

a. Lambert-Eaton syndrome
b. Myasthenia gravis
c. Myotonic dystrophy
d. Amyotrophic lateral sclerosis (ALS)
e. Normal study

25. Calibration of figure below: Each slanted line = 10 msec. Height = 100 μV. Monopolar needle electrode in the anterior tibialis.

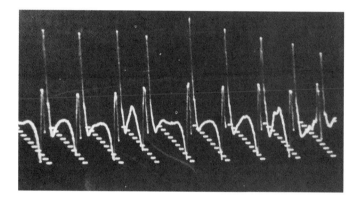

What can you infer?

a. Complex repetitive discharges
b. Cramp
c. End-plate spikes
d. Myopathic recruitment
e. Myotonic discharge

26. Calibration for figure below: 1 cm = 1 mV (vertical); 5 msec (horizontal). The surface recording is of extensor digitorum longus from peroneal nerve stimulation at the fibular head. The top trace is from the left leg; the bottom trace is from the right leg. Assume L5 radiculopathy 1 week after onset with no spontaneous activity in the muscle.

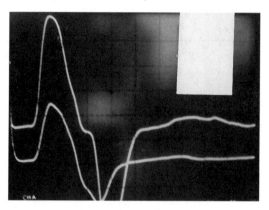

What can you infer about the severity of the lesion in relation to recovery of function?

a. Relatively poor prognosis
b. Relatively good prognosis
c. Too early to tell
d. Cannot predict prognosis from this study
e. This is a normal phenomenon

27. Calibration on the tracing below: Distance between dots = 1 msec (horizontal); 20 μV (vertical). Filter setting is 20 Hz to 2 KHz. The tracings represent antidromic SNAP to long finger at midpalm (top), wrist (middle), and elbow (bottom).

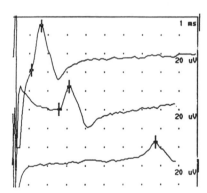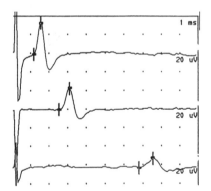

What has happened between the traces on the left and the traces on the right?

a. Change in stimulation intensity
b. Change in hand temperature
c. Movement artifact
d. Interelectrode (G1 to G2) distance shortened
e. Distance between G1 and stimulation site shortened

28. Calibration of figure below: 1 cm = 10 μV (vertical); 1 msec (horizontal). Tracing represents antidromic SNAP to digit 4. Stimulation of median nerve at 7 cm (palm, *bottom trace*) and 14 cm (wrist, *top trace*).

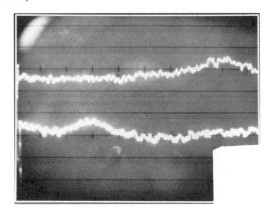

What can you infer?

a. Normal study
b. Cold hand
c. Diabetic neuropathy
d. Severe CTS
e. Diabetic neuropathy and CTS

29. Calibration for figure below: 1 cm = 5 mV. Trace interrupted at 5-msec intervals. Surface recording of soleus muscle. Stimulation of tibial nerve in the popliteal space in a 5'10" adult with a 1-week history of pain in the right buttocks and thigh. The top trace is the left; the bottom trace is the right.

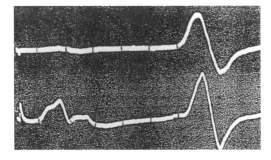

What diagnosis is suggested?

a. Left S1 radiculopathy
b. Right S1 radiculopathy
c. Normal study
d. Peripheral neuropathy
e. None of the above

30. Refer to the above figure. Assume the upper trace is normal, and the distance between the popliteal space and the medial malleolus = 40 cm. What is the patient's predicted age?

a. 25
b. 35
c. 55
d. 70
e. Cannot calculate

31. Calibration of figure below: Each slanted line = 1 msec; height = 5 mV. Surface recording of hypothenar. Ulnar nerve stimulation at the wrist.

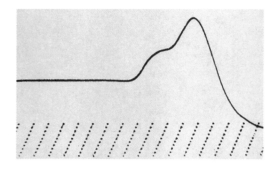

What accounts for the shape of the CMAP?

a. Volume conduction from median innervate muscles
b. Submaximal stimulation
c. Slowed conduction and temporal dispersion
d. G1 over two muscles
e. G1 not over the motor point

32. Calibration on figure below: Trigger/delay line. SFEMG electrode in the extensor digitorum communis.

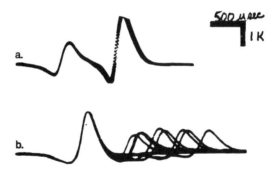

What can you infer from tracing *A*?

a. Mild Myasthenia gravis is presented
b. Normal tracing
c. Increased jitter and blocking is demonstrated
d. Fiber density is increased
e. Neurogenic blocking is demonstrated

33. Refer to the figure above. What can you infer from tracing *B*?

a. Normal muscle
b. Jitter is mildly prolonged without blocking
c. Blocking and prolonged jitter are present
d. Jitter is severely prolonged without blocking
e. Neurogenic blocking is demonstrated

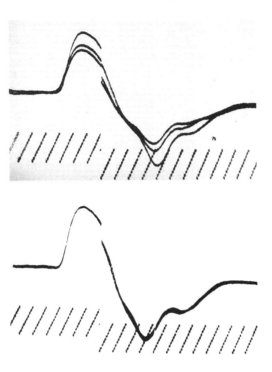

34. Calibration of figures below: Each slanted line = 1 msec; height = 2 mV. A 2-Hz repetitive stimulation was applied at Erb's point with the recording over the deltoid muscle. The upper figure represents a decremental response at 2 Hz; diagnosis is myasthenia gravis.

What happened between the upper figure and the lower figure?

a. Rest for 3 mins
b. Exercise for 10 sec
c. Exercise for 1 min
d. 1/20 curarizing dose
e. None of the above

35. Calibration is on the figure below: the distance between dots = 5 mV (vertical); 10 msec (horizontal). Needle electrode is in the pronator teres. Trace begins at the top.

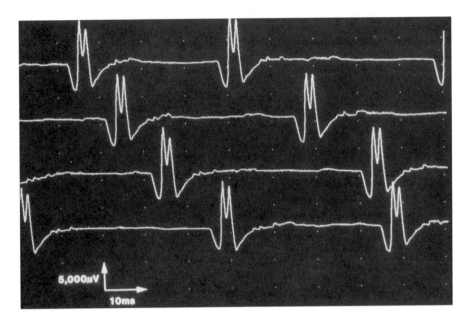

(Reprinted with permission of Pease WS: Recording of motor unit potentials and spontaneous activity. In: Kraft G, MacLean I, eds. Electromyography: A Guide for the Referring Physician. Phys Med Rehabil Clin NA 1990;1(1):27–42. Courtesy of W. B. Saunders Co.)

In which of the following conditions was this recorded?

a. Acute polymyositis
b. Pompe disease
c. Remote poliomyelitis
d. ALS
e. Type II muscle atrophy

36. What is the firing rate?

a. 5 Hz
b. 10 Hz
c. 25 Hz
d. 35 Hz
e. 45 Hz

37. Identify the peripheral nerve and nerve root innervation of muscle indicated by the arrow.

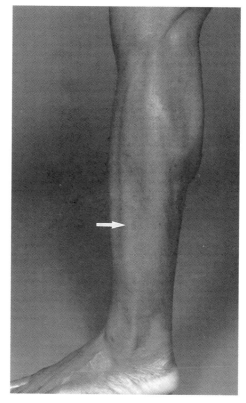

    a. L5, S1; peroneal nerve, deep branch
    b. L4, L5; peroneal nerve, deep branch
    c. L5, S1; peroneal nerve, superficial branch
    d. L5, S1, S2; tibial nerve
    e. L5, S1; tibial nerve

38. Refer to the figure below. Each slanted line is 1 msec; height = 20 μV. The trace represents antidromic median sensory SNAP at 7 cm and 14 cm to digit 3.

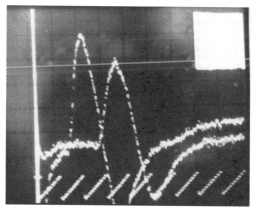

    What is the diagnosis?

    a. Mild CTS
    b. Acute CTS
    c. Diabetic neuropathy
    d. Normal study
    e. Cold hand

39. Calibration of figure below: 1 cm = 50 µV; 100 msec across the screen. Needle electrode is moved in the first dorsal interosseous.

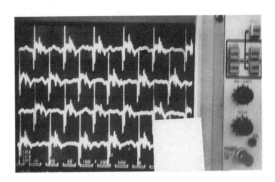

What is the origin of the electrical activity?

a. Normal insertional activity
b. Few positive waves, indicating pathology
c. Myotonic discharges
d. Complex repetitive discharges (high frequency)
e. Needle in the end-plate zone

40. The figure below represents a monopolar needle in the soleus muscle. Calibration is on the picture.

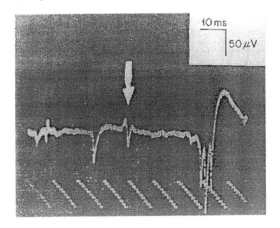

What is the electrical activity under the arrow?

a. Fibrillation potential
b. End-plate spike
c. Polyphasic MUAP
d. Motor unit potential
e. Positive sharp wave

41. The figure below represents stimulation of radial (top trace) and median (middle trace) SNAP using a bipolar surface stimulator at 10 cm with surface ring electrodes recording at digit 1. Each slanted line represents 1 msec; height = 20 μV.

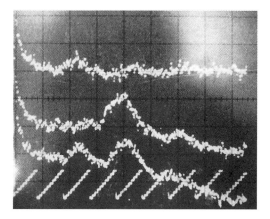

What can you infer from the bottom tracing?

a. Normal study of radial and median nerves
b. Volume conducted CMAP (lumbrical 1)
c. Accidental stimulation of the ulnar nerve
d. Carpal tunnel syndrome
e. None of the above

42. Calibration for diagram below: 1 msec/20 μV between dots. Tracing represents antidromic ulnar SNAP from the ring finger at 14 cm.

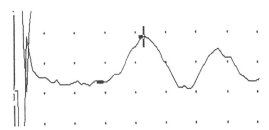

What can you infer about the potential farthest to the right in the trace?

a. Technique artifact
b. Volume conducted ulnar innervated compound muscle action potential
c. 60 Hz interference
d. Normal SNAP
e. None of the above

43. Which electrodiagnostic finding best differentiates a C8 from a C7 radiculopathy?

a. Membrane irritability in the triceps
b. Fibrillations and positive waves in the pronator quadratus
c. Fibrillations and positive waves in the flexor digiti sublimis
d. Fibrillations and positive waves in the abductor pollicis brevis
e. Fibrillations and positive waves in the sternal portion of the pectoralis major

44. The figure below represents monopolar needle in the lumbar paraspinal muscles. Calibration is on the picture.

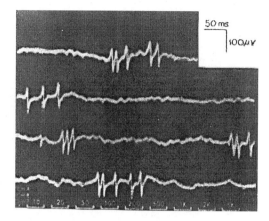

What is the electrical activity?

a. End-plate spikes
b. Cramp
c. Normal firing MUAPs
d. Myokymic discharges
e. Artifact from poor electrode contact

45. The calibration is on the figure below. Monopolar needle in the anterior tibialis muscle.

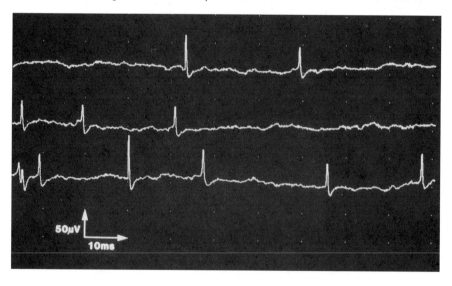

(Reprinted with permission of Pease WS: Recording of motor unit potentials and spontaneous activity. In: Kraft G, MacLean I, eds. Electromyography: A Guide for the Referring Physician. Phys Med Rehabil Clin NA 1990;1(1):27–42. Courtesy of W. B. Saunders Co.)

In which of the following conditions was this likely recorded?

a. Late-stage Duchenne muscular dystrophy
b. L5 radiculopathy, 1 month after onset
c. Type II muscular atrophy
d. End-plate from normal muscle
e. Remote polio

46. Calibration of figure below: 1 cm = 10 msec; 50 μV. Monopolar needle electrode in the first dorsal interosseous (hand).

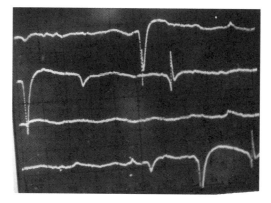

In which of the following conditions was this likely recorded?

a. Mild CTS
b. C8 radiculopathy (10 days after onset)
c. Acute polymyositis
d. Cubital tunnel syndrome (1 month after onset)
e. Needle in the end-plate zone

47. The figure below is a study of the median motor nerve in a 28-year-old-male. Needle EMG is normal. Calibration is on the picture.

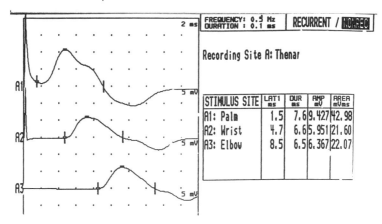

STIMULUS SITE	LAT1 ms	DUR ms	AMP mV	AREA mVms
A1: Palm	1.5	7.6	9.427	42.98
A2: Wrist	4.7	6.6	5.951	21.60
A3: Elbow	8.5	6.5	6.367	22.07

Describe the electrodiagnostic finding.

a. Normal
b. Conduction slowing
c. Conduction block
d. Probable submaximal stimulation at the wrist
e. B and D are correct

48. Refer to the figure above. Why is the shape of the CMAP different at palm stimulation?

a. Submaximal stimulation at the wrist
b. Stimulus spread to ulnar nerve at the palm
c. Palm stimulation is closer to the Thenar muscle
d. There is no substantial difference
e. This is normal CMAP

49. Calibration of picture below: Each square = 2 msec (horizontal); 2 mV (vertical). The top trace is median nerve stimulation in the distal forearm. The middle trace is median nerve stimulation just distal to pronator teres. The bottom trace is median nerve stimulation proximal to pronator teres. Patient complains of pain in forearm without numbness.

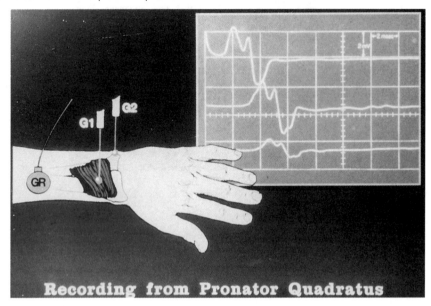

Recording from Pronator Quadratus

(Picture contributed by Drs. Mysiw and Colachis from a poster presentation that leads to the following referenced article: Am J Phys Med Rehab 1988;67(2):50–54).

What is the suggested diagnosis?

a. Pronator syndrome
b. Anterior interosseus syndrome
c. Diabetic peripheral neuropathy
d. CTS
e. None of the above

50. Calibration of figure below: Each slanted line = 1 msec; height = 20 μV. Each potential represents a SNAP of digit 3 from each hand; stimulation of Median Nerve at the wrist (14 cm). The electrode placement is similar in the two hands. Trace to the left = left hand; trace to the right = right hand.

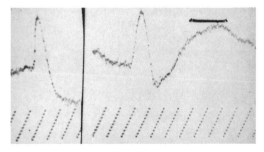

What accounts for the differences?

a. Left hand is colder
b. Right hand is colder
c. Mild CTS on the right
d. Insignificant differences
e. None of the above

ANSWERS TO QUESTIONS

1. B. Stimulation of S1 spinal nerve produces a direct S1 latency of the soleus and a central loop H wave. The first action potential is the M wave; the second action potential is the H wave (H reflex).

2. B. An increase in the low frequency filter will produce a decrease in amplitude, a decrease in the duration of the negative spike, and no change in the onset latency. The negative component will decay and lose its normal contour.

3. D. The figure illustrates a mild increase in the median motor onset latency at the wrist, a falsely elevated nerve conduction velocity of 100 m/s, and an increase in the action potential at the elbow with a positive deflection at elbow stimulation. This indicates a Martin-Gruber anomaly in the presence of mild CTS.

4. A. Conduction block at the elbow is producing a significant decrease in the ulnar nerve CMAP on proximal stimulation. Normal CMAP amplitude at the wrist indicates that there is no axonal loss.

5. E. The first two choices (a, b) are present in Martin-Gruber anastomosis in the presence of CTS and are absent in healthy individuals. The only findings present, in a normal nerve conduction study of the median nerve, are a larger CMAP at elbow stimulation and a smaller CMAP at wrist stimulation. This is because the surface electrode is recording ulnar innervated muscles in the thenar area on elbow stimulation; the wrist stimulation recording is restricted to median innervated muscles.

6. B. The figure illustrates a positive wave, which arises from a single muscle fiber discharge.

7. C. An endplate spike may be recorded as a positive wave when the tip of the needle is in the end-plate zone.

8. C. Because the bottom trace is first, the motor unit is appearing earlier in each subsequent trace, indicating a firing rate greater than 10 Hz. The motor unit would appear at the same place in each trace at a frequency of 10 Hz.

9. D.

10. C. The H reflex is elicited with submaximal intensity stimulation, low voltage (50–100 V), a stimulation frequency of 0.2–0.5 Hz, and an increased stimulation duration of 0.5 to 1.0 msec.

11. D. The top trace was obtained with a filter setting of 2 Hz to 2 KHz. The high frequency filter was reduced from 10 KHz to 2 KHz, eliminating the high frequency noise and smoothing the trace baseline.

12. C. A fibrillation potential would be most affected by this filter change. Setting the high frequency at 2 KHz would facilitate a more defined waveform that would otherwise be masked by high frequency noise.

13. A. Noise is an unwanted signal within the system; interference is an unwanted signal from outside the system.

14. A. Fibrillation potentials fire at 2 Hz to 20 Hz and have an amplitude of 50–300 μV and a duration of 0.5–1.5 msec with a biphasic or triphasic waveform. The initial phase is usually positive but may be negative if the tip of the electrode is at the point of depolarization.

15. C. The earliest electrodiagnostic findings in L5 radiculopathy include decreased recruitment interval or increased recruitment frequency, a reduced number of motor units, a reduced number of F waves during the first week, and an increase in special polyphasic units. However, in minimal L5 radiculopathy, the earliest significant abnormality is positive waves found in the paraspinals. Weakness would not be evident clinically and one would not see a decrease in the number of motor units on maximum contraction.

16. B. The picture illustrates only positive waves obtained from the abductor pollicis brevis on day 10 of a C8 radiculopathy. Fibrillation potentials would be present on day 18 of a pronator teres syndrome. The anterior interosseous nerve does not innervate any intrinsic hand muscles.

17. D. The distal motor latency is most affected by conduction slowing along a small-diameter myelinated axon as it tapers and branches distally. Note that myelin is absent in the distal portion of the axon branches. Other physiologic contributing factors include a delay between the actual initiation of the electrical discharge and the actual transmission of the impulse along the axon; slowed conduction along nonmyelinated fibers; and a delay in transmission of the signal across the myoneural junction (0.2–0.5 msec).

18. E. The technique illustrates an antidromic surface stimulation of the dorsal cutaneous branch of the ulnar nerve. This is a sensory nerve that does not cross Guyon's canal. An abnormal nerve conduction study (increased latency, decreased amplitude, and/or increased duration) would be most consistent with an ulnar nerve entrapment proximal to the wrist. In contrast,

an entrapment at Guyon's canal would affect the deep and superficial branches of the ulnar nerve, with sparing of the dorsal cutaneous branch. The nerve conduction study shown here would then be normal.

19. C. The figure represents re-innervating polyphasic motor units of increased duration, which could appear in nerve injury as early as 5 weeks following nerve injury.

20. B. The SNAP peak latency difference of the median to ulnar nerve is 0.8 msec, which indicates a mild carpal tunnel syndrome. Normal values are less than or equal to 0.3 msec. Normal ulnar nerve amplitude and latency are arguments against diabetic peripheral neuropathy and a cold hand.

21. C. The duration of a nerve fiber action potential averages 1.0–3.0 msec. This is considerably shorter than a compound muscle action potential (CMAP) that has a negative spike duration of 5–9 msec.

22. A. There is a 50% reduction in the nerve conduction velocity and a 33% reduction in the amplitude of the CMAP across the elbow. This represents conduction block and slowing from an entrapment syndrome. The normal amplitude, duration, and latency at wrist stimulation are arguments against axonal loss.

23. C. The technique pictured represents a CTS study from mixed nerve stimulation of the median nerve at 8 cm. This results in a mixed nerve action potential from stimulation of sensory and motor nerve fibers (lumbrical muscle).

24. A. The diagram represents a recording of the motor response to repetitive stimulation at a variable frequency from 2–30 Hz. Note the incremental response of up to 700% of the resting muscle with repetitive stimulation at high rates. Also note the small amplitude of the motor response at rest. This is classic for Eaton-Lambert syndrome.

25. B. The recording was obtained in the presence of a cramp and illustrates high frequency synchronous discharge of motor units at 90 Hz.

26. B. There is a 50% reduction in the amplitude of the CMAP on the right (lower trace) at week one, indicating some axonal loss. After 5 days, axons undergoing Wallerian degeneration fail to conduct. However, with 50% sparing the long-term prognosis for strength is good because collateral innervation results. The prognosis for strength is poor with less than 10% axonal sparing.

27. D. The phenomenon of interelectrode separation is demonstrated. The traces to the right demonstrate a decrease in median SNAP amplitude and a decrease in peak latency with no change in onset latency. This is due to a change in interelectrode distance from 4 cm to 1 cm. A change in hand temperature would produce a more noticeable change in onset latency and SNAP amplitude. A change in stimulus intensity would affect the total area of the action potential without changing the peak latency.

28. E. The palm and wrist median nerve SNAPs both have a marked decrease in amplitude and prolonged latency, indicating a peripheral neuropathy. The marked increase in the duration of the median nerve SNAP at the wrist indicates temporal dispersion and slowing across the carpal tunnel. In severe CTS, the median sensory response is absent.

29. B. The onset latency on the bottom trace to the right is 1.5 msec longer than that on the left, suggesting a right S1 radiculopathy.

30. A. The predicted age is calculated by converting a well-known formula: Latency = 0.46 × length (cm) + 0.1 × age (years) + 9.14. Correct substitutions give the answer of 25 years using a latency of 30 msec.

31. D. The indentation of the action potential on the ascending portion of the waveform results from placing the G1 electrode over the motor point of two hypothenar muscles.

32. B. Tracing A represents normal jitter.

33. C. Tracing B represents abnormal jitter and blocking.

34. B. The bottom trace illustrates post-activation facilitation seen after 10 seconds of exercise, which reversed the decremental response. Repetitive stimulation after one minute of exercise would produce post-activation exhaustion. Repetitive stimulation after a period of rest could produce varying decrements. Eight minutes of rest are necessary to reproduce the initial state.

35. C. The tracing was obtained from a patient with remote polio. It illustrates large-amplitude motor units (8 K to 10 K) of increased duration with serrated peaks, indicating reinnervation in a neuropathic process. Absence of membrane instability suggests a relatively inactive process.

36. C. Because the motor units appear later in each trace, the frequency is less than 30 Hz but greater than 20 Hz. Three motor units are seen on the top and bottom traces with a frequency of 30 Hz; two motor units are seen in the middle traces with a frequency of 20 Hz. The average frequency is therefore 25 Hz.

37. A. The arrow identifies the extensor digitorum longus innervated by the deep branch of the peroneal nerve from the L5, S1 nerve root. Note that the tendon does not cross behind the lateral malleolus (as does the peroneal longus' tendon).

38. E. The diagram illustrates 7 cm and 14 cm antidromic median nerve sensory studies in a cold hand at 28°C. Note the increased duration of the negative spike, increased latency, and increased amplitude of 80 μV; these factors argue against CTS.

39. D. The figure illustrates single muscle fiber complexes discharging from an ephaptic transmission. The complexes repeat themselves at 60 Hz and are therefore high-frequency discharges because the rate is higher than that of a motor unit at 45 Hz.

40. D. The arrow points to a 4-msec, triphasic motor unit firing in the presence of other waveforms that are spontaneous discharges.

41. D. The bottom trace in the figure illustrates the Bactrian sign that results from simultaneous stimulation of both the medial and radial nerves in the presence of CTS when recording from the thumb. The second potential of the "double hump" appears from conduction slowing of the median nerve as it crosses the carpal tunnel.

42. B. The potential to the right represents a motor artifact. The duration of the SNAP is prolonged because it was obtained from a cold hand.

43. D. The muscles mentioned in choices (b) and (c) receive innervation from both C7 and C8 nerve roots. Electromyographic evaluation should include the thenar, hypothenar, intrinsic, or thumb flexor musculature that are not C7 innervated. This will fully differentiate C8 from C7 radiculopathy. The latter is more frequent.

44. D. The figure illustrates myokymic discharges resulting from ephaptic activation at the injured nerve root level. They occur in an irregular pattern at a low frequency.

45. D. The figure illustrates end-plate spikes with an amplitude of 40–75 μV, a duration of 1–3 msec, and an irregular rate of discharge.

46. D. The presence of spontaneous activity in the first dorsal interosseous of the hand and absent reinnervation potentials indicate a 3–4 week nerve injury process affecting the ulnar nerve.

47. E. The diagram illustrates conduction slowing across the carpal tunnel and reduced CMAP (5.9 K) of the abductor pollicis brevis at wrist stimulation. The increase in CMAP amplitude at midpalm stimulation is not measurable because the difference in shape indicates a spread of stimulation to the ulnar nerve. The small increase in amplitude from wrist to elbow stimulation probably represents submaximal stimulation at the wrist.

48. B. There is volume conduction from stimulation of the ulnar nerve in the palm, producing a change in the shape of the CMAP, probably from the ulnar branch to the deep head of the flexor pollicius brevis.

49. B. The G1 electrode is over the pronator quadratus muscle, which is innervated by the anterior interosseous nerve. This syndrome is initially manifested as forearm pain without numbness, which progresses to weakness of muscles supplied by the nerve. Note the greater than 50% drop in amplitude with stimulation of the median nerve proximal to the pronator teres. Branching occurs at the two heads of this muscle.

50. B. The right hand is colder as indicated by the larger amplitude, duration, and peak latency.

Glossary of Terms

Stuart Reiner

Active Elements. The components of a circuit that provide amplification or that control the direction of current flow; e.g., diodes, transistors, and vacuum tubes.

Address. In digital data storage systems, the description of a location (stated in system notation) where information is stored. Also, as a verb, to select or to designate the location of information in a storage system.

Alternating Current (AC). A flow of current in which the direction of current flow reverses periodically. When the reversal occurs cyclically, two current reversals are termed one cycle. The number of complete cycles per second is the frequency, and it is stated in Hertz.

Amplifier. A device that multiplies its input voltage, current, or power by a fixed or controllable factor, usually without altering its waveform.

Amplifier, AC. This amplifier responds to alternating current (AC) signals only and not to an input potential that does not vary. This type of amplifier is used in EMG apparatus. Sometimes termed RC- or AC-coupled amplifier.

Amplifier, DC (or Direct Coupled). This amplifier responds to direct current (DC) signals, pulsating DC signals, and alternating current signals. This type of amplifier is not used in clinical EMG. It is used in force and tension measurements, as well as in the recording of intracellular resting potentials in which fixed, slowly, and rapidly changing phenomena are measured.

Amplifier, Differential. An amplifier used in EMG preamplifiers. It has two recording electrode input terminals (instead of the single input terminal of a conventional amplifier) and a ground or zero-potential terminal. It rejects unwanted potentials originating at a distance and presenting at both input terminals (common-mode or in-phase potentials).

Amplitude Modulation (AM). Systems of signal transmission, recording, or processing that utilize an alternating current carrier potential of peak amplitude that varies proportionally with the instantaneous amplitude of the signal.

Analog. A term applied to signals and devices capable of accommodating continuous change and assuming an infinite number of values with finite limits.

An analog signal may be a current or a voltage that varies in time continuously, simulating and representing a natural phenomenon.

Analog-to-Digital Converter (A/D Converter). A device that converts an analog signal, usually a varying voltage or current, to a digital output (See Digital System.)

Anode. A positive terminal. The terminal through which "electron current" enters a device. "Conventional current" flow, however, is said to be away from the anode and toward the cathode (opposite or negative) terminal.

Artifact. All unwanted potentials that originate outside the tissues examined. They are also called "noise" when they appear in measurement. An artifact may arise from biological activity, the electrode or apparatus used in the examination, the power line, or the extrinsic electricity surrounding the apparatus or patient. (See Noise.)

Attenuator. In electrical circuits, an arrangement that introduces a definite reduction in the magnitude of a voltage current or power. Attenuators may be fixed or adjustable either continuously or in steps.

Averager Signal. A signal-processing method that aids in the recording of small-stimulus evoked potentials that are obscured by noise or artifact. The stimulus is repeated a number of times, and the responses are subjected to a special summation technique that causes the random noise portion of the response to become smaller in proportion to the evoked potentials that are coherent in time with each stimulus.

Bandwidth. The amplifier frequency response limits, defined by the high and low frequency filters, in which the amplification falls to 70% of full power. (See Frequency Response.)

Beam Switching. A technique for producing a multitrace display on a single beam cathode ray tube by rapidly commutating the beam to a number of signal sources. This system is also called chopped display and electron switched display.

Bias. A fixed electrical or mechanical input to a device or a system that is distinct from the input signal. The bias brings the system to a desired operating range.

Binary Coded Decimal (BCD). A binary numbering system coding decimal numbers in groups of four bits for each decimal digit.

Binary Logic. A digital logic system that operates with two distinct states variously called "one and zero," "high and low," and "on and off."

Bit. A binary numeral, the "one and zero" or "high and low," and so on, of binary logic. A group of bits comprise a binary word.

Editors' note: This Glossary of Terms, created by the late Stuart Reiner, appeared in the first edition of Practical Electromyography. The text was so well composed that it continues to be of value. It stands as a statement of and tribute to the brilliance of this leader in the development of instrumentation for electrodiagnostic medicine.

375

Blocking. An effect that results when a large transient input potential is applied to an amplifier, temporarily causing the disappearance or severe distortion of the output signal.

Calibrator. A device that identifies units of measurement by reference to a known standard.

Calibrator, Amplitude. An accurate source of voltage of known amplitude, usually within the range of EMG motor activity—for example, between 10 μV and 1000 μV—that can be applied or switched to the input terminals of the apparatus.

Calibrator, Time. An alternating or pulsatile waveform of an accurately known frequency that can be applied to the cathode ray display of an EMG so as to permit accurate adjustment of "time per division" on the horizontal graticule scale of the EMG screen.

Capacitance. A measure of electric charge that can be stored within the insulation separating two conductors when a given voltage is applied to the conductors. A capacitor or a condenser uses conductors of large surface area separated by air or by various insulators (dielectrics) that enhance capacitative effects. The unit capacitance is the farad. Direct current is not conducted by capacitors; alternating current or pulsating direct current signals are conducted to an extent proportional to frequency.

Carrier. A potential, usually alternating current, of sine or pulse waveform used in signal transmission, recording, or processing systems that in itself carries no information, but is modified most commonly in amplitude (amplitude modulation), frequency (frequency modulation), or timing by the signal. The carrier is at least a number of times higher in frequency than the highest frequency component in the signal.

Cathode. A negative terminal. The terminal through which "electron current" leaves a device. Conventional current flow is said to be toward the cathode or away from the anode (positive) terminal.

Cathode Ray Tube (CRT). A vacuum tube used to visualize electrical waveforms. It generates X-Y traces on its screen by means of a moving fluorescent spot on its screen.

Clipping (Limiting). This occurs when signals of excessive amplitude are applied to an amplifier, with a resultant waveform at the amplifier output that faithfully reproduces the shape of the input waveform only up to a level at which the signal becomes excessive (clipping level). All portions of the waveform that exceed the clipping level appear at the output at a fixed level that does not vary with time and are therefore seriously distorted.

Common Mode Rejection. An important property of differential amplifiers that expresses their ability to discriminate against artifact potentials that appear equally at both amplifier input terminals (common mode signals) and to amplify the desired potentials (differential or series mode signals) that appear as different signals at the two input terminals.

Common Mode Rejection Ratio. A calculation performed to measure the effectiveness of the differential amplifier.

Commutation. A system that cyclically switches a number of signals sequentially to a single device amplifier, transmission, or recording channel. Also termed multiplexing.

Conduction Time Indicator. A moveable time index on the trace of the cathode ray tube that is arranged to be positioned on the screen by a dial accurately calibrated in time; it is measured either from the start of the sweep or from a shock artifact to the index position.

Crosstalk. The incursion of information from one channel into any other channel of a multichannel information-handling system. The presence of crosstalk in a multichannel EMG study can be seriously misleading.

Cycle. A complete sequence of values of an alternating quantity repeated as a unit. Cycles per second (CPS) is also called Hertz.

Decibel (dB). A dimension-less unit for comparing the ratio of signal levels on a logarithmic scale. Positive decibel values represent a signal increase with respect to a reference. Negative decibel values represent signal decrement with respect to a reference signal.

Delay Line. A short-term electrical dynamic storage device that delays potentials applied to its input so that they appear at its output as if they had occurred (1 msec to 20 msec) later in time. This permits events preceding action potentials to be seen on the cathode ray tube screen when the sweeps are triggered by the potentials.

Differentiator. A device or circuit with an output waveform that is proportional to the rate of change (speed, velocity, etc.) of the input waveform.

Digital System. A system or circuit for handing or processing information in terms of numbers and utilizing circuits that operate in the manner of switches, having two (on–off) or more discrete positions. The simplest and most common digital system is the binary system.

Digital-to-Analog Converter (D/A Converter). A circuit that accepts the discrete coded signal voltages of a digital system and generates, at its output, voltages of amplitudes analogous to the numbers represented by the digital codes at its input. The analog output may then be directly interpreted by viewing a cathode ray tube, reading a meter, or graphic recording.

Diode. A two-terminal device that permits the flow of electric current in one direction only.

Direct Current (DC). A unidirectional current. An intermittent or time-varying current that has a net flow in one direction is called pulsating direct current or direct current with an alternating current component.

Dynamic Range. The ratio of the maximum input signal capability of a system without overloading to the minimum usable signal (noise level).

Electrode. A conductor of electricity. In electrodiagnostic medicine, it is generally a metal device that introduces or picks up electricity from tissue.

Electrodes, Recording. Electrodes used to measure electrical activity from tissue.

Bipolar, Bifilar Needle Electrodes. With these electrodes, variations in voltage are measured between the bared tips of two insulated wires cemented side by side in a steel cannula. The bare tips of the electrodes are flush with the bevel of the cannula. The latter may be grounded.

Concentric (Coaxial) Needle Electrode. With this electrode, variations in voltage are measured between the bare tip of an insulated wire, usually stainless steel, silver, or platinum, and the bare shaft of a steel cannula through which it is inserted. The bare tip of the central wire (the exploring electrode) is flush with the bevel at the end of the cannula (the reference electrode).

Macro EMG Electrode. A modified single-fiber EMG needle exposing only a measured portion of its cannula. A trigger potential from the single fiber electromyography (SFEMG) synchronizes the acquisition by the cannula of a compound potential arising from the other muscle fibers of its motor unit.

Monopolar Needle Electrode. A solid wire, usually stainless steel, coated except at its tip with an insulating varnish or plastic. Variations in voltage between the tip of the needle (the exploring electrode) in the muscle and a metal plate on the skin surface or bare needle in subcutaneous tissue (the reference electrode) are measured.

Multilead Electrode. Three or more insulated wires inserted through a common steel cannula have their bared tips arranged linearly at an aperture in the wall of the cannula that is parallel with its axis. The bare tips are flush with the outer circumference of the cannula.

Single Fiber EMG Electrode. A very small wire is exposed through an aperture in the side of the needle cannula. The bare tip is flush with the surface.

Surface Electrodes. Metal plate or pad electrodes placed on the skin surface. Various sizes, shapes, and materials are used.

EMG Analyzer. A term applied to a wide range of EMG computer processing techniques that attempt to display one or a number of attributes of the EMG waveform in a more explicit manner than the conventional voltage-time graph of the usual EMG trace.

Feedback. An effect that occurs when a portion of the output of a system or a circuit is connected back to the input. When the fed-back signal reinforces the original input, the feedback is positive; when the fed-back signal tends to reduce the input signal, the feedback is negative.

Negative feedback acts to stabilize the performance of electronic instrument systems and to make the operation and calibration of such systems stable and independent of changes in many of the system components.

Positive feedback appears in oscillating circuits. Unintentional positive feedback occurs, for example, when a microphone, which is the input to an amplification systems, is brought too close to the loudspeaker output. When this occurs, positive feedback often produces an oscillatory howl. Similar undesirable positive feedback may occur when the input electrodes of an EMG system are brought too close to the loudspeaker output or the cathode ray tube output of an EMG system.

Filter. In an EMG system, these are circuits, usually comprised of capacitors and resistors, that modify or adjust the high and low frequency limits of the amplifier frequency response curve.

Frequency. The rate in cycles per second that an alternating current signal alternates. The unit of frequency is the Hertz.

Frequency Analyzer. This analyzes the EMG to produce a spectrum of sine wave frequencies (harmonics) that will uniquely describe the original EMG waveform.

Frequency Modulation (FM). Systems of signal transmission, recording, or processing that utilize a constant amplitude carrier potential with an instantaneous frequency proportional to the instantaneous amplitude of the signal.

Frequency Response. Describes the speed range (slowest to fastest) of potential waveform changes that will be displayed by the EMG apparatus. Stated as a range (band) of frequencies of sine wave test signals for which the amplification will be uniform. Amplification decreases progressively for sine wave test signals at frequencies above and below the frequency response band. The frequency between the lower and upper frequency is called the bandwidth. The amplifier frequency response bandwidth is often defined by two frequencies, one at the low end and the other at the high end, where the amplification falls to 70% of its midband value.

Gain. The increase at the output of an amplifier in voltage, current, or power of the signal applied to its input is called the amplifier voltage, current or power gain, or amplification.

Gate. A circuit used in digital systems as a decision element and having two or more inputs and one output. The output depends upon the combination of digital states of the signals at the input. A gate circuit in an analog system acts like a switch that permits or stops the flow of signals. The gate opens or closes in response to a control voltage (or gating signal).

Graticule. The ruled scale on the face of the cathode ray tube. Time and voltage display calibrations are usually adjusted with reference to the X and Y rulings on the graticule.

Ground. The neutral electrical potential reference terminal in a system. In power distribution systems, a terminal that is usually physically connected to a conductor in intimate contact with the earth. Sometimes referred to as the earth terminal. Frame and chassis portions of electrical systems are almost always connected to ground to avoid the possibility of their assuming other random potentials that might be either dangerous or cause electrical interference within the system.

Ground Loop. The condition that sometimes exists when the ground connections of two interconnected electronic instruments or circuits are not at the same potential. This may result in power line interference.

Hertz (Hz). Cycles per second.

High Pass Filter. A low-frequency filter that does not significantly impede higher frequencies.

Impedance. The hindrance to electrical current flow in an alternating current circuit; hence, it is comparable in simplified terms to resistance in DC circuits. It includes the effects of resistance, capacitance, inductance, and frequency.

Integrated EMG. The integrated EMG is a time-varying potential with instantaneous amplitude equal to the total area (voltage × time) accumulated from a designated start point under an EMG waveform. It provides a measure of total electrical activity.

Interface. An expression or device that embodies all technical considerations in interconnecting two portions of a system, such as proper mating connectors, shielding of connecting leads, establishment of compatible voltage and impedance levels, and such problems as ground cops.

Interference. A term generally applied to unwanted signals outside the system. Power line frequency is the most common form of interference. (See Artifact.)

Linear Circuit. A circuit, the output of which is congruent with its input, with the exception of possible amplification or attenuation.

Low Pass Filter. A high-frequency filter that does not significantly impede lower frequencies.

Microphonics. An effect noted in sensitive electronic systems and their connecting cables in which incidental mechanical vibration applied to portions of the system gives rise to spurious electrical outputs.

Monitor. A specialized CRT used with digital displays for computers.

Noise. Any potential other than that being measured. Commonly applied to spurious potentials originating within the apparatus of electrodes. (See Artifact, Interference, and Root Mean Square Voltage.)

Off Line. Any signal or data-processing function that is deferred with respect to the original recording or generation of signal or data.

On Line. Any signal or data-processing function that occurs simultaneously with the original recording or generation of the signal or data.

Overload. A general condition in which the input to an amplifier circuit is so large that it exceeds the capability of the circuit to perform its intended function.

Parallel. Circuit elements connected in parallel (as opposed to in series) all are subjected to the same voltage. The current flow to elements connected in parallel is inversely proportional to the impedance (resistance) of the elements. The word "shunt" is sometimes used to refer to parallel connections. In digital systems, parallel refers to a technique of transmission, storage, or logical operation on all

bits of binary data words simultaneously using separate facilities. (See Serial.)

Parameter. Any specific characteristic of a device. When considered together, all of the parameters of a device describe its operation or its physical characteristics.

Peak-to-Peak Voltage (or Current). A statement of the magnitude of an alternating voltage (or current). It is the total excursion from the most negative peak of the wave to the most positive peak of the wave.

Polarity Sense, Display. Many neurophysiologic records are published with an upward deflection denoting a negative potential on the active electrode. Engineering convention dictates an upward deflection for a positive potential.

Polarization. Electrolytic effects that occur at the metal-tissue interface of electrodes that increase the resistance of the junction and give rise to direct current potentials (which may fluctuate) that can be many times larger than EMG potentials.

Potential, Action. The voltage that results from activity of a muscle or nerve. It can be spontaneous, volitional, or evoked by stimulation. Action potentials may be named for their appearance (high frequency; positive sharp; biphasic; monophasic; polyphasic; tetraphasic; triphasic) or their origin (endplate; fasciculation; fibrillation; motor unit; muscle; nerve). The term potential also refers to an action potential.

Preamplifier. The first stage or stages of an EMG amplifier system. It must have a high input impedance, a common mode rejection, and low noise, as well as a large dynamic range.

Pulse. A signal of very short duration. It can be described according to its characteristic rise, duration, and decay.

Raster. A predetermined pattern of lines generated on a cathode ray tube (CRT) display that provides uniform coverage of an area. Also, the display on the CRT screen of an EMG in which each successive sweep is displayed below or above the previous sweep, thus permitting the observer to see more information on the screen than is possible when successive sweeps are superimposed (same baseline). Also, a similar mode of graphic recording.

Rectifier Circuit. A circuit utilizing unidirectional current flow properties of diodes that convert an alternating current into a pulsating direct current.

Resistance. A property of matter that hinders the flow of electric current. Resistance is expressed in ohms and is derived by dividing the voltage impressed by the current that flows. Resistance (R) = Voltage (E) divided by the Current (I).

Ringing. A short-duration, transient, usually low-amplitude, damped oscillation that occurs in the output of certain electronic circuits, especially some filters, wideband amplifiers, and certain delay lines, immediately after the input wave suddenly changes in amplitude.

Rise Time. A term used to describe rectangular pulses and square waveforms or amplifiers or the circuits transmitting them. Rise time is the elapsed interval between the time at which the amplitude of the rapidly changing transition part of the wave reaches specified percentages of its lower and upper limits. The rise time of an amplifier is a function of its high frequency response.

Root Mean Square (RMS) Voltage or Current. The root mean square value is a means of stating numerically the magnitude of an alternating voltage or current. It equals a direct current that has the same heating effect in a resistor as an alternating current of the same RMS magnitude.

Semiconductor. A material that exhibits relatively high resistance in a pure state but much lower resistance when minute amounts of impurities are added.

Serial. A term applied to digital circuits in which each bit is acted upon sequentially. (See Parallel.).

Series. Electrical components are in series when they are connected so that a common current flows through each of them. (See Parallel.)

Shield (Shielding). An electrostatic shield is an electrically conductive sheath or an enclosure not in contact with the circuit or device shielded. It is comprised of electrically conductive material connected directly to ground or by a low impedance to ground. It is used to prevent undesirable capacitive coupling of external voltages to the elements within the shield (or to contain potentials within the shield).

Magnetic shielding requires an enclosure of iron or other magnetically permeable alloys and provides protection against interference from magnetic fields that surround nearby current-carrying conductors or permanent magnets.

Signal. Any potential, waveform, or intelligence that is communicated, detected, transmitted, or processed with a system. It is usually in the form of a voltage or current within the system.

Silence, Electrical. The absence of signals from the tissues being studied.

Solid State. Electronic devices utilizing semiconductors. Electric currents, as well as light, heat, and magnetic fields, may interact in solid state devices. The transistor and integrated circuit are solid state devices.

Stabilized Current or Voltage Generator. A source of direct current or alternating current or voltage in which the output current or voltage remains at a predetermined, usually adjustable value independent of wide variations of load resistance or impedance or of variations of power supply voltages. The stabilized current source exhibits wide fluctuations in output voltage in response to changing load conditions, whereas the stabilized voltage source exhibits wide variations in output current in response to load changes.

*Stimulator, Ground-*Free (Isolated). Used in nerve conduction studies to minimize stimulus artifact. A ground-free stimulus output circuit has no connection to the common system ground, thereby removing a possible path for injection of undesirable artifact via the patient to the EMG amplifier input terminals.

Storage, Display. A means for retaining, usually on the screen of a cathode ray tube, a transient waveform for study or analysis, together with a means for erasing such information to permit the storage of new data. Such storage can be accomplished by means of special cathode ray tubes (CRTs) that have, in addition to other design features, special screens with electrostatic storage surfaces that store the desired waveform as a pattern of electric charges on their surfaces. The pattern is then visualized by flooding the storage screen with an unfocused beam of electrons that pass through the storage screen and strike the phosphor screen on the face of the CRT only at those points where charge was stored. Transient waveforms may also be displayed on conventional CRTs by electrically storing the transient wave in some signal storage means, such as digital storage circuits or magnetic recording systems. The signal is then displayed by rapid, repetitive read-out of the storage device and superimposed display on a conventional CRT.

Strain Gauge. An electrical transducer that generates or modifies an electrical signal proportional to a mechanical deformation owing to application of a mechanical load.

Strain Relief. A mechanical restraint, usually applied to the jacket of insulated cables where they join fixed mechanical assemblies or connectors or other terminations, especially where the cable might be subjected to repeated flexing or mechanical stress. The purpose of the strain relief is to minimize the possibility of failure of the electrical conductors within the cable or connector.

Sweep. The horizontal (X-axis) linear time axis of a cathode ray tube display generated by the left-to-right movement of the trace spot at constant preselected speeds across the face of the cathode ray tube. Sweep velocities are usually specified in reciprocals of speed: time per division on the graticule.

Telemetry. The transmission of data, typically from preamplifiers located on a subject (free to move about the laboratory) via a radio link to a receiver and then to the remainder of the recording system.

Time Constant. A factor that is an index to a speed with which voltage and currents respond to changes in the input to resistor-capacitor circuits. This term is used to describe the dynamic performance of EMG amplifiers (which contain resistor-capacitor coupling networks).

Time Scale, Electronic. A discontinuous waveform, usually in short pulses, spaced in time at 1 msec, 0.1 msec, or some other convenient time interval, applied to a trace of a cathode ray tube along with the EMG information to provide an independent timing reference.

Trace. The line of light on the face of a cathode ray tube that is generated by the moving spot of light, which is generated by the electron beam striking the phosphor-coated screen.

Transducer. A device that changes the energy form applied to its input to another form of energy at its output, such that a proportionality exists between the input and output. Transducers include loudspeakers, microphones, strain gauges, and photo-cells.

Transistor. An active semiconductor device used as an amplifier or switching device.

Trigger. A short pulse used to initiate some action within an electronic system. Also used as a verb. (See Sweep.)

Wave (Waveform). A generic term loosely applied to a time-varying voltage, current, or other quantity, the amplitude of which varies with time.

Z-Axis Modulation (Intensity Modulation). Applies to cathode ray displays in which information is applied to the beam-generating electrodes so as to vary instantaneously the brightness of the trace during the course of the sweep.

Index

Note: Page numbers followed by a "t" denote tables; those followed by "f" denote figures.

A wave, 230–231, 231f
Abdominal muscles
  anterior
    in T10 radiculopathy, 124, 125t
  electromyography of, 11
Abductor digiti minimi
  in ulnar neuropathy, 247
Abductor pollicis brevis
  in carpal tunnel syndrome, 197, 197f
Acetylcholine
  in neuromuscular junction, 344, 345f
Action potential. (see also Motor unit action potential)
  muscle fiber membrane, 2
  propagation of, 131
    anode in, 81
Adductor pollicis
  in ulnar neuropathy, 243
Age
  in carpal tunnel syndrome, 196–197
  in conduction velocity, 145–146, 147f
  in neuronal loss, 145–146
Alcohol
  neuropathy from, 331–332, 332t
Alkalosis
  fasciculation potential in, 4
ALS. (see Amyotrophic lateral sclerosis)
Amiodarone
  neuropathy from, 322
Amplification, 69–70, 70f
  differential, 71–72, 72f
  gain in, 69–70
  sensitivity in, 69–70, 70f
Amplifiers, 69–71
  in electrophysiologic exam, 63, 64f
  impedance of, 70–71
  negative, 71
  positive, 71
Amplitude
  in electromyography, 42, 43f
  in signal-to-noise ratio, 79–80
  temperature and, 145, 146f
Amyotrophic lateral sclerosis, 339, 340, 340f
  F wave in, 227–228
  macro electromyography in, 105–106
  motor unit action potential in, 340, 341f
Amyotrophy
  neuralgic
    anterior interosseous nerve syndrome from, 258
    vs. upper supraclavicular brachial plexopathy, 292–293

Anal sphincter
  external
    electromyography of, 11
Anesthesia
  paralysis after, 290–291
Anode
  block of, 81
  needle, 82
  rotation of
    stimulus artifact reduction by, 83, 83f
  in stimulator, 81
Antebrachial nerve
  lateral cutaneous
    sensory conduction study of, 287, 288f
Anterior interosseous nerve syndrome, 177, 256–259
  clinical presentation of, 258
  denervation in, 258
  differential diagnosis of, 257–258
  electrodiagnosis of, 258–259, 259t
  etiology of, 258
  history in, 256–257
  nerve conduction studies of, 259t
  neuralgic amyotrophy and, 258
  physical examination of, 256–257
  sites of, 256f
Anterior interosseus nerve, 174f, 177
Arsenic
  neuropathy from, 326f, 327
Artifacts
  stimulus, 82–83, 83f
Atrophy
  progressive, 339
Averaging, 79–80, 80f
Axilla
  trauma to
    brachial plexopathy from, 303
Axillary nerve, 159–160
  conduction studies of, 159f, 160
  injury to, 160
Axon(s), 132
  activation of
    motor nerve root inflammation and, 123
  atrophy of, 312
  blocking of, 97, 98f
  cell membrane of
    characteristics of, 135–136
    concentration gradient at, 132–133, 133f
    depolarization wave propagation in, 132, 133, 134

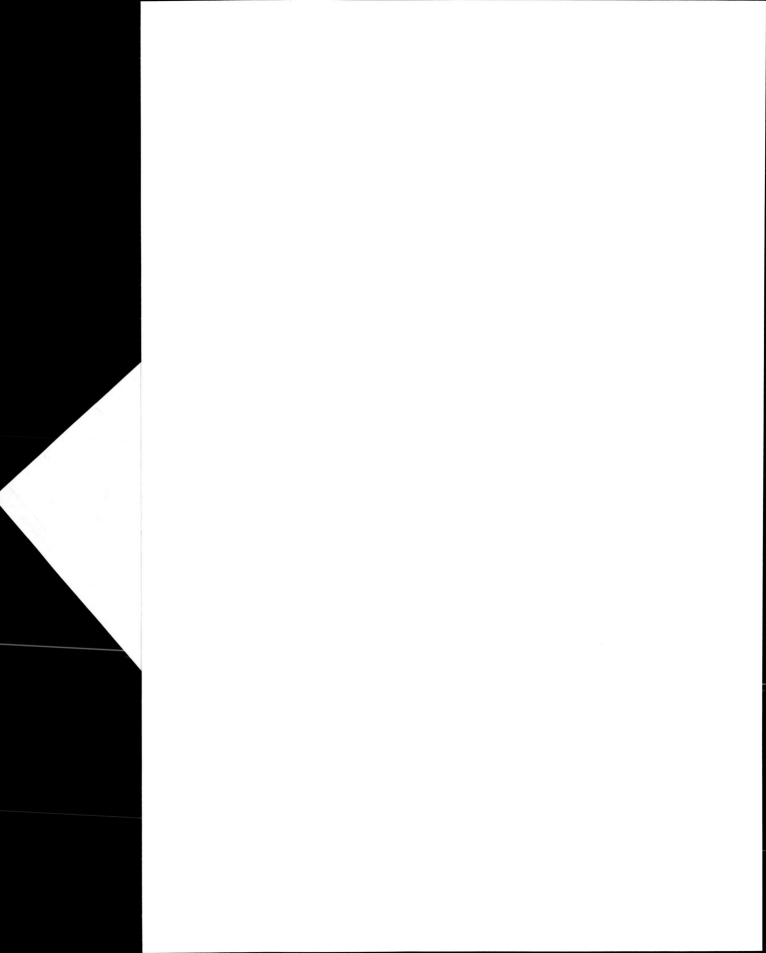

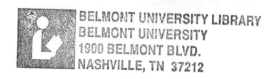
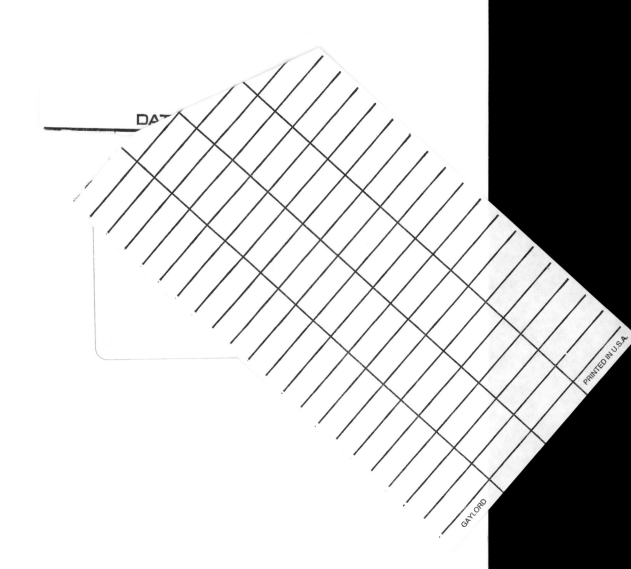

DAT

GAYLORD

PRINTED IN U.S.A.